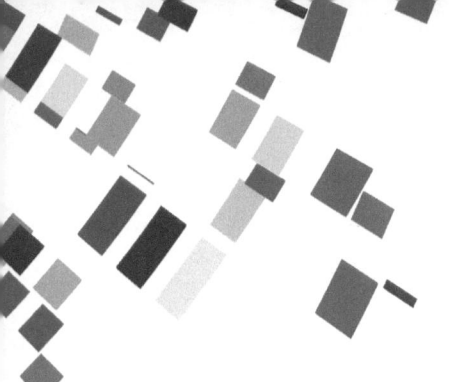

Contents

List of Boxes, Tables, and Figures v
Frequently Used Terms and Abbreviations.. x
About the Editors xii
Contributors xiii
Reviewers xvi
Foreword xviii
Preface xx
Acknowledgments xxii

SECTION 1 — Foundations of Treatment: The Human Element

CHAPTER 1	Obesity as a Disease	2
CHAPTER 2	Health Inequities in the Development, Management, and Treatment of Obesity	26
CHAPTER 3	Weight Bias and Stigma	44
CHAPTER 4	Evidence-Based Guidelines for Treatment of Overweight and Obesity	59
CHAPTER 5	Patient-Centered Care and Shared Decision-Making	67

SECTION 2 — Interprofessional Assessment of Overweight and Obesity

CHAPTER 6	Medical and Physical Assessment	80
CHAPTER 7	Nutrition Assessment	98
CHAPTER 8	Physical Activity Assessment	116
CHAPTER 9	Behavioral Health Assessment	145

SECTION 3 — Interventions for the Treatment of Overweight and Obesity

CHAPTER 10	Multicomponent Lifestyle Interventions	166
CHAPTER 11	Dietary Interventions	182
CHAPTER 12	Physical Activity Interventions	195
CHAPTER 13	Counseling Approaches for Health Behavior Change	220
CHAPTER 14	Medical and Surgical Interventions	253
CHAPTER 15	Obesity as a Chronic Disease and Its Lifelong Management	270
CHAPTER 16	Treatment of Obesity and Eating Disorders	286
CHAPTER 17	The Use of Technology in the Treatment of Obesity	316

SECTION 4 — Models and Insurance Coverage for the Treatment of Obesity

CHAPTER 18	Interprofessional Teams and Models of Practice	334
CHAPTER 19	Health Care Systems, Policies, and the Coverage of Services	346

Continuing Professional Education 365
Index 366

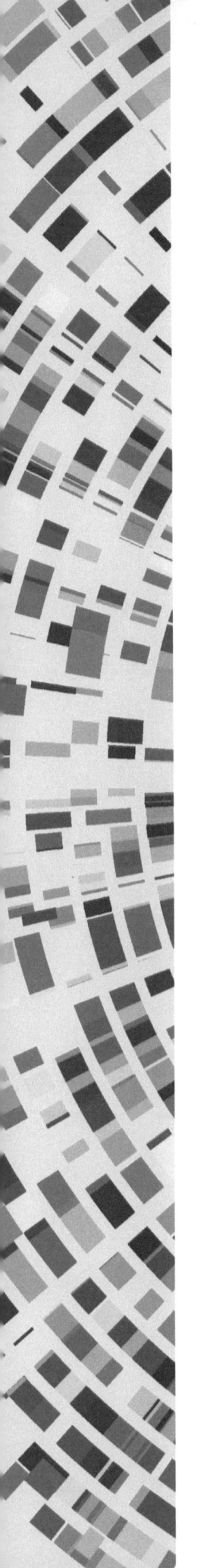

Health Professional's Guide to Treatment of Overweight and Obesity

Weight Management Dietetic Practice Group

Editors

Hollie A. Raynor, PhD, RD, LDN

Linda M. Gigliotti, MS, RDN, CDCES, CSOWM, FAND

Academy of Nutrition and Dietetics

eat right. Academy of Nutrition and Dietetics

Academy of Nutrition and Dietetics
120 S. Riverside Plaza, Suite 2190
Chicago, IL 60606

Health Professional's Guide to Treatment of Overweight and Obesity

ISBN 978-0-88091-240-2 (print)
ISBN 978-0-88091-230-3 (eBook)
Catalog Number 240224 (print)
Catalog Number 240224e (eBook)

Copyright © 2024, Academy of Nutrition and Dietetics. All rights reserved. Except for brief quotations embodied in critical articles or reviews, no part of this publication may be reproduced, stored in a retrieval system, or transmitted, in any form or by any means, electronic, mechanical, photocopying, recording, or otherwise, without the prior written consent of the publisher.

The views expressed in this publication are those of the authors and do not necessarily reflect policies and/or official positions of the Academy of Nutrition and Dietetics. Mention of product names in this publication does not constitute endorsement by the authors or the Academy of Nutrition and Dietetics. Neither the Academy nor the authors or editors assume any liability for injury and/or damage to persons or property as a matter of liability, negligence, or otherwise from use of any methods, products, instructions, or applications of information contained herein.

10 9 8 7 6 5 4 3 2 1

For more information on the Academy of Nutrition and Dietetics, visit www.eatright.org.

Library of Congress Cataloging-in-Publication Data

Names: Raynor, Hollie A, editor. | American Dietetic Association. Weight
  Management Dietetic Practice Group, editor.
Title: Health professional's guide to treatment of overweight and obesity :
  Weight Management Dietetic Practice Group / editors, Hollie A Raynor,
  PhD, RD, LDN, Linda M. Gigliotti, MS, RDN, CDCES, CSOWM, FAND.
Description: Chicago, IL : Academy of Nutrition and Dietetics, [2024] |
  Includes bibliographical references and index.
Identifiers: LCCN 2023058335 (print) | LCCN 2023058336 (ebook) | ISBN
  9780880912402 (print) | ISBN 9780880912303 (ebook)
Subjects: LCSH: Obesity--Treatment. | Reducing diets.
Classification: LCC RC628 .H416 2024 (print) | LCC RC628 (ebook) | DDC
  616.3/98--dc23/eng/20240213
LC record available at https://lccn.loc.gov/2023058335
LC ebook record available at https://lccn.loc.gov/2023058336

List of Boxes, Tables, and Figures

BOXES

BOX 1.1	Effect of Select Hormones and Neurotransmitters on Hunger	12
BOX 2.1	The Influence of Stress on Obesity	28
BOX 2.2	Economic Factors Associated With Food Insecurity	29
BOX 3.1	Recommended Dos and Don'ts for Preventing and Reducing Weight Bias and Stigma in Clinical Practice	52
BOX 4.1	Standards from the Institute of Medicine for Developing Trustworthy Clinical Practice Guidelines	60
BOX 4.2	Evidence-Based Guidelines for the Treatment of Adult Overweight and Obesity	65
BOX 5.1	Building Rapport in Patient-Centered Care	68
BOX 5.2	Steps for Health Care Practitioners in Shared Decision-Making	71
BOX 5.3	Case Study: A Patient-Centered Session With an Individual Patient	74
BOX 6.1	Sex-Specific Data Points and Considerations for the Nutrition Assessment of Transgender Patients With Overweight or Obesity	91
BOX 7.1	Total Daily Energy Expenditure for Adults	100
BOX 7.2	Advantages and Disadvantages of Commonly Used Dietary Assessment Methods	102
BOX 7.3	Additional Elements of Dietary Assessment Beyond Food Intake	106
BOX 7.4	Nutrition Focused Physical Exam for Adults with Obesity: Elements and Special Considerations	110
BOX 7.5	Social, Physical, and Laboratory Components to Integrate With Nutrition Focused Physical Exam Findings for Weight Management	111
BOX 8.1	Summary of Sedentary Behavior and Physical Activity Variables	117
BOX 8.2	Physical Behavior Domains and Examples of Associated Activity Spaces	129

v

BOX 9.1	Common Psychological Factors to Consider in a Behavioral Health Assessment for Weight Management	147
BOX 10.1	Diabetes Prevention Program Study Interventions	168
BOX 11.1	Calculators for Weight Loss Planning	183
BOX 11.2	Questions to Help Weigh and Interpret the Evidence for Popular Diets or Weight Loss Products	189
BOX 11.3	Questions to Answer About Popular Diets and Weight Loss Products	189
BOX 12.1	Guidelines and Position Stands: Physical Activity, Exercise, and Weight Management	196
BOX 12.2	Physical Activity Approaches for Weight Management in Individuals With Overweight or Obesity	206
BOX 12.3	Physical Activity Resources for Health Professionals	210
BOX 13.1	The OARS Strategy Applied to Weight Management	233
BOX 13.2	The DARN Strategy Applied to Weight Management	234
BOX 13.3	Guiding Principles of Intuitive Eating	238
BOX 14.1	Medications Associated With Weight Gain and Examples of Weight-Neutral Alternatives	260
BOX 14.2	Common Medications Used Off Label for Weight Management	261
BOX 14.3	Preoperative Checklist for Bariatric Surgery	264
BOX 14.4	Recommendations for Postoperative Care Following Bariatric Surgery	266
BOX 15.1	NOVA Food Classification System	273
BOX 15.2	Hyperpalatable Food Clusters	274
BOX 15.3	Dietary Behaviors Associated With Weight Loss Maintenance	277
BOX 15.4	Components of the Chronic Care Model and Examples of Their Application for the Management of Obesity	280
BOX 16.1	Diagnostic Criteria for the Main Types of Eating Disorders	287
BOX 16.2	Distinguishing Characteristics of Eating Disorders and Obesity	289
BOX 16.3	Shared Risk Factors for Excess Weight and Binge-Spectrum Eating Disorders in Adults	289
BOX 16.4	Correlates and Features of Co-Occurrence of Overweight or Obesity and Eating Disorders	290

	BOX 16.5	Efficacy of Existing Treatments for Binge Eating Disorder in Adults 300
	BOX 16.6	Initial Screening, Monthly Assessment, and Session Monitoring for Eating Disorders 306
	BOX 16.7	Weight Management and Disordered Eating: Practice Tips for Providers 308
	BOX 17.1	Summary of Technologies for Weight Management Interventions 327
	BOX 18.1	Ways to Establish Weight Management Expertise Within the Interprofessional Team 339
	BOX 19.1	Estimated Revenues for Registered Dietitian Nutritionist–Provided Medical Nutrition Therapy for Obesity or Overweight 353
	BOX 19.2	Estimated Revenues for Intensive Behavioral Therapy for Obesity Services for Medicare Beneficiaries 354
	BOX 19.3	Business Models for Registered Dietitian Nutritionists in Multidisciplinary Practices 356
	BOX 19.4	Solutions for Overcoming Barriers to Accessing Weight Management Services 359

TABLES

	TABLE 8.1	Characteristics of Physical Behavior Assessment Methods 120
	TABLE 9.1	Summary of Behavioral Health Assessment Questionnaires 156
	TABLE 10.1	Key Findings of the Diabetes Prevention Program Outcomes Study at 10 Years and 15 Years 173
	TABLE 10.2	Look AHEAD: Key Results at 4 Years 178
	TABLE 14.1	Obesity Treatment Options 254
	TABLE 14.2	Medications Approved by the US Food and Drug Administration for Obesity Treatment 255
	TABLE 14.3	Surgical Interventions for Obesity Treatment 262

FIGURES

	FIGURE 1.1	Defining obesity using BMI and waist circumference 3
	FIGURE 1.2	Regulation of body weight in animal studies 4
	FIGURE 1.3	Predicted BMI trajectories by race and ethnicity 5
	FIGURE 1.4	Weight regulation in humans ....
	FIGURE 1.5	Does the body get "used to" the reduced obese state? Body weights and the rate of weight regain in animal studies 6

FIGURE 1.6	Components of energy expenditure	7
FIGURE 1.7	Overview of energy homeostasis	10
FIGURE 1.8	Regions of the hypothalamus that regulate energy balance	11
FIGURE 1.9	Energy expenditure before and after weight loss	15
FIGURE 1.10	Mean (±SE) fasting and postprandial levels of ghrelin, peptide YY, amylin, and cholecystokinin at baseline, 10 weeks, and 62 weeks	15
FIGURE 1.11	Trends in age-adjusted obesity and severe obesity prevalence among adults aged 20 years and older from 1999–2000 through 2017–2018 in the United States	17
FIGURE 1.12	Age-adjusted prevalence of obesity among adults aged 20 years and older, by sex, race, and Hispanic origin, in 2017–2018 in the United States	17
FIGURE 1.13	Medical complications of obesity	21
FIGURE 1.14	Relationship between BMI and cardiovascular disease mortality	21
FIGURE 1.15	Relationship between BMI and risk of developing type 2 diabetes	22
FIGURE 3.1	Health consequences of weight stigma	47
FIGURE 6.1	Clinical and environmental risk factors for obesity	81
FIGURE 6.2	BMI and all-cause mortality in individuals with a BMI greater than 25 (never-smokers)	86
FIGURE 6.3	Select physical examination findings	87
FIGURE 7.1	Sample use of the Body Weight Planner	101
FIGURE 8.1	Decision matrix for selecting a method of physical activity measurement	126
FIGURE 8.2	Continuum of trade-offs in choosing a physical behavior assessment tool	127
FIGURE 8.3	Adapted ecological model of the determinants of physical behaviors, illustrating how environmental influences change over the life course	133
FIGURE 10.1	Cumulative incidence of diabetes according to study group	171
FIGURE 10.2	Diabetes incidence rates by ethnicity	171
FIGURE 10.3	Prevention of type 2 diabetes by changing lifestyle: the Finnish study	175
FIGURE 10.4	Look AHEAD results: weight loss at 1 year	177
FIGURE 12.1	Comparative models of energy expenditure	201
FIGURE 12.2	Energy balance predictions in constrained vs additive models of energy expenditure	201

FIGURE 13.1	The overlap between the three nondiet approaches to health	239
FIGURE 14.1	Sleeve gastrectomy	261
FIGURE 14.2	Roux-en-Y gastric bypass	262
FIGURE 15.1	Treatment algorithm: chronic disease management model for primary care of patients with overweight and obesity	281
FIGURE 16.1	Psychobehavioral paradigm of dieting	294
FIGURE 16.2	Recommended procedures for screening and monitoring for eating disorder risk	305
FIGURE 18.1	Types of interprofessional team members and specific examples	335

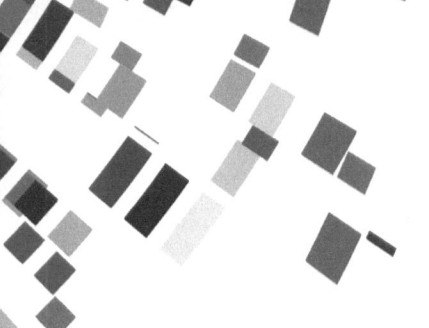

Frequently Used Terms and Abbreviations

ACTH	adrenocorticotropic hormone
ABOM	American Board of Obesity Medicine
ASMBS	American Society for Metabolic and Bariatric Surgery
ASA24	Automated Self-Administered 24-Hour Dietary Assessment Tool
BMR	basal metabolic rate
BAI	Beck Anxiety Inventory
BDI-II	Beck Depression Inventory-II
BRFSS	Behavioral Risk Factor Surveillance System
BWL	behavioral weight loss
BPD-DS	biliopancreatic diversion with duodenal switch
BED	binge eating disorder
BN	bulimia nervosa
CMS	Centers for Medicare and Medicaid Services
CCM	Chronic Care Model
CBT	cognitive-behavioral therapy
CDR	Commission on Dietetic Registration
CPT	Current Procedural Terminology
DVT	deep vein thrombosis
DPP	Diabetes Prevention Program
DPPOS	Diabetes Prevention Program Outcomes Study
DSM-5	*Diagnostic and Statistical Manual of Mental Disorders*, Fifth Edition
DASH	Dietary Approaches to Stop Hypertension
EDE	Eating Disorder Examination
EDE-Q	Eating Disorder Examination Questionnaire
EMA	ecological momentary assessment
FNDDS	Food and Nutrient Database for Dietary Studies
FFQ	food frequency questionnaire
GABA	γ-aminobutyric acid
GERD	gastroesophageal reflux disease
GAD-7	Generalized Anxiety Disorder-7
GPAQ	Global Physical Activity Questionnaire
HAES	Health at Every Size
IBT	intensive behavioral therapy
IPAQ	International Physical Activity Questionnaire
IPT	interpersonal psychotherapy

LGBTQIA	lesbian, gay, bisexual, transgender, queer (or questioning), intersex, asexual
Look AHEAD study	Action for Health in Diabetes
MNT	medical nutrition therapy
MC4R	melanocortin-4 receptor
MSH	melanocyte-stimulating hormone
MBSAQIP	Metabolic and Bariatric Surgery Accreditation and Quality Improvement Program
METs	metabolic equivalents
MB-EAT	mindfulness-based eating awareness training
mHealth	mobile health
MAUP	modifiable areal unit problem
NCHPAD	National Center on Health, Physical Activity and Disability
National DPP	National Diabetes Prevention Program
NIDDK	National Institute of Diabetes and Digestive and Kidney Diseases
NWCR	National Weight Control Registry
NSAID	nonsteroidal anti-inflammatory drug
TOS	The Obesity Society
PHQ-9	Patient Health Questionnaire-9
PAEE	physical activity energy expenditure
POMC	pro-opiomelanocortin
REE	resting energy expenditure
SSRI	selective serotonin reuptake inhibitor
SMS	Short Message Service
SGLT2	sodium-glucose cotransporter-2
STOP Obesity Alliance	Strategies to Overcome and Prevent Obesity Alliance
TDF	theoretical domains framework
TEF	thermic effect of food
TSH	thyroid-stimulating hormone
TDEE	total daily energy expenditure
USPSTF	US Preventive Services Task Force

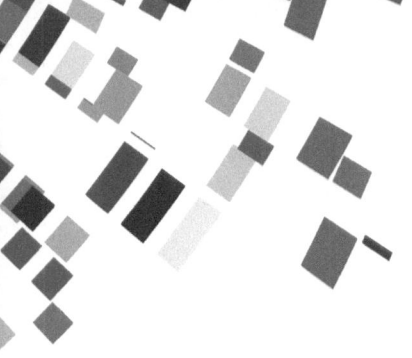

About the Editors

Hollie A. Raynor, PhD, RD, LDN, is a professor in the Department of Nutrition and the Associate Dean of Research in the College of Education, Health, and Human Sciences at the University of Tennessee. She holds a master's degree in public health nutrition and a PhD in clinical psychology. She conducts research in lifestyle interventions for pediatric and adult overweight and obesity treatment, has published over 150 peer-reviewed articles, and has received research funding from the National Institutes of Health, American Diabetes Association, and the Academy of Nutrition and Dietetics Foundation. Hollie served on the American Psychological Association's National Committee for Clinical Guidelines for Obesity and the Academy of Nutrition and Dietetics Prediabetes and Adult Obesity Treatment Evidence Analysis Library Committee. She received the Excellence in Weight Management Outcomes Research Award from the Weight Management Dietetics Practice Group in 2012 and the Excellence in Practice Dietetic Research Award from the Academy of Nutrition and Dietetics in 2018. Hollie believes in dancing for physical activity.

Linda M. Gigliotti, MS, RDN, CDCES, CSOWM, FAND, is a registered dietitian nutritionist with a master's degree in nutrition education from the University of Delaware. She has extensive experience in the clinical practice of adult weight management and multidisciplinary obesity treatment teams, serving for 20 years as the director of the Weight Management Program at the University of California, Irvine. Linda has been recognized for her leadership in program development, particularly in the areas of medically supervised weight management and worksite wellness weight management. She has extensive experience in outpatient and community education, specifically in weight management and lifestyle modification, and enjoys working with clients to make choices to manage their health. Linda has held numerous roles within the Academy of Nutrition and Dietetics and the Commission on Dietetic Registration and was engaged in the development of the interprofessional Certified Specialist in Obesity and Weight Management (CSOWM) credential. In 2021, she was awarded the Medallion Award by the Academy of Nutrition and Dietetics. She also received the Excellence in Weight Management Practice Award from the Weight Management Dietetics Practice Group in 2017 and the California Outstanding Dietitian of the Year Award in 2018. In her spare time, Linda likes to cook and entertain while embracing healthy eating!

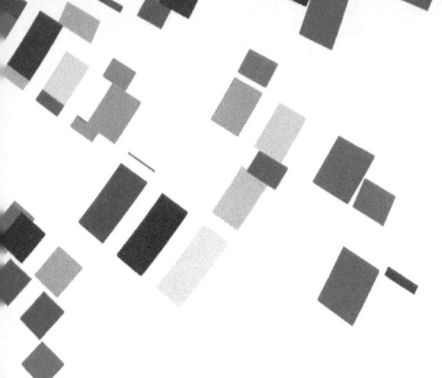

Contributors

Kelly C. Allison, PhD
Professor, Perelman School of Medicine,
University of Pennsylvania
Philadelphia, PA

Jessica Bartfield, MD, DABOM
Assistant Professor, Department of Surgery,
Obesity Medicine Specialist,
Atrium Health Wake Forest Baptist
Greensboro, NC

Daniel Bessesen, MD
Professor of Medicine, Division of Endocrinology,
Metabolism and Diabetes, University of Colorado,
School of Medicine
Director, Anschutz Health and Wellness Center, Anschutz
Foundation Endowed Chair in Health and Wellness
Denver, CO

Alena C. Borgatti, MA
Graduate Student, University of Alabama at Birmingham
Birmingham, AL

Michelle I. Cardel, PhD, MS, RD, FTOS
Head of Clinical Research & Nutrition, WeightWatchers
Adjunct Professor, University of Florida College of
Medicine
Gainesville, FL

Tiffany L. Carson, PhD, MPH
Program Co-Leader and Associate Member,
Moffitt Cancer Center
Tampa, FL

Scott E. Crouter, PhD, FACSM
Professor, University of Tennessee Knoxville
Knoxville, TN

Laura D'Adamo, MS
Doctoral Student, Drexel University
Philadelphia, PA

Andrea L. Davis, MA
Graduate Student, University of Alabama at Birmingham
Birmingham, AL

Brenda Davy, PhD, RDN
Professor, Virginia Tech
Blacksburg, VA

Kevin P. Davy, PhD
Professor, Virginia Tech
Blacksburg, VA

Gareth R. Dutton, PhD
Professor of Medicine, University of
Alabama at Birmingham
Birmingham, AL

Molly Fennig, MA
Doctoral Student, Washington University in St Louis
St Louis, MO

Ellen E. Fitzsimmons-Craft, PhD
Associate Professor of Psychiatry, Washington University
School of Medicine in St Louis
St Louis, MO

Anne Claire Grammer, MA
PhD Candidate, Clinical Psychology, Department of
Psychological and Brain Sciences and Psychiatry
Washington University in St Louis
St Louis, MO

Clarence C. Gravlee, PhD
Associate Professor, University of Florida
Gainesville, FL

Paul R. Hibbing, PhD
Assistant Professor, University of Illinois Chicago,
Department of Kinesiology and Nutrition
Chicago, IL

xiii

Christina M. Hopkins, PhD
Clinical Psychologist, Main Line Therapy
and Psychological Services
Wayne, PA

Kristen Howard, MSN, ARNP, CBN
Graduate Research Assistant, Virginia Tech
Blacksburg, VA

Hiba Jebeile, APD, PhD
Senior Research Fellow, The University of Sydney
Sydney, Australia

Crystal N. Johnson-Mann, MD, MPH, FACS, FASMBS
Clinical Assistant Professor, Department of Surgery,
University of Florida
Gainesville, FL

Bonnie Tamis Jortberg, PhD, RDN, CDCES
Associate Professor, University of Colorado School of
Medicine, Department of Family Medicine
Boulder, CO

Kathryn P. King, MA
Psychology Graduate Student Trainee, University of
Alabama at Birmingham
Birmingham, AL

Samuel R. LaMunion, PhD
Postdoctoral Fellow, National Institutes of Health
Intramural Research Program, National Institute of
Diabetes, Digestive, and Kidney Diseases; Diabetes,
Endocrinology, and Obesity Branch, Energy Metabolism
Section, Human Energy and Body Weight Regulation Core
Bethesda, MD

Alexandra M. Lee, PhD
Manager, Clinical Research, WW International, Inc
New York, NY

Chloe Panizza Lozano, PhD, MHlthProm, GradDip Dietetics
Postdoctoral Research Fellow, Department of Human
Nutrition, Food and Animal Sciences,
College of Tropical Agriculture and Human Resources,
University of Hawaii at Manoa
Honolulu, HI

Corby K. Martin, PhD, FTOS
Professor, Pennington Biomedical Research Center
Baton Rouge, LA

Hannah E. Martin, MPH, RDN
Director of Advocacy, Association of Diabetes Care &
Education Specialists
Washington, DC

Caitlin Martinez, MS, RD
Department of Nutrition, University of North
Carolina Chapel Hill
Chapel Hill, NC

Courtney McCuen-Wurst, PsyD, LCSW
Assistant Professor, Perelman School of Medicine,
University of Pennsylvania
Philadelphia, PA

Alyssa M. Minnick, PhD
Clinical Program Associate, InBody BWA
Audubon, PA
Former Postdoctoral Research Fellow, Center for Weight
and Eating Disorders, Perelman School of Medicine,
University of Pennsylvania
Philadelphia, PA

Eileen S. Myers, MPH, RDN
Consultant, Eileen Myers, LLC
Fernandina Beach, FL

Faith Anne Newsome
Doctoral Candidate, University of Florida
Gainesville, FL

Vivian Ortiz, MD
Assistant Professor of Medicine, Washington University
School of Medicine
St Louis, MO

Rebecca L. Pearl, PhD
Assistant Professor, University of Florida
Gainesville, FL

Octavia Pickett-Blakely, MD, MHS
Associate Professor of Clinical Medicine,
University of Pennsylvania Perelman School of Medicine
Philadelphia, PA

Hollie A. Raynor, PhD, RD, LDN
Associate Dean of Research,
University of Tennessee Knoxville
Knoxville, TN

Shannon M. Robson, PhD, MPH, RD
Associate Professor, University of Delaware
Newark, DE

Marsha Schofield, MS, RD, LD, FAND
Owner, Marsha Schofield & Associates LLC
Stow, OH

Fatima Cody Stanford, MD, MPH, MPA, MBA, FAAP, FACP, FAHA, FAMWA, FTOS
Obesity Medicine Physician Scientist, Massachusetts General Hospital; Associate Professor of Medicine and Pediatrics, Harvard Medical School
Boston, MA

Deborah F. Tate, PhD
Professor of Nutrition, University of
North Carolina Chapel Hill
Chapel Hill, NC

Colleen Tewskbury, PhD, RD
Assistant Professor in Nutrition Science, School of Nursing, University of Pennsylvania
Philadelphia, PA

Maya K. Vadiveloo, PhD, RD, FAHA
Associate Professor of Nutrition, University of Rhode Island
Kingston, RI

Denise E. Wilfley, PhD
Scott Rudolph University Professor of Psychiatry, Medicine, Pediatrics, and Psychological & Brain Sciences;
Washington University School of Medicine, Department of Psychiatry
St Louis, MO

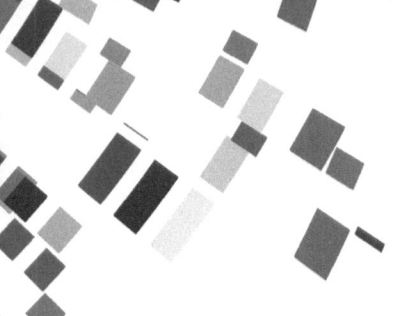

Reviewers

Laura Andromalos, MS, RD, RN, CSOWM, CDCES
Staff Nurse, Hennepin Healthcare
Minneapolis, MN

Jamy Ard, MD, FTOS
Professor, Departments of Epidemiology & Prevention and Internal Medicine
Vice Dean for Clinical Research, Wake Forest School of Medicine
Winston-Salem, NC

Melanie K. Bean, PhD
Professor of Pediatrics and Psychiatry, Division of Endocrinology and Metabolism
Co-Director, Healthy Lifestyles Center, Children's Hospital of Richmond at Virginia Commonwealth University
Richmond, VA

Britney Beatrice, MS, RDN, LDN
Instructor, University of Pittsburgh
Pittsburgh, PA

Dale S. Bond, PhD
Director of Research Integration,
Hartford Hospital/HealthCare
Hartford, CT

Mikel Bryant, MS, RDN, CSOWM, CD, LDN
Senior Dietitian, Leadership and Development,
Sensibly Sprouted
Bellingham, WA

W. Scott Butsch, MD, MSc, FTOS
Director of Obesity Medicine, Cleveland Clinic
Cleveland, OH

Catherine M. Champagne, PhD, RDN, LDN, FADA, FAND, FTOS, FAHA
Professor/Dietary Assessment and Nutrition Counseling,
Pennington Biomedical Research Center
Baton Rouge, LA

Nina Crowley, PhD, RDN, LD
Professional Affiliations and Education Manager,
seca Medical Body Composition
Mt Pleasant, SC

Connie Diekman, MEd, RD, LD FADA, FAND
Food and Nutrition Consultant, CBDiekman
Webster Groves, MO

Troy Donahoo, MD
Professor and Chief, Division of Endocrinology,
University of Florida,
Gainesville, FL

Kelli Friedman, PhD
Assistant Professor, Departments of Psychiatry and Behavioral Sciences and Surgery,
Duke University Medical Center
Durham, NC

Zachary I. Grunewald, PhD, MS, RDN, LD
Quality Manager, Emory Healthcare
Atlanta, GA

Kellene A. Isom, PhD, MS, RD, CAGS
Assistant Professor, California State Polytechnic University, Pomona
Pomona, CA

Craig Johnson, PhD
Associate Professor, University of Houston
Houston, TX

Scott Kahan, MD, MPH
Director, National Center for Weight and Wellness
Faculty, George Washington University School of Medicine
Washington, DC

Manju Karkare, MS, RDN, LDN, CLT, FAND
President/CEO, Nutritionally Yours, LLC
Wake Forest, NC

Sarah Keadle, PhD
Associate Professor, California Polytechnic State University
San Luis Obispo, CA

Robert Kushner, MD
Professor, Departments of Medicine and Medical Education,
Northwestern Feinberg School of Medicine
Chicago, IL

Melissa Majumdar, MS, RD, CSOWM, LDN
Metabolic and Bariatric Surgery Coordinator, Emory
University Hospital Midtown
Atlanta, GA

Anne Mathews, PhD, RDN
Associate Professor, University of Florida
Gainesville, FL

Jacob T. Mey, PhD, RD
Assistant Professor, Pennington Biomedical Research Center
Baton Rouge, LA

Maria Morgan-Bathke, MBA, PhD, RD, CD, LD, FAND
Associate Professor, Viterbo University
La Crosse, WI

Robin Nwankwo, MPH, RDN, CDCES
Diabetes Educator Registered Dietitian at
Department of Learning Health Sciences, Retired,
University of Michigan Medical School
Sandy Springs, GA

Melissa M. Page, MS, RDN, CSOWM, LDN
Senior Bariatric Dietitian, Maine Health Weight and
Wellness Program
Portland, ME

Rebecca Reeves, DrPH
Nutrition Consultant, Retired
Fredericksburg, TX

Julie Schwartz, MS, RDN, CSOWM, LD, ACSM-EP, NBC-HWC
Obesity Medicine Registered Dietitian Nutritionist Case
Manager, Intellihealth, Inc
New York, NY

Rebecca Skotek, RDN, LDN
Registered Dietitian, FORM
Houston, TX

Cicely Thomas, DCN, MEd, RDN, LD
WIC Nutrition Service Director,
Department of Public Health
Rome, GA

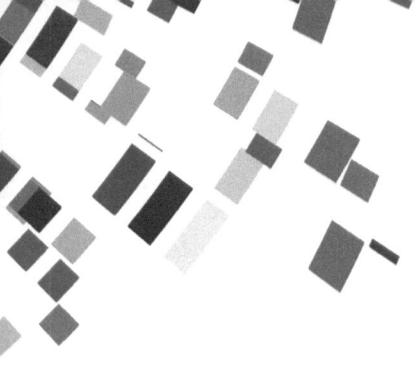

Foreword

Conversations about obesity are ever present these days—particularly given all of the emerging treatment options. As the din of voices adding perspectives and opinions on the subject grows louder, it is imperative to equip health care professionals with the knowledge and tools to effectively address this complex issue. The timeliness of the *Health Professional's Guide to Treatment of Overweight and Obesity*, a groundbreaking compilation edited by Hollie A. Raynor, PhD, RDN, LDN, and Linda M. Gigliotti, MS, RDN, CDCES, CSOWM, FAND, is just one of the features that makes this book so special. This text provides a clear guiding voice for health care professionals of all types through the collaborative efforts of esteemed experts who have devoted their careers to combating the multifaceted challenges posed by overweight and obesity.

A review of the first few chapters of the guide grounds you in some foundational knowledge and concepts that are central to a patient-centric model of care. From defining obesity as a chronic progressive disease to exploring the adverse health consequences of obesity, the initial chapter sets the foundation for the subsequent chapters that explore health disparities, weight bias, evidence-based guidelines, and patient-centered care. The interplay of these chapters will help you develop a science-based yet empathetic approach when working with patients. The initial chapters also foster a deeper understanding of the social determinants of health that drive outcomes and treatment engagement.

Through its 19 enlightening chapters, this guide provides a deep understanding of the complexities surrounding obesity as a disease, while offering evidence-based strategies for effective treatment and management. By addressing a broad range of topics, from the physiological aspects of body weight regulation to the impact of health care systems and policies on access to care, this comprehensive resource endeavors to foster a holistic perspective on patient care that emphasizes the role of myriad systems that must be considered in the patient journey.

Inherent in the holistic approach to care and management of obesity is the recognition that interdisciplinary team engagement is critical to delivering the highest quality care. Editors Raynor and Gigliotti have given you a superb guide that delves into interprofessional teams and models of practice, emphasizing the importance of teamwork and the diverse skill sets needed to address the complexities of overweight and obesity. In addition, it examines the impact of health care systems, policies, and insurance coverage on the accessibility of weight-management services, providing insights and proposing solutions to improve patient access and outcomes. As the field of comprehensive weight management continues to evolve, this text will stand as a blueprint for how collaboration in care can be implemented.

The *Health Professional's Guide to Treatment of Overweight and Obesity* stands as a testament to the dedication and expertise of its contributing authors, whose collective knowledge will undoubtedly transform the way health professionals approach and manage overweight and obesity. I fully expect that this guide will become an indispensable resource for those seeking to make a lasting impact on the health and well-being of individuals with overweight and obesity.

Jamy D. Ard, MD, FTOS
Professor and Vice Dean for Clinical Research, Wake Forest School of Medicine
Co-Director, Weight Management Center, Advocate Health Wake Forest Baptist
Winston-Salem, NC

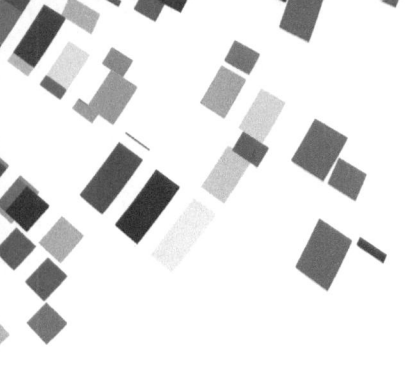

Preface

The treatment of overweight and obesity is a relatively new practice area in the health care field. While the incidence of overweight and obesity increased in the 1980s and 1990s, and the National Institutes of Health recognized obesity as a chronic disease in 1998, it was not until 2013 that the American Medical Association classified obesity as a chronic disease. For too long the health risks associated with excess adipose tissue were ignored. Obesity was attributed to individual choices and lack of self-control, and the focus of care was on changing body shape. Historically, the expectation was that calorie restriction would cure the problem of extra pounds. The landscape is still evolving today as we continue to learn about the complex nature of this chronic disease, its associated health concerns, and its management.

The *Health Professional's Guide to Treatment of Overweight and Obesity* provides a resource for clinicians involved in the care of adults with overweight and obesity. (Treatment of children and adolescents with overweight and obesity is a separate and highly nuanced topic—a subspecialty in its own right—and is not included in the scope of this book.) We begin by looking at the "big picture." Chapter 1 describes the physiological components of weight regulation, addressing genetics and life stages associated with the risk of increased adiposity. Chapters 2 and 3 incorporate the human element, describing social determinants of health, bias, and stigma, which can impact our perceptions of the disease and the care that is provided. With greater recognition of obesity as a disease, evidence-based standards for treatment have emerged, as outlined in Chapter 4. While the similarities in the guidelines outline a clearer direction for treatment, Chapter 5 reminds us that the patient is a member of the team. It is important to acknowledge the individual's goals and include them in the decision-making process; this can include whether treatment should even occur, and if it does, what it should look like.

Given the complexity of overweight and obesity, it is understandable that an interprofessional approach is now associated with comprehensive treatment. Clinicians generally tend to first look at the conditions through the lens of their own professional orientation. Chapters 6 through 14 review assessment, followed by interventions from the perspectives of medicine, nutrition, physical activity, and behavioral health. Chapter 10 highlights the strength of multicomponent lifestyle interventions, which are also part of the more intensive medical and surgical interventions described in Chapter 14. Personalized nutrition therapy from a registered dietitian nutritionist is a vital part of comprehensive obesity care, whether the approach includes lifestyle intervention, antiobesity medication, metabolic and bariatric surgery, or a combination of approaches to lose weight or maintain weight loss. As we develop greater appreciation for obesity as a chronic condition, it is important to acknowledge that it requires ongoing intervention and attention, as discussed in Chapter 15. Because obesity treatment is sometimes criticized for triggering eating disorders, Chapter 16 discusses the evidence between obesity treatment and eating pathology.

Several factors will affect how we implement interventions for overweight and obesity. We no longer rely solely on face-to-face interactions with our clients. Telehealth, remote monitoring, apps, and other technologies offer advantages—and disadvantages—for treatment plans, as discussed in Chapter 17. Chapter 18 identifies health care disciplines that may be part of an interprofessional team involved in weight management practice; each team member brings skills and expertise to the team while respecting the boundaries of their scope of practice. Though we recognize obesity as a disease and significant progress has been made to develop interventions to manage health-related risks, payment structures remain barriers to many services. Chapter 19 summarizes current health care policies and payment structures, with insight on how to advocate for enhanced policies.

The Health Professional's Guide to Treatment of Overweight and Obesity is intended for registered dietitian nutritionists; nutrition and dietetic technicians, registered; diabetes care and education specialists; physicians; nurses; pharmacists; and other allied health professionals. While obesity medicine is now recognized as a specialty practice area, given the prevalence of overweight and obesity, most of us will work with clients with overweight and obesity regardless of our area of practice. Irrespective of where one practices or who one works with, understanding the key concepts about obesity, its assessment, and its management will provide a practice foundation that is crucial for all health professionals.

Hollie A. Raynor, PhD, RD, LDN
Linda M. Gigliotti, MS, RDN, CDCES, CSOWM, FAND

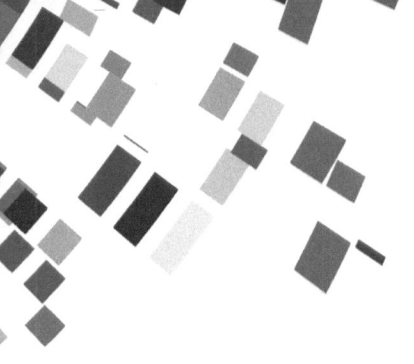

Acknowledgments

We would like to thank the Weight Management Dietetic Practice Group of the Academy of Nutrition and Dietetics for identifying the need for this book and supporting its development. A special thank you goes to the 44 authors from the fields of nutrition, medicine, psychology, behavioral health, exercise physiology, nursing, and social work who contributed their time and expertise to creating 19 excellent and informative chapters—truly an interprofessional effort!

Hollie A. Raynor, PhD, RD, LDN
Linda M. Gigliotti, MS, RDN, CDCES, CSOWM, FAND

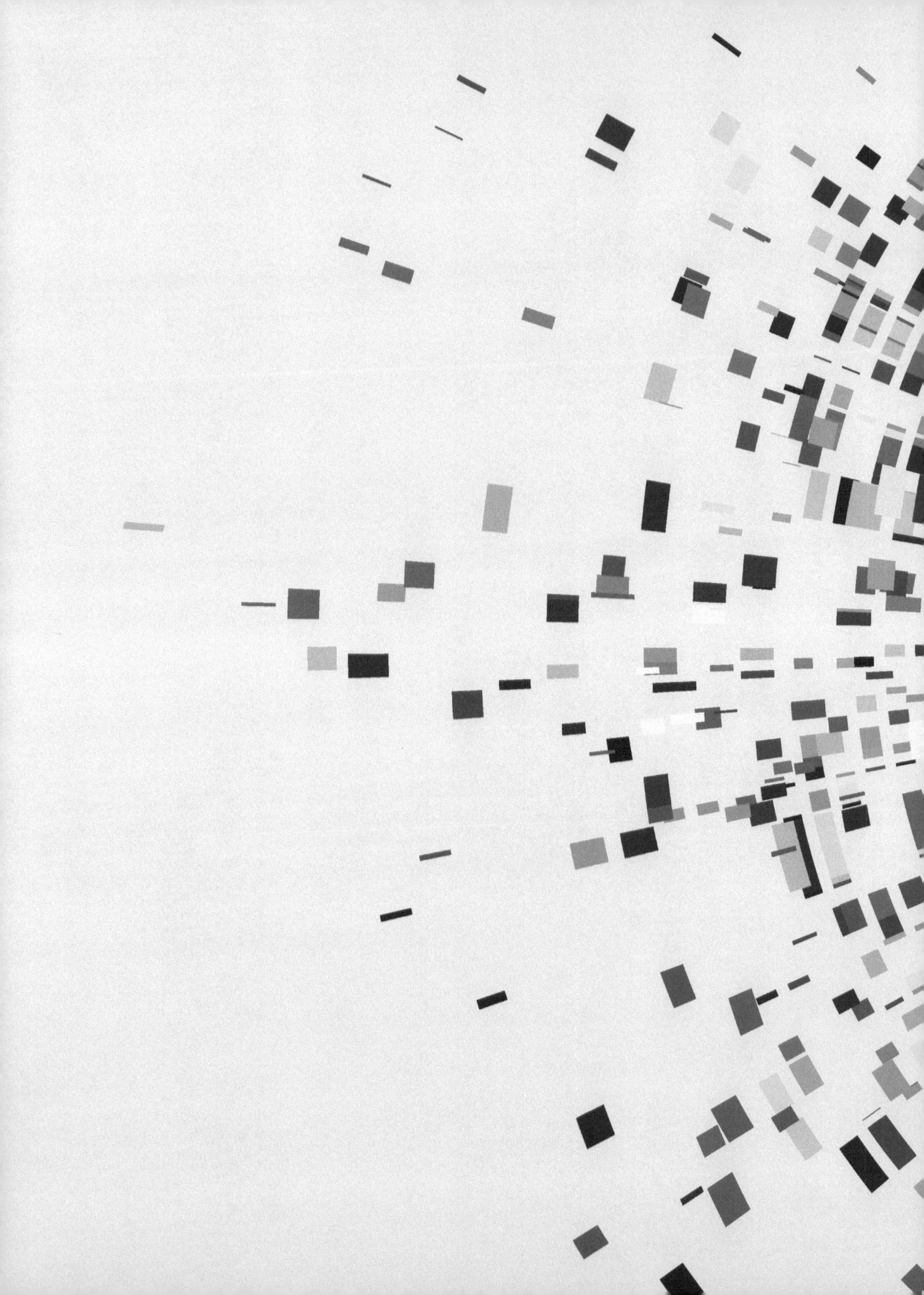

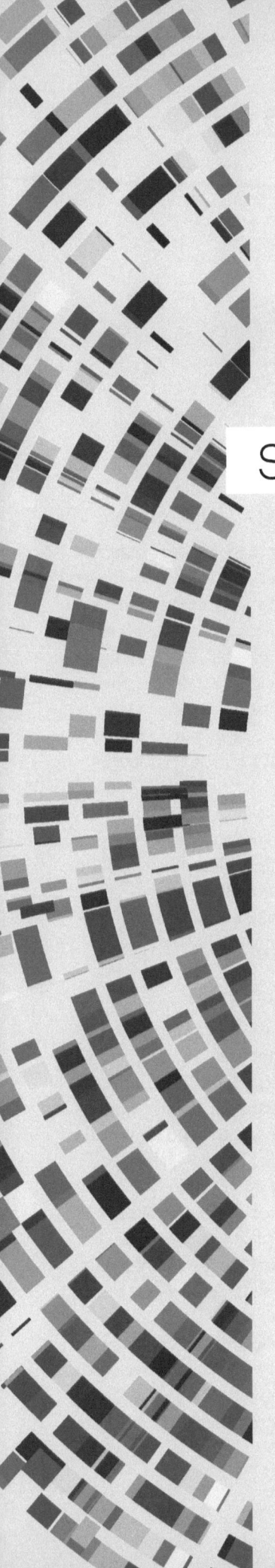

SECTION 1

Foundations of Treatment: The Human Element

CHAPTER 1 — Obesity as a Disease | 2

CHAPTER 2 — Health Inequities in the Development, Management, and Treatment of Obesity | 26

CHAPTER 3 — Weight Bias and Stigma | 44

CHAPTER 4 — Evidence-Based Guidelines for Treatment of Overweight and Obesity | 59

CHAPTER 5 — Patient-Centered Care and Shared Decision-Making | 67

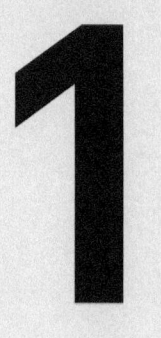

CHAPTER 1

Obesity as a Disease

Daniel Bessesen, MD

CHAPTER OBJECTIVES

- Define obesity as a chronic progressive disease.
- Summarize the physiological components of body weight regulation.
- Describe the prevalence of overweight and obesity, including the life stages during which people are at the greatest risk for increased adiposity.
- Discuss adverse health consequences of being overweight or obese.

Introduction

Obesity: A Disease of Body Weight Regulation

Many health care providers and patients believe that body weight is the product of lifestyle choices independent of any physiological regulation. On the contrary, over the last 20 years, it has become increasingly clear that body weight is carefully regulated by complex integrated physiological systems involving appetite, metabolism, the autonomic nervous system, endocrine systems, and several important brain regions.[1] This understanding has led medical professionals to conclude that obesity is a disease of body weight regulation, much the way diabetes is a disease of glucose homeostasis and hypertension is a disorder of blood pressure regulation.[2] Like these other chronic metabolic conditions, obesity is the product of a genetic predisposition to weight gain combined with an environment that promotes positive energy balance. An appreciation of the regulation of body weight and the challenges that individuals face when trying to lose weight provides health care workers and patients with a more realistic view, and better understanding, of the condition. This framework also informs key aspects of treatment. This chapter discusses body weight regulation, the adaptive responses to weight loss that promote weight regain, the definition of obesity, the prevalence of obesity, and weight changes throughout the life span.

Obesity Defined

Obesity is a level of excess adiposity associated with adverse health consequences. The most commonly used method for quantifying excess body fat is BMI calculated as a person's height, in meters squared, divided by their weight in kilograms.[3] The categories of weight based on BMI per the Centers for Disease Control and Prevention (CDC) are: overweight (BMI 25–29.9), class 1 obesity (BMI 30–34.9), class 2 obesity (BMI 35–39.9), and class 3 (severe) obesity (BMI of 40 or higher). BMI was initially developed as a population metric for estimating the risk of morbidity and mortality. Actual health risks for individuals vary substantially, independent of BMI, according to factors such as genetics, habitual physical activity levels, dietary quality, and others. BMI also has its limitations for categorizing weight, because some individuals may weigh more than others due to their having a greater lean body mass. BMI is not a direct measure of body fat but correlates well with percent body fat in populations. Because metabolic complications of obesity are related to regional fat deposition—with increased fat in the abdominal region being more associated with adverse health consequences—waist circumference can supplement BMI in the assessment of obesity-related health risks. BMI cutoff points to categorize individuals as overweight or obese differ among the various ethnic groups, as seen in Figure 1.1.[4]

The Regulation of Body Weight

Central to the understanding of obesity as a disease is the idea that body weight is regulated the same way as other important physiological variables, such as blood glucose or blood pressure. To maintain a stable body weight, energy intake must be balanced over time against energy expenditure. Stored nutrients within the body—including fat, glucose, and protein—buffer metabolic and energetic needs against hour-to-hour and day-to-day changes in energy balance. When one considers the amount of energy a person consumes and burns over the course of a lifetime, it becomes clear that body weight must be physiologically regulated. From age 20 years to age 60 years, a hypothetical cisgender male of average size might consume almost 30 million kcal of food. With certain assumptions being made about dietary composition, this represents more than 5,100 kg (11,220 lb) of food. Because of the long period of time (40 years) and the degree of daily energy flux, an increase in body weight from 66 kg (145 lb) at age 20 years to 100 kg (220 lb) at age 60 reflects an energy imbalance of only 13 kcal/d. Because energy expenditure declines with age, even in this hypothetical individual who gains 34 kg (75 lb) over 40 years, his predicted energy intake will actually decline from 2,911 kcal/d at age 20 years to 2,500 kcal/d at age 60 years, despite the increase in weight. Although people have the subjective experience that they choose what they eat and select their habitual level of physical activity, consideration of the energetics of weight balance quickly reveals how choice alone cannot produce the level of precision observed in this regulatory system, even when an individual gains weight.

Studies in animals also support the idea that body weight is physiologically regulated. Rats living in an environment with palatable food and reduced access to physical activity will gradually gain weight throughout their lives. If a researcher places a feeding tube into the rat's stomach and overfeeds it, the rat will gradually gain weight if the overfeeding is continued. When the overfeeding stops, the rat's weight will gradually decline, not to where it was but to where it would have been had the overfeeding not occurred. This is shown in Figure 1.2 on page 4.[5]

FIGURE 1.1 Defining obesity using BMI and waist circumference[4]

Populations	Classification	BMI, kg/m²	Co-morbidity risk	Waist circumference, cm	
				males < 94; females < 80	males ≥ 94; females ≥ 80
General population (Caucasian, Europid, Middle-Eastern, Sub-Saharan African)	underweight normal weight overweight obese class I obese class II obese class III	<18.5 18.5–24.9 25.0–29.9 30.0–34.9 35.0–39.9 ≥40	low but with other problems average increased moderate severe very severe	– – increased high very high extremely high	– – high very high very high extremely high
				Waist circumference, cm	
				males < 85; females < 74	males ≥ 85; females ≥ 74
East Asian, South Asian and Southeast Asian populations	normal weight overweight obese	<23 ≥23 ≥27.5	– increased high	– increased high	– high very high

Reproduced with permission from Abusnana S, Fargaly M, Alfardan SH, et al. Clinical practice recommendations for the management of obesity in the United Arab Emirates. *Obes Facts*. 2018;11(5):413-428. doi:10.1159/000491796.[4]

FIGURE 1.2 Regulation of body weight in animal studies[5]

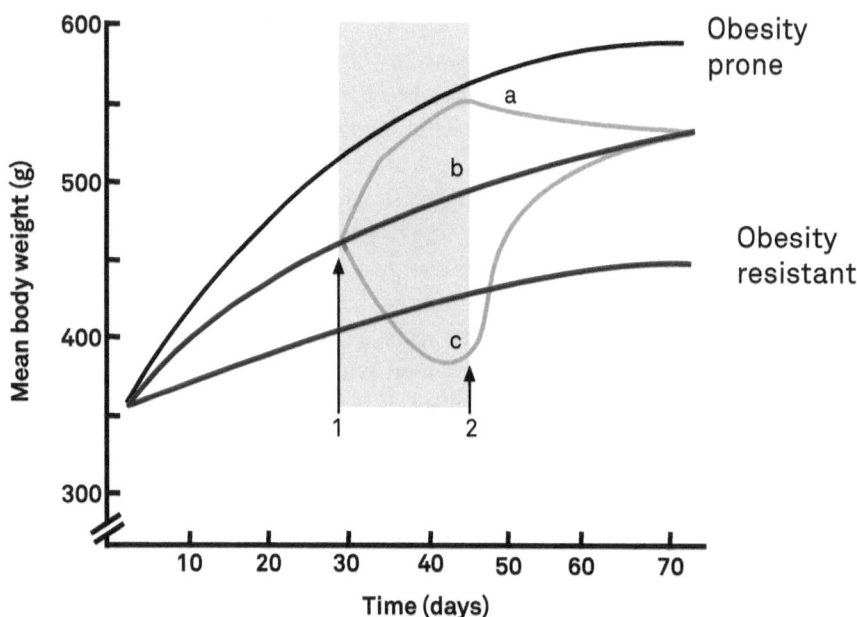

Animals tend to adjust their food intake to achieve a normal body weight. The graph shows a schematized growth curve for three groups of rats that were either force-fed (a), allowed free access to food (b), or food-restricted (c) for the period of time between the arrows. Note that the animals slowly returned to normal weight when allowed free access to food.
Reproduced with permission from Bessesen DH. Regulation of body weight: what is the regulated parameter? *Physiol Behav.* 2011;104(4):599-607. doi:10.1016/j.physbeh.2011.05.006.[5]

Alternatively, the researcher can restrict energy intake in an adult rat, and the rat's weight will gradually fall until it reaches a new plateau. If energy restriction is stopped, the rat's weight will increase, not to where it was but to where it would have been if energy restriction had not been imposed. These results suggest that weight is not regulated around a "set point" but rather around a trajectory of gradual weight gain across the life span.

Is this also true for human beings? Epidemiological data suggest that body weight gradually increases over the life span in human beings until roughly age 65 years, after which body weight gradually declines, as illustrated in Figure 1.3.[6]

Clinicians frequently see patients who experience progressive weight gain over their lifetime. When these patients adopt new lifestyle habits that produce weight loss, if the lifestyle habits are not sustained, their weight increases—not to where it was, but to an even higher level; this is consistent with what has been seen in animal studies (refer to Figure 1.4).[5] Even when an individual maintains consistent lifestyle habits or continues the use of an anti-obesity medication, weight often gradually increases over time. This increase in weight may reflect adaptive responses to weight loss that promote weight regain, but it may also reflect the natural tendency of body weight to increase over time.

This type of regulation is called *homeorhesis*.[5] Unlike a system regulated by homeostasis, where the system maintains stability in a particular physiological parameter, a system regulated by homeorhesis is regulated around a trajectory rather than a steady state. In animal studies, the trajectory of weight gain over the life span reflects both genetics and the environment. Rats that are genetically prone to weight gain display a steeper trajectory of weight gain over the course of their lives. Alternatively, rats or mice that are genetically resistant to obesity

FIGURE 1.3 Predicted BMI trajectories by race and ethnicity[a,6]

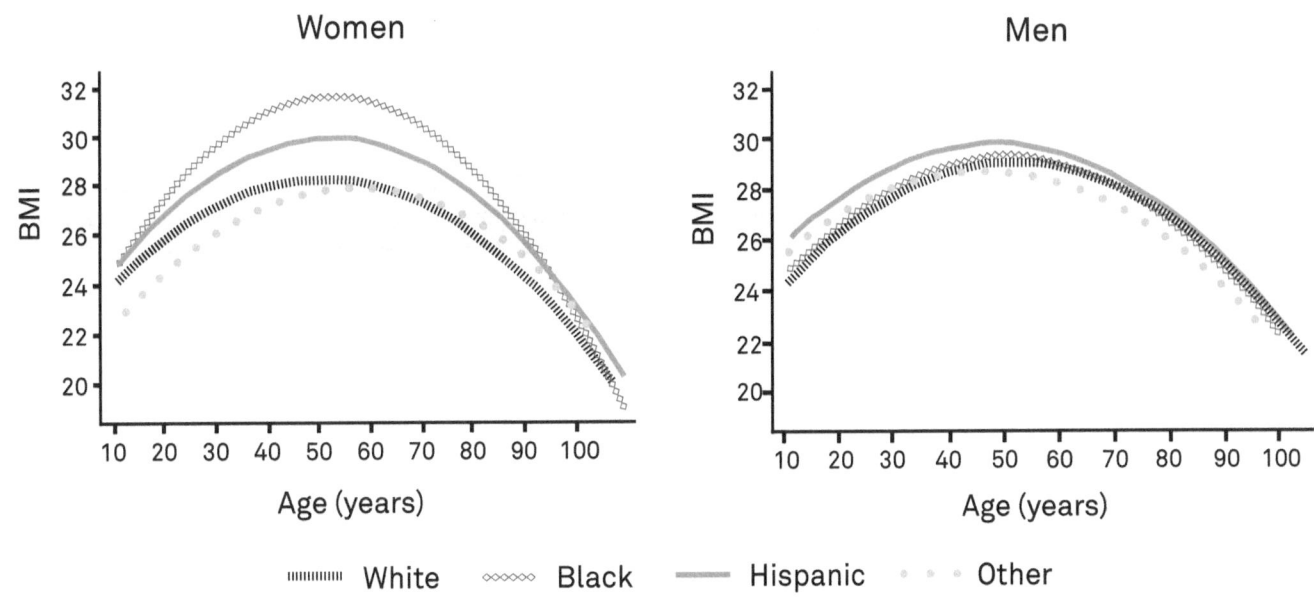

[a] Study participants were described as men and women. Gender was not further specified.
Adapted with permission from Yang YC, Walsh CE, Johnson MP, et al. Life-course trajectories of body mass index from adolescence to old age: racial and educational disparities. *Proc Natl Acad Sci U S A*. 2021;118(17):e2020167118. doi:10.1073/pnas.2020167118.[6]

FIGURE 1.4 Weight regulation in humans[5]

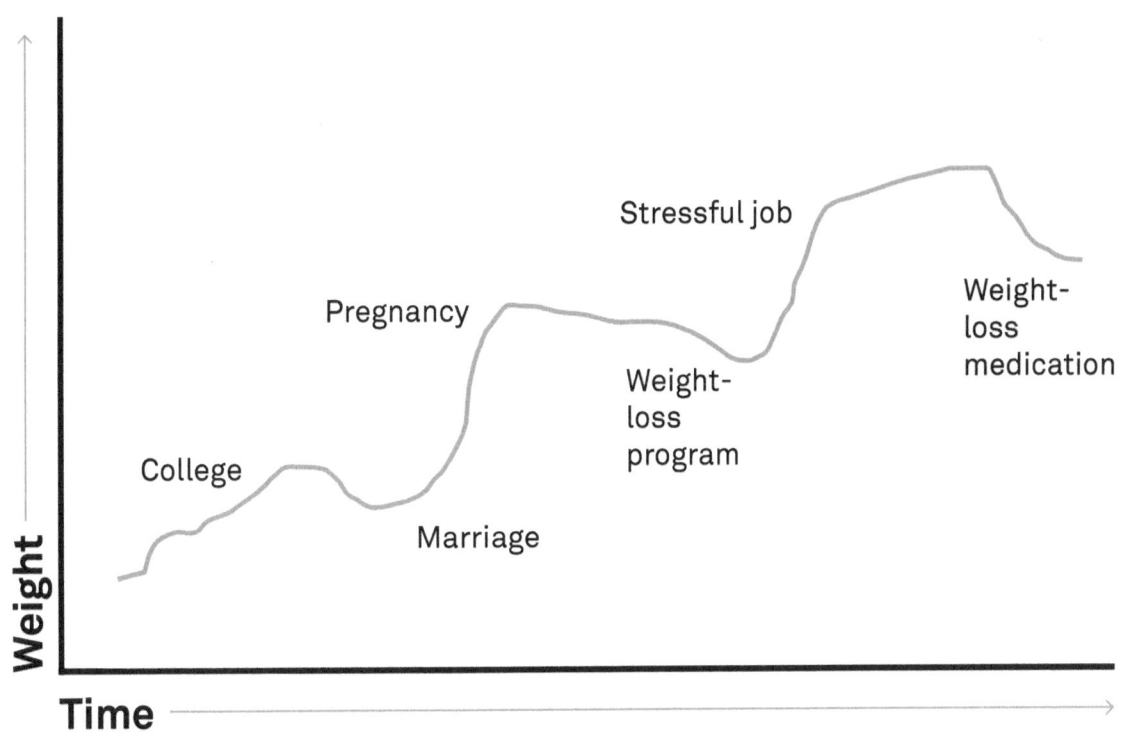

CHAPTER 1: Obesity as a Disease 5

gain less weight over their lives. An animal living in an environment where food is constantly available and highly palatable will gain more weight than the same animal living in an environment in which food is less available or less appetizing. The opportunity to exercise, made possible by the availability of a running wheel, reduces the rate of weight gain over time. All rodent models show weight gain over time; they just vary in the rate and degree of weight gain. This is similar to the situation with human beings, who vary in their weight gain based on genetic predisposition and environmental factors.

One might ask whether the trajectory of weight gain can be modified by long-term changes in lifestyle. Animal studies in which rats were placed on a hypocaloric diet for varying lengths of time and then were allowed to consume an ad libitum diet showed that the longer the animal was subjected to energy restriction, the more rapid and substantial their weight regain. Weight inevitably returned to where it would have been in control animals, not to where it was prior to energy restriction.[7] Because an animal's "defended weight" (the natural weight seen in the absence of an energy-restricted diet) continues to increase as time passes, the weight of rats subjected to prolonged energy restriction was farther away from the defended weight, resulting in a larger increase in weight when free choice of dietary intake was reintroduced (Figure 1.5).[8]

FIGURE 1.5 Does the body get used to the reduced obese state? Body weights and the rate of weight regain in animal studies[8]

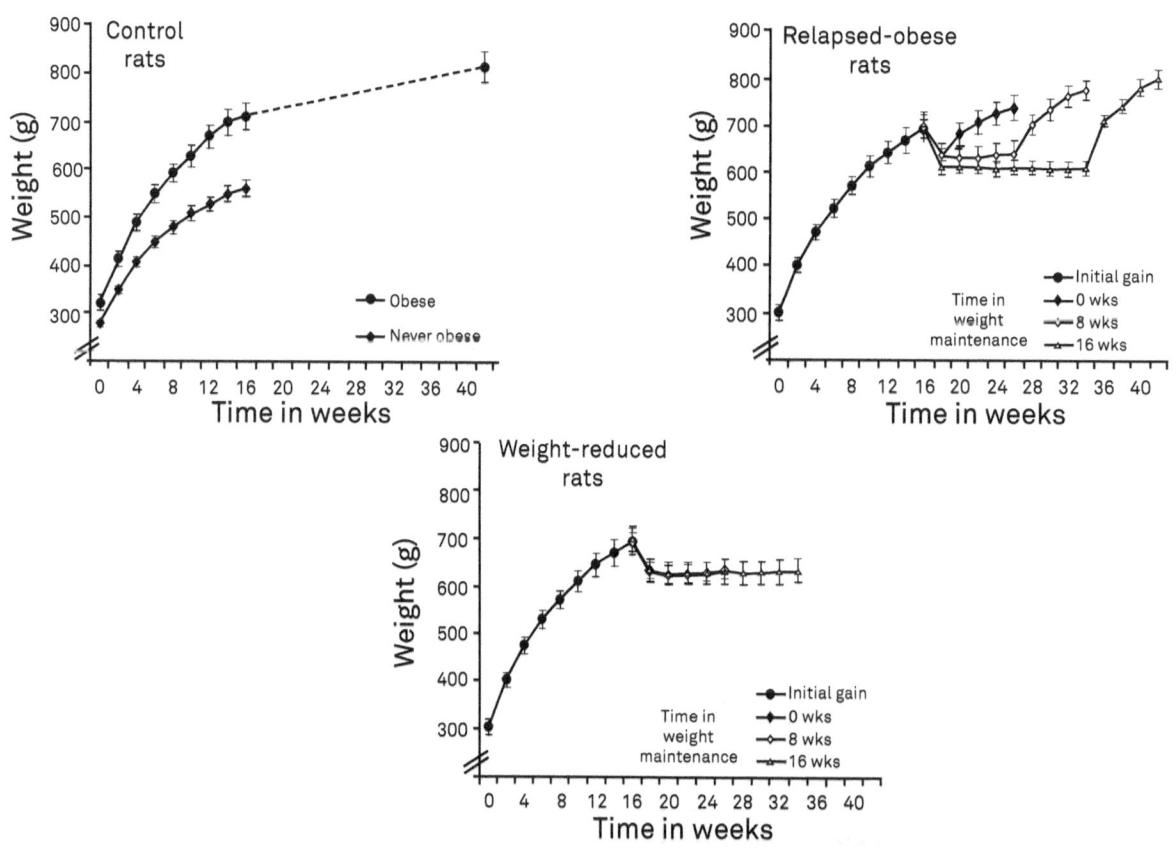

Reproduced with permission from MacLean PS, Higgins JA, Johnson GC, et al. Enhanced metabolic efficiency contributes to weight regain after weight loss in obesity-prone rats. *Am J Physiol Regul Integr Comp Physiol.* 2004;287(6):R1306-R1315. doi:10.1152/ajpregu.00463.2004.[8]

Body weight, then, is a reflection of long-term energy balance, with weight gain occurring when intake exceeds expenditure, weight loss occurring when expenditure exceeds intake, and weight stability occurring when intake equals expenditure. To gain a deeper understanding of energy balance, one must understand its components—energy expenditure and energy intake.

Energy Expenditure

Total daily energy expenditure (TDEE) is equal to the amount of energy (in kilocalories) per day that a person can consume to maintain energy balance. The three main components of TDEE are:

- basal metabolic rate (BMR),
- thermic effect of food (TEF), and
- physical activity energy expenditure (PAEE).

These are illustrated in Figure 1.6.

BMR is the largest component of TDEE, accounting for roughly 70% of TDEE in most individuals. It reflects the amount of energy consumed per day to maintain body temperature, electrolyte gradients across cell membranes, kidney function, and other vital bodily functions. BMR can be determined by measuring oxygen consumption with indirect calorimetry while an individual is awake but at rest. BMR can also be estimated using formulas, such as the Mifflin-St Jeor equation[9]:

$$\text{Male: } (10 \times \text{weight [kg]}) + (6.25 \times \text{height [cm]}) - (5 \times \text{age [y]}) + 5$$
$$\text{Female: } (10 \times \text{weight [kg]}) + (6.25 \times \text{height [cm]}) - (5 \times \text{age [y]}) - 161$$

FIGURE 1.6 Components of energy expenditure

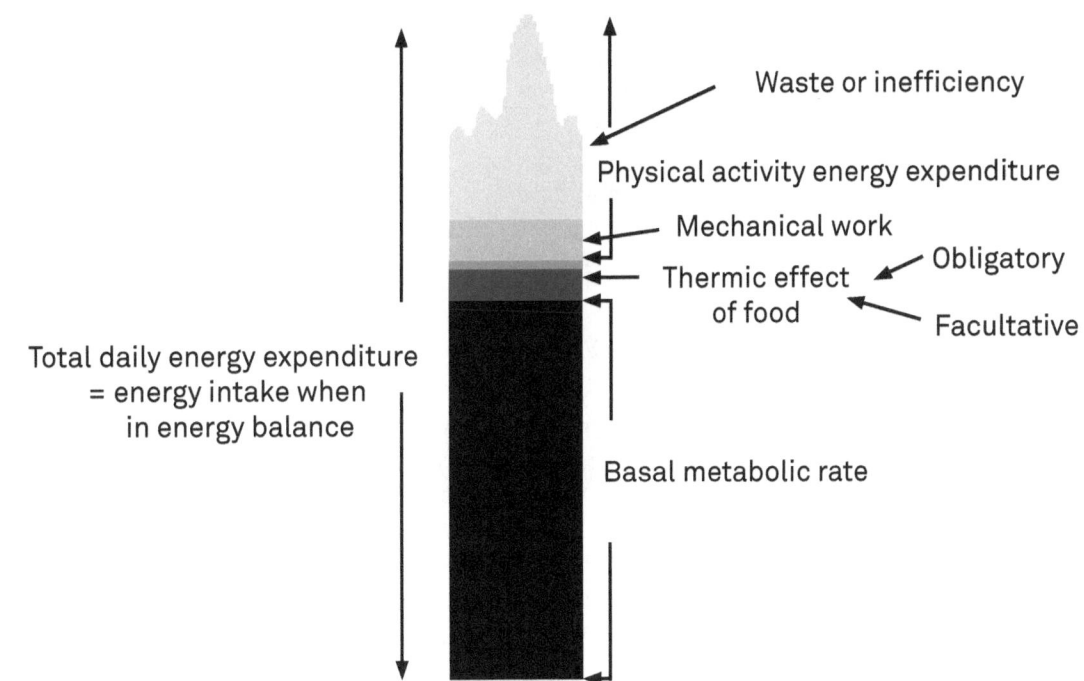

These equations reflect the observed effect of body size, sex, and age on BMR. The formula predicts that BMR will fall with age, and as a result, so will TDEE. This fall in TDEE was recently demonstrated by a large study of more than 12,000 individuals as part of the Framingham Heart Study.[10] Because of this decline, people gain weight as they age unless they reduce their energy intake or increase their physical activity over time.

BMR is linearly related to lean body mass with a nonzero intercept.[11] That is, TDEE increases linearly as lean body mass increases, but if this relationship is extrapolated to a lean body mass of zero, there will still be some level of energy expenditure. This demonstrates that a certain minimal level of energy expenditure is associated with the energy requirements of core organs such as the brain, heart, and kidneys. There is some variability in the energy expended by people with the same lean body mass. Interestingly, though, recent evidence suggests that people with slightly elevated energy expenditure are at risk for weight gain. This somewhat counterintuitive idea will need confirmation by ongoing research, but it reflects what has been called a "thrifty phenotype."

TEF is the second component of energy expenditure. It is the energy required to digest food and distribute nutrients to tissues. The portion of TEF that represents the actual chemical energy involved in these biochemical reactions is called obligatory TEF. The other portion, called the facultative TEF, reflects the inefficiency of the system; in other words, more energy is expended in the process of assimilating dietary nutrients than would be predicted simply by the chemical reactions. TEF represents 8% to 10% of TDEE and varies between individuals. Some researchers have hypothesized that people with more efficient TEF might be predisposed to weight gain, yet the evidence for this is not conclusive.

The third and most variable component of TDEE is the PAEE. As was true for TEF, some of the energy expended in physical activity is the result of the actual mechanical work done during the activity, and some of the energy expended in physical activity is wasted due to the inefficiencies of movement. That is, it takes more energy to execute the activity than is needed just for the mechanical work of the activity. People vary in their exercise efficiency, and a person can become more efficient with experience. For example, suppose an amateur swimmer and an elite swimmer swim the same 100 m at the same speed. If both swimmers weigh the same, one might expect them to burn the same amount of energy because each must move the same amount of weight through the water for the same distance at the same speed. However, the elite athlete is a highly efficient swimmer and so burns less energy at the same workload compared to the amateur (of course the amateur is not able to generate the workload that the elite swimmer can). PAEE is a function of the intensity of the activity, the duration of the activity, and the size of the person if the activity is weight-bearing.

Physical Activity

Physical activity can occur in planned bouts or might occur through the activities of daily living. Energy generated by the latter is called nonexercise activity thermogenesis, or NEAT. There is evidence that, with overfeeding, some individuals increase their NEAT, leading to increased PAEE and a protection against weight gain.[12] The implications of this finding are that physical activity levels are biologically regulated. Most people can understand how food intake might be biologically regulated, because they experience hunger and satiety. However, people do not generally think of exercise bouts in the same way they think about meals. They understand hunger as stimulating food intake, satiety as promoting meal termination, and rising hunger as affecting the length of time between meals. In contrast, what makes a person want to initiate an exercise bout? What makes them end the bout? What physiological parameters determine the interval between bouts of exercise? Ongoing research suggests that areas of the hypothalamus are involved in the regulation of physical activity in much the same way this region of the brain regulates appetite.

The observed relationship between TDEE and body size means that larger individuals have higher levels of TDEE than smaller individuals. This makes sense, as it would require more energy to sustain a larger body than a smaller body. This means that larger people who are maintaining weight must be eating more than smaller people. However, many people with obesity report very low levels of energy intake. These individuals wonder if they might have a "metabolic disorder" causing their obesity. This issue has been addressed in studies examining energy expenditure and food intake in people who are obese but report low levels of energy intake. These studies have demonstrated that energy expenditure in these people is what would be predicted based on their age, sex, and body size. These studies show that, although there is some variability in TDEE between individuals of a particular body size, the primary explanation for the discrepancy between reported energy intake and predicted TDEE is substantial underreporting of dietary intake.[13] These studies do not support the idea that very low levels of energy expenditure are a primary cause of weight gain.

While experimental evidence is firm on this point, it is rarely productive to discuss this data with patients in a clinical setting. Although it might be easy to think that the person with obesity who reports eating very little is not being entirely truthful, another view is that the basic pathophysiological problem leading to weight gain is a malfunction of the system that should allow them to get a realistic view of how much they are eating. The frequently heard comment "I'm eating almost nothing" may be more a reflection of the person's cognitive effort to restrict energy intake than an accurate assessment of what they are eating. In these situations, it may be more productive to say something such as, "It sounds like you're working hard to limit how much you are eating and trying your best to consume a good diet." In fact, this inability to accurately assess energy intake is one of the greatest barriers to effective lifestyle treatment of obesity and is the reason dietary self-monitoring is so important for those embarking on dietary restriction for weight loss.

Energy Intake

The brain is the primary regulator of energy homeostasis. Since the 1950s, following observations in human beings with tumors of the hypothalamus and studies in rodents in which brain regions were lesioned, scientists have known that the hypothalamus plays an important role in regulating body weight. To maintain body weight, the brain must receive information about energy consumed, energy expended, and nutrient stores within the body (refer to Figure 1.7 on page 10). For many years, the dominant theory of body weight regulation was the lipostatic theory, which posited that the brain regulated adipose tissue mass. It was not clear, however, how the brain knew what total-body adipose-tissue energy storage was.

In 1994, leptin was discovered as the likely hormone from adipose tissue signaling the brain on the status of total-body lipid stores. Ten years of experiments followed that revealed the underlying mechanisms by which leptin signaling in the hypothalamus affects energy balance.

It has become clear that the hypothalamus regulates energy intake through two parallel pathways: an anabolic pathway that promotes food intake and reduces

FIGURE 1.7 Overview of energy homeostasis

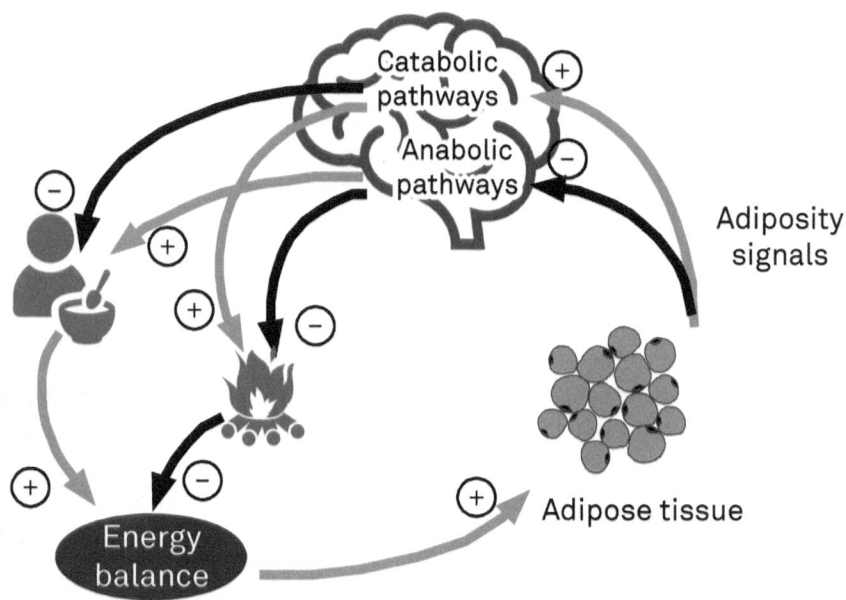

Figure 1.7 depicts the hypothalamic regulation of energy balance. The catabolic pathway from the hypothalamus inhibits food intake and stimulates energy expenditure when the body is in positive energy balance (increased fat mass). Conversely, the anabolic pathways stimulate food intake and inhibit energy expenditure when the body is in negative energy balance (decrease in fat mass). These systems work coordinately to help maintain energy homeostasis.

energy expenditure, and a catabolic pathway that reduces food intake and increases energy expenditure.[14] Changes in leptin and insulin levels signal these two pathways in a coordinate manner, stimulating the anabolic pathway in states of negative energy balance, and stimulating the catabolic pathway in states of energy excess. These two pathways live within the arcuate nucleus of the hypothalamus, as illustrated in Figure 1.8.

Cells expressing neuropeptide Y and agouti-related peptide are the first step in the anabolic pathway. Another population of cells in the arcuate nucleus express pro-opiomelanocortin and cocaine and amphetamine–regulated transcript. These cells are the first step in the catabolic pathway. Both populations of cells have receptors for leptin and insulin, although the effects of these hormones on the two cell populations are opposite. Leptin and insulin, which are increased in states of positive energy balance, stimulate the catabolic pathway and inhibit the anabolic pathway. The neurons that are downstream from these two cell populations are in the paraventricular nucleus and the lateral hypothalamus. Neuropeptide Y from the arcuate nucleus binds to receptors on cells in the paraventricular nucleus to stimulate food intake and reduce energy expenditure. A fragment of pro-opiomelanocortin, α-melanocyte-stimulating hormone, binds to downstream neurons, which express melanocortin receptors to reduce food intake and increase energy expenditure. Interestingly, agouti-related peptide made by cells in the anabolic pathway inhibits the catabolic pathway.

FIGURE 1.8 Regions of the hypothalamus that regulate energy balance

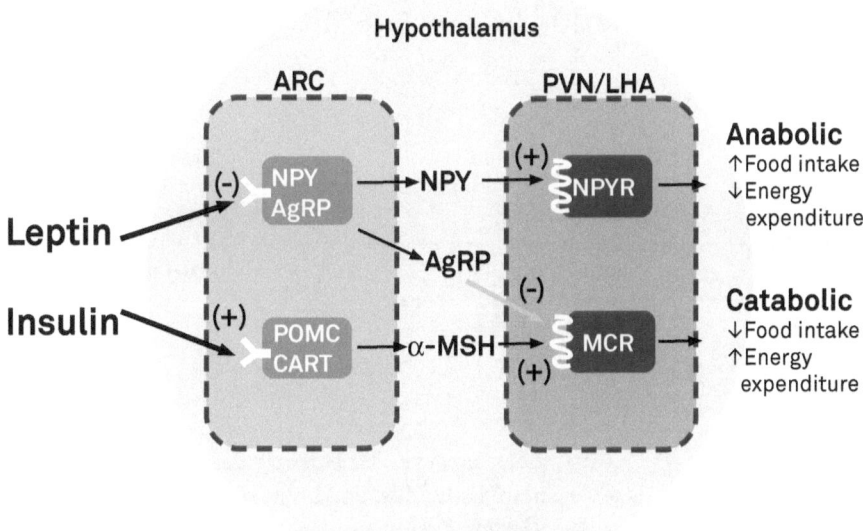

Abbreviations: AgRP, agouti-related peptide; α-MSH, α-melanocyte-stimulating hormone; ARC, arcuate nucleus; CART, cocaine and amphetamine–regulated transcript; MCR, melanocortin receptor; NPY, neuropeptide Y; NPYR, neuropeptide Y receptor; POMC, pro-opiomelanocortin; PVN/LHA, paraventricular nucleus/lateral hypothalamic area.

The Role of Appetite in Energy Intake

On closer consideration, the task of regulating appetite over time is incredibly complex. Although energy balance is generally depicted as a scale, balancing intake with expenditure, the body is rarely in energy balance. When a person wakes up in the morning, that person will not have eaten for, perhaps, 10 hours. The body is in negative energy balance and is using stored nutrients. Insulin level is low, appetite is increased, and satiety is reduced—all of which prompt the person to eat. In the hour after eating, the gastrointestinal tract is in a state of positive energy balance, but the nutrients consumed have not yet been delivered to peripheral tissues, such as skeletal muscle and adipose tissue, which remain in a state of negative energy balance. Over the course of the day, the body gradually moves into a state of positive energy balance through the ingestion of multiple meals and subsequent rising insulin levels, assimilation of ingested nutrients, and refilling of glycogen stores in the liver and muscle. Then, overnight during sleep, the body uses those stored nutrients as it transitions back to a state of negative energy balance. Thus, the body must make adjustments in energy intake on timescales shorter than what is needed for changes in levels of total body fat. The gastrointestinal tract sends out several signals that provide information on these shorter timescales. Ghrelin is a hormone made by the stomach and proximal intestine that increases with fasting and stimulates appetite. Peptide YY and glucagon-like peptide 1 are intestinal hormones whose levels increase after meal ingestion and that stimulate satiety. Many hormones are involved with regulation of hunger. The impact of these major hormones is summarized in Box 1.1 on page 12. The previously discussed cells in the hypothalamus also have receptors for and respond to these hormones. In this manner, both short-term and long-term signals of energy balance are conveyed to the hypothalamus to precisely regulate energy intake and expenditure. This system has come to be known as the *homeostatic regulatory system*.

BOX 1.1

Effect of Select Hormones and Neurotransmitters on Hunger

Hormone/neurotransmitter	Source	Effect on hunger
Leptin	Adipose tissue	Reduces
Ghrelin	Stomach	Increases
Peptide YY	Ileum and colon	Reduces
Glucagon-like peptide 1	Small intestine	Reduces

It is clear, however, that people eat not only because they are hungry. Food is a pleasurable stimulus, and brain regions that are involved in reward and pleasure are also involved in regulating food intake. The ventral striatum is one such region, and the neurotransmitter dopamine plays an important role in the process of reward and pleasure in relation to food. Some investigators have wondered whether alterations in dopamine signaling in brain regions associated with reward might be involved in the development of obesity. Studies have suggested that the density of dopamine receptors in these brain regions in people with obesity may differ from receptor density in people without obesity.[15] Whether these changes are the cause of, or the result of, obesity is not clear.

Although reward plays an important role in behavior, human beings do not always respond to rewarding stimuli. Certain regions of the brain, including the prefrontal cortex, modulate responses to rewarding stimuli in the environment. These brain regions modulate impulsivity and facilitate long-term planning. Activity in these regions has been found to be dramatically increased in individuals with eating disorders, such as anorexia nervosa, and reduced in individuals with obesity.[16] It is unclear whether these alterations in brain functioning are a cause of, or a consequence of, obesity.

Social and Cultural Influences on Intake

Food intake, physical activity, and other lifestyle behaviors are also subject to myriad social and cultural influences, which likely work through the cerebral cortex to modify behavior. Many people find that they overeat in social settings where it is encouraged, such as at holiday gatherings with family and friends. And individuals respond to a range of environmental stimuli—from the promotion of fast-food consumption to the praise of organic or natural food—that shape their behaviors. In addition, the importance of social relationships in body weight regulation has been demonstrated in studies of social networks. One such study, of people who were monitored over many years as part of the Framingham Heart Study, evaluated the available data on body weight measured longitudinally, as well as the data on the social relationships among people living in Framingham, MA.[17] The study found that social connections were strongly correlated with longitudinally measured weight gain. People in some groups gained weight together over time, and people in other groups maintained a normal weight over time. It is likely that social groups facilitated lifestyle behaviors that promoted weight gain or weight maintenance. It is not clear whether social networks can be leveraged to alter body weight; however, it is certain that social support is important in helping people adhere to a lifestyle program.

Genetics

Studies of twins raised in different households suggest that 40% to 70% of BMI is genetically determined.[18] There are several rare conditions in which single gene mutations cause obesity. Examples are mutations of leptin, the leptin receptor, pro-opiomelanocortin, and the melanocortin receptor. There are also syndromic forms of obesity, the most common of which is the Prader-Willi syndrome. These monogenic and syndromic forms of obesity are characterized by early-onset severe obesity and are often associated with other findings, such as developmental delay, short stature, and hypogonadism. Currently, genetic testing is available to make specific diagnoses for many of these conditions.[19] The development of newer therapeutic approaches to some of these genetic and syndromic conditions means that knowledge of a specific genetic problem in an individual with early-onset severe obesity may allow for specific treatment to be delivered, resulting in an improved outcome.[20]

Common obesity is explained by not one but many genes. Genome-wide association studies have identified more than 100 genetic loci that are associated with obesity. However, together these genes only explain 3% to 5% of the variance in BMI in a population. A number of gene panels have been developed that allow for the prediction of weight-gain risk, but these tests are not yet precise enough to advocate for their use in clinical practice. The most common gene associated with obesity is the fat mass and obesity associated (*FTO*) gene.[21] Variants of *FTO* appear to be associated with differences in appetite and differences in the development of thermogenic fat (beige fat). Although the *FTO* gene is the most common gene variant associated with weight gain, the effect size is small. Individuals who are homozygous for the risk allele weigh, on average, only a few more pounds than those with low-risk alleles.

Implications of Thinking of Obesity as a Disease of Body Weight Regulation

Thinking about obesity as a chronic, often progressive metabolic disease rather than as a problem of lifestyle choices changes the way health care professionals communicate with patients about it and how they treat it. First, people who undertake a lifestyle change with the goal of losing weight often become frustrated when, despite continuing the new lifestyle program, their rate of weight loss—while initially rapid—slows and reaches a new plateau. Many people become discouraged with this plateau and feel that treatment plan is no longer working. This frustration can lead to discontinuation of the lifestyle intervention and weight regain. It is important to explain to patients that TDEE declines with weight loss for a number of reasons and, as a result, a new steady state is reached in which the reduced energy intake becomes equal to a reduced TDEE. What causes the reduction in TDEE with weight loss? The most important factor is the weight loss itself. Recall that energy expenditure is linearly related to lean body mass. As a person loses weight, that person's basal metabolic rate declines. In addition, energy expended in physical activity declines because the person weighs less. Walking a mile at a body weight of 68 kg (150 lb) uses less energy than walking a mile at a weight of 102 kg (225 lb). When discussing lifestyle interventions, clinicians should make clear to patients that, while continuing the lifestyle program, they can expect their weight to plateau at a new level, and that continued adherence to the program will be required to maintain their new weight over time.

Adaptive Responses to Weight Loss That Promote Weight Regain

If weight is a physiologically regulated parameter, then when a person loses weight, it would stand to reason that the body would recruit regulatory systems to try to restore body weight to the defended (natural) trajectory. Evidence supports this hypothesis. Accumulating evidence in studies of people who have lost weight demonstrates that a person's energy expenditure falls more than one would expect based simply on the amount of weight lost, and that the person's appetite increases.[22] These responses to weight loss reduce energy needs and increase the drive for energy intake, predisposing the individual to positive energy balance and weight regain.

As noted previously, energy expenditure is linearly related to body mass. With weight loss, a person's energy expenditure would be expected to fall as a result of the reduction in body size. But studies measuring energy expenditure before and after weight loss have shown that the fall in energy expenditure is greater than what would be predicted simply by the loss in body weight.[22] This means that someone who has lost weight needs to consume less energy than a person of the same body size who has not lost weight. This disproportionate reduction in energy expenditure in relation to weight loss occurs both in the BMR and the PAEE. It is associated with a fall in leptin and thyroid hormone levels and a fall in sympathetic nervous system activity.[23] Studies examining work efficiency during low-level exercise have shown that, after weight loss, the amount of energy expended during a fixed exercise workload is lower than the amount expended at the same workload before weight loss. There is some evidence that replacing leptin to levels before weight loss restores exercise efficiency to levels before weight loss.[24] Several long-term follow-up studies have been done to see whether this reduction in energy expenditure persists over time. These studies have consistently shown that, indeed, the reduction in energy expenditure persists for years following weight loss, with no evidence that it goes into remission.[25] This means that energy intake needs to remain at a low level in order to sustain a reduced-weight state unless habitual levels of physical activity are increased to close the "energy gap." See the example in Figure 1.9.

Appetite increases with weight reduction. Studies have measured hunger and satiety in people before and after weight loss and shown, not surprisingly, that hunger increases and postmeal satiety falls. Appetite is regulated in part by levels of hormones, as discussed earlier. Levels of leptin and insulin, both satiety hormones, fall as fat mass declines with weight loss. Levels of ghrelin, the intestinal hormone that is associated with increased hunger, rise with weight loss. Levels of peptide YY, a satiety hormone from the intestine, fall with weight loss. These changes in appetite and hormonal modulators of eating behavior persist for at least a year after weight loss, the longest anyone has monitored patients for these changes (refer to Figure 1.10).[26]

Other studies have examined regional brain activity in response to food-related stimuli before and after weight loss. A wide variety of brain regions show increased blood flow in response to pictures of highly palatable food when these images are presented to patients during magnetic resonance imaging. When a normal-weight person is overfed for 3 days, these brain responses to palatable food images are markedly attenuated. However, when individuals who were previously obese and lost weight are overfed for 3 days, they continue to show robust

FIGURE 1.9 Energy expenditure before and after weight loss

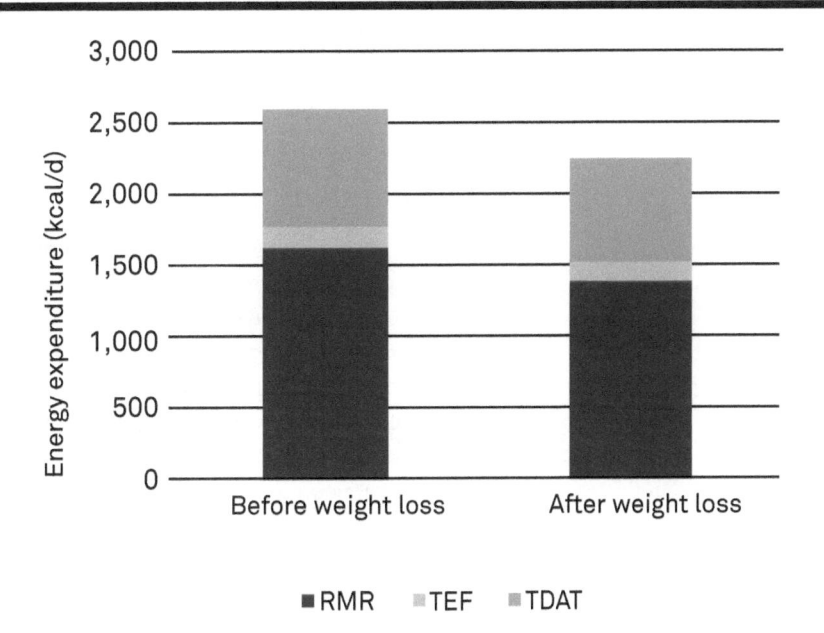

Example: A 91-kg (200-lb) female losing 11 kg (25 lb) would experience a 350 kcal/d reduction in TDEE as a result of weight loss.
Abbreviations: TDAT, total daily activity thermogenesis; TDEE, total daily energy expenditure; TEF, thermic effect of food; RMR, resting metabolic rate.

FIGURE 1.10 Mean (±SE) fasting and postprandial levels of ghrelin, peptide YY, amylin, and cholecystokinin at baseline, 10 weeks, and 62 weeks[26]

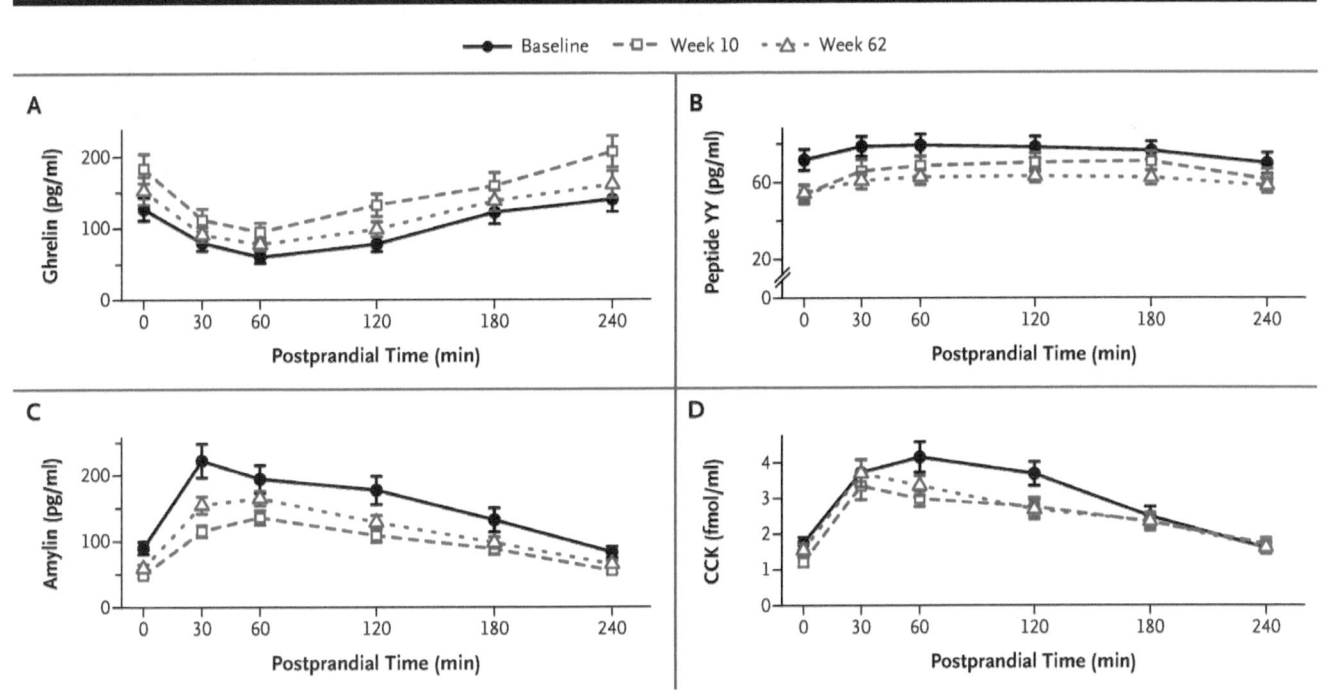

Figure 1.10 depicts levels of hormones that promote satiety (peptide YY, amylin, and cholecystokinin) and the hormone that promotes hunger (ghrelin) over 4 hours following a test meal delivered to people with obesity and consumed either before weight loss (baseline), at week 10 following weight loss, or at week 62 following weight loss.
Abbreviation: CCK, cholecystokinin.
Reproduced with permission from Sumithran P, Prendergast LA, Delbridge E, et al. Long-term persistence of hormonal adaptations to weight loss. *N Engl J Med*. 2011;365(17):1597-1604. doi:10.1056/NEJMoa1105816.[26]

increases in regional brain activity in response to images of palatable food.[27] These results support the notion that the drive to eat is increased in people who have lost weight, and their perception of food-related stimuli is different from that of people of normal weight. These findings emphasize the biological nature of weight regulation and the challenges facing people who have lost weight.

Is Weight Maintenance Possible?

How, then, can anyone maintain a reduced state in the face of all the biological mechanisms that promote weight regain? Despite what could be considered the depressing message conveyed by the data related here, many people are successful at losing weight and at maintaining that weight loss over time. The National Weight Control Registry is a group of more than 10,000 people who have lost more than 23 kg (50 lb) and maintained that weight loss for more than 5 years.[28] These individuals have been successful at pushing back against the physiologic mechanisms that drive weight regain in most people. They use cognitive strategies to counteract the biological drive for weight regain, including frequent self-weighing, high levels of physical activity, and the consumption of an energy-restricted, low-fat diet.

The Prevalence of Obesity

In the United States, two large epidemiologic studies have followed the prevalence of obesity over time. One, the Behavioral Risk Factor Surveillance System (BRFSS), is a health survey system that collects data from a large, geographically representative sample of US residents regarding their health-related risk behaviors and chronic health conditions, including obesity. BRFSS uses self-reported height and weight data to calculate BMI. Because these data are self-reported, the actual prevalence of obesity is likely underestimated. The advantage of the BRFSS data set is that it provides detailed geographic estimates of obesity prevalence over time. The second data set comes from the National Health and Nutrition Examination Survey (NHANES), which uses directly measured heights and weights from a smaller sample of people that is statistically representative but not as geographically comprehensive as the BRFSS sample.

Although some experts thought that the rising prevalence of obesity had plateaued, the most recent data suggest that the prevalence of obesity continues to rise across the United States. The most recent data from NHANES (2017–2018) showed that the prevalence of obesity among all children and adolescents aged 2 to 19 years in 2018 was 19.3%.[29] This was up from 5.2% in 1974 and from 17.2% in 2014. Among adults, the prevalence of obesity was 42.4% in 2018. From 1999–2000 to 2017–2018, the prevalence of obesity in adults increased from 30.5% to 42.4%. During the same interval, the prevalence of severe obesity increased from 4.7% to 9.2% (refer to Figure 1.11).[30]

Obesity disproportionately affects certain racial and ethnic groups. In 2017–2018, the prevalence of obesity was 49.6% in non-Hispanic Black adults and 44.8% among Hispanic adults, as shown in Figure 1.12.[30] These differences in prevalence are due in part to a number of social and environmental factors including food insecurity, aspects of the food environment, differential access to health care, financial and housing challenges, and neighborhood factors that result in barriers to physical activity. While women have more body fat at any given level of BMI, there was no difference in the prevalence of obesity in 2017–2018 between men and women.[†]

[†] Report identified participants as men and women. Gender was not further specified.

FIGURE 1.11 Trends in age-adjusted obesity and severe obesity prevalence among adults aged 20 years and older from 1999–2000 through 2017–2018 in the United States[30]

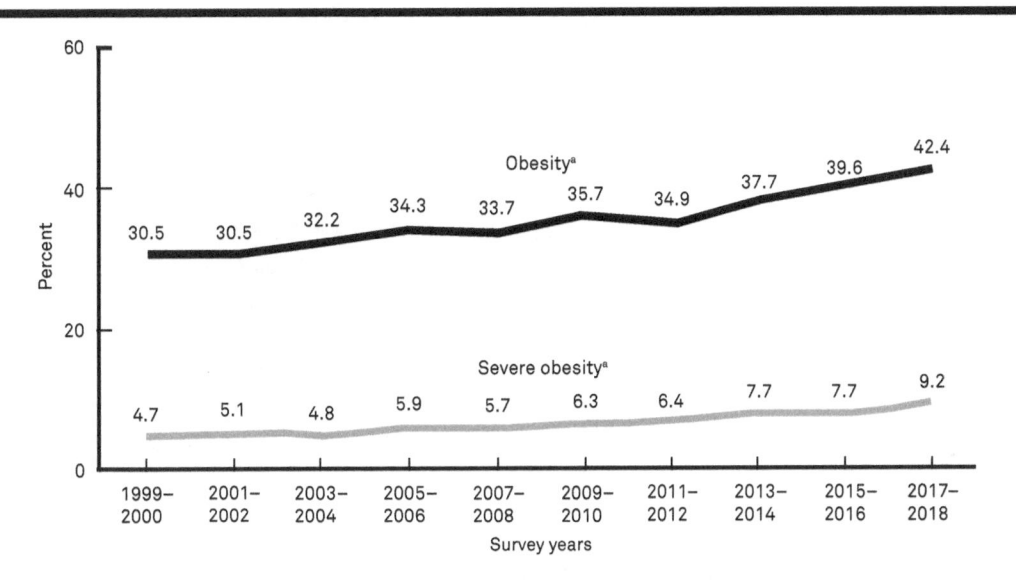

Estimates were age adjusted by the direct method to the 2000 US Census population using the age groups 20 to 39, 40 to 59, and 60 and over.

[a] Significant linear trend.
Adapted from Hales CM, Carroll MD, Fryar CD, Ogden CL. *Prevalence of Obesity and Severe Obesity Among Adults: United States, 2017-2018*. NCHS Data Brief no. 360. National Center for Health Statistics; 2020. Accessed August 22, 2022. www.cdc.gov/nchs/products/databriefs/db360.htm.[30]

FIGURE 1.12 Age-adjusted prevalence of obesity among adults aged 20 years and older, by sex, race, and Hispanic origin, in 2017–2018 in the United States[a,30]

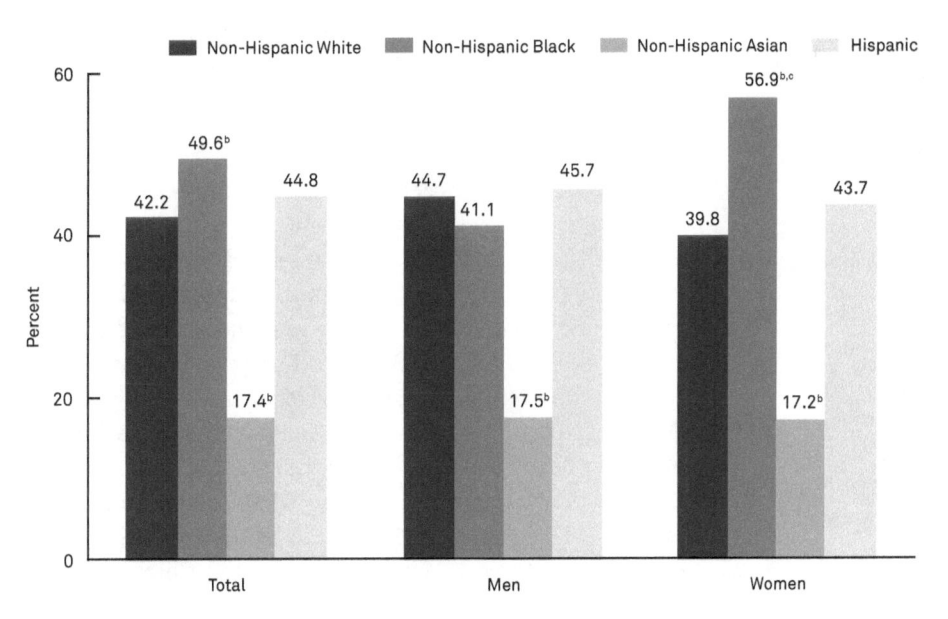

[a] Report identified participants as men and women. Gender was not further specified.
[b] Significantly different from all other race and Hispanic-origin groups.
[c] Significantly different from men for same race and Hispanic-origin group.
Estimates were age adjusted by the direct method to the 2000 US Census population using the age groups 20–39, 40–59, and 60 and over.
Adapted from Hales CM, Carroll MD, Fryar CD, Ogden CL. *Prevalence of Obesity and Severe Obesity Among Adults: United States, 2017-2018*. NCHS Data Brief no. 360. National Center for Health Statistics; 2020. Accessed August 22, 2022. www.cdc.gov/nchs/products/databriefs/db360.htm.[30]

Changes in Weight Throughout the Life Span

In Childhood

BMI is used to determine weight status among children just as it is in adults. However, in children and adolescents, BMI cutoff points defining obesity are age-specific and sex-specific in a manner that is typically referred to as BMI-for-age.[31] The CDC growth charts are commonly used to categorize children's and adolescents' weight-for-age status into corresponding percentiles. Obesity in children and adolescents is defined as a BMI at the 95th percentile or greater. Weight-for-height tends to increase in late childhood before puberty. It then falls during puberty, as linear growth accelerates. Weight then rises again in late adolescence and the period of emerging adulthood. Using BMI-for-age criteria, obesity prevalence rises with increasing age. Data from 2017–2018 show that the prevalence of obesity was 13.4% among 2- to 5-year-olds, 20.3% among 6- to 11-year-olds, and 21.2% among 12- to 19-year-olds. As is true for adults, the prevalence of obesity is higher among Hispanic children (25.6%) and non-Hispanic Black children (25.2%), as compared to non-Hispanic White children (16.1%) or non-Hispanic Asian children (8.7%).[29]

In Emerging Adulthood

Recent analyses have focused on the period of life from age 18 years to 25 years as a life stage for which obesity prevalence has been growing. This period, referred to as emerging adulthood, is characterized developmentally as a time of life when individuals transition from school to work and develop lifelong lifestyle habits along with an adult identity. An analysis of NHANES data showed that, between 1976 and 2018, the average BMI among emerging adults increased from 23.1 to 27.7. The prevalence of obesity in this group increased from 6.2% in 1976–1982 to 32.7% in 2017–2018. In contrast, the prevalence of normal weight in this group decreased from 68.7% to 37.5% over the same time. A particularly sharp rise in the prevalence of obesity occurred between 2016 and 2018.[32] Future studies should focus on the establishment of lifelong lifestyle habits in this group of young adults.

During Pregnancy

Weight gain during pregnancy is normal and important for the development of the fetus. However, excessive weight gain can lead to adverse consequences for both birth parent and child that may extend beyond pregnancy. Individuals gain an average of 14.1 kg (31 lb) during pregnancy, although those with obesity gain less weight—those with class 1 obesity gain an average of 12.2 kg (27 lb); those with class 2 obesity, 10.3 kg (23 lb); and those with class 3 obesity, 8.2 kg (18 lb).[33] In 2009, the National Academy of Medicine issued guidance on the appropriate degree of gestational weight gain. These recommendations were based on the risk of adverse health consequences to the baby and birth parent associated with excessive gestational weight gain. These guidelines suggested a range of appropriate gestational weight gain of 5 to 9 kg (11 to 20 lb) for individuals with obesity.[34] In 2019, the LifeCycle Project–Maternal Obesity and Childhood Outcomes Study Group conducted a meta-analysis of the relationship between gestational weight gain and infant and birth parent outcomes in people with obesity. They suggested that the appropriate level of gestational weight gain in those with class 1 obesity was 2 to 6 kg (4 to 13 lb); in those with class 2 obesity, it was less than 4 kg (9 lb); and in those with class 3 obesity, less than 6 kg (13 lb).[35] A more recent retrospective cohort study, using US national birth and infant death data from 2011 to 2015, examined the relationship between gestational weight gain and infant morbidity and mortality, with the goal of identifying optimal weight gain in individuals with obesity.[36] The most important finding of this study was that insufficient weight gain was associated with adverse infant outcomes, even in those with obesity. This study suggests that a goal of weight loss or even weight maintenance might be inappropriate for those with obesity during pregnancy. In addition, excessive gestational weight gain, especially during the first trimester, is strongly associated with postpartum weight gain, and subsequent adverse weight and health status later in life for the birth parent.[37]

During Menopause

During the menopausal transition, most individuals gain weight. Weight gain typically begins a year or two before the last menstrual period. The average gain during menopause is 0.45 to 0.68 kg (1 to 1.5 lb) per year, although the numbers vary a great deal. Twenty percent of people will gain a total of 4.5 kg (10 lb) during this transition. Much of the weight gain is due to increased body fat; there is a redistribution of fat from the lower body to the abdomen and a loss in lean body mass.[38] This increase in central adiposity is associated with an increased risk for metabolic diseases. The weight gain is due to a number of factors, including aging, a fall in estradiol levels, a decrease in energy expenditure, a reduction in spontaneous physical activity, and, possibly, a rise in levels of follicle-stimulating hormone. Compelling data from animal models indicate that falling estradiol levels result in a reduction in spontaneous physical activity, which predisposes one to a positive energy balance. There is growing evidence to support this phenomenon in human beings as well.[39] As a result, encouraging individuals to increase their physical activity during the menopausal transition may be an important strategy for combating weight gain. Novel data from mouse models suggest that the rise in follicle-stimulating hormone levels at menopause may have an independent effect on body weight, although data to support this effect in human beings are currently lacking.[40]

In Older Age

Weight tends to increase until the age of 65 years. After that, weight tends to gradually decline, although there is considerable interindividual variation. This is caused, in part, by a gradual reduction in skeletal muscle mass (sarcopenia), while fat mass continues to increase.[41] Weight loss may occur in older adults, in part, due to changes in taste and smell, a reduction in hunger, difficulties with eating due to dental or neurological conditions, and challenges with acquiring and preparing palatable food. Increased BMI is less associated with adverse health risks in older individuals than it is in younger individuals. The greatest health risks are associated with sarcopenic obesity (increased fat mass with reduced skeletal muscle mass) in older adults.[42] Consequently, weight loss through restriction of energy intake alone, which may promote the loss of lean body mass, may be less valuable in older individuals. The inclusion of regular physical activity in weight loss interventions for older people helps preserve lean body mass and improve functional capacity.

Recent thinking has highlighted the importance of the duration of exposure to obesity in the development of adverse health consequences. Emerging data suggests that the risk of certain complications, such as type 2 diabetes, hypertension, and lipid abnormalities, increases the longer a person has been obese.[43] These data support the concerns over the high prevalence of obesity in young people, as well as the importance of identifying and addressing obesity as early in life as possible.

The Consequences of Obesity

Obesity is defined as a degree of excess weight that predisposes an individual to adverse health consequences. Excess body fat is associated with a range of adverse health consequences, including type 2 diabetes, hypertension, coronary artery disease, metabolic dysfunction–associated steatotic liver disease, obstructive sleep apnea, reproductive dysfunction (including infertility and hypogonadism in males), degenerative arthritis, depression, and a number of cancers, to name just a few.[44,45] Some of the medical complications of obesity are shown in Figure 1.13.

Perhaps because of these associated complications, obesity is associated with increased rates of mortality. A plot of mortality vs BMI shows a curvilinear relationship (refer to Figure 1.14).[46] Individuals who are underweight have an increased risk of mortality, and those who are obese also have an increased risk of mortality. This relationship between BMI and mortality risk is the basis for the currently used cutoff points for overweight and obesity.

Researchers have raised questions about the accuracy of this relationship, as the original data showing this relationship came from the 1960s and 1970s, when fewer people were obese. In the 1990s and early 2000s, obesity became far more prevalent. This change in prevalence means that individuals with a BMI of 30 in 1970 might not be directly comparable to individuals with a BMI of 30 in 2000. People who had a BMI of 30 in 1970 would have been genetically more predisposed to gain weight in an environment that was not as obesogenic as the environment of 2000, so they may have had a greater risk for metabolic disease. In addition, the treatment of weight-related comorbidities, including hypertension, hyperlipidemia, and diabetes, has improved since these original studies were done, thus reducing the mortality risk associated with obesity in connection with comorbidities. An ideal body weight would be a level of body fat that is associated with the lowest mortality risk. In current guidelines, this ideal weight is established at a BMI of 20 to 25. There is, however, some reason to think that the ideal weight range now might be 25 to 30, especially in older individuals, in whom the relationship between weight and mortality is less than in younger people.[47]

Two of the most important contributors to morbidity in people with obesity are type 2 diabetes and insulin resistance. The risk of developing type 2 diabetes rises dramatically with increased BMI, as illustrated in Figure 1.15 on page 22.[48,49] These complications are associated with central accumulation of adipose tissue. With excess fat accumulation, circulating levels of free fatty acids rise and are thought to impair insulin action. In addition, the expanded fat tissue mass is associated with increased circulating inflammatory markers, which also interferes with normal insulin action. Finally, the inability of adipose tissue to store lipid normally because it has reached or exceeded its storage capacity results in lipid accumulation in other tissues, including skeletal muscle and pancreatic β cells. This "lipotoxicity" is associated with decreased insulin action in skeletal muscle and a reduction in insulin secretory capacity. Weight loss has been shown to reverse a number of these defects and improve insulin action, demonstrating the causal link between obesity and insulin resistance.[50]

Cardiovascular disease is more common in people with obesity.[51] This is, in part, due to changes in circulating lipid levels that favor small, dense, low-density lipoproteins, increased triglycerides, and reductions in high-density lipoprotein cholesterol. Obesity is also associated with increased rates of hypertension, which

FIGURE 1.13 Medical complications of obesity

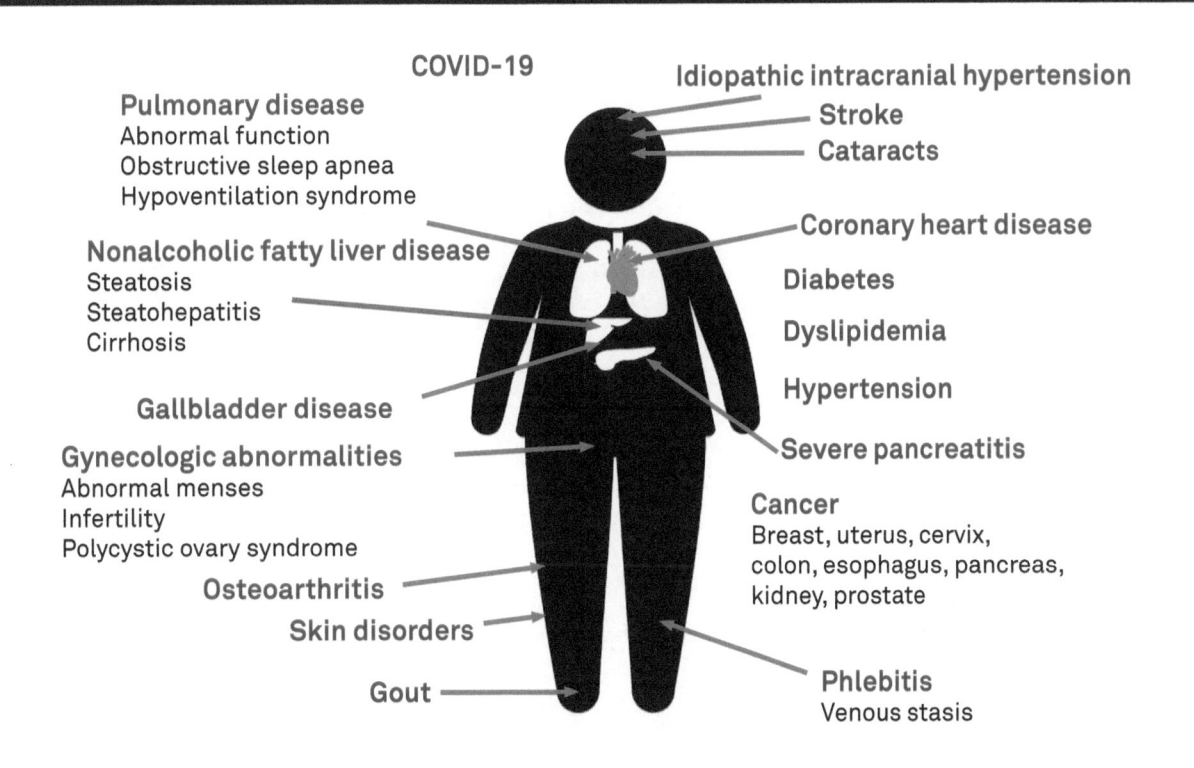

- COVID-19
- **Pulmonary disease**
  - Abnormal function
  - Obstructive sleep apnea
  - Hypoventilation syndrome
- **Nonalcoholic fatty liver disease**
  - Steatosis
  - Steatohepatitis
  - Cirrhosis
- **Gallbladder disease**
- **Gynecologic abnormalities**
  - Abnormal menses
  - Infertility
  - Polycystic ovary syndrome
- **Osteoarthritis**
- **Skin disorders**
- **Gout**
- **Idiopathic intracranial hypertension**
- **Stroke**
- **Cataracts**
- **Coronary heart disease**
- **Diabetes**
- **Dyslipidemia**
- **Hypertension**
- **Severe pancreatitis**
- **Cancer**
  - Breast, uterus, cervix, colon, esophagus, pancreas, kidney, prostate
- **Phlebitis**
  - Venous stasis

FIGURE 1.14 Relationship between BMI and cardiovascular disease mortality[a,46]

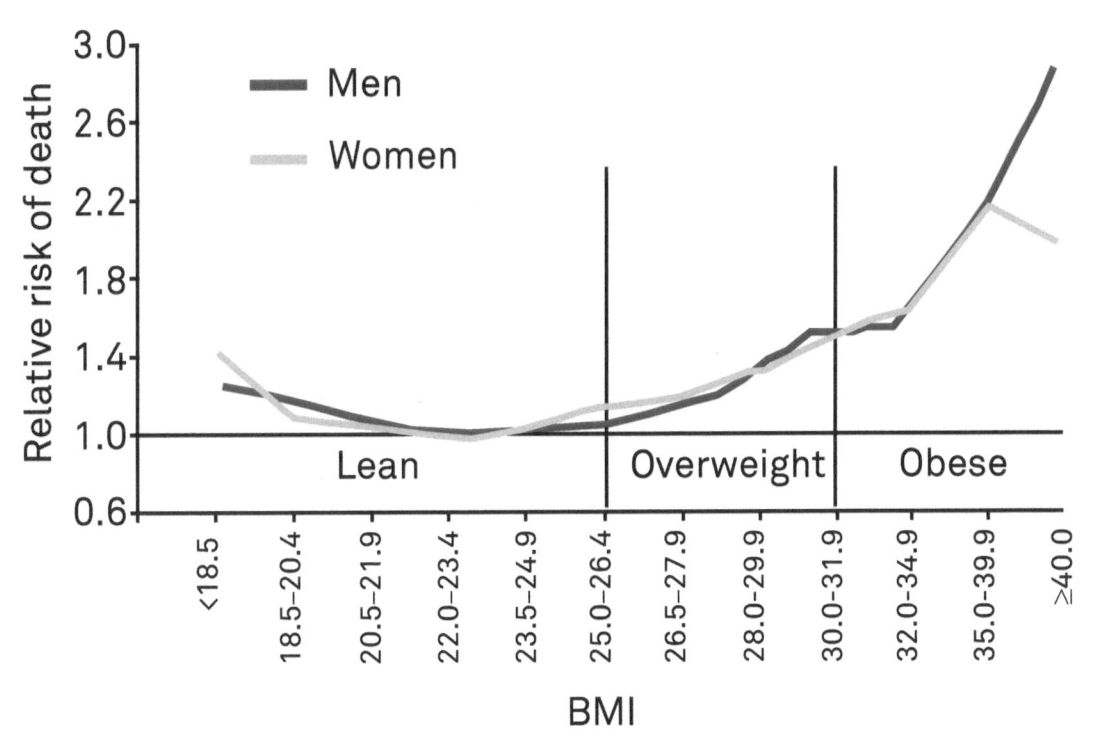

Adapted with permission from Robert Eckel, MD.
[a] Study participants were described as men and women. Gender was not further specified.

CHAPTER 1: Obesity as a Disease 21

FIGURE 1.15 Relationship between BMI and risk of developing type 2 diabetes[a,48,49]

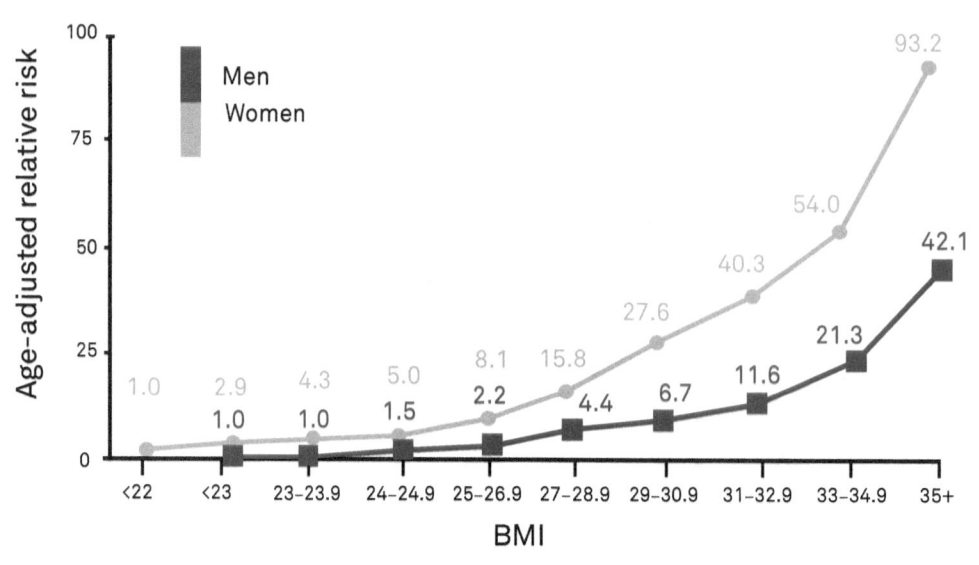

Age-adjusted relative risk vs BMI

Women: 1.0, 2.9, 4.3, 5.0, 8.1, 15.8, 27.6, 40.3, 54.0, 93.2
Men: 1.0, 1.0, 1.5, 2.2, 4.4, 6.7, 11.6, 21.3, 42.1

BMI categories: <22, <23, 23–23.9, 24–24.9, 25–26.9, 27–28.9, 29–30.9, 31–32.9, 33–34.9, 35+

Adapted with permission from Robert Eckel, MD.
[a] Study participants were described as men and women. Gender was not further specified.

also contribute to the risk for cardiovascular disease. Increased sympathetic tone, circulating blood volume, and increased cardiac output all contribute to a risk for hypertension in the setting of obesity. Insulin resistance and type 2 diabetes also contribute to the increased risk for heart disease in people with obesity.

Breast cancer and endometrial cancer are more common in females with obesity. Males with obesity have higher mortality rates from cancers of the prostate and colon. A number of other cancers have also been linked to obesity.[52] The mechanisms of these associations are not entirely clear, but increased inflammatory mediators and insulin resistance may play important roles. Although insulin is typically known for its metabolic effects, it is also a growth factor. With increasing body weight, insulin resistance occurs with compensatory increases in circulating insulin levels. The insulin resistance, however, is only in the metabolic signaling pathway within cells, while the growth-promoting effects of insulin appeared to be maintained. As a result, the increased circulating of levels of insulin may promote cell growth and division, leading to cancer in individuals at risk.

Increased fat mass can directly cause a number of problems as well. Increased body weight can lead to degenerative joint disease, especially in the hips and knees. Surgeons may be reluctant to replace joints in individuals with obesity, out of fear that the prosthetic joints may be subject to excessive stress and fail. The accumulation of adipose tissue in the abdomen can result in increased intra-abdominal pressure, leading to gastroesophageal reflux and urinary incontinence. The accumulation of fat in the retropharynx and neck can lead to obstructive sleep apnea. The ectopic storage of fat in the liver can lead to metabolic dysfunction–associated steatotic liver disease and even cirrhosis. Insulin resistance may trigger increased androgen secretion by the ovaries and the development of polycystic ovary syndrome in susceptible females, resulting in irregular menses and infertility. Males with obesity may develop hypothalamic hypogonadism. Low testosterone levels may increase with weight loss.

Although it is clear that obesity increases a person's risk for a large number of health problems, not all people with obesity have the same level of risk. Individuals with "metabolically healthy" obesity have normal serum levels of lipids and glucose, and normal blood pressure.[53] These individuals are at lower risk of developing adverse health consequences than individuals of normal weight with elevated lipid and glucose levels and hypertension. However, they are at a higher risk than individuals of normal weight with normal metabolic parameters.[54] It may be that high levels of physical activity protect some people with obesity from adverse health consequences.[55]

In addition, a growing body of literature is reporting on what has come to be known as the "obesity paradox."[56] Studies of people with heart failure surprisingly demonstrated that a number of outcomes were better in people with obesity than in people of normal weight. This unexpected observation of a protective effect of obesity has been seen in connection with several other health conditions, including renal failure, and in patients in the intensive care unit. While controversial, it may be that once a person has a serious illness, a modest increase in body fat protects them from the catabolic effects of that condition.

Summary

Although not every person with obesity suffers serious adverse consequences, excess body fat is clearly associated with a wide range of some of the most commonly seen health problems in adults. Weight loss can improve many of these adverse consequences, and greater benefits are seen with greater degrees of weight loss.

References

1. Schwartz MW, Seeley RJ, Zeltser LM, et al. Obesity pathogenesis: an Endocrine Society scientific statement. *Endocr Rev.* 2017;38(4):267-296. doi:10.1210/er.2017-00111
2. Upadhyay J, Farr O, Perakakis N, Ghaly W, Mantzoros C. Obesity as a disease. *Med Clin North Am.* 2018;102(1):13-33. doi:10.1016/j.mcna.2017.08.004
3. Jensen MD, Ryan DH, Apovian CM, et al. 2013 AHA/ACC/TOS guideline for the management of overweight and obesity in adults: a report of the American College of Cardiology/American Heart Association Task Force on Practice Guidelines and The Obesity Society. *Circulation.* 2014;129(25 suppl 2):S102-S138. doi:10.1161/01.cir.0000437739.71477.ee
4. Abusnana S, Fargaly M, Alfardan SH, et al. Clinical practice recommendations for the management of obesity in the United Arab Emirates. *Obes Facts.* 2018;11(5):413-428. doi:10.1159/000491796
5. Bessesen DH. Regulation of body weight: what is the regulated parameter? *Physiol Behav.* 2011;104(4):599-607. doi:10.1016/j.physbeh.2011.05.006
6. Yang YC, Walsh CE, Johnson MP, et al. Life-course trajectories of body mass index from adolescence to old age: racial and educational disparities. *Proc Natl Acad Sci U S A.* 2021;118(17):e2020167118. doi:10.1073/pnas.2020167118
7. Jackman MR, Steig A, Higgins JA, et al. Weight regain after sustained weight reduction is accompanied by suppressed oxidation of dietary fat and adipocyte hyperplasia. *Am J Physiol Regul Integr Comp Physiol.* 2008;294(4):R1117-R1129. doi:10.1152/ajpregu.00808.2007
8. MacLean PS, Higgins JA, Johnson GC, et al. Enhanced metabolic efficiency contributes to weight regain after weight loss in obesity-prone rats. *Am J Physiol Regul Integr Comp Physiol.* 2004;287(6):R1306-R1315. doi:10.1152/ajpregu.00463.2004
9. Madden AM, Mulrooney HM, Shah S. Estimation of energy expenditure using prediction equations in overweight and obese adults: a systematic review. *J Hum Nutr Diet.* 2016;29(4):458-476. doi:10.1111/jhn.12355

10. Pontzer H, Yamada Y, Sagayama H, et al. Daily energy expenditure through the human life course. *Science.* 2021;373(6556):808-812. doi:10.1126/science.abe5017
11. Weyer C, Snitker S, Rising R, Bogardus C, Ravussin E. Determinants of energy expenditure and fuel utilization in man: effects of body composition, age, sex, ethnicity and glucose tolerance in 916 subjects. *Int J Obes Relat Metab Disord.* 1999;23(7):715-722. doi:10.1038/sj.ijo.0800910
12. Levine JA, Eberhardt NL, Jensen MD. Role of nonexercise activity thermogenesis in resistance to fat gain in humans. *Science.* 1999;283(5399):212-214. doi:10.1126/science.283.5399.212
13. Lichtman SW, Pisarska K, Berman ER, et al. Discrepancy between self-reported and actual caloric intake and exercise in obese subjects. *N Engl J Med.* 1992;327(27):1893-1898. doi:10.1056/nejm199212313272701
14. Schwartz MW. Central nervous system regulation of food intake. *Obesity (Silver Spring).* 2006;14 suppl 1:1s-8s. doi:10.1038/oby.2006.275
15. Pak K, Seok JW, Lee MJ, Kim K, Kim IJ. Dopamine receptor and dopamine transporter in obesity: A meta-analysis. *Synapse.* 2023;77(1):e22254. doi:10.1002/syn.22254
16. Bronleigh M, Baumann O, Stapleton P. Neural correlates associated with processing food stimuli in anorexia nervosa and bulimia nervosa: an activation likelihood estimation meta-analysis of fMRI studies. *Eat Weight Disord.* 2022;27(7):2309-2320. doi:10.1007/s40519-022-01390-x
17. Christakis NA, Fowler JH. The spread of obesity in a large social network over 32 years. *N Engl J Med.* 2007;357(4):370-379. doi:10.1056/NEJMsa066082
18. Farooqi IS, O'Rahilly S. The genetics of obesity in humans. In: Feingold KR, Anawalt B, Boyce A, et al, eds. *Endotext* [internet]. MDText.com; 2000–. Updated December 23, 2017. www.ncbi.nlm.nih.gov/books/NBK279064
19. Farooqi S. Insights from the genetics of severe childhood obesity. *Horm Res.* 2007;68 suppl 5:5-7. doi:10.1159/000110462
20. Clément K, van den Akker E, Argente J, et al. Efficacy and safety of setmelanotide, an MC4R agonist, in individuals with severe obesity due to LEPR or POMC deficiency: single-arm, open-label, multicentre, phase 3 trials. *Lancet Diabetes Endocrinol.* 2020;8(12):960-970. doi:10.1016/s2213-8587(20)30364-8
21. Claussnitzer M, Dankel SN, Kim KH, et al. FTO obesity variant circuitry and adipocyte browning in humans. *N Engl J Med.* 2015;373(10):895-907. doi:10.1056/NEJMoa1502214
22. Leibel RL, Rosenbaum M, Hirsch J. Changes in energy expenditure resulting from altered body weight. *N Engl J Med.* 1995;332(10):621-628. doi:10.1056/nejm199503093321001
23. Rosenbaum M, Goldsmith RL, Haddad F, et al. Triiodothyronine and leptin repletion in humans similarly reverse weight-loss-induced changes in skeletal muscle. *Am J Physiol Endocrinol Metab.* 2018;315(5):E771-E779. doi:10.1152/ajpendo.00116.2018
24. Baldwin KM, Joanisse DR, Haddad F, et al. Effects of weight loss and leptin on skeletal muscle in human subjects *Am J Physiol Regul Integr Comp Physiol.* 2011;301(5):R1259-66. doi:10.1152/ajpregu.00397.2011
25. Fothergill E, Guo J, Howard L, et al. Persistent metabolic adaptation 6 years after "The Biggest Loser" competition. *Obesity (Silver Spring).* 2016;24(8):1612-1619. doi:10.1002/oby.21538
26. Sumithran P, Prendergast LA, Delbridge E, et al. Long-term persistence of hormonal adaptations to weight loss. *N Engl J Med.* 2011;365(17):1597-1604. doi:10.1056/NEJMoa1105816
27. Cornier MA, Salzberg AK, Endly DC, Bessesen DH, Rojas DC, Tregellas JR. The effects of overfeeding on the neuronal response to visual food cues in thin and reduced-obese individuals. *PLoS One.* 2009;4(7):e6310. doi:10.1371/journal.pone.0006310
28. National Weight Control Registry. NWCR facts. National Weight Control Registry website. Accessed February 27, 2023. http://nwcr.ws/Research/default.htm
29. Fryar CD, Carroll MD, Afful J. Prevalence of Overweight, Obesity, and Severe Obesity Among Children and Adolescents Aged 2-19 Years: United States, 1963-1965 Through 2017-2018. NCHS Health E-Stats. National Center for Health Statistics; 2020. Accessed February 1, 2022. www.cdc.gov/nchs/data/hestat/obesity-child-17-18/obesity-child.htm
30. Hales CM, Carroll MD, Fryar CD, Ogden CL. Prevalence of Obesity and Severe Obesity Among Adults: United States, 2017-2018. NCHS Data Brief no. 360. National Center for Health Statistics; 2020. Accessed August 22, 2022. www.cdc.gov/nchs/products/databriefs/db360.htm
31. Styne DM, Arslanian SA, Connor EL, et al. Pediatric obesity—assessment, treatment, and prevention: an Endocrine Society clinical practice guideline. *J Clin Endocrinol Metab.* 2017;102(3):709-757. doi:10.1210/jc.2016-2573
32. Ellison-Barnes A, Johnson S, Gudzune K. Trends in obesity prevalence among adults aged 18 through 25 years, 1976-2018. *JAMA.* 2021;326(20):2073-2074. doi:10.1001/jama.2021.16685
33. Goldstein RF, Abell SK, Ranasinha S, et al. Gestational weight gain across continents and ethnicity: systematic review and meta-analysis of maternal and infant outcomes in more than one million women. *BMC Med.* 2018;16(1):153. doi:10.1186/s12916-018-1128-1
34. Moore Simas TA, Waring ME, Sullivan GM, et al. Institute of medicine 2009 gestational weight gain guideline knowledge: survey of obstetrics/gynecology and family medicine residents of the United States. *Birth.* 2013;40(4):237-246. doi:10.1111/birt.12061

35. LifeCycle Project-Maternal Obesity and Childhood Outcomes Study Group, Voerman E, Santos S, et al. Association of gestational weight gain with adverse maternal and infant outcomes. *JAMA.* 2019;321(17):1702-1715. doi:10.1001/jama.2019.3820
36. Wang L, Zhang X, Chen T, et al. Association of gestational weight gain with infant morbidity and mortality in the United States. *JAMA Netw Open.* 2021;4(12):e2141498. doi:10.1001/jamanetworkopen.2021.41498
37. Catalano PM, Shankar K. Obesity and pregnancy: mechanisms of short term and long term adverse consequences for mother and child. *BMJ.* 2017;356:j1. doi:10.1136/bmj.j1
38. Greendale GA, Sternfeld B, Huang M, et al. Changes in body composition and weight during the menopause transition. *JCI Insight.* 2019;4(5):e124865. doi:10.1172/jci.insight.124865
39. Gavin KM, Kohrt WM, Klemm DJ, Melanson EL. Modulation of energy expenditure by estrogens and exercise in women. *Exerc Sport Sci Rev.* 2018;46(4):232-239. doi:10.1249/jes.0000000000000160
40. Liu P, Ji Y, Yuen T, et al. Blocking FSH induces thermogenic adipose tissue and reduces body fat. *Nature.* 2017;546(7656):107-112. doi:10.1038/nature22342
41. Batsis JA, Villareal DT. Sarcopenic obesity in older adults: aetiology, epidemiology and treatment strategies. *Nat Rev Endocrinol.* 2018;14(9):513-537. doi:10.1038/s41574-018-0062-9
42. Atkins JL, Whincup PH, Morris RW, Lennon LT, Papacosta O, Wannamethee SG. Sarcopenic obesity and risk of cardiovascular disease and mortality: a population-based cohort study of older men. *J Am Geriatr Soc.* 2014;62(2):253-260. doi:10.1111/jgs.12652
43. Norris T, Cole TJ, Bann D, et al. Duration of obesity exposure between ages 10 and 40 years and its relationship with cardiometabolic disease risk factors: a cohort study. *PLoS Med.* 2020;17(12):e1003387. doi:10.1371/journal.pmed.1003387
44. Bray GA, Heisel WE, Afshin A, et al. The science of obesity management: an Endocrine Society scientific statement. *Endocr Rev.* 2018;39(2):79-132. doi:10.1210/er.2017-00253
45. Afshin A, Forouzanfar MH, Reitsma MB, et al. Health effects of overweight and obesity in 195 countries over 25 years. *N Engl J Med.* 2017;377(1):13-27. doi:10.1056/NEJMoa1614362
46. Calle EE, Thun MJ, Petrelli JM, Rodriguez C, Heath CW Jr. Body-mass index and mortality in a prospective cohort of U.S. adults. *N Engl J Med.* 1999;341(15):1097-1105. doi:10.1056/NEJM199910073411501
47. Flegal KM, Kit BK, Orpana H, Graubard BI. Association of all-cause mortality with overweight and obesity using standard body mass index categories: a systematic review and meta-analysis. *JAMA.* 2013;309(1):71-82. doi:10.1001/jama.2012.113905
48. Chan JM, Rimm EB, Colditz GA, Stampfer MJ, Willett WC. Obesity, fat distribution, and weight gain as risk factors for clinical diabetes in men. *Diabetes Care.* 1994;17(9):961-969. doi:10.2337/diacare.17.9.961
49. Colditz GA, Willett WC, Rotnitzky A, Manson JE. Weight gain as a risk factor for clinical diabetes mellitus in women. *Ann Intern Med.* 1995;122(7):481-486. doi:10.7326/0003-4819-122-7-199504010-00001
50. Magkos F, Fraterrigo G, Yoshino J, et al. Effects of moderate and subsequent progressive weight loss on metabolic function and adipose tissue biology in humans with obesity. *Cell Metab.* 2016;23(4):591-601. doi:10.1016/j.cmet.2016.02.005
51. Elagizi A, Kachur S, Carbone S, Lavie CJ, Blair SN. A review of obesity, physical activity, and cardiovascular disease. *Curr Obes Rep.* 2020;9(4):571-581. doi:10.1007/s13679-020-00403-z
52. Avgerinos KI, Spyrou N, Mantzoros CS, Dalamaga M. Obesity and cancer risk: emerging biological mechanisms and perspectives. *Metabolism.* 2019;92:121-135. doi:10.1016/j.metabol.2018.11.001
53. Kramer CK, Zinman B, Retnakaran R. Are metabolically healthy overweight and obesity benign conditions? A systematic review and meta-analysis. *Ann Intern Med.* 2013;159(11):758-769. doi:10.7326/0003-4819-159-11-201312030-00008
54. Hansen L, Netterstrøm MK, Johansen NB, et al. Metabolically healthy obesity and ischemic heart disease: a 10-year follow-up of the Inter99 Study. *J Clin Endocrinol Metab.* 2017;102(6):1934-1942. doi:10.1210/jc.2016-3346
55. Ortega FB, Cadenas-Sanchez C, Migueles JH, et al. Role of physical activity and fitness in the characterization and prognosis of the metabolically healthy obesity phenotype: a systematic review and meta-analysis. *Prog Cardiovasc Dis.* 2018;61(2):190-205. doi:10.1016/j.pcad.2018.07.008
56. Lavie CJ, De Schutter A, Parto P, et al. Obesity and prevalence of cardiovascular diseases and prognosis—the obesity paradox updated. *Prog Cardiovasc Dis.* 2016;58(5):537-547. doi:10.1016/j.pcad.2016.01.008

CHAPTER 2

Health Inequities in the Development, Management, and Treatment of Obesity

Faith Anne Newsome
Clarence C. Gravlee, PhD
Alexandra M. Lee, PhD
Tiffany L. Carson, PhD, MPH
Fatima Cody Stanford, MD, MPH, MPA, MBA, FAAP, FACP, FAHA, FAMWA, FTOS
Crystal N. Johnson-Mann, MD, MPH, FACS, FASMBS
Michelle I. Cardel, PhD, MS, RD, FTOS

CHAPTER OBJECTIVES

- Describe the health disparities occurring among adults with overweight and obesity.
- Review the disparities in social determinants of health among adults with overweight and obesity.
- Describe strategies that can be used in patient care to increase health equity for patients with overweight and obesity.

Introduction

Obesity is a disease characterized by excess adiposity that negatively affects a person's physical health and impairs quality of life.[1] Several psychological, physiological, biological, environmental, and behavioral factors contribute to the risk, development, and maintenance of obesity.[2] This complex, multifactorial disease has continued to increase in prevalence in recent decades among both adult and pediatric populations.[3,4] Marginalized racial and ethnic groups include Black, Hispanic, American Indian, Pacific Islander, and Alaska Native peoples. In the United States, Black and Hispanic individuals disproportionately bear the burden of obesity prevalence.[5] Based on data from the years 2015, 2017, and 2018, the prevalence of adult obesity is 49.6% among non-Hispanic Black people, 44.8% among Hispanic people, and almost 33% among American Indian and Alaska Native individuals, compared to 42.2% among non-Hispanic White people.[5-7] Although the prevalence of obesity among American Indian and Alaska Native patients appears to be lower, these groups have a higher likelihood of having obesity.[8] Among Asian American adults, the prevalence is 17.4% and continues to rise.[9,10] These prevalence inequities may reflect a system of oppression based on race and ethnicity, shaped by the unequal distribution of social and economic barriers as well as contributing factors to the development of obesity. The disproportionate prevalence of obesity by race and ethnicity is likely influenced by social constructs that limit access to care, impact quality of life, affect the quality of care, and minimize opportunities to participate in healthy behaviors.[10-14] In addition, these social constructs increase exposure to unhealthful environments.[12,15] Awareness of these barriers and subsequent personalized treatments are imperative to effective patient-centered care. Efforts to tailor treatments to assess structural barriers and inequities are also important to further eliminate health disparities and promote equity in the treatment of obesity.

This chapter focuses on the social determinants of health that are specific to patient populations from marginalized racial and ethnic groups and offers actionable steps to aid providers in efforts to achieve equity in obesity care. Throughout this chapter, we recognize race and ethnicity as social classifications, or where one stands within a racialized system, not as a proxy for genetic or biological differences between people.[16]

Social Determinants of Health and Their Contribution to Obesity

The health-related barriers that marginalized racial and ethnic groups experience are largely attributable to social determinants of health. Social determinants of health are defined as social factors, systems, and the distribution or withholding of social resources that can directly, or indirectly, affect health.[17,18] These determinants of health contribute to changes in demographic distributions of health outcomes, such as morbidity and death.[18] It is important to note that socioeconomic status is only one of several social determinants of health.[19] Additional determinants include forces that influence daily life, such as where a person is born, where they work, and where they live, as well as gender, race, ethnicity, social class, education, income, employment status, housing, immigration status, language spoken, and disability status.[19,20] Social systems (which include classifications based on race, gender, sex, and class) are a core component of the definition of social determinants of health. These systems often influence the allocation of social resources, thereby leading to societal inequities.[18] Thus, social determinants of health contribute to racial and ethnic inequities in areas such as maternal and infant mortality, cardiovascular disease, cancer, diabetes, chronic obstructive pulmonary disease, HIV and AIDS, homicide, psychological distress, hypertension, smoking, obesity, and access to health care.[19,21]

Additional social determinants of health that are particularly salient in relation to obesity include the built environment, psychosocial factors, and sociocultural norms. Specifically, the built environment includes, but is not limited to, the location and density of fast-food restaurants, food apartheid (a reference to the structural inequities that lead to "food deserts"), and the safety of neighborhoods.[22-25] Psychosocial factors can include stress, depression, and availability of social support. Sociocultural norms refer to body weight dissatisfaction, body weight ideals, and perception of weight status.[22] These factors are all influenced by, and can differ based on, factors associated with social systems influenced by racism. The next few subsections cover specific social determinants of health pertinent to obesity in marginalized racial and ethnic groups in more depth.

Racism

It is critical that practitioners recognize the important ways that racism contributes to inequities in obesity risk and development among patients from marginalized racial and ethnic groups.[26] *Racism* is defined as a system of opportunities that provides advantages for some racialized groups and disadvantages for other racialized groups.[27,28] Racism can occur at the interpersonal, internalized, and institutional levels.[27,28] *Structural racism* occurs through housing, education, employment, and criminal justice systems, resulting in systematic disadvantage.[29,30] Closely related to structural racism, *institutional racism* affects institutional policies, clinical practice, how health care professionals are trained, and research initiatives and thus has an impact on health care spaces, such as academic medical centers, and the health care system more broadly.[31] In several ways, racism and its impact on policies, interpersonal relationships, and influential factors of society (eg, educational opportunities and factors influencing socioeconomic status attainment) is a primary social determinant of health, as it influences almost all social determinants of health mentioned in this chapter (eg, socioeconomic status, the built environment, and others). For this reason, some researchers consider racism a "fundamental cause" of health inequities.[32]

One hypothesis that has emerged to explain the effects of racism on individual health outcomes is the *weathering hypothesis*. This hypothesis states that continued exposure to social and economic disadvantage can lead to declines in physical health through biological and physiological mechanisms (eg, a high allostatic load and inflammation from chronic stress).[33] Stress itself, which can occur from chronic exposure to systematic disadvantage, has three main influences on obesity development and maintenance, as seen in Box 2.1.[34]

BOX 2.1

The Influence of Stress on Obesity[34]

Stress affects self-regulation.

Stress influences choices involving diet, physical activity, and sleep.

The experience of stress affects neurochemistry and the microbiome.

Thus, it is imperative to recognize the influence of institutional racism on inequities in the built environment, psychosocial factors, and sociocultural norms and, subsequently, its impact on the health of individuals. The instances of racism that Black, Hispanic, American Indian, Pacific Islander, and Alaska Native patients experience can result in physiological and biological changes that influence health outcomes, specifically obesity risk.[35] For example, perceived discrimination due to race has shown an association with high blood pressure, increased cortisol levels and heightened stress response, weight change, metabolic syndrome severity, and sleep disturbances that can increase cardiometabolic risk.[36-40]

Socioeconomic Status and Food Insecurity

Lower socioeconomic status is associated with increased risk for the development of obesity.[41] *Food insecurity* is one avenue through which socioeconomic status influences obesity risk and development. Food insecurity occurs when a person has insufficient resources to purchase food, which results in a disruption of eating patterns and potential alterations in energy or nutrition needs; consequently, a person experiences hunger.[42] In 2016, 12.3% of households in the United States experienced food insecurity at some point during the year.[42] Black, Hispanic, American Indian, and Alaska Native individuals experience higher rates of food insecurity than White individuals.[43,44] Specifically, 22.5% of Black households and 18.5% of Hispanic households experienced food insecurity in 2016.[42] American Indians and Alaska Natives were twice as likely as Whites to experience food insecurity between 2000 and 2010.[44] There is also a link between food security and income. The majority (58.9%) of households that experienced food insecurity were those with incomes below the 185% poverty line.[42] Based on prevalence data, it is clear that certain groups (ie, Black, Hispanic, American Indian, Alaska Native, and individuals with low incomes) experience higher levels of food insecurity compared to White and higher-income groups. There are several economic factors associated with food insecurity that demonstrate the relationship between socioeconomic status and obesity, as outlined in Box 2.2.[44-48]

BOX 2.2

Economic Factors Associated With Food Insecurity[44-48]

- Income (living below the poverty line)
- Wealth (having fewer assets)
- Employment (recently experienced job loss)
- Living expenses (having high housing costs)
- House ownership (renting a home)

Two hypotheses have emerged to explain the mechanism between food insecurity and obesity: the insurance hypothesis and the resource scarcity hypothesis.[49,50] The insurance hypothesis posits that the causal mechanism between food insecurity and obesity is physiological; the resource scarcity hypothesis postulates that unreliable access to adequate amounts of food can result in increased energy intake and fat storage.[49,50] In support of these hypotheses, studies investigating the impact of experimentally manipulated social status found that individuals who experienced food insecurity also experienced increased production of the hormone ghrelin, which regulates appetite, and they consumed substantially more of their daily energy needs at a meal than individuals who are food secure.[48,51,52] Thus, socioeconomic status and its association with food security results in inequitable risk of increased energy intake and fat storage for individuals who experience food insecurity.

Lower socioeconomic status itself has been associated with an increased prevalence of obesity in adult and pediatric populations.[53-55] Higher educational attainment and higher socioeconomic status are factors associated with lower risk of obesity.[53] The association between socioeconomic status and obesity is more consistent among females than males.[55] Socioeconomic status is an independent risk factor for the development and maintenance of obesity, as it can influence physical activity opportunities through limited availability of recreational facilities.[12,56,57] An individual's socioeconomic status can also influence their dietary choices, as energy-dense foods with less nutritional value often cost less.[57] In addition, experiencing lower socioeconomic status also influences preferences for higher-energy foods and a greater energy intake.[52]

Although socioeconomic status itself influences obesity risk, it is important to note the intersectionality of factors. Specifically, some groups are more likely to experience lower socioeconomic status, specifically marginalized racial and ethnic groups, in part due to limited opportunities for advancement.[58-60] The influence of racism and discrimination on marginalized racial and ethnic groups affects academic achievement, the decision to hire, interactions in the workplace, and wage gaps.[61-63] Thus, the bias in socioeconomic status is an important consideration in the treatment of obesity, as socioeconomic status can also result in inequitable obesity risk through aspects of the built environment, such as the availability of supermarkets, reliable transportation, and recreational centers.

The Built Environment

The most influential aspects of the built environment that contribute to obesity risk, development, and maintenance include those that affect dietary and physical activity choices. Ultimately, the decision to engage in certain health behaviors is influenced by the environment in which a person lives. Specific aspects of a built environment that can be used to quantitatively assess that environment include the location and availability of the following: street connectivity (which can be indicative of walkability), pedestrian resources, businesses, restaurants (fast-food and non–fast-food), open spaces for recreational purposes, and other resources for recreational purposes. The socioeconomic status of a neighborhood and aspects of the built environment have been shown to mediate the relationship between the prevalence of obesity and race or ethnicity.[64] Neighborhoods consisting of mainly Black and Hispanic residents have a higher density of fast-food restaurants and fewer supermarkets.[65-67] At the same time, neighborhoods with low socioeconomic status and with predominately Black and Hispanic residents have fewer recreational centers.[12] The combination of increased access to energy-dense foods, a dearth of places to engage in recreational and physical activity, and the association between the built environment and obesity risk results in an increased obesity risk for traditionally marginalized patient groups.

The issue of inequities in the built environment extends beyond differences in socioeconomic status. Race-based residential segregation also plays a substantial role. The interaction between racism and poverty can lead to reduced access to resources, such as supermarkets. Neighborhoods of lower socioeconomic status but with few Black residents have better access to supermarkets than neighborhoods of lower socioeconomic status and a majority of Black residents.[68] These areas can be described as "food deserts" because of the limited access to healthy, affordable foods.[69] Food deserts and the distance from supermarkets paired with lack of transportation result in further disadvantage for neighborhoods with a majority of Black or Hispanic residents or low-income neighborhoods.[68,70,71] This pattern, which some researchers describe as supermarket redlining or food apartheid, further emphasizes that stakeholders and other individuals in decision-making positions may act in a discriminatory manner that contributes to the overarching role of racism and its influence on social determinants of health and health outcomes among marginalized racial and ethnic groups.[24,25]

Systematic Barriers Within Health Care to Equity in Obesity Care

Beyond the broader social determinants of health—such as racism, socioeconomic status, and the built environment—several institutional pathways deeply embedded in the health care system also contribute to health inequities. Barriers to equitable care for patients with obesity include inequitable access to health care, inequities in research related to obesity treatments, inequities in treatment outcomes, as well biases exhibited by health care professionals, and a lack of cultural sensitivity in interventions and clinical care. In addition to recognizing the role of social determinants of health, clinicians must actively work to address the shortcomings of the health care system in order to offer equitable care.

Access to Health Care Resources

Access to health care, which includes access to health care coverage and evidence-based obesity treatments, is limited for certain patient groups. Broadly speaking, insurance coverage for the treatment of obesity is limited,[72] but this is further compounded by the fact that marginalized racial and ethnic groups are less likely to have insurance coverage than White patients.[73] Even when insurance is equivalent, other factors create differential access to obesity care, such as the location of clinics and physicians' differential referrals to treatment.[14,74,75] Moreover, even for those who do have insurance coverage, full coverage of evidence-based obesity care is unlikely.[72] In addition, very few clinics offer the level of intensive care recommended to comprehensively treat obesity.[75] Most clinics that do offer the recommended level of care are located in urban academic medical centers, limiting access for individuals outside the close vicinity of a college or university.[75] The location of these clinics also makes it difficult for rural populations, typically comprised of White residents but can often include American Indians, to access appropriate treatment.[76-78]

Inequities in Treatment Outcomes

The three main treatment modalities for obesity are lifestyle or behavioral interventions, pharmacotherapy, and bariatric surgery. Lifestyle or behavioral interventions are the cornerstone of all obesity treatments.[79,80] They teach patients evidence-based strategies for behavior change that aim to improve dietary patterns, achieve modest reductions in energy intake, increase physical activity, and decrease sedentary time. Specifically, behavior change techniques are based in behavioral theories, such as cognitive behavioral therapy and acceptance-based therapies.[80-82] Pharmacotherapy includes the prescription of current US Food and Drug Administration (FDA)–approved medications, such as phentermine, orlistat, combination phentermine and topiramate extended-release, combination naltrexone sustained-release and bupropion sustained-release, liraglutide, and semaglutide.[83,84] Pharmacological options are prescribed when clinically significant weight loss and maintenance cannot be achieved through lifestyle interventions alone. Finally, bariatric surgery is the most intensive and effective treatment for obesity. Surgical procedures include Roux-en-Y gastric bypass, sleeve gastrectomy, and duodenal switch.[85]

Experts have deemed these treatment modalities safe and effective; however, patient utilization and outcomes differ by race and ethnicity. Race and ethnicity can influence whether providers counsel patients on their weight and, thus, affect the potential for conversations about treatment options.[86] Prescriptions for anti-obesity medications are more common among Black, Native Hawaiian or Pacific Islander, and American Indian or Alaska Native patients[87]; however, research into differential outcomes based on race and ethnicity is lacking, and limited evidence suggests there are differences in outcomes.[11,78,88] White patients are more likely to be referred to and undergo bariatric surgery than marginalized racial and ethnic patients. In 2016, 63.9% of bariatric patients identified as White, 17.7% as Black, 13.7% as Hispanic, and 4.7% as other.[13] These values may seem proportionate to the demographics of the population, but it is important to note that the prevalence of severe obesity is higher among Black patients (11.8%) and Hispanic patients (8%) compared to White patients (7.5%).[89,90] Access to bariatric surgery itself is an issue that is complicated by insurance requirements and the location of centers that offer the intensive level of treatment.[11,14,91] In addition, for those patients able to access these options, marginalized racial and ethnic patients lose less weight than White patients do when provided with lifestyle interventions, anti-obesity medications, or bariatric surgery.[88,92-94] Among patients undergoing bariatric surgery procedures, Black patients experience higher rates of procedural complications, readmission, reintervention, and mortality; and Hispanic patients experience higher rates of postoperative complications.[95-97]

Underrepresentation of Racially and Ethnically Marginalized Health Care Providers and Researchers in Fields Related to Weight Management

The inequities in treatment outcomes can be explained, in part, by the lack of racial, ethnic, socioeconomic, and gender diversity among health care providers and researchers in fields related to obesity and weight management, in addition to the effects of societal racism and social determinants of health (eg, socioeconomic status and the built environment). Health care providers and researchers from marginalized racial and ethnic backgrounds are underrepresented in obesity-focused and nutrition-focused organizations. The Academy of Nutrition and Dietetics and the American Board of Obesity Medicine (ABOM) are two large organizations prominent in the field of obesity. Among the more than 93,000 registered dietitians and registered dietitian nutritionists credentialed by the Commission on Dietetic Registration, the overwhelming majority (81.1%) reportedly identify as White, according to a study published in 2021.[98] Only 2.6% identify as Black, 3.9% as Asian, 3.1% as Latino, 0.3% as American Indian or Alaska Native, 1.3% as Native Hawaiian or Pacific Islander, and 0.5% as multiracial (of the remaining members, 1.2% self-report as "other," 2.3% say they prefer not to identify, and 3.6% provide no response).[98] Among 4,148 certified ABOM diplomates, 6.0% identify as Black, 20.9% as Asian, 5.0% as Latino, 0.2% as Native American, and 35.5% as White (of the remaining diplomates, 2.1% identify as other, 3.8% say they prefer not to identify, and 26.5% provide no response).[98] Representation is important due to the higher obesity prevalence among marginalized communities and the fact that racial and ethnic concordance between providers and patients improves patient satisfaction and health outcomes.[99,100] In addition, health care providers and scientists who identify as belonging to marginalized racial and ethnic groups are more likely to treat or focus their research on these groups.[98] Therefore, lack of representation among leading organizations in obesity medicine may further contribute to inequities.

Inequities in Research

Most of the research on the treatment modalities (lifestyle interventions, pharmacological treatments, and bariatric surgery) has been done in majority White, cisgender female patient samples, which limits its applicability to marginalized racial and ethnic groups.[101] It is imperative that clinicians understand the inequities in the current state of research, as studies contribute to the standards for clinical care.[78] If, as previously argued, racism causes differential exposure to obesogenic environments, then interventions must be tested in such environments to assess their efficacy in the contexts in which people stand to benefit the most.

Additional research to develop culturally and context-sensitive interventions is needed to decrease differential outcomes. Not all patients respond equally to the current interventions, as they were not designed or tested in marginalized racial and ethnic groups. Culturally sensitive interventions in Black, Hispanic, American Indians, and Pacific Islander patients are sparse; however, culturally sensitive behavioral or lifestyle interventions improve weight-related outcomes.[102-104] Therefore, efforts to diversify the participants in research studies and to develop interventions that are acceptable and feasible for patients from marginalized backgrounds are necessary first steps to improve obesity treatment. It may be necessary to do needs assessments to determine future directions for research and to understand disadvantages faced by certain patient groups. One way to promote the participation of diverse groups in the research process is to employ elements of implementation science.[105] Frameworks, such as the Consolidated Framework for Implementation Research, can help researchers understand health disparities before they begin implementing interventions to reduce these disparities.[106] Additional implementation science techniques used in community-based participatory research can also encourage individuals from racial and ethnic groups to participate in research. A systematic review of clinical trials using community-based participatory research techniques found that these trials were successful in recruiting and retaining participants from marginalized groups. The trials varied in their use of community members, but common techniques included involving community partners in recruitment of research participants or delivery of the intervention. These strategies promote the participation of diverse groups in research by promoting input from the community to ensure the resulting intervention is relevant and tailored to the community's needs.[107] Thus, because research establishes standards for clinical care, research that addresses inequities can have a downstream effect on the interventions that clinicians are able to provide.

Implicit and Explicit Bias

Within the health care system, both implicit and explicit biases can influence patient care. Explicit biases are intentional beliefs that individuals willingly self-report and disclose.[108] Studies have shown explicit bias in health care providers who self-report their beliefs that Black patients are uncooperative, and that Hispanic and American Indian patients participate in more risky health behaviors.[109-111] Although explicit bias can be easier to recognize and discourage, implicit bias also negatively affects the relationship between patients and providers and may be more difficult to recognize.[112] Whereas explicit biases are beliefs that health care providers claim to have, implicit biases are not consciously recognized and thus can influence clinicians' behaviors without their knowledge. Implicit bias can contribute to health disparities via two pathways: first, through the impact of the implicit assumption on clinical judgment in regards to patient care, and second, via the impact of implicit assumptions on communication between the patient and the provider, and its implications for the patient's engagement and adherence to treatment recommendations.[111] Research has shown that health care providers exhibit more implicit bias against Black, Hispanic, and American Indian patients than they do against White patients.[111] These negative associations can also lead health care providers to associate Black and Hispanic patients with risky health behaviors and nonadherence.[111]

In addition to exhibiting implicit and explicit racial or ethnic biases, providers also exhibit weight biases, with studies reporting that clinicians can show more bias against patients with overweight and obesity.[111,113] Specifically, communication from providers may be influenced by their beliefs about whether the patient will adhere to recommendations, a bias exhibited against both patients from marginalized racial and ethnic groups and patients with obesity.[113] Therefore, the intersection of marginalized identities (eg, racial, ethnic, and weight-based) can compound negative effects, thus influencing the relationship between patient and provider and contributing to negative patient outcomes.[86] For example, fewer bariatric surgery referrals are made for for Black patients and men.†[95,114,115]

Bariatric surgery requires a high level of effort and adherence to several lifestyle and behavioral changes. Patients are required to consume an adequate amount of protein, take vitamin supplements daily, and maintain a regular physical activity routine. Thus, if a provider is concerned about adherence, they may be less likely to refer patients whom they perceive to be nonadherent for bariatric surgery. Considering existing data on referrals and concerns regarding adherence and risky behaviors among some groups, practitioners can hypothesize that explicit and implicit biases impact surgical care. However, it is important to note that no definitive studies have examined why referrals for bariatric surgery are lower for some groups compared to others. Thus, bias among providers must be fully considered and addressed.

Actionable Strategies for Achieving Equity in Obesity Care

A commitment to recognizing institutional and environmental barriers to obesity care and understanding the discrimination faced by marginalized racial and ethnic patient groups is essential for achieving equity in weight management and treatment. Awareness of structural inequities, which include racism, socioeconomic status, access to resources, the built environment, and implicit or explicit bias in the health care system, allows providers to offer tailored recommendations and to advocate for the implementation of resources that could eliminate some inequities. Various actionable strategies are recommended at both the individual and institutional level for reducing health disparities among marginalized racial and ethnic patient groups living with obesity.

Individual-Level Commitments

An overall understanding of a patient's specific, unique barriers to health care can be achieved in the clinic using quantitative and qualitative assessments. These assessments enable the clinician to offer tailored recommendations based on a patient's unique needs and circumstances.

Conduct Quantitative and Qualitative Assessments

Quantitative assessments of social determinants of health can be conducted and included in the electronic health records of patients. For example, a clinician can conduct a quantitative assessment of food insecurity by asking two questions: namely, whether the patient ever runs out of food before having money to buy more, and, if so, how long the patient's food lasts before they have money to buy more.[116] Other assessments include taking a patient's "community vital signs" to address the relevant social determinants of health and guide clinical conversations with the patient.[116,117] Addressing food insecurity in the clinic may involve connecting patients with social workers or trained volunteers who can facilitate referrals to community resources.[116-118]

---

† The literature described study participants as men. Gender was not further specified.

Qualitative assessments, conducted through conversations between patients and providers, help to personalize treatment recommendations and are another way to address disadvantages caused by structural inequities. At times, particularly in weight-management care, it may be easy for clinicians to make broad recommendations. However, it is important to ensure that patients have access to the necessary resources and equipment to make behavioral or lifestyle changes. For example, suggesting that a patient increase consumption of nutrient-dense foods such as fruits and vegetables is not helpful if the patient has no access to transportation, a local supermarket, a refrigerator to store foods safely, or a stove or other kitchen device to prepare the foods. Conversations about work, home life, and the patient's priorities may provide insights into these structural inequities. For example, if a patient experiences interpersonal discrimination at work, a referral to a specialist for stress management may aid in weight-management efforts.[119,120] Additional topics to assess qualitatively in conversations with patients include food insecurity, socioeconomic status, support systems, stress, sleep, community resources, and patient goals.[78] Questions may include, "Is there anything about your community or neighborhood that prevents you from participating in physical activity outside?" and, "Do you feel you have access to resources that will help you achieve your goals? How can we help?"[78]

Understand Patients' Goals

When discussing weight management with patients, clinicians should strive to understand their patients' goals in pursuing treatment, including their health-related and psychosocial-related motivations.[121] Some patients may hope to improve their quality of life by being able to keep up with their children, participate in activities with friends and family, or improve other psychosocial factors.[122] Whatever their motivations, it is possible that some patients will have unrealistic weight loss goals.[123] These may be driven by Western ideals about being "thin" and can lead to disordered eating behaviors in Black and Asian patients.[124-127] Part of implementing evidence-based obesity treatment is ensuring that patients have realistic expectations for treatment outcomes and can make informed treatment decisions.[128] Providers should encourage goals based on improvements in health rather than on aesthetic changes (eg, going down a dress size). For example, clinicians may choose to focus on process goals, which can include the improvement of comorbidities or behavioral or lifestyle changes.[129] In this vein, one can explain to a patient that a weight loss of 5% to 10% of body weight may not result in noticeable aesthetic changes but can lead to cardiometabolic health improvements.[130] If a patient weighs 122 kg (269 lb), a reasonable goal weight could be in the range of 116 kg (256 lb) to 110 kg (243 lb)—a loss of 5.19% to 10%. Including a discussion of patient goals and motivations in clinical conversations about weight loss treatment helps patients avoid setting unattainable goals that may promote disordered eating behaviors and promotes autonomy in the patient's decision-making process.[98-100,130,131] However, it is important to recognize the limitations of current treatment options. As previously noted, treatment outcomes differ among various patient groups, and these differences are an important area of future study.

Provide Accessible Education Materials

An additional important step to equity is to ensure the readability and accuracy of all patient health-education materials. The majority of printed materials offered to patients are written at grade levels higher than the average American eighth-grade reading level, which increases health disparities as an individual's reading level can be a strong predictor of their health status.[132] In addition, as discussed earlier, it may be difficult for some patients to attend or afford (ie, obtain insurance coverage for) treatment for weight management; therefore, they may be unable to receive any evidence-based educational materials. If unable to speak to medical professionals, patients may resolve to consult the internet, where researchers have documented disparities in accessibility to quality information. Specifically, weight loss information accessed in Spanish web searches was less comprehensive and more inaccurate than information published in English.[133] Thus, the combination of limited access to resources and printed materials from health care professionals, limited readability of available patient health-education resources, and disparities in online resources further contributes to inequities. Yet, there are some steps clinics and providers can take to improve patients' ability to access reliable information. First, providers should review any printed materials distributed by the clinic and ensure they are written at a sixth-grade reading level or lower.[134] Although the average American reading level is eighth grade, having materials written at a sixth-grade level or lower further improves readability and accessibility, as breaking information down into simpler terms and steps is more tolerable for individuals with lower literacy.[135,136] Second, clinics can invest time in teaching patients how to determine whether information is credible and comes from a reliable source, such as a registered dietitian nutritionist or reputable health care system. Access to information, in the clinic and online, combats inequities in the treatment of overweight and obesity.

This chapter has noted the influence of explicit and implicit bias on obesity treatment. There is a paucity of research on weight-bias reduction among health care professionals.[137] Even health care providers who regularly work with patients living with overweight and obesity have exhibited high levels of implicit bias.[138] However, a few interventions show promise. Among medical students, viewing a short video about weight bias in health care resulted in increased beliefs that genetic and environmental factors rather than personal choices alone contribute to the development and maintenance of obesity.[139] Other strategies to address bias and assumptions in clinical spaces include focusing on the multifactorial nature of obesity, increasing exposure to individuals who go against stereotypes, and ensuring that explicit bias is not tolerated in clinic settings.[140]

Institutional-Level Commitments

Although individual action by clinicians in the treatment of obesity is important to achieving equity, most barriers to equity are systematic and thus require large-scale systematic solutions. Serious institutional commitments are needed to advance efforts toward equitable health care. One commitment should be to increase diversity in clinical spaces. Representation is important, and patients are more satisfied with interactions and have better health outcomes when there is racial, ethnic, and linguistic concordance between the provider and the patient.[99,100] Specifically, racial and ethnic concordance increases the likelihood that patients will seek preventive care, visit their provider for new health problems, and consistently meet with providers for continued health problems.[141,142] Patients need academic and community involvement to increase diversity among health care professionals.[143] Academic and health care institutions should prioritize recruiting, retaining, and supporting trainees of diverse identities and backgrounds to promote diversity in health care fields.[144]

In addition to making serious commitment to increase diversity, institutions should make a parallel commitment to offer high-quality, evidence-based obesity care. Clinicians can achieve this goal by pursuing an obesity medicine fellowship and taking the ABOM exam. Clinicians who are ABOM diplomates (meaning they have passed the ABOM exam) offer care that aligns with evidence-based guidelines, such as the prescription of FDA-approved antiobesity medications and recommendations for nutrition, exercise, and behavioral services.[145] If institutions increase the number of providers specifically trained to treat obesity, they may improve patients' ability to access to evidence-based treatments. In addition, efforts to increase the representation of registered dietitian nutritionists who identify as racially or ethnically marginalized in organizations dedicated to providing high-quality obesity care (eg, the Academy of Nutrition and Dietetics) can also improve the quality of care.[98] However, educating care providers on weight stigma is still important because even those who specialize in obesity treatment can exhibit bias against patients with higher weights.[138] With the continued increase in obesity prevalence, the commitment of institutions to thoroughly train providers in the treatment of this chronic disease is a worthy endeavor.

Lastly, the rebuilding of the relationship between the health care system, clinicians, researchers, and patients from marginalized racial and ethnic groups should be the utmost priority. The relationship between researchers, clinicians, and diverse patient groups has been understandably strained throughout US history due to highly unethical practices conducted against systematically oppressed populations in the name of "science" and "advancing medicine."[146] Continued mistrust, a rational response to untrustworthy institutions, has been highlighted during the recent COVID-19 pandemic, specifically in the context of vaccination of marginalized racial and ethnic groups.[147,148] Because of implicit and explicit biases and the lack of appropriately tailored weight-management interventions, the distrust of health care providers likely extends to the clinical sphere of weight management. Research has shown that the stigma associated with obesity results in health care avoidance, and, thus, weight-based stigma further affects health care inequities.[149] The combination of racial, ethnic, and weight bias may, therefore, place marginalized patients at increased risk for health care avoidance. Continued commitment to patient-centered care and efforts to prioritize patient needs, goals, and desires are actionable steps that clinics and providers can take to begin to heal this relationship.

Summary

Patients from marginalized racial and ethnic groups face a range of barriers to weight management. These barriers contribute to inequitable risk for the development and maintenance of obesity. Some barriers rooted in historical and enduring structural inequalities cannot fully be addressed within clinical practice. Redressing the harms of systematic racism requires policy changes in a wide range of institutions, from housing, finance, and education to criminal justice, the food system, and more. Nevertheless, clinics and providers can still take action to address inequities and heal the historical mistrust of health care organizations. Key steps include using quantitative and qualitative assessments of social determinants of health, increasing representation of marginalized racial and ethnic groups in research and health care fields, striving to recognize cultural differences and promote patient autonomy, improving the readability and accessibility of evidence-based weight-management information, and establishing a commitment to diversity within health care institutions.

References

1. Wharton S, Lau DCW, Vallis M, et al. Obesity in adults: a clinical practice guideline. *Can Med Assoc J.* 2020;192(31):E875-E891. doi:10.1503/cmaj.191707
2. Cardel MI, Atkinson MA, Taveras EM, Holm J-C, Kelly AS. Obesity treatment among adolescents: a review of current evidence and future directions. *JAMA Pediatr.* 2020;174(6):609-617. doi:10.1001/jamapediatrics.2020.0085
3. Hales CM, Carroll MD, Fryar CD, Ogden CL. *Prevalence of Obesity and Severe Obesity Among Adults: United States, 2017-2018*. NCHS Data Brief no. 360. National Center for Health Statistics; 2020. Accessed October 2021. www.cdc.gov/nchs/products/databriefs/db360.htm
4. Fryar CD, Carroll MD, Afful J. *Prevalence of Overweight, Obesity, and Severe Obesity Among Children and Adolescents Aged 2-19 Years: United States, 1963-1965 Through 2017-2018*. NCHS Health E-Stats. National Center for Health Statistics; 2020. Accessed October 2021. www.cdc.gov/nchs/data/hestat/obesity-child-17-18/obesity-child.htm
5. Petersen R, Pan L, Blanck HM. Racial and ethnic disparities in adult obesity in the United States: CDC's tracking to inform state and local action. *Prev Chronic Dis.* 2019;16:E46. doi:10.5888/pcd16.180579
6. Ethnicity and health in America series: obesity in the Native American community. American Psychological Association Public Interest Directorate website. 2015. Accessed November 18, 2021. www.apa.org/pi/oema/resources/ethnicity-health/native-american/obesity
7. Adult obesity facts. Centers for Disease Control and Prevention website. 2021. Accessed October 2021. www.cdc.gov/obesity/data/adult.html
8. Obesity and American Indians/Alaska Natives. US Department of Health and Human Services Office of Minority Health website. Updated March 6, 2020. Accessed January 6, 2023. https://minorityhealth.hhs.gov/omh/browse.aspx?lvl=4&lvlid=40
9. Nam S. Obesity and Asian Americans in the United States: systematic literature review. *Osong Public Health Res Perspect.* 2013;4(4):187-193. doi:10.1016/j.phrp.2013.06.001
10. Akam EY, Nuako AA, Daniel AK, Stanford FC. Racial disparities and cardiometabolic risk: new horizons of intervention and prevention. *Curr Diab Rep.* 2022;22(3):129-136. doi:10.1007/s11892-022-01451-6
11. Byrd AS, Toth AT, Stanford FC. Racial disparities in obesity treatment. *Curr Obes Reports.* 2018;7(2):130-138. doi:10.1007/s13679-018-0301-3
12. Moore LV, Diez Roux AV, Evenson KR, McGinn AP, Brines SJ. Availability of recreational resources in minority and low socioeconomic status areas. *Am J Prev Med.* 2008;34(1):16-22. doi:10.1016/j.amepre.2007.09.021
13. Campos GM, Khoraki J, Browning MG, Pessoa BM, Mazzini GS, Wolfe L. Changes in utilization of bariatric surgery in the United States from 1993 to 2016. *Ann Surg.* 2020;271(2):201-209. doi:10.1097/SLA0000000000003554
14. Johnson-Mann C, Martin AN, Williams MD, Hallowell PT, Schirmer B. Investigating racial disparities in bariatric surgery referrals. *Surg Obes Relat Dis.* 2019;15(4):615-620. doi:10.1016/j.soard.2019.02.002
15. Block JP, Scribner RA, Desalvo KB. Fast food, race/ethnicity, and income. *Am J Prev Med.* 2004;27(3):211-217. doi:10.1016/j.amepre.2004.06.007
16. Duggan CP, Kurpad A, Stanford FC, Sunguya B, Wells JC. Race, ethnicity, and racism in the nutrition literature: an update for 2020. *Am J Clin Nutr.* 2020;112(6):1409-1414. doi:10.1093/ajcn/nqaa341
17. Braveman P. Health disparities and health equity: concepts and measurement. *Annu Rev Public Health.* 2006;27(1):167-194. doi:10.1146/annurev.publhealth.27.021405.102103
18. Hahn RA. What is a social determinant of health? Back to basics. *J Public Health Res.* 2021;10(4):2324. doi:10.4081/jphr.2021.2324
19. Singh GK, Daus GP, Allender M, et al. Social determinants of health in the United States: addressing major health inequality trends for the nation, 1935-2016. *Int J MCH AIDS.* 2017;6(2):139-164. doi:10.21106/ijma.236
20. Social determinants of health. Healthy People 2030 initiative. US Department of Health and Human Services, Offices of Disease Prevention and Health Promotion website. Accessed October 2021. https://health.gov/healthypeople/objectives-and-data/social-determinants-health

21. Hoyert, DL. *Maternal Mortality Rates in the United States, 2019*. NCHS Health E-Stats. National Center for Health Statistics; 2021. doi:10.15620/cdc:103855
22. Bennett GG, Wolin KY, Duncan DT. Social determinants of obesity. In: Hu F, ed. *Obesity Epidemiology*. Oxford University Press; 2008:342-376.
23. Ghosh-Dastidar B, Cohen D, Hunter G, et al. Distance to store, food prices, and obesity in urban food deserts. *Am J Prev Med*. 2014;47(5):587-595. doi:10.1016/j.amepre.2014.07.005
24. Sbicca J. Growing food justice by planting an anti-oppression foundation: opportunities and obstacles for a budding social movement. *Agric Human Values*. 2012;29(4):455-466. doi:10.1007/s10460-012-9363-0
25. Reese, Ashanté M. *Black Food Geographies: Race, Self-Reliance, and Food Access in Washington, D.C.* UNC Press Books; 2019.
26. Aaron DG, Stanford FC. Is obesity a manifestation of systemic racism? A ten-point strategy for study and intervention. *J Intern Med*. 2021;290(2):416-420. doi:10.1111/joim.13270
27. Jones CP. Levels of racism: a theoretic framework and a gardener's tale. *Am J Public Health*. 2000;90(8):1212-1215. doi:10.2105.ajph.90.8.1212
28. Jones CP. Confronting institutionalized racism. *Phylon (1960-)*. 2002;50(1/2):7-22. doi:10.2307/4149999
29. Bailey ZD, Krieger NK, Agénor M, Graves J, Linos N, Bassett MT. Structural racism and health inequities in the USA: evidence and interventions. *Lancet*. 2017;389(10077):1453-1463. doi:10.1016/s0140-6736(17)30569-X
30. Jones T. Institutional racism in the United States. *Social Work*. 1974;19(2):218-225. doi:10.1093/sw/19.2.218
31. Adkins-Jackson PB, Legha RK, Jones KA. How to measure racism in academic health centers. *AMA J Ethics*. 2021;23(2):E140-145. doi:10.1001/amajethics.2021.140
32. Phelan JC, Link BG. Is racism a fundamental cause of inequalities in health? *Annu Rev of Sociol*. 2015;41(1):311-330. doi:10.1146/annurev-soc-073014-112305
33. Forde AT, Crookes DM, Suglia SF, Demmer RT. The weathering hypothesis as an explanation for racial disparities in health: a systematic review. *Ann Epidemiol*. 2019;33:1-18.e13. doi:10.1016/j.annepidem.2019.02.011
34. Tomiyama AJ. Stress and obesity. *Annu Rev Psychol*. 2019;70:703-718. doi:10.1146/annurev-psych-010418-102936
35. Cozier YC, Yu J, Coogan PF, Bethea TN, Rosenberg L, Palmer JR. Racism, segregation, and risk of obesity in the Black women's health study. *Am J Epidemiol*. 2014;179(7):875-883. doi:10.1093/aje/kwu004
36. Goosby BJ, Straley E, Cheadle JE. Discrimination, sleep, and stress reactivity: pathways to African American-White cardiometabolic risk inequities. *Pop Res Policy Rev*. 2017;36(5):699-716. doi:10.1007/s11113-017-9439-z
37. Brondolo E, Rieppi R, Kelly K, Gerin W. Perceived racism and blood pressure: a review of the literature and conceptual and methodological critique. *Ann Behav Med*. 2003;25(1):55-65. doi:10.1207/S15324796ABM2501_08
38. Zeiders KH, Doane LD, Roosa MW. Perceived discrimination and diurnal cortisol: examining relations among Mexican American adolescents. *Horm Behav*. 2012;61(4):541-548. doi:10.1016/j.yhbeh.2012.01.018
39. Cozier YC, Wise LA, Palmer JR, Rosenberg L. Perceived racism in relation to weight change in the Black women's health study. *Ann Epidemiol*. 2009;19(6):379-387. doi:10.1016/j.annepidem.2009.01.008
40. Cardel MI, Min Y-I, Sims M, et al. Association of psychosocial stressors with metabolic syndrome severity among African Americans in the Jackson Heart Study. *Psychoneuroendocrinology*. 2018;90:141-147. doi:10.1016/j.psyneuen.2018.02.014
41. Monteiro CA, Moura EC, Conde WL, Popkin BM. Socioeconomic status and obesity in adult populations of developing countries: a review. *Public Health Rev*. 2004;82(12):940-946.
42. Coleman-Jensen A, Rabbitt MP, Gregory Ca, Singh A. *Household Food Security in the United States in 2016*. Economic Research Report no. 237 (ERR-237). US Department of Agriculture, Economic Research Service; 2017. www.ers.usda.gov/publications/pub-details/?pubid=84972
43. Odoms-Young A, Bruce MA. Examining the impact of structural racism on food insecurity: implications for addressing racial/ethnic disparities. *Fam Community Health*. 2018;41(S2):S3-S6. doi:10.1097/FCH.0000000000000183
44. Jernigan VBB, Huyser KR, Valdes J, Simonds VW. Food insecurity among American Indians and Alaska Natives: a national profile using the current population survey–food security supplement. *J Hunger Environ Nutr*. 2017;12(1):1-10. doi:10.1080/19320248.2016.1227750
45. Gorton D, Bullen CR, Mhurchu CN. Environmental influences on food security in high-income countries. *Nutr Rev*. 2010;68(1):1-29. doi:10.1111/j.1753-4887.2009.00258.x
46. Rose D. Economic determinants and dietary consequences of food insecurity in the United States. *J Nutr*. 1999;129(2):517S-520S. doi:10.1093/jn/129.2.517S
47. Ribar D, Hamrick K. *Dynamics of Poverty and Food Sufficiency*. Food Assistance and Nutrition Research Report no. 36 (FANRR-36). US Department of Agriculture, Economic Research Service; 2003. doi:10.22004/ag.econ.33851
48. Bratanova B, Loughnan S, Klein O, Claassen A, Wood R. Poverty, inequality, and increased consumption of high calorie food: experimental evidence for a causal link. *Appetite*. 2016;100:162-171. doi:10.1016/j.appet.2016.01.028

49. Nettle D, Andrews C, Bateson M. Food insecurity as a driver of obesity in humans: the insurance hypothesis. *Behav and Brain Sci.* 2017;40:e105. doi:10.1017/S0140525X16000947
50. Dhurandhar EJ. The food-insecurity obesity paradox: a resource scarcity hypothesis. *Physiol Behav.* 2016;162:88-92. doi:10.1016/j.physbeh.2016.04.025
51. Cardel M, Pavela G, Janicke D, et al. Experimentally manipulated low social status and food insecurity alter eating behavior among adolescents: a randomized controlled trial. *Obesity.* 2020;28(11):2010-2019. doi:10.1002/oby.23002
52. Cheon BK, Hong Y-Y. Mere experience of low subjective socioeconomic status stimulates appetite and food intake. *Proc Natl Acad Sci.* 2017;114(1):72-77. doi:10.1073/pnas.1607330114
53. Wang Y. Cross-national comparison of childhood obesity: the epidemic and the relationship between obesity and socioeconomic status. *Int J Epidemiol.* 2001;30(5):1129-1136. doi:10.1093/ije/30.5.1129
54. Wardle J, Waller J, Jarvis MJ. Sex differences in the association of socioeconomic status with obesity. *Am J Public Health.* 2002;92(8):1299-1304. doi:10.2105/AJPH.92.8.1299
55. Wang Y, Lim H. The global childhood obesity epidemic and the association between socio-economic status and childhood obesity. *Int Rev Psychiatry.* 2012;24(3):176-188. doi:10.3109/09540261.2012.688195
56. Pavela G, Lewis DW, Locher J, Allison DB. Socioeconomic status, risk of obesity, and the importance of Albert J. Stunkard. *Curr Obes Rep.* 2016;5(1):132-139. doi:10.1007/s13679-015-0185-4
57. Drewnowski A. Obesity, diets, and social inequalities. *Nutr Rev.* 2009;67:S36-S39. doi:10.1111/j.1753-4887.2009.00157.x
58. LaVeist TA. Disentangling race and socioeconomic status: a key to understanding health inequalities. *J Urban Health.* 2005;82(2 suppl 3):iii26-iii34. doi:10.1093/jurban/jti061
59. Rogers R, Eagle TF, Sheetz A, et al. The relationship between childhood obesity, low socioeconomic status, and race/ethnicity: lessons from Massachusetts. *Child Obes.* 2015;11(6):691-695. doi:10.1089/chi.2015.0029
60. Fradkin C, Wallander JL, Elliott MN, Tortolero S, Cuccaro P, Schuster MA. Associations between socioeconomic status and obesity in diverse, young adolescents: variation across race/ethnicity and gender. *Health Psychol.* 2015;34(1):1-9. doi:10.1037/hea0000099
61. Merolla DM, Jackson O. Structural racism as the fundamental cause of the academic achievement gap. *Sociology Compass.* 2019;13(6):e12696. doi:10.1111/soc4.12696
62. Quillian L, Pager D, Hexel O, Midtbøen AH. Meta-analysis of field experiments shows no change in racial discrimination in hiring over time. *Proc Natl Acad Sci USA.* 2017;114(41):10870-10875. doi:10.1073/pnas.1706255114
63. Watts RJ, Carter RT. Psychological aspects of racism in organizations. *Group and Organ Stud.* 1991;16(3):328-344. doi:10.1177/105960119101600307
64. Sharifi M, Sequist TD, Rifas-Shiman SL, et al. The role of neighborhood characteristics and the built environment in understanding racial/ethnic disparities in childhood obesity. *Prev Med.* 2016;91:103-109. doi:10.1016/j.ypmed.2016.07.009
65. Lamichhane AP, Warren J, Puett R, et al. Spatial patterning of supermarkets and fast food outlets with respect to neighborhood characteristics. *Health Place.* 2013;23:157-164. doi:10.1016/j.healthplace.2013.07.002
66. Powell LM, Slater S, Mirtcheva D, Bao Y, Chaloupka FJ. Food store availability and neighborhood characteristics in the United States. *Prev Med.* 2007;44(3):189-195. doi:10.1016/j.ypmed.2006.08.008
67. James P, Arcaya MC, Parker DM, Tucker-Seeley RD, Subramanian SV. Do minority and poor neighborhoods have higher access to fast-food restaurants in the United States? *Health Place.* 2014;29:10-17. doi:10.1016/j.healthplace.2014.04.011
68. Zenk SN, Schulz AJ, Israel BA, James SA, Bao S, Wilson ML. Neighborhood racial composition, neighborhood poverty, and the spatial accessibility of supermarkets in metropolitan Detroit. *Am J Public Health.* 2005;95(4):660-667. doi:10.2105/AJPH.2004.042150
69. Beaulac J, Kristjansson E, Cummins S. A systematic review of food deserts, 1966-2007. *Prev Chronic Dis.* 2009;6(3):A105. Accessed October 2021. www.cdc.gov/pcd/issues/2009/jul/08_0163.htm
70. Hendrickson D, Smith C, Eikenberry N. Fruit and vegetable access in four low-income food deserts communities in Minnesota. *Agric Human Values.* 2006;23(3):371-383. doi:10.1007/s10460-006-9002-8
71. MacNell L, Elliott S, Hardison-Moody A, Bowen S. Black and Latino urban food desert residents' perceptions of their food environment and factors that influence food shopping decisions. *J Hunger Environ Nutr.* 2017;12(3):375-393. doi:10.1080/19320248.2017.1284025
72. Jannah N, Hild J, Gallagher C, Dietz W. Coverage for obesity prevention and treatment services: analysis of Medicaid and state employee health insurance programs. *Obesity (Silver Spring).* 2018;26(12):1834-1840. doi:10.1002/oby.22307
73. Richardson LD, Norris M. Access to health and health care: how race and ethnicity matter. *Mt Sinai J Med.* 2010;77(2):166-177. doi:10.1002/msj.20174
74. Perez NP, Westfal ML, Stapleton SM, Pratt JS, Chang DC, Kelleher CM. Beyond insurance: race-based disparities in the use of metabolic and bariatric surgery for the management of severe pediatric obesity. *Surg Obes Relat Dis.* 2020;16(3):414-419. doi:10.1016/j.soard.2019.11.020
75. Newsome FA, Dilip A, Armstrong SC, Salloum RG, Cardel MI. Scaling up stage 4 pediatric obesity clinics: identifying barriers and future directions using implementation science. *Obesity (Silver Spring).* 2021;29(6):941-943. doi:10.1002/oby.23162

76. Befort CA, Nazir N, Perri MG. Prevalence of obesity among adults from rural and urban areas of the United States: findings from NHANES (2005-2008). *J Rural Health*. 2012;28(4):392-397. doi:10.1111/j.1748-0361.2012.00411.x
77. Lichter DT. Immigration and the new racial diversity in rural America. *Rural Sociol*. 2012;77(1):3-35. doi:10.1111/j.1549-0831.2012.00070.x
78. Newsome FA, Gravlee CC, Cardel MI. Systematic and environmental contributors to obesity inequities in marginalized racial and ethnic groups. *Nurs Clin North Am*. 2021;56(4):619-634. doi:10.1016/j.cnur.2021.07.003
79. Forman EM, Butryn ML, Manasse SM, et al. Acceptance-based versus standard behavioral treatment for obesity: results from the mind your health randomized controlled trial. *Obesity (Silver Spring)*. 2016;24(10):2050-2056. doi:10.1002/oby.21601
80. Cardel MI, Lee AM, Chi X, et al. Feasibility/acceptability of an acceptance based therapy intervention for diverse adolescent girls with overweight/obesity. *Obes Sci Pract*. 2021;7(3):291-301. doi:10.1002/osp4.483
81. Michie S, Richardson M, Johnston M, et al. The behavior change technique taxonomy (v1) of 93 hierarchically clustered techniques: building an international consensus for the reporting of behavior change interventions. *Ann Behav Med*. 2013;46(1):81-95. doi:10.1007/s12160-013-9486-6
82. Forman EM, Butryn ML, Juarascio AS, et al. The mind your health project: a randomized controlled trial of an innovative behavioral treatment for obesity. *Obesity (Silver Spring)*. 2013;21(6):1119-1126. doi:10.1002/oby.20169
83. Srivastava G, Apovian CM. Current pharmacotherapy for obesity. *Nat Rev Endocrinol*. 2018;14(1):12-24. doi:10.1038/nrendo.2017.122
84. Wilding JPH, Batterham RL, Calanna S, et al. Once-weekly semaglutide in adults with overweight or obesity. *N Engl J Med*. 2021;384(11):989-1002. doi:10.1056/NEJMoa2032183
85. Baptista V, Wassef W. Bariatric procedures: an update on techniques, outcomes, and complications. *Curr Opin Gastroenterol*. 2013;29(6):684-693. doi:10.1097/MOG.0b013e3283651af2
86. Bleich SN, Simon AE, Cooper LA. Impact of patient-doctor race concordance on rates of weight-related counseling in visits by Black and White obese individuals. *Obesity (Silver Spring)*. 2012;20(3):562-570. doi:10.1038/oby.2010.330
87. Saxon DR, Iwamoto SJ, Mettenbrink CJ, et al. Antiobesity medication use in 2.2 million adults across eight large health care organizations: 2009 2015. *Obesity (Silver Spring)*. 2019;27(12):1975-1981. doi:10.1002/oby.22581
88. Egan BM, White K. Weight loss pharmacotherapy: brief summary of the clinical literature and comments on racial differences. *Ethn Dis*. 2015;25(4):511-514. doi:10.18865/ed.25.4.511
89. Browning MG, Pessoa BM, Campos GM. Comment on: racial disparities may impact referrals and access to bariatric surgery. *Surg Obes Relat Dis*. 2019;15(6):E23-E24. doi:10.1016/j.soard.2019.03.024
90. Hales CM, Fryar CD, Carroll MD, Freedman DS, Aoki Y, Ogden CL. Differences in obesity prevalence by demographic characteristics and urbanization level among adults in the United States, 2013-2016. *JAMA*. 2018;319(23):2419. doi:10.1001/jama.2018.7270
91. Wallace AE, Young-Xu Y, Hartley D, Weeks WB. Racial, socioeconomic, and rural–urban disparities in obesity-related bariatric surgery. *Obes Surg*. 2010;20(10):1354-1360. doi:10.1007/s11695-009-0054-x
92. Katzmarzyk PT, Martin CK, Newton RL, et al. Weight loss in underserved patients—a cluster-randomized trial. *N Engl J Med*. 2020;383(10):909-918. doi:10.1056/NEJMoa2007448
93. Yanovski SZ, Yanovski JA. Long-term drug treatment for obesity. *JAMA*. 2014;311(1):74. doi:10.1001/jama.2013.281361
94. Osei-Assibey G, Adi Y, Kyrou I, Kumar S, Matyka K. Pharmacotherapy for overweight/obesity in ethnic minorities and White Caucasians: a systematic review and meta-analysis. *Diabetes Obes Metab*. 2011;13(5):385-393. doi:10.1111/j.1463-1326.2010.01346.x
95. Sheka A, Kizy S, Wirth K, Grams J, Leslie D, Ikramuddin S. Racial disparities in perioperative outcomes after bariatric surgery. *Surg Obes Relat Dis*. 2019;15(5):786-793. doi:10.1016/j.soard.2018.12.021
96. Welsh LK, Luhrs AR, Davalos G, et al. Racial disparities in bariatric surgery complications and mortality using the MBSAQIP data registry. *Obes Surg*. 2020;30(8):3099-3110. doi:10.1007/s11695-020-04657-3
97. Kizy S, Jahansouz C, Downey MC, Hevelone N, Ikramuddin S, Leslie D. National trends in bariatric surgery 2012–2015: demographics, procedure selection, readmissions, and cost. *Obes Surg*. 2017;27(11):2933-2939. doi:10.1007/s11695-017-2719-1
98. Carson TL, Cardel MI, Stanley TL, et al. Racial and ethnic representation among a sample of nutrition and obesity focused professional organizations in the United States. *Am J Clin Nutr*. 2021;114(6):1869-1872. doi:10.1093/acjn/nqab284
99. Fernandez A, Schillinger D, Warton ME, et al. Language barriers, physician-patient language concordance, and glycemic control among insured Latinos with diabetes: the diabetes study of northern California (DISTANCE). *J Gen Intern Med*. 2010;26(2):170-176. doi:10.1007/s11606-010-1507-6
100. Saha S, Komaromy M, Koepsell TD, Bindman AB. Patient-physician racial concordance and the perceived quality and use of health care. *Arch of Interm Med*. 1999;159(9):997-1004. doi:10.1001/archinte.159.9.997
101. Looney SM, Raynor HA. Behavioral lifestyle intervention in the treatment of obesity. *Health Serv Insights*. 2013;6:15-31. doi:10.4137/HIS.S10474

102. Lindberg N, Stevens V. Review: weight-loss interventions with Hispanic populations. *Ethn Dis.* 2007;17(2):397-402.
103. Perez LG, Arredondo EM, Elder JP, Barquera S, Nagle B, Holub CK. Evidence-based obesity treatment interventions for Latino Adults in the U.S. *Am J Prev Med.* 2013;44(5):550-560. doi:10.1016/j.amepre.2013.01.016
104. Rosas LG, Vasquez JJ, Naderi R, et al. Development and evaluation of an enhanced diabetes prevention program with psychosocial support for urban American Indians and Alaska Natives: a randomized controlled trial. *Contemp Clin Trials.* 2016;50:28-36. doi:10.1016/j.cct.2016.06.015
105. Kaiser KA, Carson TL, Dhurandhar EJ, Neumeier WH, Cardel MI. Biobehavioural approaches to prevention and treatment: a call for implementation science in obesity research. *Obes Sci Pract.* 2020;6(1):3-9. doi:10.1002/osp4.384
106. Chinman M, Woodward EN, Curran GM, Hausmann LRM. Harnessing implementation science to increase the impact of health equity research. *Med Care.* 2017;55(suppl 2):S16-S23. doi:10.1097/MLR.0000000000000769
107. Las Nueces D, Hacker K, Digirolamo A, Hicks LS. A systematic review of community-based participatory research to enhance clinical trials in racial and ethnic minority groups. *Health Serv Res.* 2012;47(3 pt 2):1363-1386. doi:10.1111/j.1475-6773.2012.01386.x
108. Boysen GA. A review of experimental studies of explicit and implicit bias among counselors. *J. Multicult Couns Devel.* 2009;37(4):240-249. doi:10.1002/j.2161-1912.2009.tb00106.x
109. Cooper LA, Roter DL, Carson KA, et al. The associations of clinicians' implicit attitudes about race with medical visit communication and patient ratings of interpersonal care. *Am J Public Health.* 2012;102(5):979-987. doi:10.2105/AJPH.2011.300558
110. Bean MG, Focella ES, Covarrubias R, Stone J, Moskowitz GB, Badger TA. Documenting nursing and medical students' stereotypes about Hispanic and American Indian patients. *J Health Dispar Res Pract.* 2014;7(4):14.
111. Zestcott CA, Blair IV, Stone J. Examining the presence, consequences, and reduction of implicit bias in health care: a narrative review. *Group Process Intergroup Relat.* 2016;19(4):528-542. doi:10.1177/1368430216642029
112. Maina IW, Belton TD, Ginzberg S, Singh A, Johnson TJ. A decade of studying implicit race/ethnic bias in healthcare providers using the implicit association test. *Soc Sci Med.* 2018;199:219-229. doi:10.1016/j.socscimed.2017.05.009
113. Phelan SM, Burgess DJ, Yeazel MW, Hellerstedt WL, Griffin JM, Ryn M. Impact of weight bias and stigma on quality of care and outcomes for patients with obesity. *Obes Rev.* 2015;16(4):319-326. doi:10.1111/obr.12266
114. Wee CC, Huskey KW, Bolcic-Jankovic D, Colten ME, Davis RB, Hamel M. Sex, race, and consideration of bariatric surgery among primary care patients with moderate to severe obesity. *J Gen Intern Med.* 2014;29(1):68-75. doi.10.1007/s11606-013-2603-1
115. Worni M, Guller U, Maciejewski ML, et al. Racial differences among patients undergoing laparoscopic gastric bypass surgery: a population-based trend analysis from 2002 to 2008. *Obes Surg.* 2013;23(2):226-233. doi:10.1007/s11695-012-0832-8
116. Lee A, Cardel M, Donahoo W. Social and environmental factors influencing obesity. In: Feingold K, Anawalt B, Boyce A, et al, eds. *Endotext* [internet]. MDText.com; 2000–. Updated October 12, 2019. www.ncbi.nlm.nih.gov/books/NBK278977
117. Bazemore AW, Cottrell EK, Gold R, et al. "Community vital signs": incorporating geocoded social determinants into electronic records to promote patient and population health. *J Am Med Inform Assoc.* 2016;23(2)407-412. doi:10.1013/jamia/ocv088
118. Barnidge E, Stenmark S, Seligman H. Clinic-to-community models to address food insecurity. *JAMA Pediatr.* 2017;171(6):507-508. doi:10.1001/jamapediatrics.2017.0067
119. Kushner R, Ryan D. Assessment and lifestyle management of patients with obesity: clinical recommendations from systematic reviews. *JAMA.* 2014;312(9):943-952. doi:10.1001/jama.2014.10432
120. Kushner RF, Foster GD. Obesity and quality of life. *Nutrition.* 2000;16(10):947-952. doi:10.1016/s0899-9007(00)00404-4
121. Strømmen M, Kulseng B, Vedul-Kjelsås E, Johnsen H, Johnsen G, Mårvik R. Bariatric surgery or lifestyle intervention? An exploratory study of severely obese patients' motivation for two different treatments. *Obes Res Clin Pract.* 2009;3(4):193-201. doi:10.1016/j.orcp.2009.04.004
122. Childerhose JE, Eneli I, Steele KE. Adolescent bariatric surgery: a qualitative exploratory study of US patient perspectives. *Clin Obes.* 2018;8(5):345-354. doi:10.1111/cob.12272
123. White DB, Bursac Z, Dilillo V, West DS. Weight loss goals among African-American women with type 2 diabetes in a behavioral weight control program. *Obesity (Silver Spring).* 2011;19(11):2283-2285. doi:10.1038/oby.2010.350
124. Witcomb G, Arcelus J, Chen J. Can cognitive dissonance methods developed in the West for combatting the "thin ideal" help slow the rapidly increasing prevalence of eating disorders in non-Western cultures? *Shanghai Arch Psychiatry.* 2013;25(6):332-340. doi:10.3969/j.issn.1002-0829.2013.06.002
125. Juarascio A, Forman E, Timko C, Herbert J, Butryn M, Lowe M. Implicit internalization of the thin ideal as a predictor of increases in weight, body dissatisfaction, and disordered eating. *Eat Behav.* 2011;12(3):207-213. doi:10.1016/j.eatbeh.2011.04.004

126. Gilbert S, Crump S, Madhere S, Schutz W. Internalization of the thin ideal as a predictor of body dissatisfaction and disordered eating in African, African-American, and Afro-Caribbean female college students. *J College Stud Psychother*. 2009;23(3):196-211. doi:10.1080/87568220902794093
127. Akoury LM, Warren CS, Culbert KM. Disordered eating in Asian American women: sociocultural and culture-specific predictors. *Front Psychol*. 2019;10:1950. doi:10.3389/fpsyg.2019.01950
128. Cardel MI, Newsome FA, Pearl RL, et al. Patient-centered care for obesity: how health care providers can treat obesity while actively addressing weight stigma and eating disorder risk. *J Acad Nutr Diet*. 2022;122(6):1089-1098. doi:10.1016/j.jand.2022.01.004
129. Cohen J, Alexander S, Signorelli C, et al. Clinician and healthcare managers' perspectives on the delivery of secondary and tertiary pediatric weight management services. *J Child Health Care*. 2021:136749352110521. doi:10.1177/13674935211052148
130. Chacko SA, Chiodi SN, Wee CC. Recognizing disordered eating in primary care patients with obesity. *Prev Med*. 2015;72:89-94. doi:10.1016/j.ypmed.2014.12.024
131. Putterman E, Linden W. Appearance versus health: does the reason for dieting affect dieting behavior? *J Behav Med*. 2004;27(2):185-204. doi:10.1023/b:jobm.0000019851.37389.a7
132. Mantwill S, Monestel-Umaña S, Schulz PJ. The relationship between health literacy and health disparities: a systematic review. *PLoS One*. 2015;10(12):e0145455. doi:10.1371/journal.pone.0145455
133. Cardel MI, Chavez S, Bian J, et al. Accuracy of weight loss information in Spanish search engine results on the internet. *Obesity (Silver Spring)*. 2016;24(11):2422-2434. doi:10.1002/oby.21646
134. Weiss B. *Health Literacy: A Manual for Clinicians*. American Medical Association Foundation and American Medical Association; 2003.
135. Doak CC, Doak LG, Root JH. *Teaching Patients With Low Literacy Skills*. 2nd ed. Lippincott; 1996.
136. Centers for Disease Control and Prevention, Office of Communication. *Scientific and Technical Information Simply Put*. 3rd ed. Centers for Disease Control and Prevention; 2009.
137. Alberga AS, Pickering BJ, Hayden KA, et al. Weight bias reduction in health professionals: a systematic review. *Clin Obes*. 2016;6(3):175-188. doi:10.1111/cob.12147
138. Schwartz MB, Chambliss HO, Brownell KD, Blair SN, Billington C. Weight bias among health professionals specializing in obesity. *Obes Res*. 2003;11(9):1033-1039. doi:10.1038/oby.2003/142
139. Poustchi Y, Saks NS, Piasecki AK, Hahn KA, Ferrante JM. Brief intervention effective in reducing weight bias in medical students. *Fam Med*. 2013;45(5):345-348.
140. Puhl RM, Phelan SM, Nadglowski J, Kyle TK. Overcoming weight bias in the management of patients with diabetes and obesity. *Clin Diabetes*. 2016;34(1):44-50. doi:10.2337/diaclin.34.1.44
141. Ma A, Sanchez A, Ma M. The impact of patient-provider race/ethnicity concordance on provider visits: updated evidence from the medical expenditure panel survey. *J Racial Ethn Health Disparities*. 2019;6(5):1011-1020. doi:10.1007/s40615-019-00602-y
142. Alsan M, Stanford FC, Banerjee A, et al. Comparison of knowledge and information-seeking behavior after general COVID-19 public health messages and messages tailored for Black and Latinx communities. *Ann Intern Med*. 2021;174(4):484-492. doi:10.7326/M20-6141
143. Goode CA, Landefeld T. The lack of diversity in healthcare: causes, consequences, and solutions. *J Best Pract Health Prof Divers*. 2018;11(2):73-95.
144. Mitchell DA, Lassiter SL. Addressing health care disparities and increasing workforce diversity: the next step for the dental, medical, and public health professions. *Am J Public Health*. 2006;96(12):2093-2097. doi:10.2105/AJPH.2005.082818
145. Gudzune KA, Wickham EP, Schmidt SL, Stanford FC. Physicians certified by the American Board of Obesity Medicine provide evidence-based care. *Clin Obes*. 2021;11(1):e12407. doi:10.1111/cob.12407
146. Brandt AM. Racism and research: the case of the Tuskegee syphilis study. *Hastings Cent Rep*. 1978;8(6):21-29. doi:10.2307/3561468
147. Johnson-Mann C, Hassan M, Johnson S. COVID-19 pandemic highlights racial health inequities. *Lancet Diabetes Endocrinol*. 2020;8(8):663-664. doi:10.1016/S2213-8587(20)30225-4
148. Bajaj SS, Stanford FC. Beyond Tuskegee—vaccine distrust and everyday racism. *N Engl J Med*. 2021;384(5):e12. doi:10.1056/NEJMpv2035827
149. Alegria Drury CA, Louis M. Exploring the association between body weight, stigma of obesity, and health care avoidance. *J Am Acad Nurse Pract*. 2002;14(12):554-561. doi:10.1111/j.1745-7599.2002.tb00089.x

CHAPTER 3

Weight Bias and Stigma

Rebecca L. Pearl, PhD

CHAPTER OBJECTIVES

- Define weight bias and weight stigma.
- Describe the health consequences of weight bias and weight stigma.
- Discuss how health care professionals may contribute to weight bias and weight stigma.
- Identify methods to reduce weight bias in patient care.

Introduction

Understanding the social consequences of overweight and obesity is critical to providing comprehensive and compassionate clinical care. Of particular importance is awareness of the pervasive and persistent stigmatization of individuals with a higher body weight (or larger body) and of how weight-based biases permeate society, including in health care settings. This chapter provides definitions and examples of weight bias and stigma and examines the health consequences of experiencing and internalizing weight stigma. The chapter focuses on the relevance of this topic to health care professionals and ends with concrete recommendations to prevent and reduce weight bias and stigma in clinical practice.

Definitions and Examples of Weight Bias and Stigma

The term *weight bias* refers to negative attitudes toward people who are perceived to have excess weight (ie, overweight or obesity).[1] Weight bias is predicated in part on the misconception that body weight is entirely within an individual's control.[2] Despite robust evidence of the powerful and complex factors that determine any individual's body weight—including genetic, biological, and socioenvironmental factors—the public continues to erroneously believe that most people could maintain a low body weight by simply eating less and exercising more.[3-5] Engaging in these health behaviors and controlling one's weight are viewed as part of an individual's "personal responsibility."[2,6] When people are perceived as being unable to control their weight, they are thus viewed as "irresponsible," which leads to blame and moralization of weight as a sign of failure.[7] Due to misperceptions about the causes of obesity, people with a higher weight are also commonly assumed (or stereotyped) to be sedentary, engaging in unhealthy eating behaviors, and in poor health. Negative stereotypes also extend to assumptions about personal characteristics, including beliefs that people with a higher weight are lazy, unintelligent, unattractive, unhappy, and lacking self-discipline.[3]

Together, negative weight attitudes, stereotypes, and blame lead to societal derogation and devaluation of people with overweight or obesity—also known as *weight stigma*. Stigmatization is the discrediting or dehumanization of a person on the basis of a particular mark, characteristic, or trait (in this case, body weight).[8] Stigmatized populations have reduced power and social status and are subject to discrimination, which involves unfair or unequal treatment (described in more detail later in the chapter).[9] Weight bias and stigma emerge in many settings and domains throughout society,[10] including in structural, interpersonal, and intrapersonal forms.[11] Examples highlighted herein include those that appear in media, laws, and policies, as well as peer victimization, discrimination, and internalization within individuals who identify as having a higher weight.

Structural Weight Stigma

Structural stigma includes societal conditions, cultural norms, or institutional policies and practices that create disadvantages and adversely affect the well-being of stigmatized individuals.[12] Popular media portrayals and news coverage of obesity are examples of contributors to a stigmatizing culture. Television shows and movies for children and adults are rife with examples of weight bias and stigma, including presentations of characters with a higher weight as villains or "comic relief" rather than as protagonists; these higher weight characters often are portrayed with stereotypical traits or behaviors (eg, eating all the time).[13] News stories that frame obesity as a simple problem of poor diet and inactivity perpetuate the narrative of personal responsibility, and images that accompany such news stories often display persons with obesity in a dehumanizing manner (eg, their heads are often not visible in videos or photos, or images zoom in on their specific body parts in an unflattering manner).[14-16] Studies show that stereotypical media depictions of obesity contribute to negative public attitudes toward individuals with a higher weight.[16,17] In addition, social media outlets such as X (formerly known as Twitter), Facebook, Instagram, and YouTube are filled with weight-stigmatizing content that mocks or disparages people with overweight or obesity, in addition to providing forums for cyberbullying and promotion of dangerous disordered eating practices.[18-20] This is of particular concern for young people, who have high exposure to social media content and may be especially vulnerable to internalizing harmful messages about weight.[21]

Laws and policies (or lack thereof) can also perpetuate stigma or fail to prevent it. In the United States and abroad, very few laws exist to protect against weight discrimination.[22,23] For example, Michigan is the only state that prohibits discrimination based on weight, and only a handful of US cities have such protections in their employment laws.[24] Similarly, despite the fact that every US state is required to have an antibullying law, only one state (Maine) enumerates weight as a protected characteristic (three additional states include physical appearance or attributes).[25] This lack of legal protection against weight-based discrimination and bullying enables mistreatment without repercussions. In health care, institutional policies often facilitate discrimination based on weight in provision of care. For example, BMI cutoffs are commonly used to determine eligibility for certain procedures, including fertility treatments and orthopedic surgeries.[26-30] The rationale for such policies is presented as attempting to mitigate health and safety risks; however, the BMI cutoffs are often made without consideration of other health factors, with the result of denied or delayed access to care that could substantially enhance health and quality of life for people with a higher weight.[24,31] Another form of health care discrimination is the lack of insurance coverage for most evidence-based obesity treatments, including lifestyle modification counseling, medications, and surgery.[32,33] This may be due in large part to weight bias and the continued conceptualization of obesity as a problem of personal responsibility that could be solved with simple diet and exercise rather than a complex disease that requires comprehensive medical care.

Interpersonal Weight Stigma

Individuals with obesity may experience weight stigma from a variety of interpersonal sources, including family members, peers, educators, coworkers, employers, community members, service workers, fitness professionals, and health care providers (the latter is discussed in more detail later).[34] Examples of interpersonal stigma may include microaggressions, such as offhanded comments about a person's weight or health behaviors (eg, criticism about food choices), as well as blatant mistreatment, including peer victimization and discrimination.

Peer victimization due to weight is highly prevalent, especially among youth. Examples include teasing, systematic bullying (verbal or physical, in person or online), social exclusion, and other forms of harassment (such as being the target of rumors).[35,36] Weight is the most common reason for victimization in adolescents—as reported by students, parents, and teachers—above all other reasons, such as race or ethnicity and sexual orientation.[37] Data suggest that children and adolescents with obesity have over two times greater odds of experiencing peer victimization as youth with lower weight.[38] Weight-based victimization is more commonly experienced by girls than boys, although weight-based victimization is also common among boys with lower weight, due in part to differences in body ideals for size and muscularity.[35,36,39]

Although weight-based victimization can be experienced throughout the life span, most research on weight-related mistreatment in adults focuses on discrimination. *Discrimination* is a broad term that can refer to unequal treatment across interpersonal relationships, education, employment, health care, and public settings, among other domains. Meta-analytic estimates suggest that 20% to 45% of women with obesity and 6% to 28% of men[†] with obesity report experiencing weight-based discrimination, with higher rates for individuals with higher BMIs.[40] Rates of weight discrimination for women[†] are comparable to rates of gender-based and race-based discrimination,[41] and weight is one of the most strongly identified reasons for mistreatment among diverse samples of adults with obesity who may experience discrimination for a variety of reasons.[42] Workplace discrimination is particularly prevalent, as it is reported in up to 28% of women with obesity and 12% of men[†] with obesity.[40] Self-reported perceptions of discriminatory experiences are supported by economic studies of unemployment and wages that show considerable weight disparities (especially for women[†]), even when controlling for other sociodemographic and health factors,[43-46] and by experimental studies that document biases in hiring, promotion, and salary decisions by employers and human resource professionals.[24,47,48] Workers with a higher weight are also ascribed more negative character traits (eg, incompetence) than lower weight workers,[47] further exemplifying how bias may contribute to unfair treatment and adverse social consequences.

Intrapersonal Weight Stigma

Stigma processes that occur within individuals with a higher body weight include anticipation of being judged or mistreated due to weight,[49] as well as the internalization of stigma (ie, self-stigma).[50] The threat or expectation of stigmatization may be present in social situations, during employment, or in health care settings. This anticipation can impair performance (eg, in a job interview) and lead to avoidance of certain settings and activities, including seeking health care.[49] The internalization of weight stigma begins with awareness among people who identify as having a higher body weight that they are devalued by others in society.[51] Negative attitudes and stereotypes may be endorsed and applied to oneself; for instance, people with obesity may blame themselves for their weight and believe that they are lazy and lack self-control. As a result, this internalization can lead to lower self-esteem or self-worth (ie, self-devaluation), based solely on weight.[51-53]

---

† Study participants were described as women and men. Gender was not further specified.

Health Consequences of Weight Bias and Stigma

Figure 3.1 provides an overview of the many ways in which weight bias and stigma affect health, including the undermining of social determinants of health and direct effects on key aspects of both mental and physical health. Notably, the relationships summarized in this figure remain significant when accounting for BMI and other health-related factors. In other words, weight stigma has a unique impact on health that is not explained by weight itself.

FIGURE 3.1 Health consequences of weight stigma

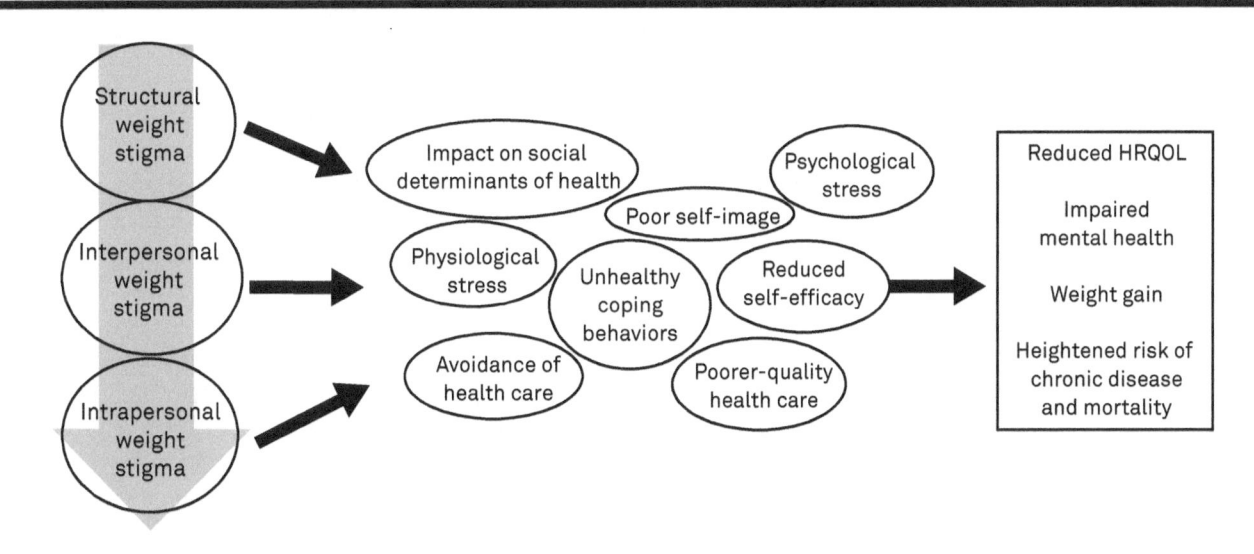

Abbreviation: HRQOL, health-related quality of life.

Social Determinants of Health

Weight bias and stigma reduce access to resources that are critical to the promotion of health. As stated earlier, weight discrimination occurs in employment and negatively affects wages for people with obesity. In addition, weight bias and stigma adversely affect educational outcomes, including grades and college enrollment.[54] This educational disparity, which remains even when accounting for relevant sociodemographic factors, may be attributable to weight bias among educators and the harmful effects of weight-based bullying on academic performance and engagement.[37] For example, studies have shown that teachers assign lower ratings of academic ability to children with obesity than to their lean peers, despite equivalent standardized test scores.[55,56] Youth who experience weight-based teasing or bullying have poorer academic performance and are more likely to report skipping school, along with other social difficulties in this environment.[38,57,58] Furthermore, experimental research has shown that students with a higher weight are discriminated against in admissions for graduate education.[59]

Education, employment, and wages are all well-established predictors of health and well-being. These factors affect the availability of resources (eg, financial, social) that have important consequences for access to healthy foods, environments, and health care.[60] Thus, by limiting educational and occupational advancement—which affect standards of living (eg, neighborhood and environmental safety) and access to health care (eg, through lack of employment-based insurance coverage)—weight bias and stigma have downstream consequences that undermine social determinants of health.[61]

Mental Health

Experiences and internalization of weight bias and stigma are robustly associated with poor mental health outcomes. Adults who report experiencing weight discrimination (compared to those who do not) have two times greater odds of having psychiatric disorders such as depression and anxiety.[62] These associations remain strong when controlling for BMI and general life stress, highlighting the unique contribution of weight discrimination to psychological distress. Weight-stigma experiences are also associated with poor body esteem and self-esteem, as well as with heightened stress and binge eating.[63] Importantly, experiences of weight-based teasing and bullying among youth are associated with increased depression, social anxiety, body dissatisfaction, poor self-esteem, loneliness, and suicidal thoughts and attempts.[36,37] These experiences also prospectively predict disordered eating and unhealthy weight-control behaviors into adulthood.[64]

As with the associations between experiences of weight stigma and mental health, *internalized* weight stigma is strongly correlated with increased symptoms for depression, anxiety, and eating disorders beyond the effects of BMI.[53] Internalized weight stigma is also associated with poorer self-esteem, body image, and mental health–related quality of life.[53] In addition, it has been shown to moderate and mediate the relationship between experiences of weight stigma and mental health, such that internalized weight stigma is often a stronger and more direct predictor of poor outcomes than experiences of stigma alone.[65-68] Both experiences and internalization of weight stigma have been found to mediate the relationship between BMI and psychological outcomes, suggesting that stigma plays a prominent role in explaining the relationship between obesity and mental health.[53,69]

Health Behaviors

Much research has focused on examining how weight stigma may affect health behaviors, with a particular focus on the behaviors that are most relevant to weight. Both experiences of weight stigma and internalization of weight stigma are associated with greater reported use of eating as a coping strategy, with emotional or disinhibited eating, and with overeating (as well as binge eating).[53,70] Experimental research in which participants are exposed to weight stigma has found increased energy consumption among women[†] with a higher weight who face weight stigma, compared to lean women or those who are not exposed to weight stigma.[71,72] Greater internalization of weight stigma is associated with lower self-efficacy or confidence to control one's eating.[53,65,68] This may be due, in part, to internalized, self-directed stereotypes that individuals with a higher weight lack willpower or self-control.

Relationships between weight stigma and reduced physical activity have also been identified, especially in relation to weight-based teasing in youth, internalized weight stigma, and experiences of weight-related microaggressions.[73] Weight stigma is associated with reduced motivation to engage in exercise, increased desire to avoid exercise, and less engagement in physical activity in youth and adulthood.[73-76] Self-application of stereotypes that people with a higher weight are lazy or inactive may, in part, explain the reduced self-efficacy to engage in physical activity that is associated with internalized weight stigma.[74]

---

† Study participants were described as women. Gender was not further specified.

Physical Health

Experiencing stigma is conceptualized as a form of chronic stress, which is accompanied by psychological distress, unhealthy coping behaviors (such as overeating or avoidance of physical activity), and physiological changes that increase risk for poor physical health, including cardiovascular and metabolic disease.[77] Experimental and large-scale epidemiological studies have found links between weight stigma and heightened markers of physiological stress. For example, laboratory studies that expose participants to weight stigma or that invoke a threat of being stigmatized produce dysregulated cortisol responses.[78,79] Observational studies have also found associations between perceived weight discrimination and heightened stress and inflammatory markers, which may be reflective of chronic hyperactivation of the hypothalamic-pituitary-adrenal axis that occurs in response to stress.[77,80-82] Importantly, cross-sectional and prospective data have linked weight discrimination to greater allostatic load (which is a summary score of dysregulated systems in the body that confers disease risk) and heightened risk for being diagnosed with a chronic disease, such as arteriosclerosis.[83-85] Internalized weight stigma has also been found to correlate with greater odds of having metabolic syndrome with dysregulated cortisol[86,87] and with poorer physical health–related quality of life,[53,88-90] which includes domains such as physical functioning and bodily pain. Perhaps of greatest concern, research has shown that perceived weight discrimination predicts increased risk of mortality in two separate, large-scale data sets.[91] As with other research on weight stigma and health, all of these findings remain after accounting for BMI and other mental and physical health risk factors. While more work is still needed to clearly define the mechanisms that link weight stigma to chronic disease, it is likely that a combination of psychological, behavioral, and physiological responses to the stress of stigma, combined with the undermining of socioeconomic advancement and resources, take a toll on health.

The effects of weight stigma on weight-related outcomes directly challenge the common misperception that shame and blame can motivate weight loss.[92] Several studies have shown prospective links between perceived weight discrimination and weight gain over time.[93,94] In a few clinical studies, internalized weight stigma has been associated with less weight loss and maintenance.[95-97] More work is needed to replicate these findings and to fully understand the impact of weight stigma on specific aspects of weight management, but it is clear that weight stigma adversely affects weight-related health and well-being.

Weight Bias and Stigma in Health Care

In addition to the aforementioned examples of structural stigma in health care and how it contributes to discrimination against people with overweight or obesity, negative attitudes about weight and stigmatizing practices by health care professionals further contribute to diminished quality of health care.

Bias Among Health Care Professionals

Weight-biased attitudes have been documented across health care professionals in medicine, nursing, dietetics, kinesiology, psychology, and even the fields of obesity and eating disorders.[98-103] Such attitudes can be explicit and blatant or implicit and subtle.[104] Explicit negative attitudes are captured by responses on measures of antifat bias in which health care professionals express negative feelings toward or beliefs about people with obesity, such as viewing them as unmotivated or unlikely to adhere to treatment recommendations.[104,105] Implicit bias is reflected in such outcomes as less time dedicated to patient visits and less use of patient-centered communication with patients with obesity compared to lean patients.[104] One study suggested that, among health care professionals who specialize in obesity, explicit weight bias increased over time (although implicit weight bias decreased).[103] These findings highlight that education about obesity alone is not enough to eliminate bias and that there is a continued need for health care professionals to become aware of their biases as a first step toward counteracting them.

Patient Experiences

Patients frequently report negative impressions of their weight-related interactions with health care professionals. In a study of more than 2,500 US adults with overweight or obesity, approximately 70% of participants reported experiencing weight stigma from a physician, and more than half reported that this happened more than once.[34] Weight-stigmatizing experiences include disrespectful or dismissive comments about weight (such as suggesting that weight should be easy to control); feeling negatively judged for their weight; receiving patronizing lectures about weight loss, even when the reason for the physician's visit is unrelated to weight; or having all health problems attributed to weight (eg, being told to lose weight to resolve difficulty breathing, instead of accurately diagnosing a respiratory infection).[104,106-109] These experiences are not limited to adult care: parents of children with obesity frequently report that providers communicate blame and use stigmatizing labels to describe their children's weight.[37,110] Other contributors to stigma in health care settings include routine weighing (even when the patient visit is unrelated to weight), lack of privacy for weighing, inappropriately sized equipment that cannot accommodate larger bodies (including not having high-capacity scales), and waiting rooms that are difficult for patients with larger bodies to maneuver in (eg, small chairs and narrow spaces to walk through) and that display magazines promoting thin ideals (eg, tabloids featuring headlines about "beach bodies").[24,104,106,109] Together, these structural examples of weight stigma create environments that are not inclusive and that increase discomfort in a setting in which patients may already feel anxious or vulnerable.

Weight bias and stigma directly affect care, particularly when providers do not explore underlying causes of health problems that are unrelated to weight and fail to treat these conditions.[104] These experiences also lead patients to report avoidance of health care appointments and settings. For example, in a diverse sample of 500 women† with a higher weight, 90% reported having health insurance that would cover preventive gynecological cancer screenings, yet 40% reported delaying or avoiding use of these services due to negative health care experiences related to their weight.[106] When patients avoid health care services, opportunities for preventive care or early intervention are missed, leading to progression of disease to the point in which treatment may be more difficult or prognosis worsens.[104] Feeling judged by a provider also undermines trust in health care and can lead to poorer adherence to treatment recommendations.[111] Among other mechanisms, this may, in part, explain a finding that patients who feel judged for their weight by their physician lose less weight than patients who do not perceive judgment.[112] Discussion of weight in health care is likely motivated largely by a desire among health care professionals to improve patient health; however, when these interactions are perceived as stigmatizing, such interventions can backfire and threaten patients' health and well-being.

---

† Study participants were described as women. Gender was not further specified.

Strategies for Preventing and Reducing Weight Bias and Stigma in Clinical Practice

In a survey of more than 500 members of the Obesity Action Coalition (a patient-oriented advocacy group) who identified as having overweight or obesity, 79% indicated that health care professionals should play a leading role in reducing weight stigma.[113] In addition, more than 90% of participants indicated that policy changes in health care to reduce weight stigma were of high importance, including comprehensive education and training in compassionate care for obesity.[113] The remainder of this chapter is devoted to discussing concrete actions that health care professionals can take to reduce the likelihood that patients will feel stigmatized and that the quality of their care will be diminished due to practitioner weight bias. The recommendations provided are based on those issued by such organizations as the Strategies to Overcome and Prevent (STOP) Obesity Alliance (with endorsement from 11 health care societies), the American Academy of Pediatrics, the Obesity Action Coalition, Obesity Canada, and the Rudd Center for Food Policy and Health.[37,114-116]

First, discriminatory policies in insurance coverage and in clinic practices (eg, BMI cutoffs) need to be eliminated in order to provide equitable health care to individuals with obesity. Structural weight stigma can also be addressed by ensuring that:

- all furniture and equipment is appropriately sized for patients with a higher weight;
- all patients can comfortably and safely move through the clinic;
- private spaces are available for weighing and discussing weight; and
- clinic reading materials and wall decorations promote size inclusivity and do not convey harmful messages about sociocultural body ideals, weight stereotypes, or misinformation about weight loss.

Addressing weight bias early in clinical training is also important to prevent negative attitudes from becoming more ingrained and to train the next generation of health care professionals to create more inclusive environments for patients of all sizes. Several research studies have tested strategies for reducing weight bias in trainees, including through such techniques as enhanced obesity education (such as learning about the complex etiology of obesity), interactions with standardized patients (individuals trained to portray patient scenarios for the instruction and assessment of clinical skills), watching educational videos, or receiving lesson plans about weight bias and stigma.[109,117,118] These strategies have yielded modest short-term effects on some aspects of weight bias (such as reduced belief in the controllability of weight), but reasearchers and practitioners need to do more work to determine the most effective ways to reduce negative attitudes. Perhaps more importantly, practitioners need to pay attention to ensure that negative attitudes or beliefs do not translate into behaviors that affect patient care. Weight-sensitivity trainings are routinely provided in some specialties (such as bariatrics) but may be beneficial across all realms of health care, considering the high proportion of patients with a higher weight seen by all providers. Such trainings should emphasize specific behaviors that are and are not recommended, as behaviors may be more feasible to assess and change than implicit biases.[119]

Box 3.1 on page 52 summarizes recommendations for weight-related clinical care interactions. These guidelines emphasize the importance of patient-centered care, which involves treating each patient as an individual person with unique needs (rather than making assumptions based on generalizations) and honoring patient preferences regarding how weight is addressed. Forming a collaborative relationship with patients that communicates respect and autonomy may prevent inadvertent stigmatization or patients' perceptions of judgment by providers.

In addition to these guidelines, studies have provided preliminary evidence that supports the use of psychological intervention to reduce internalized weight stigma,

BOX 3.1

Recommended Dos and Don'ts for Preventing and Reducing Weight Bias and Stigma in Clinical Practice

Do	Don't
Consider whether or not it is necessary to weigh a patient and if doing so may cause harm	Make assumptions about a patient's health or health habits based on weight alone
Ask patients for permission to weigh and to discuss weight	Give unsolicited advice to lose weight
Assess and consider metrics of health beyond weight	Attribute all health problems to weight
Ask open-ended questions about health habits	Lecture patients about their weight or accuse them of engaging in poor health habits
Use "people-first" and respectful language to describe and discuss weight	Use stigmatizing terms to describe weight (eg, *morbidly obese*)
Ask patients how their weight might affect their health and well-being	Base advice to patients on your own experience without considering how their needs or priorities may differ from yours
Listen to patients in order to better understand their weight-related experiences	Make derogatory or dismissive comments about weight or weight loss
Focus predominantly on health rather than on weight or appearance	Convey negative judgment about a patient's weight or appearance
Work collaboratively with patients to identify realistic goals and strategies for health behavior change	Assume that patients are unmotivated or do not care about their health based on their weight
Provide validation and encouragement	Discriminate in the delivery of clinical services based on weight or BMI
Ask for feedback from patients about weight-related discussions	Become defensive when given feedback about how your words or actions may have affected a patient
Set up a weight-inclusive space, including a private room for weighing and equipment that is comfortable and safe for people of all sizes	Display content in the clinic that promotes a thin ideal or derogates people with a higher body weight
Examine your own biases related to weight	Assume that you are immune to bias

delivered separately from or in combination with weight loss treatment.[120-124] Strategies such as helping patients challenge negative weight stereotypes through cognitive techniques, enhancing coping and assertiveness skills, and practicing self-compassion and acceptance may help to improve psychological and behavioral outcomes for patients who have experienced and internalized weight stigma. (Of note, patients who receive standard weight loss treatment without a targeted stigma intervention also report decreases in internalized weight stigma when treatment is delivered in a group setting and with compassionate care).[121,125-127]

It is also important to recognize that weight loss may not be appropriate or advisable for all patients with a higher weight, and insisting on weight loss without considering patients' individual needs contributes to stigmatization. For example, patients with a history of eating disorders, substantial distress related to body image, or who simply do not wish to lose weight should not be pressured to do so.

For such patients, an alternative approach to weight loss treatment that has gained increasing attention in recent years is known as "weight-neutral" care (also sometimes described as weight-inclusive or nondieting interventions),[128] with the Health at Every Size approach being the most prominent example.[129] Weight-inclusive or weight-neutral approaches promote healthy behaviors (such as nutritious eating and physical activity) for the goal of improving health and well-being without focusing on weight loss. They also strive to dispel myths related to weight, to reject sociocultural body ideals, and to increase body acceptance and self-acceptance. Within clinical settings, weight-neutral interventions have shown benefits for internalized weight stigma in some but not all studies,[125,130] along with improvements in related aspects of psychological well-being and health.[128,130-134] At the societal level, weight-inclusive messages combat weight stigma by advocating for equal access to high-quality care and the right (and ability) to be healthy and live life fully at any size.[129] Experts need more research to fully understand this approach's long-term impact on weight stigma among patients and the general public.

Ultimately, experts recommend patient-centered care to determine the appropriate treatment approach for patients based on their individual needs and health goals. Listening to patients, appreciating that different patients may benefit from different treatments, and presenting the various evidence-based options for them to choose from are all critical practices in patient-centered care. Regardless of the treatment approach, health care professionals can prevent weight stigma by focusing primarily on health and changing health behaviors (rather than on body weight, which patients cannot completely or directly control), promoting positive body image, and ensuring that all patients in their practice are treated with dignity and equal respect. Interventions designed to reduce weight stigma and promote weight inclusivity have been delivered by a range of health professionals, including those in psychology, dietetics, and nursing.[121-123,125,129] For providers who do not feel confident in their ability to address psychosocial aspects of weight, however, when a patient reports serious distress related to weight, referral to a mental health professional or a specialist in weight-inclusive care may be appropriate.

Summary

Weight bias and weight stigma are insidious in our society and appear at structural, interpersonal, and intrapersonal levels. The harms of weight bias and stigma for mental and physical health are well established and of high relevance to health care professionals. Unintentional expressions of weight bias by health care providers and perceived stigmatization among patients in health care settings can lead to avoidance of health care and exacerbate health disparities and inequities. Health care professionals must be willing to reflect on their own biases and be aware of how their words and actions may affect patients with a higher body weight. Patient-centered care is critical to ensuring that the treatment approach meets the patient's needs and does not cause harm. Health care professionals also have a responsibility to advocate for their patients to ensure equal treatment and access to high-quality health care for people of all sizes.

References

1. Puhl R, Brownell KD. Bias, discrimination, and obesity. *Obes Res*. 2001;9(12):788-805. doi:10.1038/oby.2001.108
2. Crandall CS. Prejudice against fat people: ideology and self-interest. *J Pers Soc Psychol*. 1994;66(5):882-894. doi:10.1037//0022-3514.66.5.882

3. Puhl RM, Brownell KD. Psychosocial origins of obesity stigma: toward changing a powerful and pervasive bias. *Obes Rev*. 2003;4(4):213-227. doi:10.1046/j.1467-789x.2003.00122.x
4. McFerran B, Mukhopadhyay A. Lay theories of obesity predict actual body mass. *Psychol Sci*. 2013;24(8):1428-1436. doi:10.1177/0956797612473121
5. von dem Knesebeck O, Ludecke D, Luck-Sikorski C, Kim TJ. Public beliefs about causes of obesity in the USA and in Germany. *Int J Public Health*. 2019;64:1139-1146. doi:10.1007/s00038-019-01295-0
6. Brownell KD, Kersh R, Ludwig DS, et al. Personal responsibility and obesity: a constructive approach to a controversial issue. *Health Aff (Millwood)*. 2010;29(3):378-386. doi:10.1377/hlthaff.2009.0739
7. Crandall CS, Reser AH. Attributions and weight-based prejudices. In: Brownell KD, Puhl RM, Schwartz MB, Rudd L, eds. *Weight Bias: Nature, Consequences, and Remedies*. Guilford Press; 2005:83-96.
8. Goffman E. *Stigma: Notes on the Management of a Spoiled Identity*. Prentice Hall; 1963.
9. Link BG, Phelan JC. Conceptualizing stigma. *Annu Rev Sociol*. 2001;27:363-385.
10. Puhl RM, Heuer CA. The stigma of obesity: a review and update. *Obesity*. 2009;17(5):941-964. doi:10.1038/oby.2008.636
11. Cook JE, Purdie-Vaughns V, Meyer IH, Busch JTA. Intervening within and across levels: a multilevel approach to stigma and public health. *Soc Sci Med*. 2014;103:101-109. doi:10.1016/j.socscimed.2013.09.023
12. Smart Richman L, Hatzenbuehler ML. A multilevel analysis of stigma and health: implications for research and policy. *Policy Insights Behav Brain Sci*. 2014;1(1):213-221. doi:10.1177/2372732214548862
13. Ata RN, Thompson JK. Weight bias in the media: a review of recent research. *Obes Facts*. 2010;3:41-46. doi:10.1159/000276547
14. Heuer CA, McClure KJ, Puhl RM. Obesity stigma in online news: a visual content analysis. *J Health Commun*. 2011;16(9):976-987. doi:10.1080/10810730.2011.561915
15. Puhl RM, Peterson JL, DePierre JA, Luedicke J. Headless, hungry, and unhealthy: a video content analysis of obese persons portrayed in online news. *J Health Commun*. 2013;18(6):686-702. doi:10.1080/10810730.2012.743631
16. Frederick DA, Saguy AC, Sandhu G, Mann T. Effects of competing news media frames of weight on antifat stigma, beliefs about weight and support for obesity-related public policies. *Int J Obes*. 2016;40(3):543-549. doi:10.1038/ijo.2015.195
17. Pearl RL, Puhl RM, Brownell KD. Positive media portrayals of obese persons: impact on attitudes and image preferences. *Health Psychol*. 2012;31(6):821-829. doi:10.1037/a0027189
18. Yoo JH, Kim J. Obesity in the news media: a content analysis of obesity videos on YouTube. *Health Commun*. 2011;27(1):86-97. doi:10.1080/10410236.2011.569003
19. Chou WS, Prestin A, Kunath S. Obesity in social media: a mixed methods analysis. *Transl Behav Med*. 2014;4(3):314-323. doi:10.1007/s13142-014-0256-1
20. Pearl RL. Weight stigma and the "quarantine-15." *Obesity*. 2020;28(7):1180-1181. doi:10.1002//oby.22850
21. Wells G, Horwitz J, Seetharaman D. Facebook knows Instagram is toxic for teen girls, company documents show. *Wall Street Journal*. September 14, 2021. Accessed November 12, 2021. www.wsj.com/articles/facebook-knows-instagram-is-toxic-for-teen-girls-company-documents-show-11631620739
22. Pomeranz JL, Puhl RM. New developments in the law for obesity discrimination protection. *Obesity*. 2013;21(3):469-471. doi:10.1002/oby.20094
23. Puhl RM, Lessard LM, Pearl RL, Grupski A, Foster GD. Policies to address weight discrimination and bullying: perspectives of adults engaged in weight management from six nations. *Obesity*. 2021;29(11):1787-1798. doi:10.1002/oby.23275
24. Pearl RL. Weight bias and stigma: public health implications and structural solutions. *Soc Issues Policy Rev*. 2018;12(1):146-182. doi:10.1111/sipr.12043
25. Hatzenbuehler ML, Flores JE, Cavanaugh JE, Onwuachi-Willig A, Ramirez MR. Anti-bullying policies and disparities in bullying: a state-level analysis. *Am J Prev Med*. 2017;53(2):184-191. doi:10.1016/j.amepre.2017.02.004
26. Bombak AE, McPhail D, Ward P. Reproducing stigma: interpreting "overweight" and "obese" women's experiences of weight-based discrimination in reproductive healthcare. *Soc Sci Med*. 2016;166:94-101. doi:10.1016/j.socscimed.2016.08.015
27. Brochu PM, Pearl RL, Puhl RM, Brownell KD. Do media portrayals of obesity influence support for weight-related medical policy? *Health Psychol*. 2014;33(2):197-200. doi:10.1037/a0032592
28. Sole-Smith V. When You're Told You're Too Fat to Get Pregnant. *New York Times*. 2019. Accessed November 12, 2021. www.nytimes.com/2019/06/18/magazine/fertility-weight-obesity-ivf.html
29. Lui M, Jones CA, Westby MD. Effect of non-surgical, non-pharmacological weight loss interventions in patients who are obese prior to hip and knee arthroplasty surgery: a rapid review. *Syst Rev*. 2015;4:121. doi:10.1186/s13643-015-0107-2
30. Tewksbury C, Williams NN, Dumon KR, Sarwer DB. Preoperative medical weight management in bariatric surgery: a review and reconsideration. *Obes Surg*. 2017;27(1):208-214. doi:10.1007/s11695-016-2422-7
31. Pillutla V, Maslen H, Savulescu J. Rationing elective surgery for smokers and obese patients: responsibility or prognosis? *BMC Med Ethics*. 2018;19(1):28. doi:10.1186/s12910-018-0272-7
32. Wilson ER, Kyle TK, Nadglowski JF, Stanford FC. Obesity coverage gap: consumers perceive low coverage for obesity treatments even when workplace wellness programs target BMI. *Obesity*. 2017;25(2):370-377. doi:10.1002/oby.21746

33. Yang YT, Pomeranz JL. States variations in the provision of bariatric surgery under affordable care act exchanges. *Surg Obes Relat Disord*. 2015;11(3):715-720. doi:10.1016/j.soard.2014.09.014
34. Puhl RM, Brownell KD. Confronting and coping with weight stigma: an investigation of overweight and obese adults. *Obesity*. 2006;14(10):1802-1815. doi:10.1038/oby.2006.208
35. Puhl RM, Latner JD. Stigma, obesity, and the health of the nation's children. *Psychol Bull*. 2007;133(4):557-580. doi:10.1037/0033-2909.133.4.557
36. Puhl RM, Lessard LM. Weight stigma in youth: prevalence, consequences, and considerations for clinical practice. *Curr Obes Rep*. 2020;9(4):402-411. doi:10.1007/s13679-020-00408-8
37. Pont SJ, Puhl R, Cook SR, Slusser W; Section on Obesity; Obesity Society. Stigma experienced by children and adolescents with obesity. *Pediatrics*. 2017;140(6):e20173034. doi:10.1542/peds.2017-3034
38. Rupp K, McCoy SM. Bullying perpetration and victimization among adolescents with overweight and obesity in a nationally representative sample. *Child Obes*. 2019;15(5):323-330. doi:10.1089/chi.2018.0233
39. Bucchianeri MM, Eisenberg ME, Wall MM, Piran N, Neumark-Sztainer D. Multiple types of harassment: associations with emotional well-being and unhealthy behaviors in adolescents. *J Adolesc Health*. 2014;54(6):724-729. doi:10.1016/j.jadohealth.2013.10.205
40. Spahlholz J, Baer N, Konig HH, Riedel-Heller S, Luck-Sikorski C. Obesity and discrimination—a systematic review and meta-analysis of observational studies. *Obes Rev*. 2016;17(1):43-55. doi:10.1111/obr.12343
41. Puhl RM, Andreyeva T, Brownell KD. Perceptions of weight discrimination: prevalence and comparison to race and gender discrimination in America. *Int J Obes*. 2008;32(6):992-1000. doi:10.1038/ijo.2008.22
42. Pearl RL, Wadden TA, Tronieri JS, Chao AM, Alamuddin N, Berkowitz RI. Everyday discrimination in a racially diverse sample of patients with obesity. *Clin Obes*. 2018;8(2):140-146. doi:10.1111/cob.12235
43. Baum CL, Ford WF. The wage effects of obesity: a longitudinal study. *Health Econ*. 2004;13(9):885-899. doi:10.1002/hec.881
44. Pinkston JC. The dynamic effects of obesity on the wages of young workers. *Econ Hum Biol*. 2017;27 (Pt A):154-166. doi:10.1016/j.ehb.2017.05.006
45. Shinall, Jennifer Bennett, Occupational Characteristics and the Obesity Wage Penalty (October 7, 2015). Vanderbilt Law and Economics Research Paper No. 16-12, Vanderbilt Public Law Research Paper No. 16-23. doi:10.2139/ssrn.2379575
46. Huang CY, Chen DR. Association of weight change patterns in late adolescence with young adult wage differentials: a longitudinal study. *PLos ONE*. 2019;14(7):e20219123. doi:10.1371/journal.pone.0219123
47. Roehling MV, Choi MG, Roehling PV. Weight discrimination in the workplace. In: Stone DL, Dulebohn JH, eds. *The Only Constant in HRM Today Is Change: Research in Human Resource Management*. Information Age Publishing; 2019:97-137.
48. Flint SW, Cadek M, Codreanu SC, Ivic V, Zomer C, Gomoiu A. Obesity discrimination in the recruitment process: "You're not hired!" *Front Psychol*. 2016;7:647. doi:10.3389/fpsyg.2017.00647
49. Hunger JM, Major B, Blodorn A, Miller CT. Weighed down by stigma: how weight-based social identity threat contributes to weight gain and poor health. *Soc Personal Psychol Compass*. 2015;9(6):255-268. doi:10.1111/spc3.12172
50. Durso LE, Latner JD. Understanding self-directed stigma: development of the Weight Bias Internalization Scale. *Obesity*. 2008;16:S80-S86. doi:10.1038/oby.2008.448
51. Corrigan PW, Larson JE, Rusch N. Self-stigma and the "why try" effect: impact on life goals and evidence-based practices. *World Psychiatry*. 2009;8(2):75-81. doi:10.1002/j.2051-5545.2009.tb00218.x
52. Corrigan PW, Watson AC, Barr L. The self-stigma of mental illness: implications for self-esteem and self-efficacy. *J Soc Clin Psychol*. 2006;25(9):875-884. doi:10.1521/jscp.2006.25.8.875
53. Pearl RL, Puhl RM. Weight bias internalization and health: a systematic review. *Obes Rev*. 2018;19(8):1141-1163. doi:10.1111/obr.12701
54. Crosnoe R. Gender, obesity, and education. *Sociol Educ*. 2007;80:241-260. doi:10.1177/0038040707080003
55. Zavodny M. Does weight affect children's test scores and teacher assessments differently? *Econ Educ Rev*. 2013;34:135-145. doi:10.1016/j.econedurev.2013.02.003
56. Kenney EL, Gortmaker SL, Davison KK, Austin SB. The academic penalty for gaining weight: a longitudinal change-in-change analysis of BMI and perceived academic ability in middle school students. *Int J Obes*. 2015;39:1408-1413. doi:10.1038/ijo.2015.88
57. Puhl RM, Luedicke J. Weight-based victimization among adolescents in the school setting: emotional reactions and coping behaviors. *J Youth Adolesc*. 2012;41(1):27-40. doi:10.1007/s10964-011-9713-z
58. Krukowski RA, West DS, Perez AP, Bursac Z, Phillips MM, Raczynski JM. Overweight children, weight-based teasing and academic performance. *Int J Pediatr Obes*. 2009;4(4):274-280. doi:10.3109/17477160902846203
59. Burmeister JM, Kiefner AE, Carels RA, Musher-Eizenman D. Weight bias in graduate school admissions. *Obesity*. 2013;21:918-920. doi:10.1002/oby.20171
60. Healthy People 2030: social determinants of health. US Department of Health and Human Services website. Accessed November 12, 2021. https://health.gov/healthypeople/objectives-and-data/social-determinants-health
61. Hatzenbuehler ML, Phelan JC, Link BG. Stigma as a fundamental cause of population health disparities. *Am J Public Health*. 2013;103(5):813-821. doi:10.2105/AJPH.2012.301069

62. Hatzenbuehler ML, Keyes KM, Hasin DS. Associations between perceived weight discrimination and prevalence of psychiatric disorders in the general population. *Obesity*. 2009;17(11):2033-2039. doi:10.1038/oby.2009.131

63. Papadopoulos S, Brennan L. Correlates of weight stigma in adults with overweight and obesity: a systematic literature review. *Obesity*. 2015;23(9):1743-1760. doi:10.1002/oby.21187

64. Haines J, Neumark-Sztainer D, Eisenberg ME, Hannan PJ. Weight teasing and disordered eating behaviors in adolescents: longitudinal findings from Project EAT (Eating Among Teens). *Pediatrics*. 2006;117(2):e209-e215. doi:10.1542/peds.2005-1242

65. Pearl RL, Puhl RM, Himmelstein MS, Pinto AM, Foster GD. Weight stigma and weight-related health: associations of self-report measures among adults in weight management. *Ann Behav Med*. 2020;54(11):904-914. doi:10.1093/abm/kaaa026

66. Latner JD, Barile JP, Durso LE, O'Brien KS. Weight and health-related quality of life: the moderating role of weight discrimination and internalized weight bias. *Eat Behav*. 2014;15(4):586-590. doi:10.1016/j.eatbeh.2014.08.014

67. O'Brien KS, Latner JD, Puhl RM, et al. The relationship between weight stigma and eating behavior is explained by weight bias internalization and psychological distress. *Appetite*. 2016;102:70-76. doi:10.1016/j.appet.2016.02.032

68. Pearl RL, Puhl RM, Lessard LM, Himmelstein MS, Foster GD. Prevalence and correlates of weight bias internalization in weight management: a multinational study. *Soc Sci Med Popul Health*. 2021;13:100755. doi:10.1016/j.ssmph.2021.100755

69. Hunger JM, Major B. Weight stigma mediates the association between BMI and self-reported health. *Health Psychol*. 2015;34(2):172-175. doi:10.1037/hea0000106

70. Vartanian LR, Porter AM. Weight stigma and eating behavior: a review of the literature. *Appetite*. 2016;102:3-14. doi:10.1016/j.appet.2016.01.034

71. Schvey NA, Puhl RM, Brownell KD. The impact of weight stigma on caloric consumption. *Obesity*. 2011;19(10):1957-1962. doi:10.1038/oby.2011.204

72. Major B, Hunger JM, Bunyan DP, Miller CT. The ironic effects of weight stigma. *J Exp Soc Psychol*. 2014;51:74-80. doi:10.1016/j.jesp.2013.11.009

73. Pearl RL, Wadden TA, Jakicic JM. Is weight stigma associated with physical activity? A systematic review. *Obesity*. 2021;29(12):1994-2012. doi:10.1002/oby.23274

74. Pearl RL, Puhl RM, Dovidio JF. Differential effects of weight bias experiences and internalization on exercise among women with overweight and obesity. *J Health Psychol*. 2015;20(12):1626-1632. doi:10.1177/1359105313520338

75. Vartanian LR, Novak SA. Internalized societal attitudes moderate the impact of weight stigma on avoidance of exercise. *Obesity*. 2011;19(4):757-762. doi:10.1038/oby.2010.234

76. Vartanian LR, Shaprow JG. Effects of weight stigma on exercise motivation and behavior: a preliminary investigation among college-aged females. *J Health Psychol*. 2008;13(1):131-138. doi:10.1177/1359105307084318

77. Tomiyama AJ. Weight stigma is stressful: a review of evidence for the Cyclic Obesity/Weight-Based Stigma model. *Appetite*. 2014;82:8-15. doi:10.1016/j.appet.2014.06.108

78. Schvey NA, Puhl RM, Brownell KD. The stress of stigma: exploring the effects of weight stigma on cortisol reactivity. *Psychosom Med*. 2014;76(2):156-162. doi:10.1097/PSY.0000000000000031

79. Himmelstein MS, Belsky ACI, Tomiyama AJ. The weight of stigma: cortisol reactivity to manipulated weight stigma. *Obesity*. 2015;23(2):368-374. doi:10.1002/oby.20959

80. Jackson SE, Kirschbaum C, Steptoe A. Perceived weight discrimination and chronic biochemical stress: a population-based study using cortisol in scalp hair. *Obesity*. 2016;24(12):2515-2521. doi:10.1002/oby.21657

81. Tomiyama AJ, Epel ES, McClatchey TM, et al. Associations of weight stigma with cortisol and oxidative stress independent of adiposity. *Health Psychol*. 2014;33(8):862-867. doi:10.1037/hea0000107

82. Sutin AR, Stephan Y, Luchetti M, Terracciano A. Perceived weight discrimination and C-reactive protein. *Obesity*. 2014;22(9):1959-1961. doi:10.1002/oby.20789

83. Vadiveloo M, Mattei J. Perceived weight discrimination and 10-year risk of allostatic load among US adults. *Ann Behav Med*. 2017;51(1):94-104. doi:10.1007/s12160-016-9831-7

84. Udo T, Purcell K, Grilo CM. Perceived weight discrimination and chronic medical conditions in adults with overweight and obesity. *Int J Clin Pract*. 2016;70:1003-1011. doi:10.1111/ijcp.12902

85. Udo T, Grilo CM. Cardiovascular disease and perceived weight, race, and gender discrimination in US adults. *J Psychosom Res*. 2017;100:82-88. doi:10.1016/j.jpsychores.2017.07.007

86. Pearl RL, Wadden TA, Hopkins CM, et al. Association between weight bias internalization and metabolic syndrome among treatment-seeking individuals with obesity. *Obesity*. 2017;25(2):317-322. doi:10.1002/oby.21716

87. Jung FU, Bae YJ, Kratzsch J, Riedel-Heller SG, Luck-Sikorski C. Internalized weight bias and cortisol reactivity in social stress. *Cogn Affect Behav Neurosci*. 2020;20(1):49-58. doi:10.3758/s13415-019-00750-y

88. Pearl RL, White MA, Grilo CM. Weight bias internalization, depression, and self-reported health among overweight binge eating disorder patients. *Obesity*. 2014;22(5):E142-E148. doi:10.1002/oby.20617

89. Olson KL, Landers JD, Thaxton TT, Emery CF. The pain of weight-related stigma among women with overweight or obesity. *Stigma Health*. 2019;4(3):243-246. doi:10.1037/sah0000137

90. Walsh OA, Wadden TA, Tronieri JS, Chao AM, Pearl RL. Weight bias internalization is negatively associated with weight-related quality of life in persons seeking weight loss. *Front Psychol*. 2018;9:2576. doi:10.3389/fpsyg.2018.02576
91. Sutin AR, Stephan Y, Terracciano A. Weight discrimination and risk of mortality. *Psychol Sci*. 2015;26(11):1803-1811. doi:10.1177/0956797615601103
92. Callahan D. Obesity: Chasing an elusive epidemic. *Hastings Cent Rep*. 2013;43(1):34-40. doi:10.1002/hast.114
93. Sutin AR, Terracciano A. Perceived weight discrimination and obesity. *PLos ONE*. 2013;8(7). doi:10.1371/journal.pone.0070048
94. Jackson SE, Beeken RJ, Wardle J. Perceived weight discrimination and changes in weight, waist circumference, and weight status. *Obesity*. 2014;22:2485-2488. doi:10.1002/oby.20891
95. Pearl RL, Wadden TA, Chao AM, et al. Association between causal attributions for obesity and long-term weight loss. *Behav Med*. 2020;46(2):87-91. doi:10.1080/08964289.2018.1556202
96. Olson KL, Lillis J, Thomas JG, Wing RR. Prospective evaluation of internalized weight bias and weight change among successful weight-loss maintainers. *Obesity*. 2018;26(12):1888-1892. doi:10.1002/oby.22283
97. Puhl RM, Quinn DM, Weisz BM, Suh YJ. The role of stigma in weight loss maintenance among U.S. adults. *Ann Behav Med*. 2017;51(5):754-763. doi:10.1007/s12160-017-9898-9
98. Budd GM, Mariotti M, Graff D, Falkenstein K. Health care professionals' attitudes about obesity: an integrative review. *Appl Nurs Res*. 2011;24(3):127-137. doi:10.1016/j.apnr.2009.05.001
99. Davis-Coelho K, Waltz J, Davis-Coelho B. Awareness and prevention of bias against fat clients in psychotherapy. *Prof Psychol Res Pract*. 2000;31(6):682-684. doi:10.1037/0735-7028.31.6.682
100. Phelan SM, Dovidio JF, Puhl RM, et al. Implicit and explicit weight bias in a national sample of 4732 medical students: the medical student CHANGES study. *Obesity*. 2014;22(4):1201-1208. doi:10.1002/oby.20687
101. Puhl RM, Latner JD, King KM, Luedicke J. Weight bias among professionals treating eating disorders: attitudes about treatment and perceived patient outcomes. *Int J Eat Disord*. 2014;47(1):65-75. doi:10.1002/eat.22186
102. Swift JA, Hanlon S, El-Redy L, Puhl RM, Glazebrook C. Weight bias among UK trainee dietitians, doctors, nurses, and nutritionists. *J Hum Nutr Diet*. 2013;26(4):395-402. doi:10.1111/jhn.12019
103. Tomiyama AJ, Finch LE, Belsky AC, et al. Weight bias in 2001 versus 2013: contradictor attitudes among researchers and health professionals. *Obesity*. 2015;23(1):46-53. doi:10.1002/oby.20910
104. Phelan SM, Burgess DJ, Yeazel MW, Hellerstedt WL, Griffin JM, Ryn M. Impact of weight bias and stigma on quality of care and outcomes for patients with obesity. *Obes Rev*. 2015;16(4):319-326. doi:10.1111/obr.12266
105. Puhl RM, Phelan SM, Nadglowski J, Kyle TK. Overcoming weight bias in the management of patients with diabetes and obesity. *Clin Diabetes*. 2016;34(1):44-50. doi:10.2337/diaclin.34.1.44
106. Amy NK, Aalborg A, Lyons P, Keranen L. Barriers to routine gynecological cancer screenings for White and African-American obese women. *Int J Obes*. 2006;30:147-155. doi:10.1038/sj.ijo.0803105
107. Drury CAA, Louis M. Exploring the association between body weight, stigma of obesity, and health care avoidance. *J Am Acad Nurse Pract*. 2002;14(12):554-561. doi:10.1111/j.1745-7599.2002.tb00089.x
108. Mensinger JL, Tylka TL, Calamari ME. Mechanisms underlying weight status and healthcare avoidance in women: a study of weight stigma, body-related shame and guilt, and healthcare stress. *Body Image*. 2018;25:139-147. doi:10.1016/j.bodyim.2018.03.001
109. Alberga AS, Edache IY, Forhan M, Russell-Mayhew S. Weight bias and health care utilization: a scoping review. *Prim Health Care Res Dev*. 2019;20:e116. doi:10.1017/S1463423619000227
110. Puhl RM, Peterson JL, Luedicke J. Parental perceptions of weight terminology that providers use with youth. *Pediatrics*. 2011;128(4):786. doi:10.1542/peds.2010-3841
111. Gudzune KA, Bennett WL, Cooper LA, Bleich SN. Patients who feel judged about their weight have lower trust in their primary care providers. *Patient Educ Couns*. 2014;97:128-131. doi:10.1016/j.pec.2014.06.019
112. Gudzune KA, Bennett WL, Cooper LA, Bleich SN. Perceived judgment about weight can negatively influence weight loss: a cross-sectional study of overweight and obese patients. *Prev Med*. 2014;62:103-107. doi:10.1016/j.ypmed.2014.02.001
113. Puhl RM, Himmelstein MS, Gorin AA, Suh YJ. Missing the target: including perspectives of women with overweight and obesity to inform stigma-reduction strategies. *Obes Sci Pract*. 2017;3(1):25-35. doi:10.1002/osp4.101
114. Strategies to Overcome and Prevent (STOP) Obesity Alliance. *Weight Can't Wait: Guide for the Management of Obesity in the Primary Care Setting*. STOP Obesity Alliance; October 2020. Accessed November 12, 2021. https://stop.publichealth.gwu.edu/sites/g/files/zaxdzs4356/files/2022-02/wcw-guide-for-the-management-of-obesity-in-the-primary-care-setting.pdf
115. Canadian adult obesity clinical practice guidelines. Obesity Canada website. 2020. Accessed November 12, 2021. https://obesitycanada.ca/guidelines
116. Healthcare providers: informational handouts and resources. UConn Rudd Center for Food Policy and Health website. Accessed November 21, 2021. https://uconnruddcenter.org/research/weight-bias-stigma/healthcare-providers
117. Kushner RF, Zeiss DM, Feinglass JM, Yelen M. An obesity educational intervention for medical students addressing weight bias and communication skills using standardized patients. *BMC Med Educ*. 2014;14(1):53. doi:10.1186/1472-6920-14-53

118. Oliver TL, Qi BB, Shenkman R, Diewald L, Smeltzer SC. Weight sensitivity training among undergraduate nursing students. *J Nurs Educ*. 2020;59(8):453-456. doi:10.3928/01484834-20200723-06
119. Hagiwara N, Dovidio JF, Stone J, Penner LA. Applied research/ethnic healthcare disparities research using implicit measures. *Soc Cogn*. 2020;38:S68-S97. doi:10.1521/soco.2020.38.supp.s68
120. Pearl RL, Hopkins CM, Berkowitz RI, Wadden TA. Group cognitive-behavioral treatment for internalized weight stigma: a pilot study. *Eat Weight Disord*. 2018;23(3):357-362. doi:10.1007/s40519-016-0336-y
121. Pearl RL, Wadden TA, Bach C, et al. Effects of a cognitive-behavioral intervention targeting weight stigma: a randomized controlled trial. *J Consult Clin Psychol*. 2020;88(5):470-480. doi:10.1037/ccp0000480
122. Levin ME, Potts S, Haeger J, Lillis J. Delivering acceptance and commitment therapy for weight self-stigma through guided self-help: results from an open pilot trial. *Cogn Behav Pract*. 2018;25(1):87-104. doi:10.1016/j.cbpra/2017.02.002
123. Palmeira L, Pinto-Gouveia J, Cunha M. Exploring the efficacy of an acceptance, mindfulness and compassionate-based group intervention for women struggling with their weight (Kg-Free): a randomized controlled trial. *Appetite*. 2017;112:107-116. doi:10.1016/j.appet.2017.01.027
124. Davies AE, Burnette CB, Ravyts SG, Mazzeo SE. A randomized control trial of Expand Your Horizon: an intervention for women with weight bias internalization. *Body Image*. 2022;40:138-145. doi:10.1016/j.bodyim.2021.12.006
125. Mensinger JL, Calogero RM, Tylka TL. Internalized weight stigma moderates eating behavior outcomes in women with high BMI participating in a healthy living program. *Appetite*. 2016;102:32-43. doi:10.1016/j.appet.2016.01.033
126. Pearl RL, Wadden TA, Bach C, Tronieri JS, Berkowitz RI. Six-month follow-up from a randomized controlled trial of the Weight BIAS Program. *Obesity*. 2020;28(10):1878-1888. doi:10.1002/oby.22931
127. Pearl RL, Wadden TA, Chao AM, et al. Weight bias internalization and long-term weight loss in patients with obesity. *Ann Behav Med*. 2019;53(8):782-787. doi:10.1093/abm/kay084
128. Tylka TL, Annunziato RA, Burgard D, et al. The weight-inclusive versus weight-normative approach to health: evaluating the evidence for prioritizing well-being over weight loss. *J Obes*. 2014;2014:983495. doi:10.1155/2014/983495
129. HAES [Health at Every Size] principles. Association for Size Diversity and Health website. Last updated 2013. Accessed November 12, 2021. www.sizediversityandhealth.org/health-at-every-size-haes-approach
130. O'Hara L, Ahmed H, Elashie S. Evaluating the impact of a brief Health at Every Size-informed health promotion activity on body positivity and internalized weight-based oppression. *Body Image*. 2021;37:225-237. doi:10.1016/j.bodyim.2021.02.006
131. King C. Health at Every Size approach to health management: the evidence is weighed. *Top Clin Nutr*. 2007;22(3):272-285. doi:10.1097/01.TIN.0000285381.24089.84
132. Mensinger JL, Calogero RM, Stranges S, Tylka TL. A weight-neutral versus weight-loss approach for health promotion in women with high BMI: a randomized-controlled trial. *Appetite*. 2016;105:364-374. doi:10.1016/j.appet.2016.06.006
133. Clifford D, Ozier A, Bundros J, Moore J, Kreiser A, Morris AN. Impact of non-diet approaches on attitudes, behaviors, and health outcomes: a systematic review. *J Nutr Educ Behav*. 2015;47(2):143-155. doi:10.1016/j.jneb.2014.12.002
134. Wilson RE, Marshall RD, Murakami JM, Latner JD. Brief non-dieting intervention increases intuitive eating and reduces dieting intention, body image dissatisfaction, and anti-fat attitudes: a randomized controlled trial. *Appetite*. 2020;148:104556. doi:10.1016/j.appet.2019.104556

CHAPTER 4

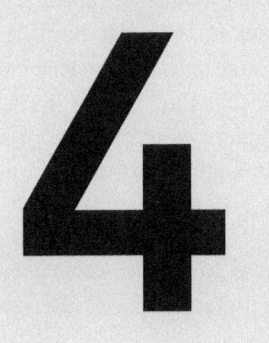

Evidence-Based Guidelines for Treatment of Overweight and Obesity

Hollie A. Raynor, PhD, RD, LDN

CHAPTER OBJECTIVES

- Define evidence-based guidelines and their use in practice.
- Review the commonly used evidence-based guidelines for the treatment of overweight and obesity.
- Outline online resources for evidence-based guidelines for the treatment of overweight and obesity.

Introduction

Applying evidence from research studies to clinical practice is essential for achieving evidence-based practice. To engage in evidence-based practice is to combine graded recommendations developed from systematic literature reviews with individual patient or client values and preferences to inform care. This approach, which integrates a patient- or client-centered focus with research, is believed to result in optimal health care.[1] This chapter provides an overview of the history of evidence-based practice, defines how graded recommendations and evidence-based guidelines are developed, explains how guidelines are to be used in evidence-based practice, and reviews commonly used evidence-based guidelines for the treatment of adult overweight and obesity.

The History of Evidence-Based Practice

Evidence-based practice has its roots in the concept of evidence-based medicine. In 1992, the idea of examining clinical research to assist with clinical decision-making was introduced as "evidence-based medicine."[2] At this time, researchers were changing methodological designs used for clinical research and placing greater emphasis on the randomized clinical trial and the ability to infer causation from the results of such trials. Furthermore, researchers developed the capacity to conduct meta-analyses, in which the outcomes of multiple studies using similar study designs were statistically analyzed to draw conclusions.[3] When evidence-based medicine was introduced, experts acknowledged that there could be some challenges with its implementation. Specifically, they noted that practitioners would need to have the skills to critically evaluate methodologically rigorous research, have access to all available scientific literature, and have the time to review it in order to draw appropriate conclusions.[2]

To address these implementation challenges, the Institute of Medicine (now the National Academy of Medicine), at the request of the US Congress, established standardized procedures by which evidence-based guidelines could be developed from research literature.[4] These procedures, now widely used by many health care-focused professional organizations to develop evidence-based guidelines, are based on eight standards (summarized in Box 4.1).[3,4] Evidence-based guidelines provide practitioners with graded recommendations in the areas of assessment, diagnosis, and treatment. The graded recommendations summarize critically evaluated scientific literature and are designed so that they can be immediately implemented in practice. Thus, evidence-based guidelines reduce the previously identified barriers to implementing evidence-based medicine effectively.[3]

Developing Evidence-Based Guidelines

Creating graded recommendations for evidence-based guidelines involves utilizing the skills of content and methodology experts and implementing a clearly defined, reproducible process.

Development of Clinical Questions

Once experts have been identified to form a guideline development group (which should also include a current or former patient or patient advocate[4]), they work to develop appropriate clinical questions for the guideline. These questions often follow a population, intervention, comparison intervention, and outcome (PICO) format.[1,5] This format helps establish the study eligibility criteria to be used in the systematic literature search for each clinical question. How the four areas of the PICO format are defined for each clinical question determines the specificity of the recommendations that are ultimately developed.[1] For example, if the population defined in the question is adults with obesity rather than adults with overweight, the final recommendation may not be generalizable to adults with overweight. However, if the population is defined as adults with overweight and obesity, the recommendation will be generalizable to both groups. Due to time and resource constraints, not all questions developed by the guideline development group may be addressed (the constraints are often established by the organization supporting

---

BOX 4.1

Standards from the Institute of Medicine for Developing Trustworthy Clinical Practice Guidelines[a,3,4]

Standard 1: Establishing transparency

The processes of guideline development and funding should be detailed explicitly and made publicly accessible.

Standard 2: Management of conflict of interest (COI)

Prior to selection of the guideline development group, individuals being considered for membership should declare all interests and activities potentially resulting in a COI with development group activity, by written disclosure.

All COIs of members should be discussed by the prospective guideline development group.

Members should divest of financial investments affected by recommendations.

When possible, members should not have COIs (ie, chair of the development group should have no COIs; funders should have no role in the group).

Box continues

BOX 4.1 (CONTINUED)

Standard 3: Guideline development group composition

The guideline development group should be multidisciplinary and include a variety of methodological experts, clinicians, and representatives of populations expected to be affected by guidelines.

Patient and public involvement should be facilitated by including a current or former patient and a patient advocate or patient organization representative in the group.

Strategies to increase effective participation of patient representatives, including training in appraisal of evidence, should be adopted.

Standard 4: Clinical practice guideline–systematic review intersection

The development group should use systematic reviews that meet standards set by the Institute of Medicine's Committee on Standards for Systematic Reviews of Comparative Effectiveness Research.

When systematic reviews are conducted specifically to inform particular guidelines, the development group and systematic review team should interact regarding the scope, approach, and output of both processes.

Standard 5: Establishing evidence foundations for and rating strength of recommendations

For each guideline recommendation, the following should be provided:
- an explanation of the reasoning underlying the recommendation (ie, benefits; harms; summary of evidence; description of the quality, quantity, and consistency of evidence; description of values, opinion, theory, and clinical experience that are part of the recommendation)
- a rating of certainty regarding the evidence underpinning the recommendation
- a rating of the strength of the recommendation
- a description and explanation of any differences of opinion regarding the recommendation

Standard 6: Articulation of recommendations

Recommendations should be communicated in a standardized form with detail regarding what the recommended action is and when it should occur.

Strong recommendations should be worded so that compliance can be evaluated.

Standard 7: External review

External reviewers should comprise a spectrum of relevant stakeholders.

External reviews submitted should be kept confidential unless that protection has been waived.

The guideline development group should consider all external reviewer comments and keep a written record of the rationale for modifying or not modifying a guideline in response to comments.

A draft of the guideline at the external review stage, or immediately following it, should be made available to the general public for comment.

Standard 8: Updating

The guideline publication date, date of pertinent systematic evidence review, and proposed date for future guideline review should be documented.

Literature should be monitored to identify new, potentially relevant evidence and evaluate the continued validity of the guideline.

Guidelines should be updated when new evidence suggests the need for modification.

[a] The Institute of Medicine is now the National Academy of Medicine.
Adapted with permission from Graham R, Mancher M, Miller Wolman D, Greenfield S, Steinberg E, eds. Clinical Practice Guidelines We Can Trust. National Academies Press; 2011.[4]

the development of the guidelines). For this reason, the questions developed are often prioritized by their importance to clinical practice, potential influence on patients, potential impact on health care costs, potential ability to reduce controversy or confusion, and whether enough new research exists.[5]

Systematic Literature Search

The guideline development group then creates a plan to systematically search the literature relevant to each question.[1,5] This plan lays out the eligibility and ineligibility criteria for the type of studies to include for each question. These criteria often stipulate the type of study design to be included in each literature search, which strongly influences the quality of the literature included for each question. Common eligibility criteria for systematic searches used in developing evidence-based guidelines are that the studies included must be peer-reviewed and published in English and that they must be human studies (meaning molecular, cellular, and animal research studies are not included).[5] Each search is usually conducted by trained methodology experts using a comprehensive search strategy. The process of each literature search is reported in detail so that it can be reproduced if needed. Databases used in searches are described and may include MEDLINE (from the National Library of Medicine), Embase, the Cochrane Library, and the Cumulative Index to Nursing and Allied Health Literature.[1,5] The guideline development group reviews the results of each search to ensure that only studies meeting the eligibility criteria are included. When articles are excluded, documentation must outline the reason for exclusion and at what point the exclusion occurred during the review process. This documentation usually follows the Preferred Reporting Items for Systematic Reviews and Meta-Analyses, or PRISMA, flow chart for each search.[6]

Literature Assessment and Summary of Results

Following a search, the guideline development group assesses all included articles for study execution and methodologic quality, mainly to assess for scientific rigor and validity.[5] Then, the results of the included studies are briefly summarized, combining relevant and valid information.[1,5]

Summary Statements and Grading

Development group members then draft a summary statement for each clinical question from the included studies and assign a grade to that statement, indicating the strength of the evidence to support it.[1,5] There is no single, consistent way to grade the strength of evidence for the summary statement, but usually the methodological quality, consistency of findings, the number of studies, the clinical impact of the findings, and the generalizability of the outcomes are included in the grading.[5] Summary statements based on evidence of high-quality methodology, with consistent findings from several studies that demonstrate high clinical impact and generalize well to the population of interest, receive a high evidence grading. Summary statements with evidence that is limited in any of these areas receive a lower evidence grading.

Recommendations and Ratings

The guideline development group then drafts evidence-based recommendations from the graded summary statements.[7] At least one recommendation should be created from each summary statement, but some summary statements may result in more than one recommendation. In developing recommendations, the benefits, risks, inconvenience, and costs associated with each recommendation are considered, along with the strength of the evidence. Each recommendation is given a rating that reflects a balance of the factors that were included in its development. A rating, rather than grading, is given to the recommendation to separate the process of evaluating the quality of the literature (grading) from the overall evaluation of the recommendation (rating), which includes more than just the quality of the literature. Stronger or higher ratings reflect recommendations that have greater benefits and stronger evidence to support them.

Final Guidelines

Finally, these graded, evidence-based recommendations are incorporated into guidelines. Guidelines describe the population to which they apply and explain the process by which the component evidence-based recommendations were developed. The recommendations are also organized in such a way as to assist practitioners in assessing, diagnosing, and treating the health condition of interest.[7]

Implementing Evidence-Based Guidelines

Practitioners can implement evidence-based guidelines through the process of shared decision-making with a patient or client (refer to Chapter 5). In this approach, practitioners inform their patients or clients about available treatment options according to evidence-based guidelines and the grading of the various options. This allows clients to make informed decisions while taking into account other important factors in their lives.[8] Clients may choose the option with the strongest rating or one with a weak rating or, perhaps, no rating. What is important is that the patient or client is informed and educated on the graded strength of each recommendation and its associated risks and benefits. The practitioner then supports the patient or client in making an informed decision while appropriately documenting the process.

As part of the process, practitioners should continually monitor and evaluate treatment outcomes and keep their patients or clients informed.[3] Presenting outcomes to patients or clients provides valuable information that helps their understanding of how a chosen treatment has influenced their health. When patients or clients see their health outcomes improve, this positive feedback can reinforce adherence to the chosen plan and help motivate the patient or client. If health outcomes do not improve, this can indicate that the chosen option is having no effect, which may prompt the patient or client to choose an option with a higher evidence grading.

One evidence-based practice guideline for weight management is the 2014 Adult Weight Management Evidence-Based Nutrition Practice Guideline from the Evidence Analysis Library (EAL) of the Academy of Nutrition and Dietetics.[9] As an example of how to implement this guideline, consider the following nutrition-intervention recommendation for weight loss, which has a strong rating: "For weight loss, the registered dietitian nutritionist (RDN) should advise overweight or obese adults that as long as the target reduction in calorie level is achieved, many different dietary approaches are effective. There is strong and consistent evidence that when calorie intake is controlled, macronutrient proportion, glycemic index, and glycemic load of the diet are not related to losing weight."[10] If a patient or client chooses the option of reducing energy (calorie) intake in order to lose weight, the RDN should provide the patient or client with several methods for achieving this, such as removing foods from the diet, reducing portion sizes, substituting lower-energy foods for higher-energy foods (to help create a 500 to 750 kcal daily energy deficit), and consuming a low-carbohydrate diet. As there is no single recommended strategy, the patient or client can choose from these options based on individual preference and values. The practitioner should support the patient's/client's decision.

Patients or clients may sometimes opt to implement a dietary strategy that has minimal evidence to support its effectiveness.[3] For example, a patient or client may choose to set a goal of eating more fruit and vegetable servings to assist with weight loss. No statement in the 2014 guideline supports this strategy on its own as a method for losing weight.[9] From the standpoint of evidence-based practice, therefore, the practitioner should inform the patient or client that although increasing fruit and vegetable consumption is a healthy choice and part of the US Dietary Guidelines for Americans,[11] this dietary strategy alone is not supported by the evidence as being effective for weight loss. Even when told that a strategy may not be effective (ie, that it has a low rating or no rating) according to available evidence, the patient or client may still choose the strategy. In such cases, the practitioner should support the patient or client's decision. What is important is that the patient or client has been well informed.

In evidence-based practice, if various treatment options are presented as having equal gradings when they do not, or if highly graded options are not presented to a patient or client (ie, are absent from the discussion), the practitioner has failed to inform the patient or client of the potential effectiveness of the available options.[3] When this occurs, patients or clients are denied the opportunity to make informed decisions, which breaks the shared decision-making tenet of evidence-based practice.

Evidence-Based Guidelines for the Treatment of Adult Overweight and Obesity

Professional organizations with a focus on the treatment of adult overweight and obesity commonly develop evidence-based guidelines for use by their members and other health care providers. Examples of these organizations and their respective guidelines are summarized in Box 4.2.[9,12-15] The frequency with which guidelines are updated varies tremendously among these organizations, with the American Diabetes Association producing the most frequent updates (ie, annually).[14] Thus, it is important that health care providers regularly check the websites and journals of professional organizations for the most current guidelines to use in practice.

For the most part, the guidelines agree in their recommendations for the treatment of adult overweight and obesity. The slight variations between guidelines from different organizations is usually due to the scope of practice that the organization targets for its key membership. For treatment, a multicomponent intervention (consisting of diet, activity, and cognitive behavioral therapy), pharmacotherapy, or bariatric and metabolic surgery is recommended, alone or in combination. Some guidelines also provide algorithms to assist practitioners with determining treatment options based on data obtained from patient or client assessments. Evidence-based guidelines are the basis for the recommendations regarding client assessments described in Chapters 6 through 9, and for the recommended interventions detailed in Chapters 10 through 14.

BOX 4.2

Evidence-Based Guidelines for the Treatment of Adult Overweight and Obesity[9,12-15]

Issuing organization(s)	Guideline
Academy of Nutrition and Dietetics	Adult Weight Management (AWM) Guideline (2014)[9]
American Association of Clinical Endocrinologists/ American College of Endocrinology	Comprehensive Clinical Practice Guidelines for Medical Care of Patients With Obesity (2016)[12]
American Association of Clinical Endocrinologists/ American College of Endocrinology, The Obesity Society, American Society for Metabolic and Bariatric Surgery, Obesity Medicine Association, and American Society of Anesthesiologists	Clinical Practice Guidelines for the Perioperative Nutrition, Metabolic, and Nonsurgical Support of Patients Undergoing Bariatric Procedures—2019 Update[13]
American Diabetes Association	Standards of Medical Care in Diabetes—2022[14]
American Heart Association, American College of Cardiology, and The Obesity Society	2013 AHA/ACC/TOS Guideline for the Management of Overweight and Obesity in Adults[15]

Summary

Evidence-based guidelines for all manner of health conditions are developed using a systematic approach and are designed to summarize and grade research and recommendations to support the implementation of research evidence in practice. The use of evidence-based guidelines provides a foundation for clinicians to engage in evidence-based practice. Evidence-based guidelines for the treatment of obesity are developed by several professional organizations and are regularly updated, incorporating new evidence, for clinicians to use.

References

1. Lim W, Arnold DM, Bachanova V, et al. Evidence-based guidelines—an introduction. *Hematology Am Soc Hematol Educ Program*. 2008;2008:26-30. doi:10.1182/asheducation-2008.1.26
2. Guyatt G, Cairns J, Churchill D, et al. Evidence-based medicine: a new approach to teaching the practice of medicine. *JAMA*. 1992;268(17):2420-2425. doi:10.1001/jama.1992.03490170092032
3. Raynor HA, Beto JA, Zoellner J. Achieving evidence-based practice in dietetics by using evidence-based practice guidelines. *J Acad Nutr Diet*. 2020;120(5):751-756. doi:10.1016/j.jand.2019.10.011
4. Graham R, Mancher M, Miller Wolman D, Greenfield S, Steinberg E, eds. *Clinical Practice Guidelines We Can Trust*. National Academies Press; 2011.
5. Handu D, Moloney L, Wolfram T, Ziegler P, Acosta A, Steiber A. Academy of Nutrition and Dietetics methodology for conducting systematic reviews for the Evidence Analysis Library. *J Acad Nutr Diet*. 2016;116(2):311-318. doi:10.1016/j.jand.2015.11.008
6. Preferred Reporting Items for Systematic Reviews and Meta-Analyses (PRISMA). Accessed May 24, 2015. www.prisma-statement.org

7. Papoutsakis C, Moloney L, Sinley RC, Acosta A, Handu D, Steiber AL. Academy of Nutrition and Dietetics methodology for developing evidence-based nutrition practice guidelines. *J Acad Nutr Diet.* 2017;117(5):794-804. doi:10.1016/j.jand.2016.07.011

8. Elwyn G, Frosch DL, Kobrin S. Implementing shared decision-making: consider all the consequences. *Implementation Sci.* 2016;11:114. doi:10.1186/s13012-016-0480-9

9. Academy of Nutrition and Dietetics. Adult weight management (AWM) guideline (2014). Evidence Analysis Library. Accessed January 8, 2022. www.andeal.org/topic.cfm?menu=5276&cat=4688

10. Academy of Nutrition and Dietetics. AWM: executive summary of recommendations (2014). Evidence Analysis Library. Accessed December 8, 2017. www.andeal.org/topic.cfm?menu=5276&cat=4690

11. US Department of Agriculture, US Department of Health and Human Services. *Dietary Guidelines for Americans, 2020-2025*. 9th ed. US Department of Agriculture and US Department of Health and Human Services; 2020. www.dietaryguidelines.gov/resources/2020-2025-dietary-guidelines-online-materials

12. Garvey WT, Mechanick JI, Brett EM, et al; reviewers of the AACE/ACE obesity clinical practice guidelines. American Association of Clinical Endocrinologists and American College of Endocrinology comprehensive clinical practice guidelines for medical care of patients with obesity. *Endocrine Practice.* 2016;22(Suppl 3):1-203. doi:10.4158/EP161365.GL

13. Mechanick JI, Apovian C, Brethauer S, et al. Clinical practice guidelines for the perioperative nutrition, metabolic, and nonsurgical support of patients undergoing bariatric procedures—2019 update: cosponsored by American Association of Clinical Endocrinologists/American College of Endocrinology, The Obesity Society, American Society for Metabolic and Bariatric Surgery, Obesity Medicine Association, and American Society of Anesthesiologists. *Surg Obes Relat Dis.* 2020;16(2):175-247. doi:10.1016/j.soard.2019.10.025

14. American Diabetes Association. Standards of medical care in diabetes—2022. *Diabetes Care.* 2022;45(Suppl 1):S1-S59. doi:10.2337/dc22-Srev

15. Jensen MD, Ryan DH, Apovian CM, et al. 2013 AHA/ACC/TOS guideline for the management of overweight and obesity in adults: a report of the American College of Cardiology/American Heart Association Task Force on Practice Guidelines, and The Obesity Society. *Circulation.* 2014;129(25 Suppl 2):S102-S138. doi:10.1161/01.cir.0000437739.71477.ee

CHAPTER 5

Patient-Centered Care and Shared Decision-Making

Eileen S. Myers, MPH, RDN

CHAPTER OBJECTIVES

- Define patient-centered care and shared decision-making.
- Review how patient-centered care can be applied in individual and group education sessions.
- Describe how shared decision-making can be used in patient care for the treatment of overweight and obesity.

Introduction

In 2019, a proposed standard of care for all health care providers and payers was published for the purpose of developing actionable statements reflecting minimum standards of care for the treatment of adults with obesity. Among the core principles and standards discussed in the article, shared decision-making and patient-centered bidirectional communication within evidence-based care were emphasized.[1] This chapter defines and explains how to employ patient-centered care and shared decision-making when working with patients for the treatment of overweight and obesity. The word *patient* will be used instead of *client* in this chapter, for much of the literature on this topic uses the term *patient-centered care*.

What Is Patient-Centered Care?

Health care professionals who work with patients must first understand their own needs and values if they plan to establish a healthy relationship with patients.[2] Practitioners should ask themselves the following questions:

- Do I need to be seen as an expert, giving too much advice and taking too much control?
- Do I need to be liked?
- Do I need to be depended on and seen as competent, and do I become upset when patients do not change?
- Do I have my own dietary health beliefs that cause me to become blind to whatever problems patients may find important?

In 1988, the Picker/Commonwealth Program for Patient-Centered Care (now the Picker Institute) coined the term *patient-centered care* to call attention to the need for health care professionals, staff, and health care systems to shift focus away from diseases and back to the patient and family. Their multiyear research revealed that patient-centered care encompasses seven dimensions from the patient perspective: (1) respect for patients' values, preferences, and expressed needs; (2) coordination and integration of care; (3) information, communication, and education; (4) physical comfort; (5) emotional support and alleviation of fear and anxiety; (6) involvement of family and friends; and (7) transition and continuity of care.[3]

In the Institute of Medicine's 2001 landmark publication, *Crossing the Quality Chasm: A New Health System for the 21st Century*, patient-centeredness is identified as one of the fundamental attributes of quality health care alongside safety, effectiveness, timeliness, efficiency, and equity. The Institute of Medicine (now the National Academy of Medicine) defines patient-centeredness as "providing care that is respectful for and responsive to individual patient preferences, needs and values and ensuring that patient values guide all clinical decisions."[4] Studies have shown that this concept of patient-centeredness improves health care quality and safety, increases patient satisfaction, improves adherence, and reduces health care costs.[5]

Building Rapport and Trust

Patient-centered care has been positively associated with both patients' trust in health care providers and evaluation of health care quality.[6] Building rapport and trust includes appropriate verbal and nonverbal communication. Health care professionals can make sure they build rapport using the items listed in Box 5.1.

BOX 5.1

Building Rapport in Patient-Centered Care

Look directly at patients.

Reach out a hand to patients in greeting.

Ask patients to have a seat.

Ask if the chair is comfortable.

Ask patients if it is okay to ask questions.

Ask patients if they want to work on the concern that brought them to the office.

Ask if it is okay to start talking about the concern together.

Ask patients what type of feedback they prefer.

Ask patients to let me know which words they are comfortable with and which words they would like me to avoid (eg, obesity, fat, weight).

Ask patients how I am doing in meeting their needs.

Remind patients of their progress and learnings.

Use appropriate facial expressions, eye contact, and body language.

Patient-centered care means patients are educated about the essential role *they* play in decision-making. Patients are given effective tools to help them understand their options and the consequences of their decisions. Patients should receive support to express their values and preferences and be able to ask questions without censure. The practitioner's role is not to be the single, paternalistic authority but to become a more effective coach or partner, learning how to ask, "What matters to you?" as well as "What is the matter?" Viewing the health care experience through the patient's eyes helps the provider be more responsive to the patient's needs.[7]

Respecting a patient's values, preferences, and expressed needs is fundamental to an effective patient–provider encounter. In a counseling relationship, there are two people involved, each with their own feelings, needs, values, experiences, and expectations. If counseling is to be successful, health care professionals must understand these differences as well as the concerns of patients. By understanding a patient's feelings, needs, values, experiences, and expectations, as well as their immediate concerns, the practitioner can connect the problem to the patient, which is important for an effective counseling relationship. Practitioners must be able to communicate this understanding to patients and determine whether their understanding is accurate. Rapport is developed when there is a mutual understanding that makes communication possible. Until rapport is developed, everything else, including information-giving and goal setting, is premature.[2]

Approaches to Patient-Centered Care

Motivational Interviewing

Motivational interviewing is a style of behavior-change counseling. It has been studied in a variety of settings in which behavior change is known to improve health outcomes.[8,9] This style of counseling will be discussed in greater detail in Chapter 13, but for the purposes of developing patient-centered relationships, practitioners should understand that motivational interviewing involves showing compassion and acceptance. Expressing empathy is an essential step in motivational interviewing and an essential component of patient-centered care. It involves showing warmth and practicing reflective listening. Health care professionals must strive to understand their patients' feelings and perspectives without judging, criticizing, or blaming. They can show respect by remaining unbiased and expressing a desire to understand the patient's perspective. Showing empathy helps practitioners build alliances and support their patients' self-esteem.

Motivational interviewing helps assure patients that their health care professional is listening and also facilitates patients' exploration of their motivations and values. Important skills of the motivational interviewer include asking, reflecting, and informing. Open-ended questions and reflections help the provider discover a patient's values, fears, and hopes.[10]

Shared Decision-Making

Considered the keystone of patient-centered care, shared decision-making involves mutual collaboration between patient and practitioner and a thorough discussion of the patient's preferences.[11] It is a process of communication in which the practitioner and patient work together to make informed health care decisions that align with what matters most to the patient. In shared decision-making, the practitioner informs patients about treatment options that are available according to evidence-based guidelines and discusses the grading of these options. With this information in hand, patients can weigh their options against what is important in their lives. A decision made by the patient in this manner is, thus, both informed and preferred.[12] This approach ensures that the right treatment is matched to the right patient at the right time.

In 2017, the National Quality Forum published a national call to action encouraging providers to embrace and integrate shared decision-making into clinical practice as a standard of patient-centered care.[13] Developed in response to a fundamental need for health care to be safe, effective, patient-centered, timely, efficient, and equitable, shared decision-making is a vital method for strengthening the patient-centered approach to health care.

The three essential components of shared decision-making are as follows[14]:

- Information provided must be accurate, impartial, and understandable, and must include the option for the patient to refuse any intervention.
- Information must be communicated by the health care professional in an individualized way, taking into consideration the patient's particular situation.
- The patient's values, goals, informed preferences, and concerns must be incorporated in the communications.

The goal of shared decision-making is to help patients make informed health decisions. A mismatch between the treatment the patient receives and the treatment the patient prefers (due to a lack of discussion of the patient's concerns and goals or the patient's not being fully informed about their options) is called a preference misdiagnosis.[15]

Shared decision-making is used primarily for making major decisions, such as decisions about cancer treatment, whether or not to have a screening, or whether to have surgery. However, it is also appropriate for managing chronic conditions, as it has been shown to improve both adherence to medications in patients with chronic conditions and patient engagement and diabetes prevention outcomes.[16,17]

Patient Decision Aids

Patient decision aids are structured tools that help facilitate shared decision-making. Although not essential to the process, in a systematic review including more than 31,000 patients, they have been shown to improve medical decisions, increase patient involvement, and increase the alignment of preferences and treatment.[18] A patient decision aid can be an easy-to-read document, a video, an interactive website, or a visual aid that incorporates the evidence-based, unbiased information about the patient's condition and treatment options along with the risks and benefits of each option as they apply to each patient. High-quality decision aids present information in a neutral way, offering information to patients and supporting them in making the decision that best aligns with their individual needs but not pushing them toward a particular decision.[19] Currently, there are no national certifications for patient decision aids and no specific aids for the condition of obesity. However, examples of patient decision aids are available for use as templates for creating aids for chronic care management.[20-22]

When using a patient decision aid, the health care professional summarizes all the key options as well as the corresponding research, allows the patient time to read and think about these options, and assesses how each option relates to what is important to the patient.

There is an important distinction between patient decision aids and educational materials that are not patient decision aids. A decision aid supports a patient in making a decision by fully exploring *all* of their relevant options, whereas non-aid educational materials typically provide detailed information about a single possible approach.[19]

Steps in Shared Decision-Making

Several implementation models for the shared decision-making process exist; however, they all contain similar core steps. The following model, described in more detail in Box 5.2, is taken from the Agency for Healthcare Research and Quality. It includes five steps for health care practitioners to follow and goes by the acronym SHARE.[23,24]

1. **Seek** your patient's participation: Invite the patient to participate and communicate that a choice exists.
2. **Help** your patient explore and compare treatment options: Present the options, including the option to do nothing. Use evidence-based resources to compare the treatment options. Present the patient decision aid, if available.
3. **Assess** your patient's values and preferences: Stop and listen to what matters most to the patient.
4. **Reach** a decision with your patient: Guide the patient to express whether any of the presented options is consistent with what matters to them most

and ask whether they are ready to make a decision. Give the patient the option to speak with significant others if they choose. Ask whether more time is needed. Schedule a follow-up visit.
5. **Evaluate** your patient's decision: Reconnect with the patient to monitor and offer support for purposes of clarification, further discussion, and implementation.

BOX 5.2

Steps for Health Care Practitioners in Shared Decision-Making[23,24]

Step	Purpose	How to achieve the purpose	Examples of what to say
1. Seek your patient's participation.	Summarize the health problem and ask the patient to participate in the process of reviewing treatment options.	Show empathy and interest. Ask permission.	"There are options I can present. If you agree, I can go over the options."
2. Help your patient explore and compare treatment options.	Provide the patient with evidence-based, unbiased information on each of the options, along with the benefits and risks of each.	Show empathy and interest.	"Here are some choices to consider." "I'd like to go over what we know about the pros and cons of the options."
3. Assess your patient's values and preferences.	Encourage the patient to talk about values and preferences, and come to an agreement on what is important to the patient.	Ask open-ended questions. Use active listening, reflecting, and summarizing.	"When you think about these options, what matters most to you?"
4. Reach a decision with your patient.	Discern whether the patient is ready to make a decision, needs more information, or needs to speak with a family member before making a decision. Also, schedule another session and confirm the decision.	Ask open-ended questions. Use active listening, reflecting, and summarizing.	"I get that this is a tough decision to make." "Given what we talked about, are you leaning toward any one option?" "Would you like to talk with someone else before making a decision?"
5. Evaluate your patient's decision.	Follow up with the patient and help the patient with decision implementation, which is important for success.	Ask open-ended questions. Use active listening, reflecting, and summarizing.	"When can we talk again?" "How can I help with the next steps?"

Incorporating Motivational Interviewing and Shared Decision-Making Into Practice

Both motivational interviewing and shared decision-making focus on encouraging patients to explore their views and opinions about options for treatment or approaches to management of their condition. Both are used in patient-centered care and enhance the provider-patient relationship through understanding, respect, and curiosity about the patient as a person. Finally, both of these tools rely on the core communications skills of establishing trust and empathy, reflective listening, and responding to emotions. As will be discussed further in Chapter 13, motivational interviewing is more than an engaging technique; it is a behavior-change technique used throughout an intervention. The primary purpose of shared decision-making, however, is to invite, present, and clarify treatment or management options and to facilitate a collaborative discussion of those options.[25]

Patient-Centered Care for Individuals and Groups

Working With an Individual Patient

Joe Smith was told he needs to lose weight, as he now has prediabetes. He has tried many diets throughout his life but cannot keep the weight off. Box 5.3 provides a sample case study of a health care professional working with Joe and using the components of motivational interviewing and shared decision-making to provide patient-centered care.

Working in a Group Setting

Working in a group setting can be more challenging than working one-on-one with individuals because health care professionals often think of their role in a group as "leader and teacher," rather than "partner and collaborator," as discussed in the previous section. To achieve the outcomes of patient-centered care in a group setting, the practitioner must be skillful in establishing group cohesion facilitating personalized solutions, managing group dynamics, and teaching a particular component of a curriculum.

In a group setting, the verbal and nonverbal skills needed to provide patient-centered care still apply. What most likely does not apply when working with groups is the use of shared decision-making, as everyone in the group likely went through the shared decision-making process already and opted to join the group. To incorporate patient-centered care in the group setting, practitioners can do the following[26]:

- Inform participants of the style of the group and ask for permission to proceed. For example, one could say, "I'd like to go around the room so that everyone has a chance to respond. Is this approach okay, or does anyone have another suggestion?"
- Ask each participant about their reason for joining the group and what they hope to achieve through the group. This will help the health care professional know whether a shared decision-making process was involved or if participants joined because they were told that they should.
- Learn what matters to each individual group participant by asking open-ended questions and using reflections to help understand their motivations and values.
- Inform participants of what to expect if they are taking up too much of the group's time or going off track. One can say, "I'd like everyone to have a

BOX 5.3

Case Study: A Patient-Centered Session With an Individual Patient

Joe Smith enters the office. The health care provider greets Joe and offers him a seat. The provider asks Joe what brought him to the office and what he hopes to get out of their time together.

Joe says he was recently diagnosed with prediabetes and that it scared him. He doesn't want to develop diabetes, as he witnessed his father losing the ability to walk because of the complications related to the disease. Joe has not been successful at losing weight in the past and questions trying again. He admits he doesn't know the best approach. He hasn't been feeling good with the excess weight and gets tired playing a round of golf. He was always active in the past, loves golf, and wants to feel good like he did at a lower weight. He doesn't know what he'll do if he becomes like his father and can no longer walk. He'd feel more hopeful about succeeding if he knew what he needed to do. He hopes he doesn't have to stop eating all his favorite foods.

Features of motivational interviewing	Showing empathy
	Building trust
	Asking open-ended questions
	Reflecting
Features of shared decision-making	Exploring the patient's understanding of their situation

The health care provider nods and confirms understanding of Joe's frustration, as there are so many diets out there that promise success. The provider asks if it is okay to explain what the research currently states about weight loss and weight loss diets. Joe nods yes, and the provider explains that weight loss is complicated, and that some people have more success than others. The provider tells Joe that he has some options he can consider and invites him to be involved in the decision-making process.

The health care provider asks to share a few documents with Joe that may help him understand his options, stating that the information will help ensure that what Joe chooses fits best with what matters to him most. The provider shows Joe an example of a patient decision aid that the provider admits is not a validated tool but hopes will help Joe make a decision.

The health care provider reviews the patient decision aid with Joe. The aid presents the different options Joe might consider for weight loss and the pros and cons of each option. It also presents the question of what is most important to Joe as he considers the various options.

The health care provider reviews three options with Joe:

- Make no changes at this time.
- Make changes to his diet and exercise level without focusing on weight loss.
- Increase physical activity and reduce dietary intake by 500 to 1,000 kcal/d to accomplish a 5% to 10% weight loss. The provider explains that there are many dietary approaches that can accomplish weight loss, such as Mediterranean, low-fat, low-carbohydrate, and portion-controlled diets; the key feature is that there is an energy deficit. The most important aspect of this option is the decision to reduce total energy intake and increase physical activity.

The provider reviews the pros and cons of each option based on the available evidence from randomized clinical trials.

Features of motivational interviewing	Showing empathy
	Asking permission
Features of shared decision-making	Inviting the patient to participate
	Helping the patient explore options
	Providing information on the benefits and risks of the various options

Box continues

BOX 5.3 (CONTINUED)

The health care provider asks Joe to review and consider the options, add any of his own pros and cons, and then rate what matters most to him.

Once Joe is finished, the provider asks him if he is comfortable talking about his ratings. After this discussion, the provider nods in respect of Joe's reasoning and asks if he is leaning toward one of the options. Joe states that he really needs to feel better and avoid diabetes, so he wants to try diet and exercise, hoping to lose 5% to 10% of his body weight (option 3).

Features of motivational interviewing	Collaborating
	Asking permission
Features of shared decision-making	Eliciting patient values and preferences for positive and negative outcomes
	Facilitating deliberation and decision-making

The health care provider asks Joe if he wants to talk this over with his wife before deciding. Joe says no, as he knows his wife is on board and will be supportive.

Features of motivational interviewing	Asking
Features of shared decision-making	Providing the opportunity to involve trusted others

The health care provider acknowledges the work Joe put into this decision and restates that many dietary approaches are effective for weight loss, as long as the approach involves an energy deficit. The provider states that there will be more options to discuss next time, and wants to take time to better understand Joe's food preferences, eating patterns, work schedule, and lifestyle before revisiting the decision of which type of diet he should follow.

Features of motivational interviewing	Reflecting
	Affirming
	Asking

Joe says he is excited to start but admits that he fears that giving up some of his current habits will be difficult, as he loves to eat. He is happy to know that the health care provider understands and will follow Joe's lead on what type of diet will work best for him, and he says he is willing to make changes if one approach isn't working.

Features of motivational interviewing	Showing empathy
Features of shared decision-making	Assisting with implementation

SECTION 1: Foundations of Treatment: The Human Element

chance to speak," or, "I'm going to ask each of you to take no more than 3 minutes to go around the room to talk about your successes of the previous week. Would it be okay if I cut you off if you go into someone else's time?" When an individual does go off track, the practitioner can acknowledge the importance of what the person is saying by stating, "I hear that this is very important to you, and yet, if you are okay with it, I'd like the group to hear how you might use this approach in your upcoming week."

- Observe body language to assess how well one is engaging the group. Practitioners can assess if someone is agreeing too much, has lowered their head and is not maintaining eye contact, or is off topic and whether any of these behaviors reflect that the session has moved from participant-focused (patient-centered) to leader- or teacher-focused (practitioner-centered).

Steps in Applying a Patient-Centered Approach in Groups

In a group setting, the group leader (health care practitioner) and participants (patients) introduce themselves in a welcoming and empathetic atmosphere that facilitates interaction. The program objectives, approaches, and expectations are presented by the leader and discussed by the participants. Steps for a patient-centered group may proceed as follows[24,27]:

1. **Welcome**: The leader works to develop empathy within the group, discusses the importance of participation in the group, and stresses the need for confidentiality.
2. **Ask**: The leader asks participants how they feel about sharing situations and behaviors related to their eating and also about what types of questions participants feel are acceptable to ask and what types are not. The leader also asks each participant to state what benefit they hope to get from being in the group and what they hope to accomplish (their goals and dreams) after a certain number of weeks in the program.
3. **Explore**: The group leader asks open-ended questions about lifestyle, habits, and ambivalence about change and uses reflections to ensure that what was heard is accurate and to let the participants know they are being heard. The leader empathizes with feelings of ambivalence and assures participants that ambivalence is normal and the group is meant to help reduce ambivalence.
4. **Evoke**: The group leader elicits "change talk" using a "confidence and importance ruler" (refer to Chapter 13 for more on this concept) to explore values, with a goal of having patients become more aware of the inconsistencies between their present behaviors and personal values.
5. **Plan**: The group leader poses open-ended questions and uses reflections to help participants identify feasible strategies and become more aware of their internal and external resources for making change possible.

Challenges in Delivering Patient-Centered Care

When asked if one delivers patient-centered care, most health care professionals will say yes. Yet, there are differing perceptions of what defines patient-centered care. For some, patient-centered care is simply allowing the patient to drive the conversation and make decisions without the shared decision-making process. A lack of clarity about what actually constitutes patient-centered care creates a challenge for practitioners. Challenges in delivering patient-centered care include the time pressures of seeing more patients per day and inadequate reimbursement for the extra time spent with patients. Within the organizational setting, support from leadership may be lacking for the delivery of patient-centered care; and evaluating effectiveness is difficult, as there are currently no tools for measuring whether the treatment a patient receives matches their preference for the management of their condition.[28] Finally, academic and professional education on this topic has, to date, been inadequate.[29-31]

Summary

There is broad agreement that patient-centered care is an essential component of health care.[3-5] It is fundamental to the safety, cost-effectiveness, and quality of health care. It is also associated with improved clinical care, increased patient engagement, and improved satisfaction and quality of life. A patient-centered approach aims to provide care that is respectful and responsive to patients' needs and preferences and requires different methods based on the clinical situation. Motivational interviewing and shared decision-making are styles and methods of interacting that help achieve patient-centered care. To reduce barriers to implementation and increase utilization of a patient-centered model of care, access to standardized training and adequate resources are needed for both health care leaders and health care professionals.

References

1. Dietz WH, Gallagher C. A proposed standard of obesity care for all providers and payors. *J Obes*. 2019;27(7):1059-1062. doi:10.1002/oby.22507
2. Danish SJ, Laquatra I. *Working With Challenging Clients: When Giving Information Isn't Enough*. American Dietetic Association; 2004.
3. Gerteis M, Edgman-Levitan S, Daley J, et al. *Through the Patient's Eyes: Understanding and Promoting Patient-Centered Care*. Jossey-Bass Publishers; 1993.
4. Institute of Medicine. *Crossing the Quality Chasm: A New Health System for the 21st Century*. National Academies Press; 2001.
5. Rathert C, Wyrwich MD, Boren SA. Patient-centeredness care and outcomes: a systematic review of the literature. *Med Care Res Rev*. 2013;70(4):351-379. doi:10.1177/1077558712465774
6. Hyehyun H, Hyun JO. The effects of patient-centered communication: exploring the mediating role of trust in healthcare providers. *Health Commun*. 2020;35(4):502-511. doi:10.1080/10410236.2019.1570427
7. Tonelli MR, Sullivan MD. Person-centered shared decision making. *J Eval Clin Pract*. 2019;25(6):1057-1062. doi:10.1111/jep.13260
8. Rollnick S, Miller WR, Butler CC. *Motivational Interviewing in Health Care*. Guilford Press; 2008.
9. Hettema J, Steele J, Miller WR. Motivational interviewing. *Annu Rev Clin Psychol*. 2005;1:91-111. doi:10.1146/annurev.clinpsy.1.102803.143833
10. Miller WR, Rollnick S. *Motivational Interviewing: Helping People Change*. 3rd ed. Guilford Press; 2012.
11. Barry MJ, Edgman-Levitan S. Shared decision making—pinnacle of patient-centered care. *N Engl J Med*. 2012;366(9):780-781. doi:10.1056/NEJMp1109283
12. Raynor HA, Beto JA, Zoellner J. Achieving evidence-based practice in dietetics using evidence-based practice guidelines. *J Acad Nutr Diet*. 2020;120(5):751-756. doi:10.1016/j.jand.2019.10.011
13. National Quality Forum. *Shared Decision Making: A Standard of Care for All Patients*. National Partners Action Brief. October 2017. Accessed December 12, 2021. www.qualityforum.org/Publications/2017/10/NQP_Shared_Decision_Making_Action_Brief.aspx
14. Cypher RL. Shared decision-making: a model for effective communication and patient satisfaction. *J Perinat Neonatal Nurs*. 2019;33(4):285-287. doi:10.1097/JPN.0000000000000441

15. Mulley AG, Trimble C, Elwyn G. Stop the silent misdiagnosis: patients' preferences matter. *BMJ*. 2012;345:e6572. doi:10.1136/bmj.e6572
16. Wilson SR, Strub P, Buist AS, et al. Shared treatment decision making improves adherence and outcome in poorly controlled asthma. *Am J Respir Crit Med*. 2010;15(6):566-577. doi:10.1164/rccm.200906-0907OC
17. Moin T, Turk N, Mangione C, et al. Shared decision-making for diabetes prevention—one-year results from the prediabetes informed decision and education (PRIDE) study. *Diabetes*. 2018;67(suppl 1):168-OR. doi:10.2337/db18-168-OR
18. Stacey D, Legare F, Lewis K, et al. Decision aids for people facing health treatment or screening decisions. *Cochrane Database Syst Rev*. 2017;4(4):CD001431. doi:10.1002/14651858.CD001431.pub5
19. How to identify a high-quality patient decision aid (PDA). Washington Health Care Authority website. September 2021. Accessed December 12, 2021. www.hca.wa.gov/assets/program/how-to-identify-high-quality-pda.pdf
20. Patient decision aids: alphabetical list of decision aids by health topic. Ottawa Hospital Research Institute website. Updated December 3, 2021. Accessed December 12, 2021. https://decisionaid.ohri.ca/azlist.html
21. Patient decision aids. Washington State Health Care Authority website. Accessed December 12, 2021. www.hca.wa.gov/about-hca/making-informed-health-care-decisions/patient-decision-aids-pdas
22. Decision worksheets. MGH Health Decision Sciences Center website. Accessed December 12, 2021. https://mghdecisionsciences.org/tools-training/decision-worksheets
23. The SHARE approach. Agency for Healthcare Research and Quality. Created July 2014. Reviewed October 2020. Accessed December 12, 2021. www.ahrq.gov/health-literacy/professional-training/shared-decision/index.html
24. SHARE Approach Workshop Curriculum. Agency for Healthcare Research and Quality website. Created September 2014. Reviewed September 2020. Accessed December 12, 2021. www.ahrq.gov/health-literacy/professional-training/shared-decision/workshop/mod1-guide.html
25. Elwyn G, Dehlendorf C, Epstein RM, Marrin K, White J, Frosch DL. Shared decision making and motivational interviewing: achieving patient-centered care across the spectrum of health care problems. *Ann Fam Med*. 2014;12(3):270-275. doi:10.1370/afm.1615
26. Wagner CC, Ingersoll KS. *Motivational Interviewing in Groups*. Guilford Press; 2013.
27. Centis E, Petroni ML, Ghirelli V, et al. Motivational interviewing adapted to group settings for the treatment of relapse in the behavioral therapy of obesity: a clinical audit. *Nutrients*. 2020;12(12):3881. doi:10.3390/nu12123881
28. Gartner FR, Bomhof-Roordink H, Smith IP, et al. The quality of instruments to assess the process of shared decision making: a systematic review. *PLoS ONE*. 2018;13(2):e0191747. doi:10.1371/journal.pone.0191747
29. Sladdin I, Chabooyer W, Ball L. Patients' perceptions and experiences of patient-centered care in dietetic consultations. *J Hum Nutr Diet*. 2018;31(2);188-196. doi:10.1111/jhn.12507
30. Moore, L, Britten, N, Lydahl D, Naldemirci Ö, Elam M, Wolf A. Barriers and facilitators to the implementation of person-centered care in different healthcare contexts. *Scand J Caring Sci*. 2017;31(4):662-673. doi:10.1111/scs.12376
31. Levey R, Ball L, Chaboyer W, Sladdin I. Dietitians' perspectives of the barriers and enablers to delivering patient-centered care. *J Hum Nutr Diet*. 2020;33(1):106-114. doi:10.1111/jhn.12684

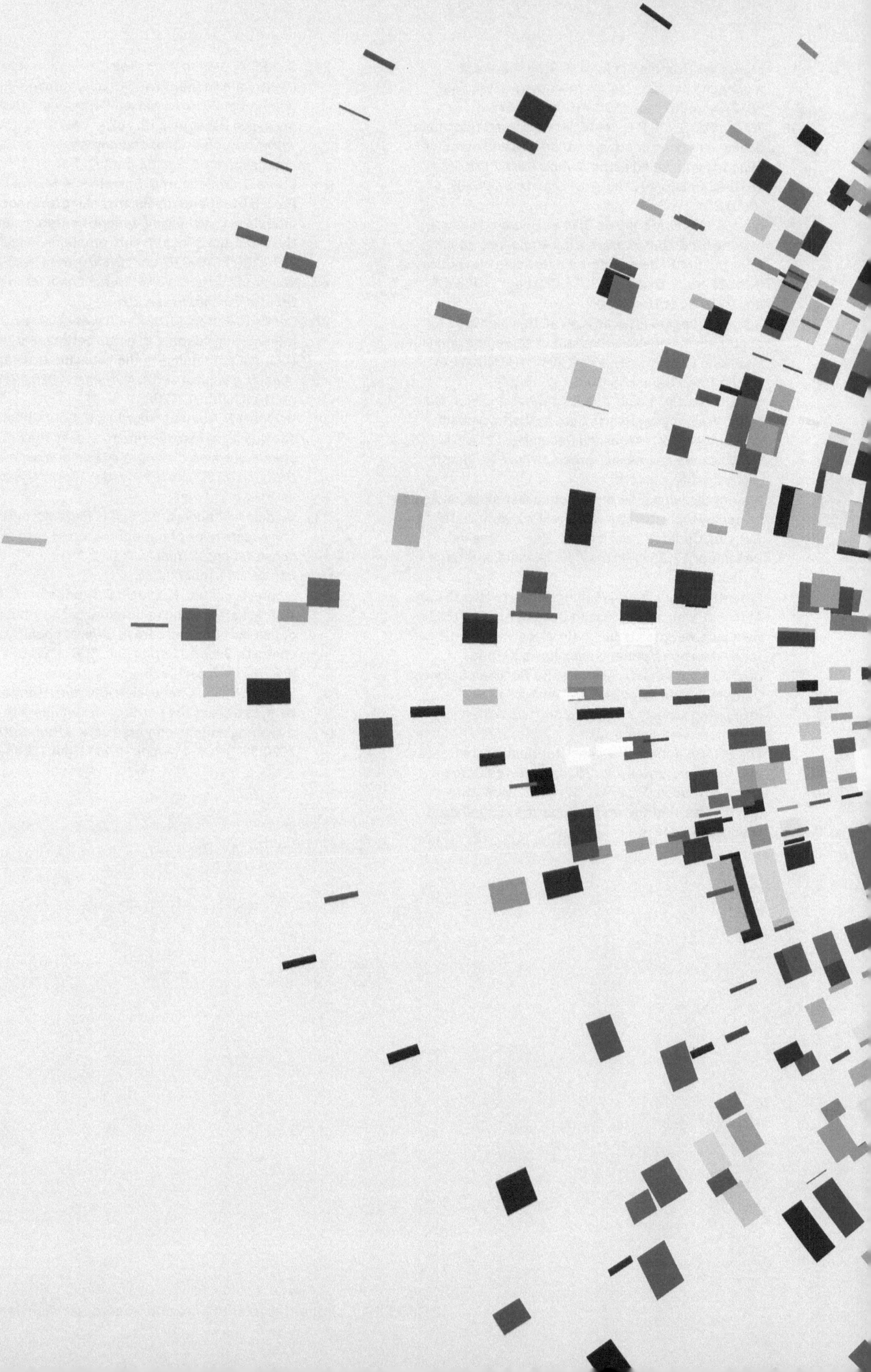

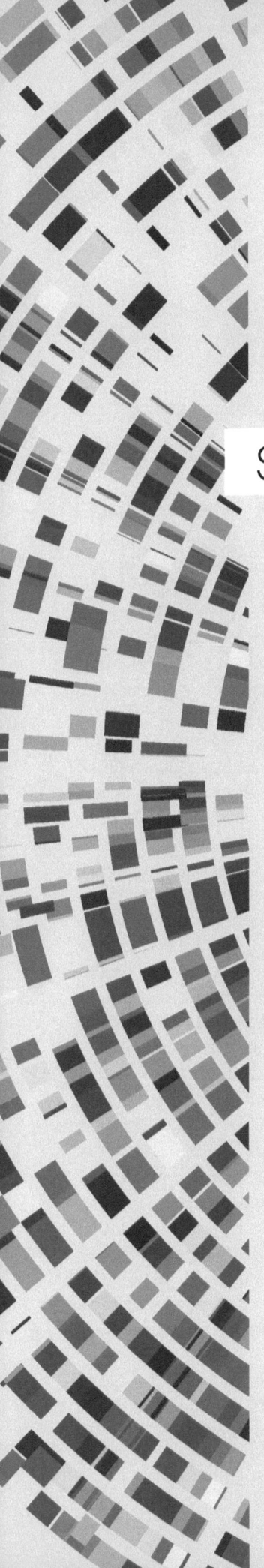

SECTION 2

Interprofessional Assessment of Overweight and Obesity

CHAPTER 6   Medical and Physical Assessment | 80

CHAPTER 7   Nutrition Assessment | 98

CHAPTER 8   Physical Activity Assessment | 116

CHAPTER 9   Behavioral Health Assessment | 145

CHAPTER 6

Medical and Physical Assessment

Vivian Ortiz, MD
Octavia Pickett-Blakely, MD, MHS

CHAPTER OBJECTIVES

- Review the medical and physical parameters related to obesity that should be collected during assessment.
- Describe how the medical and physical parameters can be brought together in an obesity-focused history.
- Define how collected parameters can assist with identifying patients who are at increased health risk.

Introduction

According to the Greek physician and philosopher Galen, people with obesity represented a "natural humoral condition," but those with *polisarkos*, or "excessive fat," had an unbalanced state that was treated with diet, exercise, massage, and baths.[1] In medieval times, larger bodies were associated with abundance and wealth. The term *obesity* was first used in 1620 by Thomas Venner in his book *Via Recta* as a distinguishing condition of the English upper class.[2] However, during the 18th and 19th centuries, obesity became associated with laziness, gluttony, and greed, and was perceived negatively. William Banting first documented the concept of dieting in 1863 in his *Letter on Corpulence, Addressed to the Public*, in which he described achieving weight loss and a healthier state through a diet low in starch and sugar. The negative stigma attached to states of excess body weight intensified amid the rise of capitalism, as it became seen as a consequence of one's behaviors rather as a medical illness. Not until 2004 was obesity recognized by the Centers for Medicare and Medicaid Services as a disease, and nearly a decade later, in 2013, the American Medical Association finally followed suit.[3] The recognition of obesity as a disease by the Centers for Medicare and Medicaid Services provided a pathway for heightened disease awareness and the subsequent establishment of screening and preventive programs, as well as reimbursement for some obesity therapies.[3,4]

Despite these milestones, obesity is underdiagnosed and undertreated. Studies from the mid-2000s report that as few as 20% of patients with obesity receive a formal diagnosis, and only 23% are provided with a management plan.[5,6] This phenomenon has been attributed to patient embarrassment, frustration, and lack of medications for the condition, while physicians lack the time and confidence to holistically address obesity.[7,8] As the definition of obesity and the data showing its substantial clinical and societal impact have evolved, so have measurement tools that stratify patients by risk in order to develop effective treatment plans.[8] Today, obesity in adults is recognized as a condition of abnormal or excessive body fat, as indicated by a BMI of 30 or higher, elevated body fat (defined as a body fat percentage of 25% or more in males and 32% or more in females), or elevated waist circumference (varies based on sex and racial background).

A thorough approach to treating individuals with overweight or obesity has never been more important. Just over one-third of adults in the United States are obese, with almost one-fourth of children fitting this category,[9] and the prevalence is growing.[10] Obesity is associated with higher socioeconomic status in developing countries, whereas it is associated with lower socioeconomic status in developed nations.[11] While a large component of the obesity epidemic is attributed to the pervasive "Western diet" and consumption of energy in excess of expenditure, obesity warrants a holistic approach wherein assessment extends beyond discussions focused solely on diet and exercise. The medical assessment of patients with obesity should involve a comprehensive evaluation of potential endocrine, hereditary, and psychological etiologies that may underlie obesity. Physicians and health care professionals across fields appreciate that the evaluation relies on a multidisciplinary team whose goal is to prevent and manage obesity and its complications, including type 2 diabetes, cardiovascular disease, cancer, and metabolic dysfunction–associated steatotic liver disease.[12] At the societal level, obesity is associated with lower work productivity and higher unemployment and disability, which can perpetuate suboptimal physical health. Furthermore, obesity is more difficult to address in low socioeconomic settings where resources are scarce.[11,13] This chapter outlines a standard approach to the evaluation of the patient with obesity, from the history and physical examination to anthropometric measurements and diagnostic testing that can be used to devise an individualized therapeutic plan.

Assessment for Obesity

Weight History

As with most medical visits, an evaluation for obesity starts with a comprehensive clinical history that enhances the clinician's understanding of the factors contributing to the patient's current weight status and the impact on their overall health. The medical interview for the patient with obesity is complex because it accounts for an array of physical and environmental factors that contribute to disease (refer to Figure 6.1).

FIGURE 6.1 Clinical and environmental risk factors for obesity

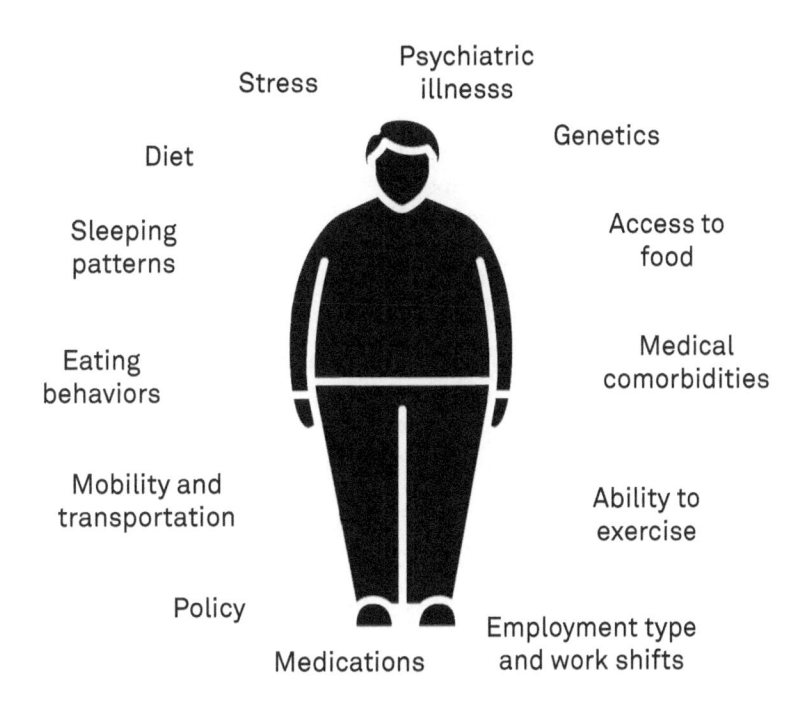

Labels surrounding figure: Stress, Psychiatric illnesss, Diet, Genetics, Sleeping patterns, Access to food, Eating behaviors, Medical comorbidities, Mobility and transportation, Ability to exercise, Policy, Medications, Employment type and work shifts

Experts recommend starting by obtaining details about an individual's body weight trajectory in association with clinically significant health and life events. The assessment should document changes in body weight throughout the patient's life cycle, including in childhood, adolescence, and early and late adulthood, as well as precipitating factors. In this context, prior therapies, including behavioral interventions, medications, endoscopic procedures, and surgeries, will give indications of resistance to therapy, behaviors that need modifications, new underlying etiologies, and additional therapies that can be offered. Obesity in childhood, adolescence, and early adulthood is associated with obesity in adulthood and adult-onset cardiovascular disease, stroke, hypertension, cancer, and type 2 diabetes.[14-18] In fact, studies suggest a linear relationship between the duration of obesity in years and elevations in glycated hemoglobin A1c (HbA1c).[16] Similarly, a cohort of participants monitored for 48 years in the Framingham Heart Study demonstrated a relationship between duration of obesity in years and all-cause mortality, with mortality doubling for every 10 years that participants had obesity.[19] Maximum BMI is also important to note, as studies have shown its association with all-cause mortality, particularly in those with class 1 and 2 obesity, even if they enter a lower BMI category after weight loss.[20,21]

Sex affects body weight throughout the life cycle: females having greater amounts of adipose tissue compared to males for a given BMI.[14] In pregnancy, birth parent weight, energy expenditure, and glucose utilization increase, while hepatic glucose production decreases.[22] Yet in pregnancy, insulin sensitivity progressively decreases toward the third trimester, and even more so in those with insulin insensitivity prior to pregnancy. The insulin resistance of pregnancy is believed to be a consequence of increased activity of inflammation markers and especially hormones (ie, human placental lactogen), which can ultimately result in gestational diabetes and type 2 diabetes later in life.[23] Understanding a patient's weight history can also inform risk stratification for future pregnancies in those who have not been pregnant. Individuals with obesity have a higher risk of reduced fertility, gestational diabetes, adverse pregnancy outcomes (preterm and still-birth deliveries), postpartum weight retention, and postpartum venous thromboembolism.[24-26] After menopause, adipose tissue increases and metabolic syndrome is more prevalent.[27] With age, hormonal alterations such as reduced estrogen result in peripheral fat shifts from the gluteal and femoral region to the abdomen.[16] Such shifts lead to increased visceral fat (fat in the central abdominal region), decreased lean muscle, and increased waist circumference and waist-to-hip ratio.[28,29]

Special considerations when working with transgender patients are discussed later in this chapter.

As people advance in age, sarcopenia (a decrease in muscle mass) ensues in the context of decreased energy expenditure and increased total body fat.[30] Fat redistribution from the subcutaneous region to the central abdomen (visceral fat) increases the risk of cardiovascular disease, type 2 diabetes, and metabolic syndrome in elderly individuals.[31] Bone and joint changes, such as decreased intervertebral height, decreased flexibility at the hip and knees, and spinal deformities, lead to height loss.[32] An understanding of these physiologic changes is essential to the assessment and treatment recommendations of the patient with obesity across life stages.

Weight Loss and Diet History

Understanding a patient's prior weight loss interventions, successes, and failures can provide insight into which therapies to consider using and which to avoid. The clinician should also take time to ask about eating behaviors: experts suggest inquiring about patient food and beverage intake, specifically the amount, type, frequency, and timing of food ingestion. In developed societies, energy-dense convenience foods are ubiquitous, and the consumption of inexpensive precooked meals with high salt content and artificial flavors has increased, while consumption of higher-priced fresh produce has decreased.[33-35] In addition to obtaining a detailed history of diet composition, it is critical that the practitioner elucidate a patient's eating behaviors during the medical evaluation. Binge eating, the rapid consumption of large portions of food over a short period of time, substantially increases one's risk of metabolic syndrome, hypertriglyceridemia, and hypertension.[36] Binge eating has been associated with higher BMI and depression and has been shown to be influenced by anxiety.[37] Nocturnal eating is also associated with an increased risk of obesity and complicated type 2 diabetes.[38] Snacking between meals often involves the intake of carbohydrate-dense and energy-dense foods that substantially increase overall energy intake. Being privy to this information can help influence treatment strategies, such as increasing the protein and fiber content of meals to promote longer periods of satiation, or substituting higher fiber, healthy snacks to facilitate weight loss.[39] Grazing, the continuous consumption of multiple small meals during the day, is associated with obesity because people who graze have a greater propensity for binge eating. This behavior may ultimately lead to lower weight loss success and should be proactively addressed.[40]

Exercise History

Increased energy intake coupled with decreased energy expenditure, driven by an involuntary and complex neurohormonal and metabolic interplay, is the pathophysiologic basis for obesity in most patients.[41,42] Routine high-intensity exercise in combination with dietary modifications (reduced energy intake) results in weight loss, including a decrease in abdominal and visceral fat.[43,44] Hence, a thorough history detailing a patient's physical activity—including baseline physical activity, recent changes in physical activity with respect to weight, and the type, duration, and intensity of structured exercise—is critical. It is important to inquire about musculoskeletal injuries and physical impediments to exercise in order to formulate a suitable exercise regimen. An appreciation of a patient's baseline activity and physical capability allows the clinician to determine whether the recommended 150 minutes of weekly moderate-intensity exercise is being met. Frequent exercise of shorter duration or at shorter intervals is associated with greater success of absolute total-body fat mass reduction than infrequent exercise of longer duration.[45,46] It is also important to discern whether the patient's exercise routine consists primarily of aerobic exercise or of strength and resistance exercise, as the former is associated with greater energy expenditure and weight loss.[42] Aerobic exercise should, however, be balanced with strength and resistance training.

Past Medical and Surgical History

Disease-Related Causes of Obesity

The patient's past medical history is of particular importance because of the interplay between obesity and related comorbidities. Genetic conditions can give rise to obesity and should be considered when a patient describes childhood obesity. Those conditions that involve the leptin pathway and mutations in melanocortin-4 receptor are rare causes of infant and early childhood obesity.[47] Prader-Willi syndrome, WAGR syndrome (a syndrome of Wilms tumor, aniridia, genitourinary anomalies, and intellectual disability), Albright hereditary osteodystrophy, and Bardet-Biedl syndrome also give rise to early-onset obesity.[48]

Hormonal alterations are also implicated in the pathogenesis of obesity, and a history of such alterations may be elicited while obtaining a medical history. Hypersecretion of insulin leads to insulin resistance and metabolic syndrome.[23] Growth hormone deficiency leads to visceral and truncal fat accumulation; and hypercortisolism, such as that seen in Cushing syndrome, leads to insulin insensitivity and visceral fat accumulation from decreased lipolysis.[49] Decreased metabolic rate and thermogenesis occur in patients with hypothyroidism and have been related to abnormalities in the feedback mechanism of thyrotropin, leading to higher thyrotropin levels and lower thyroxine levels. The exact mechanism, however, is poorly understood.[49-51] In addition, polycystic ovary syndrome is associated with obesity and insulin secretion, leading to excess production of androgens by the ovaries.[52]

Iatrogenic causes of obesity should also be explored during the medical visit. Several medications, including thiazolidinediones for type 2 diabetes, antidepressants, HIV antiretrovirals, and psychotropics such as risperidone and olanzapine, cause weight gain (antiretrovirals against HIV lead to fat redistribution).[53,54] Corticosteroid therapy is a common offender that increases appetite, alters lipid metabolism, and, consequently, increases fat accumulation and dysregulated glucose metabolism.[53] Cranial surgery or radiation can damage the hypothalamic neural circuits involved in appetite and cause vagal-driven insulin hypersecretion and insulin resistance.[55]

Obesity-Related Disease

When assessing a patient for obesity therapies, it is important to assess comorbidities that may exist as a consequence of obesity. Type 2 diabetes is 20 times more common in people with obesity.[56] Hypertension risk is also higher in those with a BMI of more than 25.[57] Obstructive sleep apnea is prevalent in individuals with obesity due to the relaxation of enlarged muscles surrounding the airway, which contributes to airway narrowing and subsequent hypoxia. These chronic hypoxic episodes are linked to the metabolic syndrome and dyslipidemia.[58]

Family History

A family history of obesity is a risk factor for both childhood-onset and adult-onset obesity.[59] In addition, a family history of type 2 diabetes, hypertension, and coronary artery disease are also risk factors for obesity. Studies show that a family history of obesity leads to earlier age of onset of obesity, and the class of obesity in the family is correlated with progressive metabolic syndrome.[60] The effect of a family history of type 2 diabetes has been attributed to hereditary conditions, as well as environmental factors such as family eating behaviors, urbanization, and access to healthy food.[59] Obtaining this information from the patient can allow for risk stratification of children of parents with obesity and empower clinicians to adopt early interventions.

Social History

The typical elements of the social history should no doubt be included in the assessment of patients with obesity. Obtaining information about an individual's upbringing, with a specific focus on eating behaviors in childhood—including family and cultural mores around food, health, weight, and body image that can influence adult behaviors—is extremely important. For example, a German study showed that several childhood environmental factors, including single-parent households, parental smoking and obesity, low physical activity, and low socioeconomic status, were risk factors for obesity.[61] Practitioners may also find it useful to ask patients about important or traumatic life events that may be linked to weight-related behaviors.

Occupation is a particularly important element of the social history. A person's occupation, in many instances, can be a surrogate marker of their activity level, with sedentary occupations being associated more often with obesity than high-mobility occupations. Indeed, the rising obesity prevalence has been exacerbated by the rise in technology-based jobs and home-office environments, which inherently decrease individual mobility.[12,62]

People with professions that lead to sleep disruption and frequent changes in their sleep-wake cycle (eg, shift workers, such as nurses or flight attendants) are at greater risk for obesity and metabolic syndrome.[63] Sleep patterns are an important component of the assessment of patients with obesity prior to treatment. Research has shown that getting less than 6 hours of sleep per night is associated with increased risk of obesity related to reward-eating behavior, increased perception of hunger, and emotional stress associated with increased food intake.[64-67]

In addition, professions with long work hours can hamper opportunities for structured exercise, and those paying low wages may necessitate an individual's working multiple jobs, which leaves less time for exercise.[68,69] Lastly, income often dictates food and resource accessibility. Amid the obesity epidemic, the growing income inequality gap has illuminated disparities in food security, which is certainly a contributor to obesity.[41,70,71]

The patient's social history should also include any history of substance use, especially alcohol and marijuana use, which in some patients is a driver of excess energy intake. A history of substance use may also provide insight into certain food-related behaviors, such as binge eating, poor impulse control, and emotional eating, that may ultimately inform treatment recommendations. Lastly, the presence of social stressors should be elicited in the social history.[72,73]

Physical Examination for Obesity

Anthropometrics

The physical examination of a patient with obesity should be a careful evaluation for features that may indicate the etiology and complications of excess body weight. Weight and height should be recorded at every visit for calculation of BMI and classification of obesity. The concept of BMI, weight normalized to height (kilograms per meters squared), was first used in 1872 to correlate with fat accumulation.[74,75] The US Preventive Services Task Force recommends screening for obesity in all adults and providing weight-related counseling to those who fit the criteria.[76,77] Body weight categories are defined by the World Health Organization and the Centers for Disease Control and Prevention into underweight (BMI less than 18.5), normal (BMI of 18.5–24.9), overweight (BMI of 25–29.9), class 1 obesity (BMI of 30–34.9), class 2 obesity (BMI of 35–39.9), and class 3 (severe) obesity (BMI of 40 or higher).[78,79] According to the World Health Organization, a BMI of 30 or higher is the point at which obesity has an impact on health.[80] A meta-analysis involving 10.6 million adults from 32 countries demonstrated an association between higher BMI and all-cause mortality, especially in men† (refer to Figure 6.2 on page 86) and younger adults.[81] However, the use of BMI is limited

---

† The meta-analysis uses the word men to describe study participants. Gender was not further specified.

FIGURE 6.2 BMI and all-cause mortality in individuals with a BMI greater than 25 (never-smokers)[a,81]

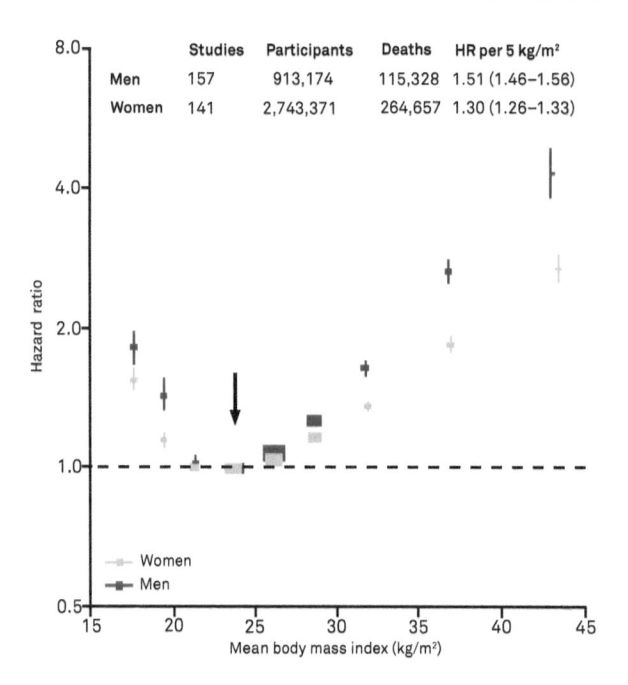

	Studies	Participants	Deaths	HR per 5 kg/m²
Men	157	913,174	115,328	1.51 (1.46–1.56)
Women	141	2,743,371	264,657	1.30 (1.26–1.33)

The reference category is shown with the arrow and is BMI 22.5–25.0.
Abbreviation: HR, heart rate.
[a] Study participants were described as men and women. Gender was not further specified.
Reproduced with permission from Di Angelantonio E, Bhupathiraju SN, Wormser D, et al. Body-mass index and all-cause mortality: individual-participant-data meta-analysis of 239 prospective studies in four continents. *Lancet*. 2016;388(10046):776-786. doi:10.1016/S0140-6736(16)30175-1.[81]

in certain body types and in those with an increased ratio of muscle vs adipose tissue composition.[78] Though it has been independently associated with ethnicity, BMI is also influenced by age and sex as a result of aforementioned physiologic changes; hence, this measurement should not be interpreted in isolation.[82,83] For example, Asian people have a higher percentage of body fat compared to White people at the same BMI and of the same age and sex, leading to a higher risk for cardiovascular disease, dyslipidemia, hypertension, and type 2 diabetes.[84]

For this reason, BMI measurement can be complemented by waist circumference, which is a strong indicator of visceral fat.[85] The use of waist circumference is appropriate for patients with a BMI between 25 and 34.9. Assessment of body habitus, specifically fat distribution, has prognostic implications: adipose concentration in the abdomen (ie, "apple shape") correlates with increased cardiometabolic risk, morbidity, and mortality, while truncal adipose distribution (ie, "pear shape") correlates with a lower risk.[86,87] A waist circumference of more than 102 cm in males and more than 88 cm in females strongly correlates with a BMI of 30 or higher.[88,89] Waist circumference values above these thresholds are associated with type 2 diabetes, metabolic syndrome, hypertension, dyslipidemia, and all-cause mortality.[90]

Blood Pressure

Elevated blood pressure measurements can indicate hypertension, and when combined with physical signs of heart failure, such as elevated jugular venous pressure and lower extremity edema, they can indicate cardiovascular compromise. Elevated resting heart rate can suggest cardiovascular deconditioning or an arrhythmia, which has implications for exercise recommendations and obesity pharmacotherapies.

Physical Findings

It is important to be mindful of the following features and findings during a physical examination for obesity.

- **Features of lipodystrophy:** Patients being treated with antiretroviral drugs for HIV may present with features of lipodystrophy. "Moon faces" and supraclavicular fat accumulation that spares extremities may suggest Cushing syndrome (refer to Figure 6.3).
- **Acanthosis nigricans:** The presence of acanthosis nigricans suggests underlying insulin resistance (refer to Figure 6.3).
- **Wide neck:** A neck circumference greater than 37.5 cm in males and greater than 32.5 cm in females can be a clue to underlying obstructive sleep apnea.[91] Clinicians can screen such patients for obstructive sleep apnea using tools such as the STOP-BANG questionnaire or the Epworth Sleepiness Scale.[92]
- **Signs of hypothyroidism:** Patients with hypothyroidism can present with hair thinning, periorbital swelling, dry skin, bradycardia, and hyporeflexia, and, when hypothyroidism is severe, pretibial edema and extreme fatigue.
- **Hirsutism and acne:** In a female, these findings can indicate the presence of polycystic ovary syndrome.

FIGURE 6.3 Select physical examination findings

"Moon face"

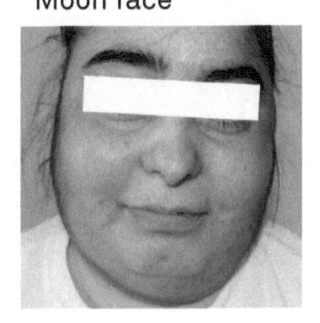

Acanthosis nigricans

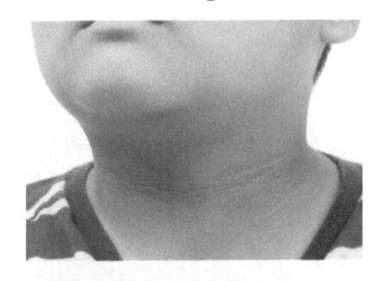

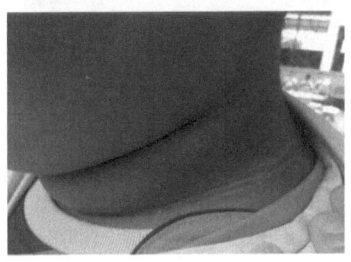

"Moon face" image reproduced under CC BY 2.5 from Celik O, Niyazoglu M, Soylu H, Kadioglu P. Iatrogenic Cushing's syndrome with inhaled steroid plus antidepressant drugs. *Multidiscip Respir Med*. 2012;7(1):26. Published 2012 Aug 29. doi:10.1186/2049-6958-7-26

CHAPTER 6: Medical and Physical Assessment **87**

- **Abdominal irregularities:** The physical examination must involve inspection for hernias, prior abdominal surgeries, and organomegaly, specifically hepatomegaly, which can be seen in metabolic dysfunction–associated steatotic liver disease.
- **Indicators of osteoarthritis:** Extremities should be assessed for edema, venous insufficiency, joint deformity, and abnormal gait that may indicate the presence of osteoarthritis, which can complicate obesity and impede mobility.[93]
- **Skin irregularities:** Examination of the skin is important, as it allows for visualization of skin infections in intertriginous areas, skin thinning, xanthomas, and excoriations.
    - Skin hyperpigmentation can be a sign of niacin deficiency.
    - Cheilitis, stomatitis, and glossitis can indicate vitamin B12 deficiency, with the latter two also being a manifestation of vitamin B6 deficiency.
    - Dermatitis can indicate niacin, vitamin A, and zinc deficiencies.
- **Motor and sensory abnormalities:** Motor and sensory abnormalities can also accompany vitamin deficiencies. Examples include a decrease in proprioception related to vitamin B12 deficiency, myopathy with vitamin E deficiency, and peripheral neuropathy with thiamin deficiency.

Laboratory Testing for Obesity

Laboratory testing aims to evaluate the patient for potential etiologies of obesity as well as obesity-related complications. The following laboratory studies and tests should be considered during the evaluation:

- **Complete blood count:** A complete blood count can reveal anemia and thrombocytopenia that may indicate underlying hepatic dysfunction.
- **Comprehensive metabolic panel:** A comprehensive metabolic panel may reveal evidence of underlying liver disease with elevated aminotransferase levels. In addition, an elevated serum blood glucose level may suggest type 2 diabetes, and an elevated creatinine level may indicate kidney dysfunction.
- **Anemia studies:** In the presence of anemia, iron studies, vitamin B12 level, and folate level can help define the type of anemia.
- **Tests for micronutrient deficiencies:** In the context of poor diet and other factors, as many as three-fourths of patients with obesity have underlying micronutrient deficiencies.[94] Revealing preexisting micronutrient deficiencies is extremely important when considering weight loss therapies that could potentially exacerbate such deficiencies. For example, fat-soluble vitamin deficiencies may be exacerbated with orlistat use and bariatric surgery.[95]
- **Thyroid function test:** Thyroid function should be assessed with a thyroid stimulating hormone (TSH) level.
- **Adrenal insufficiency screening:** When adrenal insufficiency is suspected, patients should undergo a corticotropin stimulation test.
- **Fasting lipid profile:** A fasting lipid profile can establish the presence of dyslipidemia alone or with metabolic syndrome. A diagnosis of metabolic syndrome requires the presence of at least three of the following five criteria:
    - fasting glucose level above 100 mg/dL
    - blood pressure higher than 130/85 mm Hg

- high-density lipoprotein cholesterol level below 40 mg/dL in males or below 50 mg/dL in females
- triglyceride level above 150 mg/dL
- waist circumference greater than 40 in (male) or 35 in (female)

- **Diabetes screening:** An HbA1c test can be used to screen for type 2 diabetes.[16]
- **Abdominal ultrasound:** Given the link between obesity and cholelithiasis, an abdominal ultrasound should be done in the presence of biliary symptoms. Hepatic steatosis may be incidentally detected on abdominal ultrasound for the evaluation of symptoms, and this may prompt further evaluation of the liver by modalities such as ultrasound or magnetic resonance elastography.
- **Electrocardiography:** Although not supported by evidence, in clinical practice obtaining an electrocardiogram can reveal signs of ventricular hypertrophy, arrythmias, and QTc prolongation, which are important to be aware of if the patient is considering treatment with the appetite suppressant phentermine for management of obesity.[96]
- **Polysomnography:** Polysomnography should be considered for patients in whom sleep apnea is suspected.
- **Gastric emptying assessment:** For patients considering the use of short-acting glucagon-like peptide 1 (GLP-1) receptor agonists to achieve weight loss, a gastric emptying assessment may help identify those with accelerated gastric emptying. Individuals with accelerated emptying are more likely to positively respond to short-acting GLP-1 receptor agonists via a decrease in gastric motility and decreased energy ingestion.[97]

It is important to collaborate with primary care physicians to assess for these comorbidities, so that appropriate referrals and follow-up are coordinated.[98]

Body Composition Profiling

Hydrostatic weighing is a tool for measuring body composition based on the Archimedes principle of density. This tool uses the difference between body weight in air and body weight in water to determine body density and fat composition. Hydrostatic weighing, however, is not routinely used in clinical practice, and a substantial proportion of patients with obesity have difficulty performing the water submersion.[99]

Skinfold thickness is an anthropometric measurement that can be used in the outpatient setting. To measure skinfold thickness, the clinician pinches the skin with calipers to assess regional fat composition. This technique assumes that fat content is equally distributed in the subcutaneous tissue; when thickness is low, this can indicate systemic nutritional deficiencies. It requires special competency on the part of the practitioner and needs further investigation to validate its utility.[100]

Dual-energy x-ray absorptiometry (DXA) scan is the gold standard for assessing bone density, but it is also a suitable method for assessing body fat percentage. DXA uses x-rays at two different energies to measure bone and tissue attenuation, for which it is more accurate than densitometry measurements.[101] DXA is also able to quantify lean mass and in other settings can be used for frailty assessment.[102] However, DXA is not routinely used in clinical practice because it cannot quantify visceral fat, is expensive, requires expertise, and involves radiation exposure. Fat-referenced magnetic resonance imaging, on the other hand, other than providing measurements that correspond to DXA scan measurements, can also provide quantification of visceral fat by automated image segmentation.[103] This modality is also not routinely used in clinical practice.

Bioimpedance methods are noninvasive ways to measure body cell mass and total body water, which are useful data for determining fat distribution. These methods take advantage of the flowing ions within intracellular and extracellular compartments to measure impedance or resistance by applying different frequencies.[104] These measures indicate areas containing fat and fat-sparing spaces, including visceral adipose tissue and segmental muscle mass, allowing for evaluation of both obesity and sarcopenia. Bioimpedance methods have the potential to be incorporated in clinical practice, given that they can be done quickly (in less than a minute); however, they are costly.[105]

Air-displacement plethysmography was validated in 1995 for measuring an object's volume by measuring the displacement of air volume inside a chamber.[106] In adults with obesity, this has proven to be reliable in measuring body fat percentage and was not substantially different when compared to hydrostatic weighing. However, when using air-displacement plethysmography as an assessment tool, body fat percentage was overestimated in females and underestimated in males, which may be secondary to the greater amount of hair in males than in females.[107]

Considerations When Working With Transgender Patients With Obesity

Certain aspects of physical and biochemical assessments are sex-specific and thus require unique considerations when working with patients who identify as transgender.[108] Practitioners should ask their patients the following two questions when collecting information for the patient history[109]:

1. What sex were you assigned at birth on your original birth certificate?
2. What is your current gender?

Practitioners can also inquire about the patient's preferred pronouns. If the patient's current gender differs from the sex assigned at birth, the practitioner should inquire about whether the patient is currently using masculinizing or feminizing hormone therapy, as this will affect sex-specific assessment criteria, and not everyone who identifies as transgender goes through the medical transition process using hormone therapy.

Weight gain is a common effect of hormone therapy for both transgender men (male gender identity and female birth-assigned sex) and transgender women (female gender identity and male birth-assigned sex).[110,111] Hormone therapy for transgender men tends to increase lean body mass and decrease fat mass, while hormone therapy for transgender women tends to decrease lean body mass and increase fat mass. Transgender men have greater rates of obesity and weight gain both before and during hormone therapy.

As there are no specific clinical guidelines for the assessment and treatment of transgender patients, the practitioner must use clinical judgment and sometimes consider data in ranges that combine both cisgender male and female reference values. Box 6.1 summarizes sex-specific data points to consider when assessing transgender patients seeking treatment for overweight or obesity.[108-113]

Bariatric Surgery Considerations

In the case of severe obesity, specifically in the case of patients with a BMI of 40 or higher, or a BMI of 35 to 40 with obesity-related comorbidities that are expected to improve with weight loss, bariatric surgery should be considered. Bariatric surgery is superior to medical therapy alone with respect to improvement in obesity-related comorbidities such as type 2 diabetes,[114] metabolic dysfunction–associated steatotic

BOX 6.1

Sex-Specific Data Points and Considerations for the Nutrition Assessment of Transgender Patients With Overweight or Obesity[108-113]

Assessment domain	Data points with sex-specific reference range	Considerations
Food and nutrition–related history	Energy needs	Be aware that predictive energy equations (eg, Mifflin-St Jeor) use sex as a variable.
		Use the sex assigned at birth, except when the patient has medically transitioned.
		Consider the patient's use of hormone therapy and stage of medical transition.
	Dietary Reference Intake for protein	Masculinizing hormone therapy increases muscle mass and the need for protein.
Anthropometric measures	Body fat percentage Waist circumference Waist-to-hip ratio BMI	Use the sex assigned at birth, except when the patient has medically transitioned.
		Body fat will decrease or increase with masculinizing or feminizing hormone therapy, respectively.
		It may be appropriate to use a combination of male and female ranges.
Biochemical data	Hemoglobin and hematocrit levels	Use the sex assigned at birth, except when the patient has medically transitioned.
		For patients on feminizing hormone therapy, use the female reference value for the lower limit of normal and the male reference value for the upper limit of normal.
		For patients on masculinizing hormone therapy, use the male reference value for the upper and lower limits of normal if the patient is amenorrheic.
Nutrition focused physical exam		Changes in muscle and fat mass are expected with a medical transition.

liver disease,[115] osteoarthritis, hypertension, cancer incidence, obstructive sleep apnea, and overall mortality.[116] Careful selection of patients for these procedures requires a series of assessments to ensure that the patient selected achieves durable weight loss as well as to improve mortality and ensure patient safety.[117]

The assessment of comorbidities and the physical examination in patients with obesity, as previously described, are paramount for patients considering bariatric surgery. A laboratory workup aims not only to identify etiologies of obesity but also to assess the patient's risk for surgery. In addition to the aforementioned evaluation for those with obesity, a prothrombin level, blood type and screening, urinalysis, *Helicobacter pylori* test, and age-appropriate cancer screening should also be completed prior to surgery.[117]

Evaluation by a registered dietitian nutritionist is critical, not only for assessing the patient's energy intake, level of hydration, and eating behaviors but also to help counsel the patient on healthy eating practices in order to maximize surgical outcomes. This evaluation may involve anthropometric measurements and a body fat composition examination. Because up to 76% of patients with obesity have micronutrient deficiencies that can potentially worsen postoperatively, evaluation for deficiencies in certain micronutrients (vitamin A, thiamin, vitamin D, vitamin E, vitamin K, copper, selenium, and zinc) should be undertaken.[94] Though some deficiencies may be easy to correct before surgery, a consistent pattern of vitamin deficiencies may require further workup for underlying malabsorptive conditions.[118]

Experts recommend a psychosocial evaluation to delineate the patient's motives, readiness, understanding, social support, suicide risk, and risky behaviors.[117] Tobacco history should be assessed, as smoking is associated with an extremely high risk of morbidity and mortality.[119] The psychosocial evaluation is especially helpful if there is a concern for substance abuse and underlying psychiatric illness, as it can help identify any additional therapy that the patient may need. The assessment should also include screening for eating disorders for which bariatric surgery patients are at increased risk, risk factors for postoperative weight regain, level of social support, and environmental risk factors that may contribute to negative postsurgical outcomes.[120,121]

A thorough preoperative risk assessment must be done in patients with obesity prior to bariatric and nonbariatric bariatric surgeries; however, the details of this assessment are beyond the scope of this chapter.

Summary

As the global prevalence of obesity has increased, so has that of its associated comorbid conditions. The socioeconomic dynamics surrounding the obesity epidemic include urban planning, food cost, and existing comorbidities, all of which influence the magnitude of the epidemic. Consequently, the stigma associated with obesity is increasing, yet little effort is made to address the factors that motivate weight gain.

Various medical organizations, such as the American Society for Metabolic and Bariatric Surgery, have made efforts to guide physicians and other health care practitioners in the care of patients with obesity. Their approach to assessing this patient population, as outlined in this chapter, goes beyond simply focusing on diet and exercise history and advocates for the holistic evaluation of patients. This holistic approach is accomplished through a comprehensive history and physical examination, which serves to uncover potential etiologies of obesity, characterize the degree of obesity via anthropometric measurements, and evaluate the medical impact of obesity. This assessment can also be applied to patients who qualify for bariatric surgery and, therefore, require an in-depth assessment of their nutritional status and presurgical anatomy. With a comprehensive evaluation, patients with obesity can be offered personalized treatment that can lead to a greater likelihood of success.

References

1. Warin M. The politics of disease: obesity in historical perspective. *Aust J Gen Pract*. 2019;48(10):728-731. doi:10.31128//AJGP-03-19-4878
2. Barnett R. Obesity. *Lancet*. 2005;365(9474):1843. doi:10.1016/S0140-6736(05)66604-4

3. Medicare changes policy on obesity. *Washington Post*. July 16, 2004. Accessed October 4, 2021. www.washingtonpost.com/wp-dyn/articles/A52835-2004Jul15.html
4. Kyle TK, Dhurandhar EJ, Allison DB. Regarding obesity as a disease: evolving policies and their implications. *Endocrinol Metab Clin North Am*. 2016;45(3):511. doi:10.1016/J.ECL.2016.04.004
5. Bleich SN, Pickett-Blakely O, Cooper LA. Physician practice patterns of obesity diagnosis and weight-related counseling. *Patient Educ Couns*. 2011;82(1):123-129. doi:10.1016/j.pec.2010.02.018
6. Bardia A, Holtan SG, Slezak JM, Thompson WG. Diagnosis of obesity by primary care physicians and impact on obesity management. *Mayo Clin Proc*. 2007;82(8):927-932. doi:10.4065/82.8.927
7. Galuska DA, Will JC, Serdula MK, Ford ES. Are health care professionals advising obese patients to lose weight? *J Am Med Assoc*. 1999;282(16):1576-1578. doi:10.1001/jama.282.16.1576
8. Lyznicki JM, Young DC, Riggs JA, Davis RM. Obesity: assessment and management in primary care. *Am Fam Physician*. 2001;63(11):2185-2196.
9. Hales CM, Carroll MD, Fryar CD, Ogden CL. *Prevalence of Obesity Among Adults and Youth: United States, 2015-2016*. NCHS Data Brief no. 288. National Center for Health Statistics; 2017. Accessed October 3, 2021. www.cdc.gov/nchs/products/databriefs/db288.htm
10. Hales CM, Carroll MD, Fryar CD, Ogden CL. *Prevalence of Obesity and Severe Obesity Among Adults: United States, 2017-2018*. NCHS Data Brief no. 360. National Center for Health Statistics; 2020. Accessed October 3, 2021. www.cdc.gov/nchs/products/databriefs/db360.htm
11. Dinsa G, Goryakin Y, Fumagalli E, Suhrcke M. Obesity and socioeconomic status in developing countries: a systematic review. *Obes Rev*. 2012;13(11):1067. doi:10.1111/J.1467-789X.2012.01017.X
12. Blüher M. Obesity: global epidemiology and pathogenesis. *Nat Rev Endocrinol*. 2019;15(5):288-298. doi:10.1038/s41574-019-0176-8
13. Biener A, Cawley J, Meyerhoefer C. The impact of obesity on medical care costs and labor market outcomes in the US. *Clin Chem*. 2018;64(1):108-117. doi:10.1373/CLINCHEM.2017.272450
14. Llewellyn A, Simmonds M, Owen CG, Woolacott N. Childhood obesity as a predictor of morbidity in adulthood: a systematic review and meta-analysis. *Obes Rev*. 2016;17(1):56-67. doi:10.1111/obr.12316
15. Güngör NK. Overweight and obesity in children and adolescents. *J Clin Res Pediatr Endocrinol*. 2014;6(3):129. doi:10.4274/JCRPE.1471
16. Norris T, Cole TJ, Bann D, et al. Duration of obesity exposure between ages 10 and 40 years and its relationship with cardiometabolic disease risk factors: a cohort study. *PLOS Med*. 2020;17(12):e1003387. doi:10.1371/JOURNAL.PMED.1003387
17. Lee L, Sanders RA. Metabolic syndrome. *Pediatr Rev*. 2012;33(10):459-468. doi:10.1542/pir.33-10-459
18. Owen CG, Whincup PH, Orfei L, et al. Is body mass index before middle age related to coronary heart disease risk in later life? Evidence from observational studies. *Int J Obes (Lond)*. 2009;33(8):866. doi:10.1038/IJO.2009.102
19. Abdullah A, Wolfe R, Stoelwinder JU, et al. The number of years lived with obesity and the risk of all-cause and cause-specific mortality. *Int J Epidemiol*. 2011;40(4):985-996. doi:10.1093/IJE/DYR018
20. Song M. Trajectory analysis in obesity epidemiology: a promising life course approach. *Curr Opin Endocr Metab Res*. 2019;4:37-41. doi:10.1016/J.COEMR.2018.08.002
21. Kushner RF, Batsis JA, Butsch WS, et al. Weight history in clinical practice: the state of the science and future directions. *Obesity*. 2020;28(1):9-17. doi:10.1002/oby.22642
22. Catalano PM, Tyzbir ED, Roman NM, Amini SB, Sims EAH. Longitudinal changes in insulin release and insulin resistance in nonobese pregnant women. *Am J Obstet Gynecol*. 1991;165(6 part 1):1667-1672. doi:10.1016/0002-9378(91)90012-G
23. Dennison RA, Chen ES, Green ME, et al. The absolute and relative risk of type 2 diabetes after gestational diabetes: a systematic review and meta-analysis of 129 studies. *Diabetes Res Clin Pract*. 2021;171. doi:10.1016/J.DIABRES.2020.108625

24. Catalano PM, Shankar K. Obesity and pregnancy: mechanisms of short term and long term adverse consequences for mother and child. *BMJ*. 2017;356:j1. doi:10.1136/BMJ.J1
25. Fraser A, Tilling K, Macdonald-Wallis C, et al. Associations of gestational weight gain with maternal body mass index, waist circumference, and blood pressure measured 16 y after pregnancy: the Avon Longitudinal Study of Parents and Children (ALSPAC). *Am J Clin Nutr*. 2011;93(6):1285-1292. doi:10.3945/ajcn.110.008326
26. Poston L, Caleyachetty R, Cnattingius S, et al. Preconceptional and maternal obesity: epidemiology and health consequences. *Lancet Diabetes Endocrinol*. 2016;4(12):1025-1036. doi:10.1016/S2213-8587(16)30217-0
27. Stefanska A, Bergmann K, Sypniewska G. Metabolic syndrome and menopause: pathophysiology, clinical and diagnostic significance. *Adv Clin Chem*. 2015;72:1-75. doi:10.1016/BS.ACC.2015.07.001
28. Lizcano F, Guzmán G. Estrogen deficiency and the origin of obesity during menopause. *Biomed Res Int*. 2014;2014:757461. doi:10.1155/2014/757461
29. Heine PA, Taylor JA, Iwamoto GA, Lubahn DB, Cooke PS. Increased adipose tissue in male and female estrogen receptor-α knockout mice. *Proc Natl Acad Sci U S A*. 2000;97(23):12729-12734. doi:10.1073/pnas.97.23.12729
30. Reinders I, Visser M, Schaap L. Body weight and body composition in old age and their relationship with frailty. *Curr Opin Clin Nutr Metab Care*. 2017;20(1):11-15. doi:10.1097/MCO.0000000000000332
31. Ponti F, Santoro A, Mercatelli D, et al. Aging and imaging assessment of body composition: from fat to facts. *Front Endocrinol (Lausanne)*. 2020;10:861. doi:10.3389/FENDO.2019.00861
32. Beaufrère B, Morio B. Fat and protein redistribution with aging: metabolic considerations. *Eur J Clin Nutr*. 2000;54(suppl 3):S48-S53. doi:10.1038/SJ.EJCN.1601025
33. Cutler D, Glaeser E, Shapiro J. Why have Americans become more obese? Working paper 9446. National Bureau of Economic Research. Issued January 2003. Accessed October 6, 2021. doi:10.3386/w9446
34. Moore LV, Diez Roux AV, Nettleton JA, Jacobs DR. Associations of the local food environment with diet quality—a comparison of assessments based on surveys and geographic information systems: the multi-ethnic study of atherosclerosis. *Am J Epidemiol*. 2008;167(8):917-924. doi:10.1093/aje/kwm394
35. Darmon N, Ferguson EL, Briend A. A cost constraint alone has adverse effects on food selection and nutrient density: an analysis of human diets by linear programming. *J Nutr*. 2002;132(12):3764-3771. doi:10.1093/jn/132.12.3764
36. Solmi F, Moreno AB, Lewis G, Angélica Nunes M, de Jesus Mendes da Fonseca M, Harter Griep R. Longitudinal association between binge eating and metabolic syndrome in adults: findings from the ELSA-Brasil cohort. *Acta Psychiatr Scand*. 2021;144(5):464-474. doi:10.1111/ACPS.13356
37. Duarte-Guerra LS, Kortchmar E, Maraviglia ECS, et al. Longitudinal patterns of comorbidity between anxiety, depression and binge eating symptoms among patients with obesity: a path analysis. *J Affect Disord*. 2022;303:255-263. doi:10.1016/J.JAD.2022.02.030
38. Morse SA, Ciechanowski PS, Katon WJ, Hirsch IB. Isn't this just bedtime snacking? The potential adverse effects of night-eating symptoms on treatment adherence and outcomes in patients with diabetes. *Diabetes Care*. 2006;29(8):1800-1804. doi:10.2337/dc06-0315
39. Bellisle F. Meals and snacking, diet quality and energy balance. *Physiol Behav*. 2014;134(C):38-43. doi:10.1016/j.physbeh.2014.03.010
40. Heriseanu AI, Hay P, Corbit L, Touyz S. Grazing in adults with obesity and eating disorders: a systematic review of associated clinical features and meta-analysis of prevalence. *Clin Psychol Rev*. 2017;58:16-32. doi:10.1016/J.CPR.2017.09.004
41. Swinburn BA, Sacks G, Hall KD, et al. The global obesity pandemic: shaped by global drivers and local environments. *Lancet*. 2011;378(9793):804-814. doi:10.1016/S0140-6736(11)60813-1
42. Cox AJ, West NP, Cripps AW. Obesity, inflammation, and the gut microbiota. *Lancet Diabetes Endocrinol*. 2015;3(3):207-215. doi:10.1016/S2213-8587(14)70134-2
43. Petridou A, Siopi A, Mougios V. Exercise in the management of obesity. *Metabolism*. 2019;92:163-169. doi:10.1016/j.metabol.2018.10.009
44. Verheggen RJHM, Maessen MFH, Green DJ, Hermus ARMM, Hopman MTE, Thijssen DHT. A systematic review and meta-analysis on the effects of exercise training versus hypocaloric diet: distinct effects on body weight and visceral adipose tissue. *Obes Rev*. 2016;17(8):664-690. doi:10.1111/obr.12406
45. Jakicic JM, Winters C, Lang W, Wing RR. Effects of intermittent exercise and use of home exercise equipment on adherence, weight loss, and fitness in overweight women a randomized trial. *J Am Med Assoc*. 1999;282(16):1554-1560. doi:10.1001/jama.282.16.1554
46. Zhang H, Tong TK, Kong Z, Shi Q, Liu Y, Nie J. Exercise training-induced visceral fat loss in obese women: the role of training intensity and modality. *Scand J Med Sci Sports*. 2021;31(1):30-43. doi:10.1111/sms.13803
47. Tao YX, Segaloff DL. Functional characterization of melanocortin-4 receptor mutations associated with childhood obesity. *Endocrinology*. 2003;144(10):4544-4551. doi:10.1210/en.2003-0524
48. Han JC, Lawlor DA, Kimm SY. Childhood obesity. *Lancet*. 2010;375(9727):1737-1748. doi:10.1016/S0140-6736(10)60171-7
49. Nieman LK. Diagnosis of Cushing's syndrome in the modern era. *Endocrinol Metab Clin North Am*. 2018;47(2):259-273. doi:10.1016/J.ECL.2018.02.001
50. Ventura-Aguiar P, Campistol JM, Diekmann F. Safety of mTOR inhibitors in adult solid organ transplantation. *Expert Opin Drug Saf*. 2016;15(3):303-319. doi:10.1517/14740338.2016.1132698

51. Sanyal D, Raychaudhuri M. Hypothyroidism and obesity: an intriguing link. *Indian J Endocrinol Metab*. 2016;20(4):554-557. doi:10.4103/2230-8210.183454
52. Patel S. Polycystic ovary syndrome (PCOS), an inflammatory, systemic, lifestyle endocrinopathy. *J Steroid Biochem Mol Biol*. 2018;182:27-36. doi:10.1016/j.jsbmb.2018.04.008
53. Singh S, Ricardo-Silgado ML, Bielinski SJ, Acosta A. Pharmacogenomics of medication-induced weight gain and antiobesity medications. *Obesity*. 2021;29(2):265-273. doi:10.1002/OBY.23068
54. Sax PE, Erlandson KM, Lake JE, et al. Weight gain following initiation of antiretroviral therapy: fisk factors in randomized comparative clinical trials. *Clin Infect Dis*. 2020;71(6):1379-1389. doi:10.1093/cid/ciz999
55. Lustig RH, Rose SR, Burghen GA, et al. Hypothalamic obesity caused by cranial insult in children: altered glucose and insulin dynamics and reversal by a somatostatin agonist. *J Pediatr*. 1999;135(2 pt 1):162-168. doi:10.1016/S0022-3476(99)70017-X
56. Maggio CA, Pi-Sunyer FX. Obesity and type 2 diabetes. *Endocrinol Metab Clin North Am*. 2003;32(4):805-822. doi:10.1016/S0889-8529(03)00071-9
57. Wilson PWF, D'Agostino RB, Sullivan L, Parise H, Kannel WB. Overweight and obesity as determinants of cardiovascular risk: the Framingham experience. *Arch Intern Med*. 2002;162(16):1867-1872. doi:10.1001/ARCHINTE.162.16.1867
58. Drager LF, Togeiro SM, Polotsky VY, Lorenzi-Filho G. Obstructive sleep apnea: a cardiometabolic risk in obesity and the metabolic syndrome. *J Am Coll Cardiol*. 2013;62(7):569. doi:10.1016/J.JACC.2013.05.045
59. Corica D, Aversa T, Valenzise M, et al. Does family history of obesity, cardiovascular, and metabolic diseases influence onset and severity of childhood obesity? *Front Endocrinol (Lausanne)*. 2018;9:187. doi:10.3389/fendo.2018.00187
60. Weiss R, Dziura J, Burgert TS, et al. Obesity and the metabolic syndrome in children and adolescents. *N Engl J Med*. 2004;350(23):2362-2374. doi:10.1056/nejmoa031049
61. Plachta-Danielzik S, Landsberg B, Johannsen M, Lange D, Mller MJ. Determinants of the prevalence and incidence of overweight in children and adolescents. *Public Health Nutr*. 2010;13(11):1870-1881. doi:10.1017/S1368980010000583
62. Clemmensen C, Petersen MB, Sørensen TIA. Will the COVID-19 pandemic worsen the obesity epidemic? *Nat Rev Endocrinol*. 2020;16(9):469-470. doi:10.1038/s41574-020-0387-z
63. Brondel L, Romer MA, Nougues PM, Touyarou P, Davenne D. Acute partial sleep deprivation increases food intake in healthy men. *Am J Clin Nutr*. 2010;91(6):1550-1559. doi:10.3945/ajcn.2009.28523
64. Swift DL, McGee JE, Earnest CP, Carlisle E, Nygard M, Johannsen NM. The effects of exercise and physical activity on weight loss and maintenance. *Prog Cardiovasc Dis*. 2018;61(2):206-213. doi:10.1016/j.pcad.2018.07.014
65. Patel SR, Hu FB. Short sleep duration and weight gain: a systematic review. *Obesity*. 2008;16(3):643-653. doi:10.1038/oby.2007.118
66. Zhu B, Shi C, Park CG, Zhao X, Reutrakul S. Effects of sleep restriction on metabolism-related parameters in healthy adults: a comprehensive review and meta-analysis of randomized controlled trials. *Sleep Med Rev*. 2019;45:18-30. doi:10.1016/j.smrv.2019.02.002
67. Chaput J-P. Short sleep duration promoting overconsumption of food: a reward-driven eating behavior? *Sleep*. 2010;33(9):1135-1136. doi:10.1093/SLEEP/33.9.1135
68. Nelson RJ, Chbeir S. Dark matters: effects of light at night on metabolism. *Proc Nutr Soc*. 2018;77(3):223-229. doi:10.1017/S0029665118000198
69. Ludwig J, Sanbonmatsu L, Gennetian L, et al. Neighborhoods, obesity, and diabetes—a randomized social experiment. *N Engl J Med*. 2011;365(16):1509-1519. doi:10.1056/nejmsa1103216
70. Bleich SN, Moran AJ, Vercammen KA, et al. Strengthening the public health impacts of the Supplemental Nutrition Assistance Program through policy. *Annu Rev Public Health*. 2020;41:453-480. doi:10.1146/annurev-publhealth-040119-094143
71. Kenney EL, Barrett JL, Bleich SN, Ward ZJ, Cradock AL, Gortmaker SL. Impact of the healthy, hunger-free kids act on obesity trends. *Health Aff*. 2020;39(7):1122-1129. doi:10.1377/hlthaff.2020.00133
72. Sinha R. Role of addiction and stress neurobiology on food intake and obesity. *Biol Psychol*. 2018;131:5-13. doi:10.1016/j.biopsycho.2017.05.001
73. Meule A, Reichenberger J, Blechert J. Smoking, stress eating, and body weight: the moderating role of perceived stress. *Subst Use Misuse*. 2018;53(13):2152-2156. doi:10.1080/10826084.2018.1461223
74. Banting W. Letter on corpulence, addressed to the public. *Obes Res*. 1993;1(2):153-163. doi:10.1002/J.1550-8528.1993.TB00605.X
75. Keys A, Fidanza F, Karvonen MJ, Kimura N, Taylor HL. Indices of relative weight and obesity. *J Chronic Dis*. 1972;25(6-7):329-343. doi:10.1016/0021-9681(72)90027-6
76. Anderson SE, Whitaker RC. Prevalence of obesity among US preschool children in different racial and ethnic groups. *Arch Pediatr Adolesc Med*. 2009;163(4):344-348. doi:10.1001/archpediatrics.2009.18
77. Curry SJ, Krist AH, Owens DK, et al. Behavioral weight loss interventions to prevent obesity-related morbidity and mortality in adults US Preventive Services Task Force recommendation statement. *JAMA*. 2018;320(11):1163-1171. doi:10.1001/jama.2018.13022
78. Javed AA, Aljied R, Allison DJ, Anderson LN, Ma J, Raina P. Body mass index and all-cause mortality in older adults: a scoping review of observational studies. *Obes Rev*. 2020;21(8):e13035. doi:10.1111/obr.13035
79. Defining adult overweight and obesity. Centers for Disease Control and Prevention website. Accessed October 6, 2021. www.cdc.gov/obesity/adult/defining.html

80. Physical status: the use and interpretation of anthropometry. Report of a WHO Expert Committee. *World Health Organ Tech Rep Ser*. 1995;854:1-452.

81. Di Angelantonio E, Bhupathiraju SN, Wormser D, et al. Body-mass index and all-cause mortality: individual-participant-data meta-analysis of 239 prospective studies in four continents. *Lancet*. 2016;388(10046):776-786. doi:10.1016/S0140-6736(16)30175-1

82. Gallagher D, Visser M, Sepúlveda D, Pierson RN, Harris T, Heymsfield SB. How useful is body mass index for comparison of body fatness across age, sex, and ethnic groups? *Am J Epidemiol*. 1996;143(3):228-239. doi:10.1093/oxfordjournals.aje.a008733

83. Fu J, Hofker M, Wijmenga C. Apple or pear: size and shape matter. *Cell Metab*. 2015;21(4):507-508. doi:10.1016/j.cmet.2015.03.016

84. Nishida C, Barba C, Cavalli-Sforza T, et al. Appropriate body-mass index for Asian populations and its implications for policy and intervention strategies. *Lancet*. 2004;363(9403):157-163. doi:10.1016/S0140-6736(03)15268-3

85. Snijder MB, van Dam RM, Visser M, Seidell JC. What aspects of body fat are particularly hazardous and how do we measure them? *Int J Epidemiol*. 2006;35(1):83-92. doi:10.1093/ije/dyi253

86. Després J-P. Body fat distribution and risk of cardiovascular disease. *Circulation*. 2012;126(10):1301-1313. doi:10.1161/circulationaha.111.067264

87. Bosomworth NJ. Normal-weight central obesity: unique hazard of the toxic waist. *Can Fam Physician*. 2019;65(6):399.

88. Lean ME, Han TS, Morrison CE. Waist circumference as a measure for indicating need for weight management. *BMJ*. 1995;311(6998):158-161. doi:10.1136/bmj.311.6998.158

89. Ross R, Neeland IJ, Yamashita S, et al. Waist circumference as a vital sign in clinical practice: a consensus statement from the IAS and ICCR Working Group on Visceral Obesity. *Nat Rev Endocrinol*. 2020;16(3):177-189. doi:10.1038/s41574-019-0310-7

90. Janssen I, Katzmarzyk PT, Ross R. Body mass index, waist circumference, and health risk: evidence in support of Current National Institutes of Health guidelines. *Arch Intern Med*. 2002;162(18):2074-2079. doi:10.1001/archinte.162.18.2074

91. Alzeidan R, Fayed A, Hersi AS, Elmorshedy H. Performance of neck circumference to predict obesity and metabolic syndrome among adult Saudis: a cross-sectional study. *BMC Obes*. 2019;6(1). doi:10.1186/s40608-019-0235-7

92. Chiu HY, Chen PY, Chuang LP, et al. Diagnostic accuracy of the Berlin questionnaire, STOP-BANG, STOP, and Epworth sleepiness scale in detecting obstructive sleep apnea: a bivariate meta-analysis. *Sleep Med Rev*. 2017;36:57-70. doi:10.1016/j.smrv.2016.10.004

93. Srivastava G, Kushner RF, Apovian CM. Use of the historical weight trajectory to guide an obesity-focused patient encounter. In: Feingold KR, Anawalt B, Boyce A, et al, eds. *Endotext* [internet]. MDText.com; 2000–. Updated April 16, 2019. Accessed October 6, 2021. www.ncbi.nlm.nih.gov/books/NBK541616

94. Weng TC, Chang CH, Dong YH, Chang YC, Chuang LM. Anaemia and related nutrient deficiencies after Roux-en-Y gastric bypass surgery: a systematic review and meta-analysis. *BMJ Open*. 2015;5(7):e006964. doi:10.1136/bmjopen-2014-006964

95. McDuffie JR, Calis KA, Booth SL, Uwaifo GI, Yanovski JA. Effects of orlistat on fat-soluble vitamins in obese adolescents. *Pharmacotherapy*. 2002;22(7):814-822. doi:10.1592/phco.22.11.814.33627

96. Jordan J, Astrup A, Engeli S, Narkiewicz K, Day WW, Finer N. Cardiovascular effects of phentermine and topiramate: a new drug combination for the treatment of obesity. *J Hypertens*. 2014;32(6):1178. doi:10.1097/HJH.0000000000000145

97. Acosta A, Camilleri M, Burton D, et al. Exenatide in obesity with accelerated gastric emptying: a randomized, pharmacodynamics study. *Physiol Rep*. 2015;3(11):e12610. doi:10.14814/phy2.12610

98. Kushner RF, Roth JL. Assessment of the obese patient. *Endocrinol Metab Clin North Am*. 2003;32(4):915-933. doi:10.1016/S0889-8529(03)00068-9

99. Heath EM, Adams TD, Daines MM, Hunt SC. Bioelectric impedance and hydrostatic weighing with and without head submersion in persons who are morbidly obese. *J Am Diet Assoc*. 1998;98(8):869-875. doi:10.1016/S0002-8223(98)00201-6

100. Ketel IJG, Volman MNM, Seidell JC, Stehouwer CDA, Twisk JW, Lambalk CB. Superiority of skinfold measurements and waist over waist-to-hip ratio for determination of body fat distribution in a population-based cohort of Caucasian Dutch adults. *Eur J Endocrinol*. 2007;156(6):655-661. doi:10.1530/EJE-06-0730

101. Bazzocchi A, Ponti F, Albisinni U, Battista G, Guglielmi G. DXA: technical aspects and application. *Eur J Radiol*. 2016;85(8):1481-1492. doi:10.1016/j.ejrad.2016.04.004

102. Chen LK, Woo J, Assantachai P, et al. Asian Working Group for Sarcopenia: 2019 consensus update on sarcopenia diagnosis and treatment. *J Am Med Dir Assoc*. 2020;21(3):300-307.e2. doi:10.1016/j.jamda.2019.12.012

103. Borga M, West J, Bell JD, et al. Advanced body composition assessment: from body mass index to body composition profiling. *J Investig Med*. 2018;66:887-895. doi:10.1136/jim-2018-000722

104. Jaffrin MY, Morel H. Body fluid volumes measurements by impedance: a review of bioimpedance spectroscopy (BIS) and bioimpedance analysis (BIA) methods. *Med Eng Phys*. 2008;30(10):1257-1269. doi:10.1016/j.medengphy.2008.06.009

105. Hanna DJ, Jamieson ST, Lee CS, et al. Bioelectrical impedance analysis in managing sarcopenic obesity in NAFLD. *Obes Sci Pract*. 2021;7(5):629-645. doi:10.1002/osp4.509

106. Fields DA, Goran MI, McCrory MA. Body-composition assessment via air-displacement plethysmography in adults and children: a review. *Am J Clin Nutr.* 2002;75(3):453-467. doi:10.1093/ajcn/75.3.453
107. Biaggi RR, Vollman MW, Nies MA, et al. Comparison of air-displacement plethysmography with hydrostatic weighing and bioelectrical impedance analysis for the assessment of body composition in healthy adults. *Am J Clin Nutr.* 1999;69(5):898-903. doi:10.1093/ajcn/69.5.898
108. Linsenmeyer L, Garwood S, Waters, J. An examination of the sex-specific nature of nutrition assessment within the nutrition care process: considerations for nutrition and dietetics practitioners working with transgender and gender diverse clients. *J Acad Nutr Diet.* 2022;122(6):1081-1086. doi:10.1016/j.jand.2022.02.014
109. National Academies of Sciences, Engineering, and Medicine. *Measuring Sex, Gender Identity, and Sexual Orientation.* National Academies Press; 2022. doi:10.17226/26424
110. Kyinn M, Banks K, Leemaqz SY, Sarkodie E, Goldstein D, Irwig MS. Weight gain and obesity rates in transgender and gender-diverse adults before and during hormone therapy. *Int J Obes (Lond).* 2021;45(12):2562-2569. doi:10.1038/s41366-021-00935-x
111. USCF Transgender Care, Department of Family and Community Medicine, University of California San Francisco. *Guidelines for the Primary and Gender-Affirming Care of Transgender and Gender Nonbinary People.* 2nd ed. Deutsch MB, ed. June 2016. Accessed July 19, 2022. https://transcare.ucsf.edu/guidelines
112. Academy of Nutrition and Dietetics. Transgender nutrition scoping review (2020). Evidence Analysis Library. Accessed June 30, 2022. www.andeal.org/topic.cfm?menu=6062
113. Rozga M, Linsenmeyer W, Cantwell Wood J, Darst V, Gradwell EK. Hormone therapy, health outcomes and the role of nutrition in transgender individuals: a scoping review. *Clin Nutr ESPEN.* 2020;40:42-56. doi:10.1016/j.clnesp.2020.08.011
114. Schauer PR, Bhatt DL, Kirwan JP, et al. Bariatric surgery versus intensive medical therapy for diabetes—5-year outcomes. *N Engl J Med.* 2017;376(7):641-651. doi:10.1056/nejmoa1600869
115. Lassailly G, Caiazzo R, Ntandja-Wandji LC, et al. Bariatric surgery provides long-term resolution of nonalcoholic steatohepatitis and regression of fibrosis. *Gastroenterology.* 2020;159(4):1290-1301.e5. doi:10.1053/j.gastro.2020.06.006
116. Lemanu DP, Singh PP, Rahman H, Hill AG, Babor R, MacCormick AD. Five-year results after laparoscopic sleeve gastrectomy: a prospective study. *Surg Obes Relat Dis.* 2015;11(3):518-524. doi:10.1016/J.SOARD.2014.08.019
117. Mechanick JI, Apovian C, Brethauer S, et al. Clinical practice guidelines for the perioperative nutrition, metabolic, and nonsurgical support of patients undergoing bariatric procedures—2019 update: cosponsored by American Association of Clinical Endocrinologists/American College of Endocrinology, The Obesity Society, American Society for Metabolic and Bariatric Surgery, Obesity Medicine Association, and American Society of Anesthesiologists—executive summary. *Endocr Pract.* 2019;25(12):1346-1359. doi:10.4158/GL-2019-0406
118. Cotterell AH, Fisher RA, King AL, et al. Calcineurin inhibitor-induced chronic nephrotoxicity in liver transplant patients is reversible using rapamycin as the primary immunosuppressive agent. *Clin Transplant.* 2002;16(suppl 7):49-51. doi:10.1034/j.1399-0012.16.s7.7.x
119. Haskins IN, Amdur R, Vaziri K. The effect of smoking on bariatric surgical outcomes. *Surg Endosc.* 2014;28(11):3074-3080. doi:10.1007/S00464-014-3581-Z
120. Chao AM, Wadden TA, Faulconbridge LF, et al. Binge-eating disorder and the outcome of bariatric surgery in a prospective, observational study: two-year results. *Obesity.* 2016;24(11):2327-2333. doi:10.1002/oby.21648
121. Flores CA. Psychological assessment for bariatric surgery: current practices. *Arq Bras Cir Dig.* 2014;27(suppl 1):59. doi:10.1590/S0102-6720201400S100015

CHAPTER 7

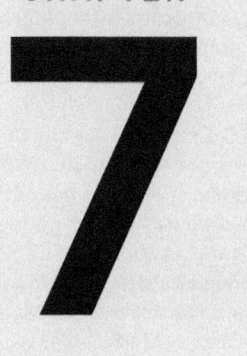

Nutrition Assessment

Maya K. Vadiveloo, PhD, RD, FAHA

CHAPTER OBJECTIVES

- Review methods used to establish energy requirements with considerations for a patient's goal of weight loss.
- Identify methods of dietary assessment and factors to consider with use in outpatient settings.
- Discuss the assessment of food access, food security, and sociocultural factors, and their relationship to dietary intake.
- Review the nutrition focused physical exam, with emphasis on the patient with overweight or obesity.

Introduction

Dietary assessment is an integral part of clinical weight management and the nutrition focused physical exam (NFPE). Although objective measures, including body composition and cardiometabolic risk factors, are critical components of clinical weight management, the overreliance on these measures can undermine the importance of dietary intake and quality, while overemphasizing the importance of weight. This chapter takes a holistic approach to clinical weight management by addressing multiple aspects of diet and weight loss. First, the chapter describes best practices for estimating individual energy requirements and how weight loss and weight loss maintenance affect the thermodynamics of energy balance. Next, the pros and cons of different dietary assessment methods are discussed, as well as considerations for selecting the best method based on an individual patient's needs and goals at the start of dietary counseling. Lastly, because diet is the complex product of many influences, this chapter addresses the impact of the broader food environment and sociocultural factors on nutrition security and how to discuss these determinants of diet quality with patients when conducting a nutrition assessment.

Establishing Energy Requirements

The accurate estimation of energy requirements is an essential aspect of weight management that can facilitate individual recommendations for achieving energy balance. The body's energy requirements are determined by three main factors: the basal metabolic rate (BMR), which can be thought of as "the cost of living"; the thermic effect of food, which accounts for roughly 10% of energy requirements; and activity thermogenesis, the most variable part of energy expenditure that encompasses both physical activity and nonexercise activity (eg, fidgeting) and accounts for approximately 20% to 40% of energy needs.[1] Notably, BMR is largely influenced by lean body mass, which may change with weight loss.

Measurement of Resting Energy Expenditure

The gold standard for measuring energy requirements under real-world conditions is the "doubly labeled water" technique, which is highly precise but also relatively expensive and places a high burden on the patient. In this method, adults who are in energy balance are given a measured amount of water that contains heavy isotopes of both oxygen and hydrogen. As these isotopes are subsequently secreted in urine and saliva over several days, measurements are taken and the patient's energy utilization is calculated using validated equations.

Indirect calorimetry is another highly precise but expensive and burdensome method for measuring resting energy expenditure (REE), which is highly correlated with BMR. Indirect calorimetry measurements are typically taken in a laboratory setting by measuring the exchange of oxygen and carbon dioxide during respiration for a specified period. Typically, this is done with metabolic carts in hospital settings or with newer portable technology in clinics and gyms.

Estimation of Resting Energy Expenditure

Alternatively, REE can be estimated using the validated Mifflin-St Jeor equation, originally validated for use in healthy normal-weight and moderately overweight individuals.[1] The Mifflin-St Jeor equation is recommended for use in adults with obesity with the caveat that certain factors may reduce the accuracy of this equation for adults with more than class 3 obesity.[2-5] The Mifflin-St Jeor equation for estimating REE is as follows[†]:

Male: (10 × weight [kg]) + (6.25 × height [cm]) − (5 × age [y]) + 5

Female: (10 × weight [kg]) + (6.25 × height [cm]) − (5 × age [y]) − 161

Although sometimes still used, the older Harris-Benedict equations are considered less accurate and, therefore, are not recommended for estimating energy needs.[1]

Estimation of Total Energy Expenditure

Estimate total daily energy expenditure (TDEE) by multiplying a patient's REE by an activity factor, such as 1.2 (sedentary), 1.55 (moderately active), or 1.725 (very active).[6] Activity factors are estimates, and specific guidelines for physical activity can vary; thus clinical judgement is warranted in applying activity factors to estimated REE. Broadly, adults are classified as moderately active if they engage in 150 min/wk of moderate-intensity physical activity (eg, brisk walking, cycling, raking leaves) or 75 min/wk of vigorous physical activity (eg, running, swimming laps, aerobic exercise classes).[1] Adults are classified as very active if they exceed those thresholds and engage in up to 300 min/wk of moderate-intensity physical activity or 150 min/wk of vigorous physical activity.[1] Overestimation of physical activity is common, so it is helpful to explain the activities associated with each factor to the patient.

In 2023 the National Academies of Sciences published updated Dietary References Intakes for Energy,[7] noting that the physical activity factors cited above do not remain constant through the life cycle. Most variation is found in the first 20 years of life. The Dietary Reference Intake equations incorporate age into the physical activity categories to provide estimates of TDEE. The National Academies of Sciences, Engineering, and Medicine emphasize identifying the correct physical activity level. While overweight and obesity can increase the risk for chronic disease states, there are no modifications outlined for those with overweight or obesity.[7] TDEE equations for adults are listed in Box 7.1 on page 100.[7]

Notably, TDEE requirements may vary by more than 100 kcal depending on the equation and physical activity level selected, so careful monitoring of body weight is warranted when using predictive energy equations to estimate energy needs.

---

† Equations for transgender individuals were not provided.

BOX 7.1

Total Daily Energy Expenditure for Adults[a,b,7]

Male, inactive	753.07 − (10.83 × age[c]) + (6.50 × height[d]) + (14.10 × weight[e])
Male, low active	581.47 − (10.83 × age) + (8.30 × height) + (14.94 × weight)
Male, active	1,004.82 − (10.83 × age) + (6.52 × height) + (15.91 × weight)
Male, very active	−517.88 − (10.83 × age) + (15.61 × height) + (19.11 × weight)
Female, inactive	584.90 − (7.01 × age) + (5.72 × height) + (11.71 × weight)
Female, low active	575.77 − (7.01 × age) + (6.60 × height) + (12.14 × weight)
Female, active	710.25 − (7.01 × age) + (6.54 × height) + (12.34 × weight)
Female, very active	511.83 − (7.01 × age) + (9.07 × height) + (12.56 × weight)

Total energy expenditure in kilocalories per day.
[a] Adults aged 19 years and above.
[b] Equations for transgender individuals were not provided
[c] Age in years
[d] Height in centimeters
[e] Weight in kilograms

Special Considerations for Energy Adjustments for Weight Change

The Mifflin-St Jeor equation plus an activity factor remain the most frequently cited predictive equations for estimating TDEE in adult patients with obesity; nevertheless, they are not ideal, and if more precision is required for dietary intervention planning, experts recommend indirect calorimetry.[2] Furthermore, if health care providers are estimating TDEE to facilitate weight loss efforts, they should attempt to use tools that incorporate more sophisticated modeling of how dynamic changes in energy balance influence body weight.[8] With growing recognition of the complex metabolic, hormonal, and neurochemical adaptations associated with obesity,[9] it is essential that providers who assess TDEE to facilitate weight loss do so as accurately as possible. In addition, registered dietitian nutritionists (RDNs) should avoid perpetuating the myth that a mere energy deficit of 500 kcal/d will produce 1 lb (0.45 kg) of weight loss per week.[10] Such gross oversimplification, particularly with respect to long-term weight loss (in which case the laws of thermodynamics modify this equation), may inhibit rapport between patients and RDNs and set unrealistic expectations that ultimately promote reduced adherence to dietary and lifestyle recommendations.

In 2011, a team at the National Institute of Diabetes and Digestive and Kidney Diseases published the research behind an online tool known as the Body Weight Planner.[8,11] This tool accounts for the dynamic changes in energy balance that occur in response to energy-expenditure adaptations that happen during weight loss and weight loss maintenance. For example, suppose a clinician is counseling a 50-year-old female patient who currently weighs 180 lb (81.8 kg) and is 5 ft 6 in (168 cm) tall (BMI 29). This patient engages in light daily activity and would like to lose 20 lb (9.1 kg) in the next 3 months. The Body Weight Planner can help balance her food and activity based on her preferences and lifestyle. If she wants to increase her physical activity by 50%, her daily energy-intake goal will be 1,733 kcal for weight loss (2,330 kcal for weight maintenance). Once she achieves her goal weight, she can maintain her weight at 160 lb (72.7 kg) by consuming 2,522 kcal/d. This example is illustrated in Figure 7.1.[11]

However, if the patient elects to maintain her current light daily activity level, her daily energy-intake goal will reduce to 1,404 kcal/d for weight loss; and once she achieves her desired weight loss, she can maintain her 160 lb weight by consuming 2,154 kcal/d. The difference in energy needs after weight loss reflects the projected changes in body composition associated with changes in fat and lean mass, which vary according to amount of energy expended in physical activity and maintenance of lean body mass.

Without more in-depth assessment of body composition, the Body Weight Planner models the expected changes to lean and fat mass and concomitant BMR associated with reductions in energy intake and increases in physical activity.[8] Precise modeling of both REE and the energy cost of physical-activity change in response to weight loss can make energy reduction and physical-activity targets for weight loss more accurate.[12] The Body Weight Planner may also be used to elicit patient goals with respect to dietary and physical-activity changes. Because reductions in energy intake compared to increases in physical activity have different effects on the predicted rate of weight loss, patients can identify what changes are feasible given their lifestyle and have a more realistic understanding of how those

FIGURE 7.1 Sample use of the Body Weight Planner[11]

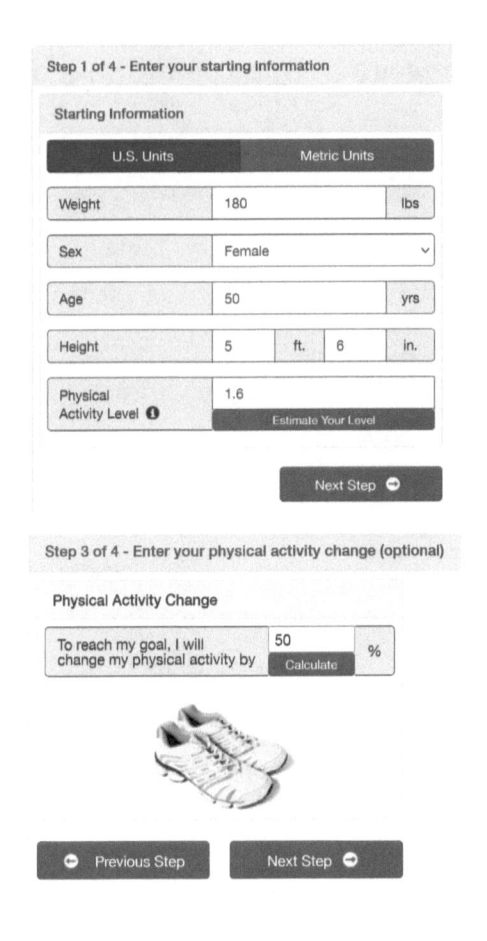

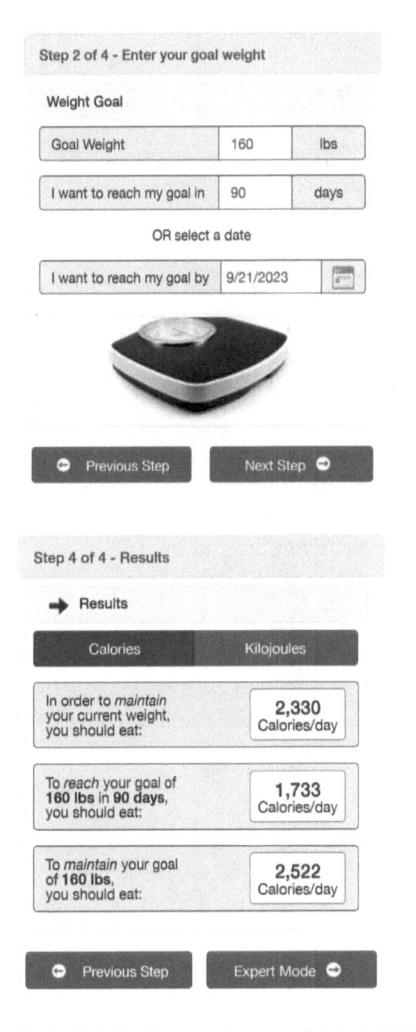

Reproduced from National Institute of Diabetes and Digestive and Kidney Diseases. Body Weight Planner. Accessed July 1, 2022. www.niddk.nih.gov/bwp.[11]

changes may affect their long-term body weight trajectory. For example, increasing physical activity can preserve or increase lean body mass, which is more metabolically active and thus helps to preserve BMR relative to energy restriction. Some research suggests that maintaining high levels of physical activity at a reduced body weight is important for long-term maintenance of weight loss.[13]

Methods of Dietary Assessment

Dietary assessment is integral to measuring dietary patterns and counseling patients about dietary approaches for weight management. Because most forms of dietary assessment rely on some degree of self-report, there are pros and cons to most established methods. These pros and cons require consideration when assessing diet in clinical and research settings. They are summarized in Box 7.2.[14-25]

BOX 7.2

Advantages and Disadvantages of Commonly Used Dietary Assessment Methods[14-25]

Dietary assessment method	Advantages	Disadvantages	Type of information collected
24-hour recall	Freely available Allows for reporting of all foods Low participant burden Low level of literacy required	Relies on memory With insufficient number of days, may not reflect usual intake Social desirability bias (desire to respond in a socially acceptable way)	Number of meals and snacks Frequency of eating Timing of meals and snacks Unique foods consumed Food and nutrient intake
24-hour recall with Automated Self-Administered 24-Hour Dietary Assessment Tool (ASA24)[17]	Uses the Automated Multiple-Pass Method, which improves accuracy of recall Automatically calculates Healthy Eating Index scores	Time-consuming for multiple days of recall Requires access to a computer or smartphone	Number of meals and snacks Frequency of eating Timing of meals and snacks Unique foods consumed Food and nutrient intake
Food diary (3-day, 4-day, or 7-day)	Eliminates reliance on memory Can be used for self-monitoring Allows for reporting of all foods	Cost of linking to a nutrient database Potential for reactivity (ie, changes in diet due to logging) Potential for forgetting to record food Social desirability bias	Number of meals and snacks Timing of meals and snacks Unique foods consumed Food, food group, and nutrient intake

Box continues

BOX 7.2 (CONTINUED)

Dietary assessment method	Pros	Cons	Type of information collected
Food frequency questionnaire[18,19]	Relatively inexpensive Measures usual intake over periods ranging from 1 month to 1 year	Relatively high level of measurement error and recall bias Burdensome to participants Finite list of foods, and may not contain all foods consumed by a target population	Food group and nutrient intake Food variety
Food photography[15]	Low participant burden Eliminates recall bias when foods are photographed at the time of consumption Can use common objects as size references to enhance portion-size estimation	Requires linkage to nutrient database Potentially poor image quality May require participants to provide additional recipe details Potential for forgetting to photograph food	Number of meals and snacks Timing of meals and snacks Unique foods consumed and composition Food, food group, and nutrient intake
Biomarkers[20-24]	Provides measure of intake and bioavailability within the body Does not rely on self-reporting	Expensive More appropriate for short-term intake More appropriate for individual nutrients rather than dietary patterns Used mainly in research settings, though the Veggie Meter skin carotenoid indicator is affordable for clinical use	Food or nutrient utilization Relative intake of nutrient-containing foods
Dietary screeners[16,25]	Inexpensive and quick Freely available (eg, the National Cancer Institute's All-Day Screener) May provide a snapshot of a few dietary behaviors	Imprecise Not possible to link to nutrient intake	Intake frequency Semiquantitative serving of included food groups

Energy intake is an essential component of energy balance that is difficult to assess accurately. Self-reported intake measured using standard methods, such as the 24-hour recall, food frequency questionnaire (FFQ), or food diary, even when supplemented with food photographs, are notoriously inaccurate with respect to measuring energy intake.[26] Nevertheless, self-reported dietary assessments can validly measure dietary quality and reveal important information about people's dietary behaviors, including the timing of when they eat and the macronutrient composition of the diet.[14] Moreover, when food, mood, and hunger logs are used, they may reveal important triggers for eating certain foods or exceeding recommendations for total energy intake.[27] With mobile technologies now in wider use, many of these tools have been adapted for smartphones and can be used with ecological momentary assessment (EMA) protocols to assist individuals in trying to adhere to reduced-energy dietary patterns.[28,29] Greater use of mobile technologies and EMA protocols may enhance the accuracy of conventional dietary assessment methods, while also reducing participant burden.[15,30]

Food diaries tend to increase people's awareness of what they are consuming, providing insights into their dietary choices and "mindless" eating.[16] Research from the National Weight Control Registry and other studies of long-term weight loss show that self-monitoring, including food tracking, can be an important component of adherence to reduced-energy diet patterns; thus, food diaries continue to be valuable with dietary interventions.[31] Despite the imperfections associated with diet assessment, it is essential to start the conversation about diet across clinical settings in a manner that minimizes weight stigma.[16]

Dietary Assessment Across Clinical Settings

The 24-hour dietary recall is considered a gold-standard method of dietary assessment, particularly when used over multiple days and with newer technologies such as the Automated Self-Administered 24-Hour Dietary Assessment Tool (ASA24).[17] The ASA24 is a freely available, validated, online tool (https://epi.grants.cancer.gov/asa24/) that can be used to collect dietary data for research studies as well as for individuals. Some benefits of the ASA24 are that it employs the Automated Multiple-Pass Method (used in the National Health and Nutrition Examination Survey), which can improve the accuracy of recall. In addition, because ASA24 food codes are linked to the US Department of Agriculture's Food and Nutrient Database for Dietary Studies (FNDDS), ASA24 data can be used to calculate Healthy Eating Index scores,[32] which are a common measure of adherence to the US Dietary Guidelines for Americans. As a free tool linked to the FNDDS, ASA24 can reduce the costs associated with dietary assessment.

Food diaries and records, whether on paper, online, or in mobile-based formats, remain useful tools for tracking diet quality.[33] Many mobile apps utilize machine learning, which can reduce participant burden over time. For example, if someone habitually drinks coffee with a quarter cup of reduced-fat milk in the morning, internet-based or mobile food diaries may prepopulate that person's list of favorite foods accordingly or confirm that the person did not drink coffee on a given day if it was not entered in the food log. Nevertheless, caution is warranted with respect to precisely estimating energy, macronutrient intake, or micronutrient intake using these methods.[34]

The method of dietary assessment selected depends on the dietary information needed. For example, 24-hour recalls and food records provide information on eating frequency, number of meals and snacks, and timing of eating—whereas FFQs and biomarkers (indicators of nutritional status often related to the intake or metabolism of foods and nutrients) do not. FFQs and biomarkers provide information about a person's usual intake and nutrient utilization, respectively, which may be necessary in some cases. Other considerations when choosing a method of dietary assessment include the available resources, patient characteristics (24-hour recall is beneficial for those with low literacy levels), patient burden, and goals of dietary assessment. Notably, food diaries support self-monitoring efforts, which is important for achieving long-term dietary changes.[35]

In addition to the more comprehensive dietary screening tools already described, brief dietary screening tools are also available that can be valuable in clinical settings. More frequent dietary screening in clinical settings can increase referrals to RDNs for individuals who require more intensive dietary counseling for weight loss. Furthermore, it can enhance recommendations for evidence-based dietary strategies that promote cardiometabolic health, potentially reducing the influence of nutrition misinformation on people's dietary habits. Though the screening tool selected may vary with practice setting, brief dietary screening in primary care settings by other clinicians and members of the health care team may enhance clinical practice for RDNs.[16] In addition, some evidence suggests that simple dietary guidance using results from a dietary screener in a mobile-health intervention can still promote positive dietary changes.[36]

Beyond food intake, many other factors related to diet and health behaviors should be assessed when evaluating a patient's diet. These elements are summarized in Box 7.3 on page 106.[37-40]

Food Access, Food Security, and Dietary Intake

Food choice, dietary intake, and diet quality are shaped by many factors in our broader food environment, making it essential for RDNs to assess various social and environmental determinants of diet quality and health. Food security is defined by the United Nations Committee on World Food Security to mean that, "all people, at all times, have physical, social, and economic access to sufficient, safe, and nutritious food that meets their food preferences and dietary needs for an active and healthy life."[41] This holistic definition underscores the global and complex nature of food security, which is influenced by climate change, agricultural practices, and global food trade and policy, as well as food prices, food availability and access, and food processing. Yet, at the personal level, this definition reminds clinicians that an individual's ability to consume a healthy dietary pattern is markedly affected by income, food availability and cost, and varied cultural preferences. Although screening tools for food insecurity, such as the US Household Food Security Survey Module are available for clinical use,[40,42] starting a conversation with patients about the broader dimensions of food access and availability may be helpful before making dietary recommendations.

Food access and availability are often overlooked dimensions of food security. More recently, the importance of assessing nutrition security ("an individual or household condition of having equitable and stable availability access, affordability, and utilization of foods and beverages that promote well-being and prevent and treat disease") rather than *food security* has gained recognition, given that diet is the leading contributor to cardiometabolic disease.[43] Processed, energy-dense foods, most of which are heavily marketed, shelf-stable, highly palatable, and inexpensive due to their subsidized production, are widely available in the broader food environment (and, hence, promote excess consumption) and are implicated in obesity.[44] In comparison, foods that are less energy-dense and more nutrient-rich, such as fruits and vegetables, are more expensive, often unavailable, perishable, and require more preparation, all of which contribute to making them less frequently consumed.

BOX 7.3

Additional Elements of Dietary Assessment Beyond Food Intake[37-40]

Factors to consider	Specific components
Food allergies and intolerances	Nine major food allergens (peanuts, tree nuts, egg, soy, milk, wheat, fish, shellfish, and sesame)
	Other food allergies or intolerances
	Celiac disease
	Lactose intolerance
Dietary restrictions	Vegan, vegetarian, pescatarian, plant-based, or other
	Intermittent fasting
	Paleo, keto, or other diet trends
Alcohol use	Frequency of alcohol consumption
	Type of alcohol consumed
	Amount of alcohol consumed
Dietary behaviors	Appetite
	Food cravings
	Dietary restraint, disinhibition, and hunger[37]
	Usual dietary patterns and typical intake
	Frequency of eating out at restaurants
	Eating competence[38]
	Support system
Nutrition knowledge and cooking skills	Nutrition self-efficacy
	Nutrition knowledge
	Cooking ability
	Fluency with reading food labels
Nutrition history	Prior diet or weight loss attempts
	Food beliefs
	Beliefs about how to successfully lose weight
Cultural preferences	Food sovereignty and availability of culturally appropriate foods[39]
Sleep habits	Average number of hours of sleep per day
Smoking and vaping	Current smoking status
	Frequency of use of tobacco products

Box continues

BOX 7.3 (CONTINUED)

Factors to consider	Specific components
Weight and health goals	Weight history
	Motivation for weight loss
	Weight loss goals
	Health goals
Food insecurity and participation in nutrition assistance programs	US Household Food Security Survey Module: Six-Item Short Form[40] (www.ers.usda.gov/topics/food-nutrition-assistance/food-security-in-the-u-s/survey-tools/#six)
	Participation in food and nutrition assistance programs, such as the Supplemental Nutrition Assistance Program (SNAP); Special Supplemental Nutrition Program for Women, Infants, and Children (WIC); and others
	Access to health care
Supplement and medication use	Protein supplements
	Multivitamin and mineral supplements
	Herbal or other over-the-counter supplements for weight loss
	Medications that affect appetite or metabolic parameters (eg, statins, oral hypoglycemic agents, insulin, semaglutide)
Readiness for change	Stage of change: precontemplation, contemplation, preparation, action, maintenance
	Patient goals and desired outcome
Physical activity	Types of physical activity enjoyed
	Average amount of time per day spent engaged in moderate and vigorous physical activity at work, school, home, and for leisure
	Screen time (computer, smartphone, television)

Impact of the Food Environment on Diet Quality

Food policies that subsidize the production and promotion of processed, energy-dense foods have direct effects in the neighborhoods where people live and work. Neighborhoods deemed "food swamps" or "food deserts" have an overabundance of retail outlets that sell shelf-stable, energy-dense, packaged foods and a limited number of grocery stores or other retailers that sell a wide variety of less energy-dense, minimally processed foods. As a result, it is challenging for many individuals to find affordable options that meet their dietary preferences and health needs. The effects of unhealthy food environments on diet quality are further exacerbated in lower-income households if access to convenient, reliable transportation and food preparation and cooking facilities are also affected. Moreover, when issues of food security intersect with varied cultural preferences among populations of color, it contributes to lower diet quality and health disparities among these groups.[39]

The pivotal role of food environments in shaping dietary choices and cardiometabolic health is gaining greater recognition.[45] Several recent reviews describe validated tools that can be used to measure multiple dimensions, ranging from geographic to individual perception of the environment.[46-48] One widely used tool, the Nutrition Environment Measures Survey (NEMS, https://nems-upenn.org), is frequently used to evaluate the availability and pricing of healthy and unhealthy foods in retail outlets and restaurants. Although health care professionals working in clinical or private-practice settings may not need to use validated food environment measures to counsel patients undergoing weight loss, greater discussion of the broader contextual factors that shape diet quality and energy intake is warranted.

Ultraprocessed Foods

Paralleling the general concern with wider availability of energy-dense, nutrient-poor foods is the growing domestic and global availability of ultraprocessed foods. The Ministry of Health of Brazil and the American Heart Association recommend choosing minimally processed foods and minimizing the intake of ultraprocessed foods to promote cardiometabolic health, based on research linking excess consumption of ultraprocessed foods with metabolic dysregulation.[49,50] Though specific assessment tools do not exist to measure the proportion of ultraprocessed foods in an individual's diet, it may be valuable for RDNs and other health care providers to discuss the level of food processing with patients seeking to lose weight.[51]

The NOVA classification system was developed to classify foods according to the extent and purpose of food processing they undergo.[52,53] While there is no widely accepted definition of *ultraprocessed*, the NOVA definition is used most frequently and refers to industrially manufactured, ready-to-eat (or ready-to-heat) formulations that contain foods with little or no whole foods and ingredients.[52,53] Concerns around the growing proportion of energy intake from ultraprocessed foods in both children and adults are detailed in a review.[54] Energy from ultraprocessed foods displaces energy from minimally processed foods that are less energy-dense and that are associated with higher diet quality, satiety, and, often, weight loss. In addition, there is some evidence that packaging materials used to produce these foods may have endocrine-disrupting chemicals that leach into foods and affect body weight, appetite, and energy balance.[54] Food processing may also disrupt characteristics of the food matrix, potentially resulting in unintended adverse health effects, including lipid dysregulation, insulin resistance, and other metabolic derangements. Some of the putative short-term and long-term health effects of ultraprocessed foods may be partly mediated by alterations to the gut microbiota, which has been increasingly implicated in appetite regulation.

Sociocultural Factors Affecting Diet

Closely related to issues of food security are dietary preferences and health behaviors and beliefs that are influenced by a person's culture or their ethnic identity, or both (eg, Asian American, Puerto Rican, African American, or other). Individuals with strong ties to cultural food traditions, particularly recent immigrants, may struggle with enjoying new, unfamiliar foods. Moreover, many readily available foods that are considered staples of the "typical American diet" may increase disease risk among these populations.[55] As such, an important component of increasing patients' adherence to healthy dietary patterns is greater cultural familiarity and humility among RDNs and health care professionals (ie, receptiveness to another person's identity and how that person's cultural background may shape diet and health practices).[56] Though there is tremendous variability within all cultures, learning more about which foods are central to a patient's food traditions is important. For example, when counseling patients of Middle Eastern or Mexican descent, RDNs should be aware that these patients may consume more red meat than advised because various meats are staple foods in the diet.[57] Thus, practitioners would be warranted to discuss portion size and frequency of intake, in addition to other strategies, to shift dietary intake to align more with dietary recommendations. Similarly, building flexibility into any dietary recommendations to make allowances for cultural food traditions facilitates the adoption and maintenance of healthy dietary patterns for weight management.[58]

Attitudes about body weight, body size, and management of health risks may also vary by culture,[59] with some evidence suggesting that greater westernization and urbanization worldwide are increasing the adoption of a "thin ideal" across socioeconomically developed populations.[60] Health care providers may develop a more effective counseling dynamic by discussing issues related to culturally preferred foods and traditions, ideals of body weight and shape, and beliefs about health practices related to diet.[39,61,62] Providers who subscribe to the Academy of Nutrition and Dietetics Nutrition Care Manual may find the available resources pertaining to cultural foods useful for assessment and counseling.[63]

Nutrition Focused Physical Exam

The NFPE is an important component of a comprehensive nutrition assessment. The exam evaluates patients for body composition and any signs and symptoms of nutrition-related deficiencies and excesses. The main elements of the NFPE are summarized in Box 7.4 on page 110, and a detailed rubric, which can be used by RDNs and other health care professionals, has been published.[64]

The overarching goal of the NFPE is to identify nutrition-related indicators of health risk, which can be used to prioritize a patient's dietary interventions. However, it is important for the clinician to integrate the findings of the NFPE with the information gathered during the medical and physical assessments, as well as the dietary assessment (summarized in Box 7.3), of the patient before discussing any dietary intervention. This is because, regardless of a patient's risk profile, if the clinician does not also understand the patient's preferences, barriers to following a healthier dietary pattern, and interest or willingness to engage in health behaviors that may promote better cardiometabolic health, the patient may not follow the proposed lifestyle recommendations in the end.

Integrating Findings From the Nutrition Focused Physical Exam

Time constraints and variability among individual patients may prevent the evaluation of all nutrition-related considerations in one office visit. Clinicians conducting an NFPE, therefore, may benefit from taking a more holistic approach to evaluating the myriad factors, outlined in Box 7.3 and Box 7.5 (refer to page 111),[1,65] that shape an individual's nutritional status. For example, body adiposity, blood pressure, blood lipids, and blood glucose or insulin levels (or both) can be helpful inputs when considering dietary recommendations. While maintaining energy balance is important for all individuals looking to achieve and maintain a healthful body weight, and although healthy dietary patterns are largely similar for both individuals with cardiometabolic risk factors and those without, clinicians may need to make further adjustments for patients at higher risk of chronic disease.[50] For example, patients with prediabetes or type 2 diabetes may especially benefit from carbohydrate-restricted dietary patterns,[66] whereas individuals with dyslipidemia may need to focus more on patterns low in saturated fat and sodium.

It is equally important to assess the patient's food allergies, intolerances, and preferences, as long-term adherence to healthier dietary patterns is contingent on the person's satisfaction with the pattern. Moreover, individuals with more restrictive dietary patterns, such as vegan and paleo diets, may require more detailed meal-planning and assessment to ensure that dietary patterns meet the macronutrient and micronutrient needs for their life stage and age. Similarly, because food cost, nutrition knowledge, nutrition self-efficacy, and cooking skills shape food availability, incorporating a discussion of these factors may help contextualize the findings from the NFPE and can be helpful for tailoring recommendations.

BOX 7.4

Nutrition Focused Physical Exam for Adults With Obesity: Elements and Special Considerations[64]

Exam component	Relevant elements	Special considerations
Micronutrient deficiencies and excesses	Evaluation of skin, hair, teeth, and nails for texture, temperature, and color; examination for clinical signs of micronutrient deficiency	Deficiencies of vitamins B12 and D are of particular importance in individuals undergoing bariatric surgery or who follow a vegan dietary pattern.
Head and face	Fat and muscle assessment of orbital fat pads and temple	
Upper body	Fat and muscle assessment of triceps, mid-axillary, and ribs; evaluation of musculature of clavicle, shoulder, scapula, and hand	Check for presence of acanthosis nigricans or "buffalo hump" on the base of the neck.
Lower body	Muscle assessment of thigh and calf Examination of ankles and feet for fluid accumulation (edema)	Check for presence of ascites or anasarca. Evaluate bone mineral density as needed.
Abdomen	Waist circumference measurement Listening for bowel sounds	
Functional status	Grip strength measurement	

BOX 7.5

Social, Physical, and Laboratory Components to Integrate With Nutrition Focused Physical Exam Findings for Weight Management[1,65]

Factors to consider	Specific components
Social, medical, and health history	
Family medical history	Cardiovascular disease
	Diabetes
	Cancer
	Hypertension
Pertinent background information	Age
	Race and ethnicity
	Sexual and cultural identity
	Socioeconomic status
	Household composition
	Education
	Language barriers
	Occupation
	Caretaking responsibilities
	Nutrition security
Patient medical history	Irritable bowel syndrome
	Crohn's disease and colitis
	Polycystic ovary syndrome
	Diabetes
	Hypertension
	Hyperlipidemia
	Metabolic syndrome
	Thyroid disease
	Surgical history (eg, bariatric surgery)
	Osteoarthritis
	Cancer
	Gastroesophageal reflux
	Sleep apnea
	Mental health

Box continues

BOX 7.5 (CONTINUED)

Factors to consider	Specific components
Laboratory and physical assessments	
Metabolic syndrome components	Waist circumference (ethnic-specific criteria established by the International Diabetes Federation[63])
	Blood lipids (triglycerides, high-density lipoprotein cholesterol, and low-density lipoprotein cholesterol)
	Blood pressure
	Blood glucose and hemoglobin A1c
Body weight and weight change	BMI
	Intentional or unintentional weight loss
Diet-related laboratory values	Serum iron, hemoglobin, and hematocrit
	Blood urea nitrogen and creatinine
	Thyroid hormones and endocrine profile
	Blood glucose and hemoglobin A1c
	Lipid profile

Summary

As our understanding of obesity pathogenesis and behavior change has evolved, nutrition assessment for weight management requires a more comprehensive assessment of sociocultural, dietary, health, and environmental factors alongside metabolic and physical assessments. A natural extension of the multidimensional nutrition assessment for weight management is growth in the skill set of practitioners. Nutrition assessment, which encompasses diet assessment, the NFPE, and other dimensions of a patient's social and medical history, is essential for comprehensively evaluating the numerous influences that shape a person's food choice, dietary quality, and nutrition-related risk factors and for developing patient-centered recommendations reflective of those factors.

References

1. Brown JE. Adult nutrition and Adult nutrition: conditions and interventions. In: *Nutrition Through the Life Cycle*. 6th ed. Cengage Learning; 2017.
2. Cancello R, Soranna D, Brunani A, et al. Analysis of predictive equations for estimating resting energy expenditure in a large cohort of morbidly obese patients. *Front Endocrinol (Lausanne)*. 2018;9:367. doi:10.3389/fendo.2018.00367
3. Frankenfield DC. Bias and accuracy of resting metabolic rate equations in non-obese and obese adults. *Clin Nutr*. 2013;32(6):976-982. doi:10.1016/j.clnu.2013.03.022

4. Bedogni G, Bertoli S, Leone A, et al. External validation of equations to estimate resting energy expenditure in 14952 adults with overweight and obesity and 1948 adults with normal weight from Italy. *Clin Nutr.* 2019;38:457-464. doi:10.1016/j.clnu.2017.11.011

5. Thom G, Gerasimidis K, Rizou E, et al. Validity of predictive equations to estimate RMR in females with varying BMI. *J Nutr Sci.* 2020;9:e17. doi:10.1017/jns.2020.11

6. Institute of Medicine. *Dietary Reference Intakes for Energy, Carbohydrate, Fiber, Fat, Fatty Acids, Cholesterol, Protein, and Amino Acids.* The National Academies Press; 2005. doi:10.17226/10490

7. National Academies of Sciences, Engineering, and Medicine. *Dietary Reference Intakes for Energy.* The National Academies Press; 2023. doi:10.17226/26818

8. Hall KD, Sacks G, Chandramohan D, et al. Quantification of the effect of energy imbalance on bodyweight. *Lancet.* 2011;378:826-837. doi:10.1016/S0140-6736(11)60812-X

9. Blüher M. Obesity: global epidemiology and pathogenesis. *Nat Rev Endocrinol.* 2019;15(5):288-298. doi:10.1038/s41574-019-0176-8

10. Webb D. Farewell to the 3,500-calorie rule. Today's Dietitian website. 2014;26(11):36. Accessed August 25, 2022. www.todaysdietitian.com/newarchives/111114p36.shtml

11. Body Weight Planner. National Institute of Diabetes and Digestive and Kidney Diseases. Accessed July 1, 2022. www.niddk.nih.gov/bwp

12. Leibel RL, Rosenbaum M, Hirsch J. Changes in energy expenditure resulting from altered body weight. *N Engl J Med.* 1995;332:621-628. doi:10.1056/NEJM199503093321001

13. Ostendorf DM, Caldwell AE, Creasy SA, et al. Physical activity energy expenditure and total daily energy expenditure in successful weight loss maintainers. *Obesity (Silver Spring).* 2019;27:496-504. doi:10.1002/oby.22373

14. Subar AF, Freedman LS, Tooze JA, et al. Addressing current criticism regarding the value of self-report dietary data. *J Nutr.* 2015;145:2639-2645. doi:10.3945/jn.115.219634

15. Boushey CJ, Spoden M, Zhu FM, Delp EJ, Kerr DA. New mobile methods for dietary assessment: review of image-assisted and image-based dietary assessment methods. *Proc Nutr Soc.* 2017;76:283-294. doi:10.1017/S0029665116002913

16. Vadiveloo M, Lichtenstein AH, Anderson C, et al. Rapid diet assessment screening tools for cardiovascular disease risk reduction across healthcare settings: a scientific statement from the American Heart Association. *Circ Cardiovasc Qual Outcomes.* 2020;13:e000094. doi:10.1161/HCQ.0000000000000094

17. Kirkpatrick SI, Subar AF, Douglass D, et al. Performance of the Automated Self-Administered 24-hour Recall relative to a measure of true intakes and to an interviewer-administered 24-h recall. *Am J Clin Nutr.* 2014;100:233-240. doi:10.3945/ajcn.114.083238

18. Kristal AR, Kolar AS, Fisher JL, et al. Evaluation of web-based, self-administered, graphical food frequency questionnaire. *J Acad Nutr Diet.* 2014;114:613-621. doi:10.1016/j.jand.2013.11.017

19. Diet History Questionnaire III (DHQ III). Epidemiology and Genomics Research Program, Division of Cancer Control and Population Sciences, National Cancer Institute. May 2022. Accessed August 17, 2022. https://epi.grants.cancer.gov/dhq3

20. Cuparencu C, Praticó G, Hemeryck LY, et al. Biomarkers of meat and seafood intake: an extensive literature review. *Genes Nutr.* 2019;14:35. doi:10.1186/s12263-019-0656-4

21. Trieu K, Bhat S, Dai Z, et al. Biomarkers of dairy fat intake, incident cardiovascular disease, and all-cause mortality: a cohort study, systematic review, and meta-analysis. *PLoS Med.* 2021;18:e1003763. doi:10.1371/journal.pmed.1003763

22. Sri Harsha PSC, Wahab RA, Garcia-Aloy M, et al. Biomarkers of legume intake in human intervention and observational studies: a systematic review. *Genes Nutr.* 2018;13:25. doi:10.1186/s12263-018-0614-6

23. Woodside JV, Draper J, Lloyd A, McKinley MC. Use of biomarkers to assess fruit and vegetable intake. *Proc Nutr Soc.* 2017;76:308-315. doi:10.1017/S0029665117000325

24. Radtke MD, Poe M, Stookey J, et al. Recommendations for the use of the Veggie Meter® for spectroscopy-based skin carotenoid measurements in the research setting. *Curr Dev Nutr.* 2021;5:nzab104. doi:10.1093/cdn/nzab104

25. Downloadable dietary assessment screeners, methodological information, and analytic files. Epidemiology and Genomics Research Program, Division of Cancer Control and Population Sciences, National Cancer Institute website. 2022. Accessed August 17, 2022. https://epi.grants.cancer.gov/diet/screeners/files.html

26. Winkler JT. The fundamental flaw in obesity research. *Obes Rev.* 2005;6:199-202. doi:10.1111/j.1467-789X.2005.00186.x

27. Papadakis T, Ferguson SG, Schüz B. Within-day variability in negative affect moderates cue responsiveness in high-calorie snacking. *Front Psychol.* 2020;11:590497. doi:10.3389/fpsyg.2020.590497

28. Maugeri A, Barchitta M. A systematic review of ecological momentary assessment of diet: implications and perspectives for nutritional epidemiology. *Nutrients.* 2019;11:2696. doi:10.3390/nu11112696

29. Dao KP, De Cocker K, Tong HL, Kocaballi AB, Chow C, Laranjo L. Smartphone-delivered ecological momentary interventions based on ecological momentary assessments to promote health behaviors: systematic review and adapted checklist for reporting ecological momentary assessment and intervention studies. *JMIR Mhealth Uhealth.* 2021;9(11):e22890. doi:10.2196/22890

30. Schembre SM, Liao Y, O'Connor SG, et al. Mobile ecological momentary diet assessment methods for behavioral research: systematic review. *JMIR Mhealth Uhealth*. 2018;6:e11170. doi:10.2196/11170
31. Harvey J, Krukowski R, Priest J, West D. Log often, lose more: electronic dietary self-monitoring for weight loss. *Obesity (Silver Spring)*. 2019;27:380-384. doi:10.1002/oby.22382
32. Kirkpatrick SI, Dodd KW, Potischman N, et al. Healthy Eating Index-2015 scores among adults based on observed vs recalled dietary intake. *J Acad Nutr Diet*. 2021;121:2233-2241.e1. doi:10.1016/j.jand.2021.06.009
33. Marcano Belisario JS, Jamsek J, Huckvale K, O'Donoghue J, Morrison CP, Car J. Comparison of self-administered survey questionnaire responses collected using mobile apps versus other methods. *Cochrane Database Syst Rev*. 2015;2015(7):MR000042. doi:10.1002/14651858.MR000042.pub2
34. Zhang L, Misir A, Boshuizen H, Ocké M. A systematic review and meta-analysis of validation studies performed on dietary record apps. *Adv Nutr*. 2021;12:2321-2332. doi:10.1093/advances/nmab058
35. Chatterjee A, Prinz A, Gerdes M, Martinez S. Digital interventions on healthy lifestyle management: systematic review. *J Med Internet Res*. 2021;23:e26931. doi:10.2196/26931
36. Young CL, Mohebbi M, Staudacher H, Berk M, Jacka FN, O'Neil A. Assessing the feasibility of an m-Health intervention for changing diet quality and mood in individuals with depression: the My Food & Mood program. *Int Rev Psychiatry*. 2021;33:266-279. doi:10.1080/09540261.2020.1854193
37. Stunkard AJ, Messick S. The three-factor eating questionnaire to measure dietary restraint, disinhibition and hunger. *Journal Psychosom Res*. 1985;29:71-83. doi:10.1016/0022-3999(85)90010-8
38. Satter E. Eating competence: definition and evidence for the Satter Eating Competence model. *J Nutr Educ Behav*. 2007;39:S142-S153. doi:10.1016/j.jneb.2007.01.006
39. Hearst MO, Yang J, Friedrichsen S, Lenk K, Caspi C, Laska MN. The availability of culturally preferred fruits, vegetables and whole grains in corner stores and non-traditional food stores. *Int J Environ Res Public Health*. 2021;18:5030. doi:10.3390/ijerph18095030
40. Food Security Survey Module: six-item short form. SNAP-Ed Connection, US Department of Agriculture; 2022. Accessed August 17, 2022. https://snaped.fns.usda.gov/library/materials/food-security-survey-module-six-item-short-form
41. Food security. International Food Policy Research Institute. 2022. Accessed August 17, 2022. www.ifpri.org/topic/food-security
42. Sahyoun N, Vaudin A. Expanded Food Security Screener. College of Agriculture and Natural Resources, Department of Nutrition and Food Science, University of Maryland; 2022. Accessed August 17, 2022. https://nfsc.umd.edu/sites/nfsc.umd.edu/files/files/images/Aging%20QuestionaireFHQ.pdf
43. Thorndike AN, Gardner CD, Kendrick KB, et al. Strengthening US food policies and programs to promote equity in nutrition security: a policy statement from the American Heart Association. *Circulation*. 2022;145:e1077-e1093. doi:10.1161/CIR.0000000000001072
44. Do WL, Bullard KM, Stein AD, Ali MK, Narayan KMV, Siegel KR. Consumption of foods derived from subsidized crops remains associated with cardiometabolic risk: an update on the evidence using the National Health and Nutrition Examination Survey 2009-2014. *Nutrients*. 2020;12:3244.
45. Vadiveloo MK, Sotos-Prieto M, Parker HW, Yao Q, Thorndike AN. Contributions of food environments to dietary quality and cardiovascular disease risk. *Curr Atheroscler Rep*. 2021;23:14. doi:10.1007/s11883-021-00912-9
46. Glanz K, Johnson L, Yaroch AL, Phillips M, Ayala GX, Davis EL. Measures of retail food store environments and sales: review and implications for healthy eating initiatives. *J Nutr Educ Behav*. 2016;48:280-288.e281. doi:10.1016/j.jneb.2016.02.003
47. Glanz K, Sallis JF, Saelens BE. Advances in physical activity and nutrition environment assessment tools and applications: recommendations. *Am J Prev Med*. 2015;48:615-619. doi:10.1016/j.amepre.2015.01.023
48. Lytle LA, Sokol RL. Measures of the food environment: a systematic review of the field, 2007-2015. *Health Place*. 2017;44:18-34. doi:10.1016/j.healthplace.2016.12.007
49. Ministry of Health of Brazil, Secretariat of Health Care, Primary Health Care Department. *Dietary Guidelines for the Brazilian Population*. Carlos Augusto Monteiro, trans. Ministry of Health of Brazil; 2015. Accessed August 17, 2022. https://bvsms.saude.gov.br/bvs/publicacoes/dietary_guidelines_brazilian_population.pdf
50. Lichtenstein AH, Appel LJ, Vadiveloo M, et al. 2021 dietary guidance to improve cardiovascular health: a scientific statement from the American Heart Association. *Circulation*. 2021;144:e472-e487. doi:10.1161/CIR.0000000000001031
51. Monteiro CA, Astrup A. Does the concept of "ultra-processed foods" help inform dietary guidelines, beyond conventional classification systems? YES. *Am J Clin Nutr*. 2022;116(6):1476-1481. doi:10.1093/ajcn/nqac122
52. Monteiro CA, Moubarac JC, Cannon G, Ng SW, Popkin B. Ultra-processed products are becoming dominant in the global food system. *Obes Rev*. 2013;14 (suppl 2):21-28. doi:10.1111/obr.12107
53. Monteiro CA, Cannon G, Levy RB, et al. Ultra-processed foods: what they are and how to identify them. *Public Health Nutr*. 2019;22:936-941. doi:10.1017/S1368980018003762
54. Juul F, Vaidean G, Parekh N. Ultra-processed foods and cardiovascular diseases: potential mechanisms of action. *Adv Nutr*. 2021;12:1673-1680. doi:10.1007/s10903-008-9120-z

55. Patil CL, Hadley C, Nahayo PD. Unpacking dietary acculturation among new Americans: results from formative research with African refugees. *J Immigr Minor Health*. 2009;11:342-358. doi:10.1007/s10903-008-9120-z
56. Khan S. Cultural humility vs. cultural competence—and why providers need both. HealthCity, Boston Medical Center Health System. March 9, 2021. Accessed August 17, 2022. https://healthcity.bmc.org/policy-and-industry/cultural-humility-vs-cultural-competence-providers-need-both
57. Nemec K. Cultural awareness of eating patterns in the health care setting. *Clin Liver Dis (Hoboken)*. 2020;16:204-207. doi:10.1002/cld.1019
58. Monterrosa EC, Frongillo EA, Drewnowski A, de Pee S, Vandevijvere S. Sociocultural influences on food choices and implications for sustainable healthy diets. *Food Nutr Bull*. 2020;41:59S-73S. doi:10.1177/0379572120975874
59. Naigaga DA, Jahanlu D, Claudius HM, Gjerlaug AK, Barikmo I, Henjum S. Body size perceptions and preferences favor overweight in adult Saharawi refugees. *Nutr J*. 2018;17:17. doi:10.1186/s12937-018-0330-5
60. Swami V. Cultural influences on body size ideals: unpacking the impact of Westernization and modernization. *Eur Psychol*. 2015;20(1):44-51. doi:10.1027/1016-9040/a000150
61. McCabe CF, O'Brien-Combs A, Anderson OS. Cultural competency training and evaluation methods across dietetics education: a narrative review. *J Acad Nutr Diet*. 2020;120:1198-1209.
62. IDEA [Inclusion, Diversity, Equity, and Access] hub. Academy of Nutrition and Dietetics. 2022. Accessed August 17, 2022. www.eatrightpro.org/practice/practice-resources/diversity-and-inclusion
63. Nutrition Care Manual. Resources: Cultural Food Practices. Academy of Nutrition and Dietetics. Accessed August 17, 2022. www.nutritioncaremanual.org/topic.cfm?ncm_category_id=11&lv1=38815&ncm_toc_id=38815&ncm_heading=Resources
64. MacQuillan E, Ford J, Baird K. Increased competency of registered dietitian nutritionists in physical examination skills after simulation-based education in the United States. *J Educ Eval Health Prof*. 2020;17:40. doi:10.3352/jeehp.2020.17.40
65. IDF consensus worldwide definition of the metabolic syndrome. International Diabetes Federation. 2006. Last updated July 29, 2020. Accessed August 17, 2022. www.idf.org/e-library/consensus-statements/60-idfconsensus-worldwide-definitionof-the-metabolic-syndrome.html
66. Goldenberg JZ, Day A, Brinkworth GD, et al. Efficacy and safety of low and very low carbohydrate diets for type 2 diabetes remission: systematic review and meta-analysis of published and unpublished randomized trial data. *BMJ*. 2021;372:m4743. doi:10.1136/bmj.m4743

CHAPTER 8

Physical Activity Assessment

Scott E. Crouter, PhD, FACSM
Paul R. Hibbing, PhD
Samuel R. LaMunion, PhD

CHAPTER OBJECTIVES

- Define metabolic equivalents and how they are used to quantify types of physical activity.
- Review methods and best practices for assessing sedentary behavior and physical activity.
- Review how to screen for medical safety when starting physical activity.
- Describe how to assess a patient's access to activity spaces and how this is related to activity.
- Review the assessment of sociocultural factors that may influence activity.

Introduction

Physical activity is defined as any bodily movement by skeletal muscles that produces an increased energy expenditure above rest.[1] Physical activity is one component of physical behavior, which also includes factors such as posture and activity intensity.[2] Physical behavior is complex and multidimensional, making it challenging to assess with any one instrument or tool.[3-5] Furthermore, several important considerations must be evaluated when determining the most appropriate method for assessing physical behavior in outpatient or free-living settings. The method and the instrument, or tool, selected for a physical behavior assessment should be dictated by the outcome or target that the researcher intends to capture.[5] This chapter provides an overview of the methods for assessing sedentary behaviors and physical activity and covers the various assessment tools available. It also reviews critical factors that affect sedentary behavior and physical activity, such as the activity space of interest and sociocultural factors.

Physical Activity Energy Expenditure

Energy expenditure is defined as the exchange of energy required to perform biological work. Numerous methods have been developed for assessing physical activity and the associated energy expenditure. Typically, energy expenditure is expressed as either a gross value (eg, resting metabolic rate plus activity energy expenditure) or a net value (eg, physical activity energy expenditure minus resting metabolic rate) and expressed in kilocalories or metabolic equivalents (METs). In adults, 1 MET is the energy cost of sitting still, which is equivalent to approximately 3.5 mL per kilogram of body mass per minute of oxygen consumption or 1 kcal per kilogram of body mass per hour.[6] Furthermore, physical activity can be assessed in several dimensions, including duration, volume, and frequency. Box 8.1 provides an overview of example variables used to assess sedentary behavior and physical activity.

MET is one of the most common expressions of activity intensity and energy expenditure. As an example, the adult and youth compendiums of physical activities provide a table for MET values of different activities.[7,8] In this case, METs are used for classifying activity intensity as follows:

- sedentary behaviors: 1.5 METs or less
- light physical activity: 1.51 to 2.99 METs
- moderate physical activity: 3 to 5.99 METs
- vigorous physical activity: 6 METs or greater

For example, an activity requiring four times the oxygen consumption of rest would be a 4-MET activity and classified as moderate.

The use of METs is not without its flaws. A limitation to this approach is that it assumes that every individual has a resting metabolic rate of 3.5 METs, but this rate can vary widely depending on age, body composition, and other physiological factors. Thus, the use of a corrected MET value has been proposed such that the measured energy cost is divided by a measured or estimated resting metabolic rate for the individual.[7,9] The corrected-MET approach is common in youth (ie, the youth MET), as it helps to account for decreases in resting metabolic rate due to aging.[8,10,11] Experts now recognize that using the standard MET definition in adults and youth can misclassify intensity and energy expenditure of activities.[9,12] In addition, employing a measured or predicted resting metabolic rate can affect the prediction of a MET value.[12] Although there is no consensus on the use of the MET, practitioners should

---

BOX 8.1

Summary of Sedentary Behavior and Physical Activity Variables

Variable	Example
Aggregate metrics	
Volume	Minutes per day
	Steps per day
	Kilocalories per day
Frequency	Bouts per day
	Days per week with at least one bout
Pattern metrics	
Continuous	Average bout duration
	Time in bouts exceeding 10 minutes
Categorical	High and low bout length (median splits)
	Movement profile (clustering-based)
Circadian timing metrics	
Absolute	Activity between 9:00 AM and 12:00 PM
Relative	Activity between 0 and 3 hours after waking

be aware of the differences between the definitions, including understanding how they are calculated as well as the strengths and limitations of their applications.

Screening for Medical Safety

Before embarking on a physical activity study or program, patients should undergo a health status screening to determine their risk of experiencing a medical event while engaging in the study or program. Numerous standardized questionnaires have been developed for this purpose. The most commonly used is the Physical Activity Readiness Questionnaire for Everyone (PAR-Q+; available at https://eparmedx.com). For further guidance and important information on preparticipation health screening and evaluation, practitioners should consult the American College of Sports Medicine guidelines for exercise testing and prescription.[13]

Methods for Assessing Physical Activity and Sedentary Behavior

Criterion Measures of Energy Expenditure

Two primary criterion measures of physical activity and sedentary behavior as they relate to the measurement of energy expenditure are doubly labeled water (DLW) and indirect calorimetry.[3,5] The DLW method is considered the gold standard for measuring total daily energy expenditure and is applicable in any environment, as it is does not interfere with daily life.[14,15] The patient is given a dose of water that contains stable isotopes (^2H and ^{18}O) to enrich the isotope concentrations in body water above background levels. Carbon dioxide production is determined by measuring the rates at which these stable isotopes are eliminated from the body. The ^{18}O isotope is eliminated from the body both as water (ie, sweat and urine) and as carbon dioxide (ie, bicarbonate exchange), and the ^2H isotope is eliminated only as water. The standard practice is to take a urine sample for isotope analysis, but methods also exist for blood and saliva samples. An initial sample is taken within a few hours after the DLW dose is administered to establish isotope enrichment levels in the body water. A sample is taken again 1 to 3 weeks after the dose to determine the differential rates of isotope elimination. DLW is ideal for measuring total daily energy expenditure in free-living individuals, as it requires no additional equipment or burden for an individual and does not interfere with the activities of everyday life. However, one of the main limitations of the DLW technique is a lack of temporal resolution to parse data in shorter time periods, such as hours or days; it is also costly to administer, collect, and analyze the data.[3]

Indirect calorimetry is based on the principle that energy intake from carbon-based food is broken down into carbon dioxide, water, and heat when oxygen is present.[16-18] It approximates heat production based on substrate utilization by determining the ratio of carbon dioxide produced by the body to oxygen consumed by the body, which is then used to calculate energy expenditure. Among the types of indirect calorimetry systems available are whole-room indirect calorimeters and metabolic systems that use hoods or facemasks; the choice of system depends on the measurement needed and the setting.[18] Whole-room indirect calorimeters, sometimes referred to as respiratory or metabolic chambers, are small rooms that can be sealed with a participant inside, thus allowing for continuous measurement of energy metabolism with sensitive flow controllers and specialized gas analyzers. These rooms typically include a bed and may also include a desk, chair, exercise equipment (eg, treadmill, cycle ergometer), toilet, and sink. Studies using whole-room indirect calorimetry can last from a few hours to several days and provide the time resolution to parse different components of energy metabolism, including sleep, rest, and activity energy expenditure, as well as the thermic effect of feeding. Though they are considered the gold standard of indirect calorimetry, whole-room calorimeters require considerable resources to operate. They are generally found in high-level research and clinical spaces and are built, operated, validated, and maintained by a multidisciplinary team of experts.

As an alternative to whole-room metabolic chambers, hoods may be used with stationary metabolic carts that are equipped with flow control to measure resting energy expenditure at the bedside. Metabolic carts can also work with face masks or mouthpieces to measure the oxygen cost during submaximal and maximal exercise, but this method is limited to mostly aerobic activities on a treadmill or cycle ergometer. Several portable indirect calorimeters are also available; they are worn in backpack-type harness systems and use a face mask to measure gas exchange. Portable systems allow for a broader range of activities to be captured and can be used in free-living applications.[18-20] However, these systems are typically reserved for research development and validation studies and are limited by cost, participant burden, and a short assessment period (less than 6 hours).[3,21] In addition, indirect calorimetry only measures the energy expended as a result of aerobic metabolism (ie, oxygen consumed) and is not able to capture the energy expenditure from anerobic metabolism.

Although both the DLW method and indirect calorimetry are considered gold standard measures of energy expenditure, they are typically only used in development and validation studies as they require a precisely structured or laboratory environment, specialized equipment, and expertise to collect, process, and analyze the data, and they can be time intensive and expensive. Two types of assessment methods for assessing free-living physical behavior more practically are report-based methods (eg, self-report questionnaires, recalls, surveys, diaries, or logs) and device-based measures (eg, wearable monitors such as pedometers or accelerometer-based devices). Both types are validated against the criterion measures previously discussed, and while they have some limitations, they are practical and the most widely applicable for many practitioners and their patients or clients. For this reason, it is important to understand their strengths and limitations so that an informed decision about the best method of assessment for a specific use case can be made. Table 8.1 on page 120 provides a general overview of the characteristics of the primary physical behavior assessment methods.

Report-Based Measures

Report-based measures include recalls (recalling physical activity or behavior from the previous day, week, year, or other time frame) and self-reported questionnaires that ask about prior or typical behavior patterns or habits, as well as diaries or logs of current behavior habits.[3] Report-based instruments are often aimed at capturing data as bouts of physical activity, which can be interpreted in terms of intensity or energy expenditure using the Compendium of Physical Activities.[7,22,23] Report-based methods are generally easy to use and inexpensive to administer, making them well suited for large-scale cross-sectional studies. However, they are susceptible to recall bias and social desirability bias because data are either self-reported or reported in a structured interview conducted via paper, internet, telephone, or in person. Common report-based instruments are the Global Physical Activity Questionnaire (GPAQ),[24] the International Physical Activity Questionnaire (IPAQ),[25] and the more recently developed Activities Completed Over Time in 24 Hours (ACT24) previous-day recall.[26] These report-based instruments work well to capture contextual and behavioral information to complement device-based data when making an assessment in an outpatient

TABLE 8.1 Characteristics of Physical Behavior Assessment Methods[a]

		Report-Based Measures	
		Surveys or questionnaires	**Diaries or logs**
	Example	IPAQ, GPAQ	Sleep log
Dimensions	Frequency of activity	X	X
	Intensity of activity	X	X
	Time (duration) of activity	X	X
	Type (mode) of activity	X	X
	Total activity (volume)	X	X
Domains	Domestic (household) activity	X	X
	Leisure time activity	X	X
	Occupational activity	X	X
	Transportation activity	X	X
	Overall physical activity	X	X
	Energy expenditure	Estimated	Estimated
	Cost	$	$
	Participant burden	Low	Moderate
	Researcher burden	Low	Moderate
	Potential biases	Recall; social desirability	Recall; social desirability
	Duration of assessment	Single time point	Days to weeks
	Group size	Large	Large

Abbreviations: GPAQ, Global Physical Activity Questionnaire; IPAQ, International Physical Activity Questionnaire.
[a] This table breaks down the three broad methods of physical behavior assessment (report-based, device-based, and criterion) into subtypes, giving examples of each tool subtype and what it is best suited for. This can aid in the selection of a specific tool and can act as a guide for comparing tools from different categories.

	Device-Based Measures				Criterion Measures	
	Pedometers	Heart rate monitors	Consumer-grade wearables	Research-grade wearables	Indirect calorimetry	Doubly labeled water
	Yamax DigiWalker SW-200	Polar H10	Fitbit, Apple Watch, Garmin, Samsung	ActiGraph, activPAL, GENEActiv, Axivity	Parvo Medics TrueOne 2400, Cosmed K5	
	-	X	X	X	-	-
	-	X	X	X	X	-
	-	X	X	X	-	-
	-	-	X	X	-	-
	X	X	X	X	X	X
	-	-	X	X	-	-
	-	-	X	X	-	-
	-	-	X	X	-	-
	-	-	X	X	-	-
	X	X	X	X	X	-
	-	Estimated	Estimated	Estimated	Measured	Measured
	$	$-$$	$$-$$$	$$-$$$	$$$$$	$$$$$
	Low	Moderate	Moderate	Moderate	High	Low
	Low	Moderate	Moderate	High	High	High
	Reactivity	Reactivity	Reactivity	Reactivity	Reactivity	-
	Hours to weeks	Hours to days	Hours to weeks	Hours to weeks	Hours	Days to weeks
	Large	Moderate	Moderate	Moderate	Small	Small

CHAPTER 8: Physical Activity Assessment 121

or free-living environment. Typically, these instruments take a cross-sectional snapshot of behavior, making them best suited for looking at differences in behavior between individuals. A recent development in the daily diary or log format is the use of ecological momentary assessment (EMA) surveys that can capture more instantaneous data about physical behaviors over short periods of time (eg, 4 hours), which can help reduce recall bias and improve ecological validity (ie, how generalizable results are to real-world settings).[27] The EMA surveys can be delivered electronically at preset time points or be event-based and adaptive, using a respondent's answers to a previous survey. The frequency and repetition of EMA emphasizes the temporally and spatially varying characteristics of behavior that fluctuate at an individual level to generate intensive longitudinal data for a single patient. In addition, EMA works well in tandem with device-based measures to capture both continuous-movement data, taking frequent snapshots of the environment in which behaviors naturally occur, and the psychological aspects of these behaviors, including attitude, mood, belief, and perception.[27]

The majority of evidence about the relationship between physical behaviors and health outcomes comes from report-based measures. These tools are used in large-scale population-based studies of physical behaviors due to their low cost, ease of use, and low time burden.[28] However, several notable population surveillance studies have also incorporated a device-based measure, including the National Health and Nutrition Examination Survey during specific cycles (NHANES 2003–2006, 2011–2014),[29,30] the UK Biobank study,[31] and the German National Cohort (NAKO).[32] This number of new population surveillance and prospective cohort studies incorporating a device-based measure continues to increase[33] and will support objectives identified by the second edition of the *Physical Activity Guidelines for Americans* (2018)[34,35] and the 2020 World Health Organization physical activity guidelines.[36]

Report-based measures are often used to obtain cross-sectional data on physical behavior in a standardized way. At the group level, self-report instruments capture the necessary information to obtain population-based estimates of generic physical behaviors; however, these estimates do not adequately capture the individual differences in behavior and lack sufficient time resolution to characterize any temporal aspects of physical behavior. Report-based instruments can be used alone but also work well in conjunction with device-based measures to obtain contextual information about behavior.

Device-Based Measures

Compared to the criterion measures of energy expenditure, device-based measures are lower in cost and noninvasive, which can potentially capture continuous physical behavior data over time intervals ranging from a few hours to more than a month.[3] They provide sufficient temporal resolution (ie, amount of data captured with respect to time) for capturing variation and change in physical behaviors such as physical activity, sedentary behavior, and sleep.[3,37,38] Though device-based measures are objective, they can induce reactivity bias and, as a stand-alone tool, only capture movement data without any contextual information.[3]

Wearable devices include pedometers, heart rate monitors, single-sensor devices (eg, accelerometers), multimodal devices (multiple sensors in a single device at a single attachment site), and multisensor arrays (one or more different sensor types at multiple attachment sites). These devices can be broadly categorized as either research-grade (eg, ActiGraph, activPAL, GENEActiv, and Axivity) or consumer-grade (eg, Fitbit, Apple, Garmin, and Samsung), according to their level of data availability and outcome transparency.

Pedometers

Step counting has been in use since the mid-1900s, and it remains relevant in health research today, largely because of the somewhat universal understanding of what a step is and the prevalence of walking.[39] Pedometers are among the longest-standing device-based measures of physical behavior and are a relatively basic technology.[39] The simplest pedometers use a lever arm in a housing worn at the waist; when the lever arm moves beyond a specified threshold, a step is counted.[39] However, the spring-lever arm mechanisms are affected by slow walking and external factors such as obesity and pedometer tilt can cause underestimation of steps. In contrast, newer pedometers with accelerometer mechanisms are less susceptible to tilting and other factors.[40] A 2018 study evaluated several pedometers and research-grade step counters under free-living conditions. The StepWatch, a research-grade step counter worn on the ankle, achieved the highest criterion validity and counted between 95.3% and 102.8% of hand-counted steps over the course of a day. Generally, most waist-worn devices undercounted steps (by 20%–30%) and most wrist-worn devices overcounted steps (by 20%–30%) compared to hand-counted steps over the course of a day, although this was dependent on the settings used for the most advanced devices.[41] If used in a healthy adult population with a typical movement profile, a validated pedometer is an inexpensive and easy-to-use tool for quickly capturing stepping behavior or to jump-start behavior change for a physical behavior promotion, such as a couch to 5K program.[42,43]

Heart Rate Monitors

Most device-based measures use a single sensor—an accelerometer—to capture movement. Although these movement data can be translated to intensity and energy, devices using an accelerometer have limited utility for certain types of activities; for example, a device placed on the hip or wrist of a cyclist will not record much movement, yet the cyclist's activity intensity may be high. Independently, heart rate sensors provide a physiological signal that can robustly capture intensity and be used to estimate energy expenditure. Heart rate monitors straddle the line between research-grade and consumer-grade devices, as some devices, such as a Holter monitor, capture raw electrocardiogram data that are suitable for clinical and research purposes. More commonly in free-living situations, a chest strap with a transmitter, such as the Polar H10, can be used to measure the electrical activity in the heart and record the number of beats per minute. This information can be transmitted to a paired smartphone application or to exercise equipment, such as stationary bikes and treadmills in gyms and group fitness classes.

A more recent advancement in free-living heart rate measurement is photoplethysmography (PPG), which captures heart rate by measuring the volumetric changes in blood circulation using an infrared light source and a photodetector placed against the skin.[44] PPG sensors are often a feature of multimodal, wrist-worn, consumer-grade wearables and are used to measure heart rate and estimate heart rate variability. Though PPG sensors are noninvasive, they do have some limitations; for instance, they require consistent skin contact and can be sensitive to motion artifact (voluntary or involuntary movement of the sensor that comes about due to shaking with movement of the body) during activity, especially at higher intensities.[45] Overall, PPG provides a reasonable estimate of free-living heart rate trends in most individuals, especially with the newest-model consumer-grade devices. A 2020 systematic review and meta-analysis found that the use of heart rate data coupled with accelerometer sensor data yielded better energy expenditure estimates than using accelerometer sensor data alone.[46] Guidelines for evaluating wrist-worn, consumer-grade devices that measure heart rate were recently published.[47]

Research-Grade Wearables

Research-grade devices provide access to raw sensor data, which may be collected under structured laboratory conditions, semistructured conditions, or simulated free-living conditions. Researchers use these data in conjunction with a criterion measure of energy expenditure (indirect calorimetry) and activity (direct observation) to develop analytical methods for estimating energy expenditure, quantifying activity intensity, and classifying physical activity type. In most cases, these methods are peer-reviewed and published, which allows for independent validation. In a recent trend, researchers have been publishing raw data and open-source code in order to improve the validation process; however, some research-grade devices (eg, activPAL) have proprietary algorithms included in their software. The development process as outlined results in analytical methods that are valid for the population used in collecting the original data, for the activities performed in the original data collection, and for data collected using the same parameters (eg, device attachment site, sampling frequency, device brand).[2] The use of research-grade devices for assessing physical activity is always evolving. While these data provide a great deal of analytical flexibility, they require technical expertise to process and interpret. Health care practitioners should consult an expert in the field before implementing research-grade wearable devices in a project in order to ensure that the most current devices and methods are being employed.

Although the hip and wrist are the most common attachment sites, several others are effective; thigh-worn devices, such as the activPAL, are rapidly gaining in popularity.[48] The latter trend is especially notable, given the differences between sedentary behavior and physical activity, which must be considered when deciding how to measure the two. Specifically, sedentary behavior involves both an energy expenditure component (energy expenditure of 1.5 METs or less) and a postural component (seated or lying posture, excluding sleep),[49,50] whereas physical activity has only an energy expenditure component (eg, energy expenditure of 3 METs or more for moderate-to-vigorous physical activity). Thus, the assessment of sedentary behavior generally requires more detail than the assessment of physical activity, and this can lead to challenges when deciding which device to use.

Posture detection is most accurate with thigh-worn devices,[51,52] whereas energy expenditure is more accurately captured by monitors worn on other parts of the body (eg, ActiGraph devices worn on the hip or wrist).[53,54] Multiple monitors can be worn simultaneously to ensure that both variables are adequately captured, but doing so places a greater burden on the patient; thus, trade-offs may need to be made between logistical and empirical factors.[55]

Multiple-monitor arrays are not the only promising path toward optimizing the assessment of both posture and energy expenditure. Algorithms such as the Convolutional Neural Network (CNN) Hip Accelerometer Posture, or CHAP, method have shown that deep learning can be useful for increasing the convergence of posture estimates from hip-worn and thigh-worn monitors.[56] Gyroscope sensors may also hold unique promise for assessing sedentary behavior, beyond what has been achieved to date with traditional accelerometer data.[57] However, gyroscopes have a short battery life that currently precludes their large-scale use, again requiring trade-offs between logistical and empirical factors.

Consumer-Grade Wearables

Consumer-grade devices are designed to provide immediate feedback and summary measures of physical behaviors directly to the wearer via the device itself or through an app on a smartphone or tablet. These devices can estimate steps, energy expenditure (in kilocalories per day), flights of stairs climbed, distance walked, active time, sitting time, sleep time, recovery time, and more. Individualized summary data are made available to the wearer, but the raw data are generally unavailable, and the processing methods for calculating the summary data are proprietary and unpublished. This is further compounded by how frequently consumer-grade devices are updated. The major device manufacturers release an updated version of a flagship device approximately once a year and debut a completely new device every 2 to 4 years. These devices usually include updated user features and the latest hardware; however, it is unclear how these hardware updates factor into the summary measures provided by the devices.[46,58]

The other factor contributing to the calculation of summary measures is the device firmware. Firmware updates are released periodically for both the individual devices and their accompanying smartphone apps. These updates can be pushed to multiple generations of the same device despite hardware differences, but users often do not know the data that is part of the updates and whether there is any effect on the summary measures generated.

These limitations just described—the frequency with which change occurs and the lack of transparency surrounding the data and generated outcomes—make it challenging to perform rigorous validations of consumer-grade devices. Despite these limitations, consumer-grade devices have been recognized as valuable tools for stimulating behavior change through self-management and accountability. Though imperfect, the physical behavior estimates they provide can generate immediate individualized feedback, which can be an effective behavior change technique for placing the focus on health habits as they relate to physical behaviors.[42,43]

In addition, although research-grade devices are the preferred method for many studies, third-party platforms such as Fitabase can act as a bridge for researchers or practitioners using consumer-grade devices.[59] Fitabase is a data management platform that connects users with the application programming interface (API) provided by the consumer-grade device manufacturers as a paid service. Accessing the API allows Fitabase users to communicate with the consumer-grade device platforms and pull data as they are synced. This provides a way for researchers and practitioners to view data in near real time and also export the summary data at the day, hour, and minute level. Although the raw data remain unavailable and data processing methods remain proprietary, third-party data management services do help bridge a gap for researchers aiming to use consumer-grade devices, which can provide sufficient data for some use cases.

Selecting an Assessment Method

Given the complexity and multidimensional nature of measuring physical behavior, several important factors must be considered when selecting an assessment method. To facilitate the decision-making process, practitioners can use a systematic approach like the decision matrix shown in Figure 8.1 on page 126.[5] This resource identifies four critical components: (1) target outcomes to be assessed, (2) feasibility and practicality of the method, (3) resources needed, and (4) method of delivery or administration.[5]

FIGURE 8.1 Decision matrix for selecting a method of physical activity measurement[a,5]

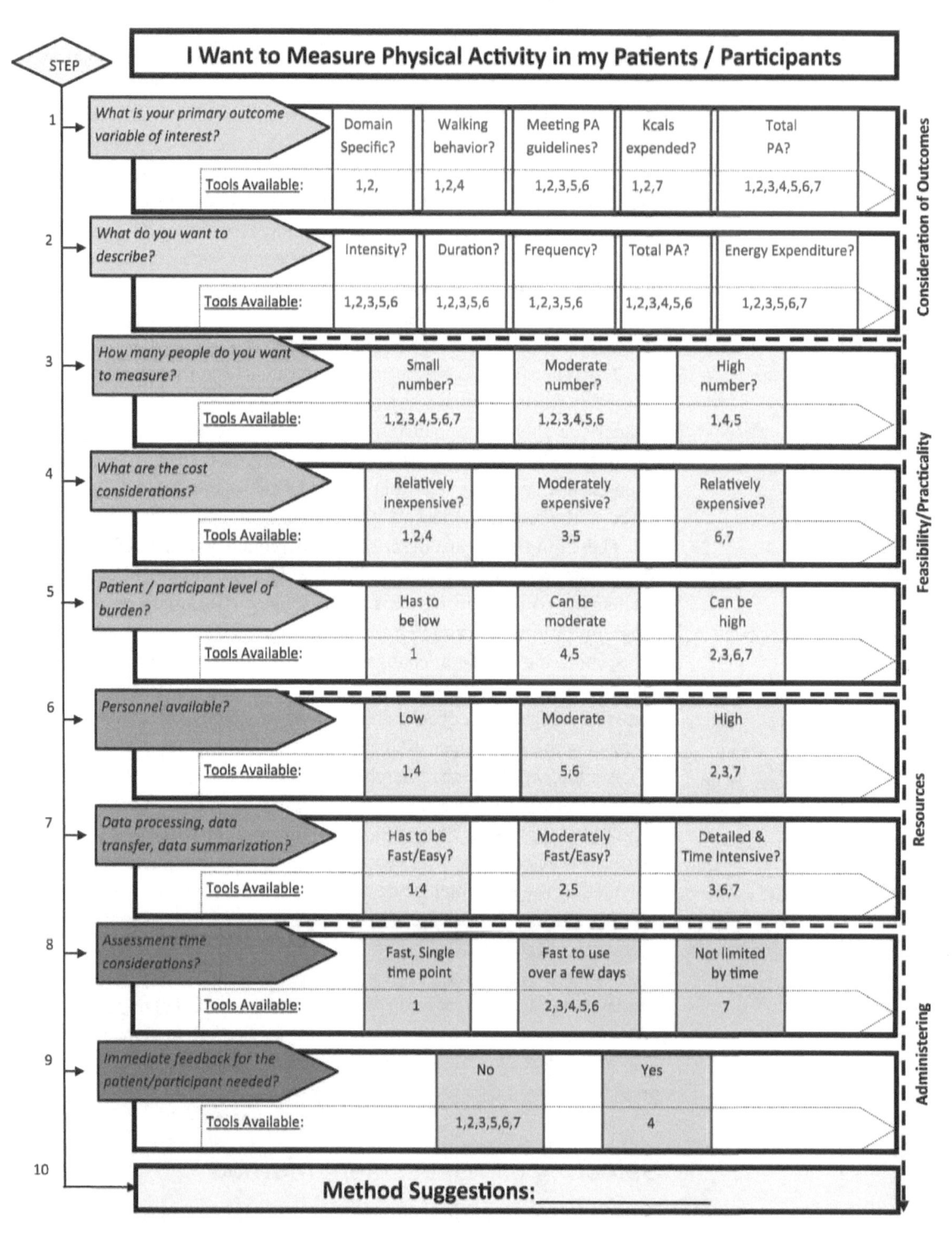

I Want to Measure Physical Activity in my Patients / Participants

STEP 1 — What is your primary outcome variable of interest?

	Domain Specific?	Walking behavior?	Meeting PA guidelines?	Kcals expended?	Total PA?
Tools Available:	1,2	1,2,4	1,2,3,5,6	1,2,7	1,2,3,4,5,6,7

STEP 2 — What do you want to describe?

	Intensity?	Duration?	Frequency?	Total PA?	Energy Expenditure?
Tools Available:	1,2,3,5,6	1,2,3,5,6	1,2,3,5,6	1,2,3,4,5,6	1,2,3,5,6,7

Consideration of Outcomes

STEP 3 — How many people do you want to measure?

	Small number?	Moderate number?	High number?
Tools Available:	1,2,3,4,5,6,7	1,2,3,4,5,6	1,4,5

STEP 4 — What are the cost considerations?

	Relatively inexpensive?	Moderately expensive?	Relatively expensive?
Tools Available:	1,2,4	3,5	6,7

STEP 5 — Patient / participant level of burden?

	Has to be low	Can be moderate	Can be high
Tools Available:	1	4,5	2,3,6,7

Feasibility/Practicality

STEP 6 — Personnel available?

	Low	Moderate	High
Tools Available:	1,4	5,6	2,3,7

STEP 7 — Data processing, data transfer, data summarization?

	Has to be Fast/Easy?	Moderately Fast/Easy?	Detailed & Time Intensive?
Tools Available:	1,4	2,5	3,6,7

Resources

STEP 8 — Assessment time considerations?

	Fast, Single time point	Fast to use over a few days	Not limited by time
Tools Available:	1	2,3,4,5,6	7

STEP 9 — Immediate feedback for the patient/participant needed?

	No	Yes
Tools Available:	1,2,3,5,6,7	4

Administering

STEP 10 — **Method Suggestions:** _____

Note: 1=Physical activity questionnaires; 2=Physical activity logs/diaries; 3=Heart Rate Monitoring; 4=Pedometers; 5=Accelerometer; 6=Multi-unit Sensors; 7=Doubly Labeled Water

Abbreviation: PA, physical activity.
[a]The practitioner can work through this decision matrix by answering the questions at each step for a specific use case, and an assessment tool will be suggested.
Reproduced with permission from Strath SJ, Kaminsky LA, Ainsworth BE, et al. Guide to the assessment of physical activity: clinical and research applications: a scientific statement from the American Heart Association. *Circulation*. 2013;128(20):2259-2279. doi:10.1161/01.cir.0000435708.67487.da.[5]

When defining the target outcomes, typically a good place to start is with an outline of the dimensions of physical behavior (frequency, intensity, type, and duration) and domains of physical behavior (domestic, occupational, transportation, and leisure time) that need to be captured.[3,5,60] From there, the practitioner can determine whether a particular method is suitable for assessing those components. To do this, one must understand what each method of measurement provides, the potential sources of error, and the purpose or population for which the method of measurement is validated.[3,5,60] The decision matrix in Figure 8.1 provides a guide for these specific content areas of the decision-making process. The continuum shown in Figure 8.2 illustrates the trade-offs to consider when selecting a method of physical behavior assessment based on validity, patient burden, cost, and practicality and feasibility.[61]

As is evident from the preceding discussions, the landscape of physical behavior assessment is vast, and numerous tools are available. This can make choosing a tool challenging. In addition to the selection strategies highlighted thus far, resources such as the Digital Clinical Measures Playbook, better known as *The Playbook* by the Digital Medicine Society, can aid in the selection process (https://playbook.dimesociety.org). This guide synthesizes the available evidence and

FIGURE 8.2 Continuum of trade-offs in choosing a physical behavior assessment tool[a,61]

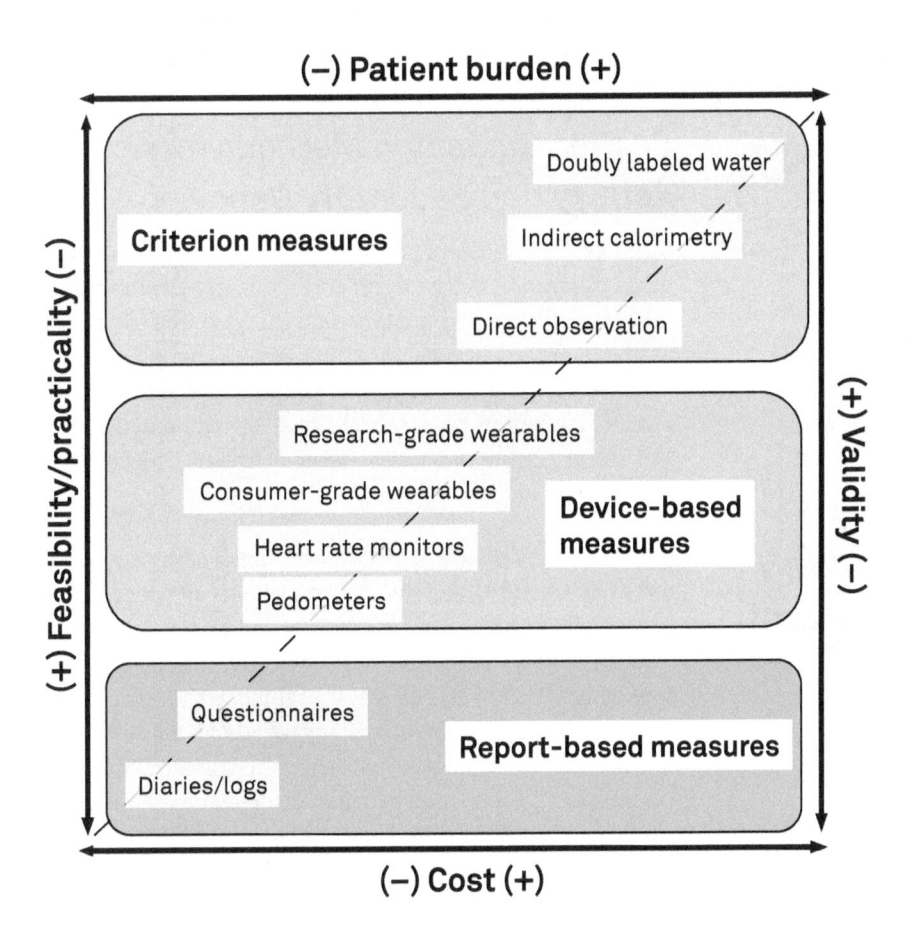

[a] This continuum illustrates the trade-offs in the decision-making process for selecting a physical behavior assessment tool. Adapted from Welk G, Morrow J, Saint-Maurice P. Overview of physical activity assessment tools. In: *Measures Registry User Guide: Individual Physical Activity*. National Collaborative on Childhood Obesity Research; 2017:section 5. www.nccor.org/tools-mruserguides/individual-physical-activity/overview-of-physical-activity-assessment-tools.[61]

provides a methodical way to select the right tool based on specific use cases. *The Playbook* functions on verification, analytical validation, and clinical validation (the V3 principle), which is a standardized approach for evaluating digitally connected technologies and the quality of the supporting evidence for the use of specific devices.[62,63] *The Playbook* is a collaborative resource designed to serve as a guide for using remote connected technologies for remote patient monitoring. It synthesizes best-practice recommendations for using digitally connected technologies for physical behavior assessment. In addition, published studies compare benchmarks for consumer-grade summary measures set forth in the Consumer Technology Association standards for heart rate[64] and step counting.[65]

A 2018 systematic literature review provides additional information on the quality of available evidence for and the general performance of the various categories of physical activity assessment methods. The authors summarized the available evidence on criterion validity, concurrent validity, test-retest reliability, interinstrument reliability, and sensitivity for self-report instruments and wearable devices compared to criterion measures of energy expenditure using DLW. In general, both self-report instruments and wearable devices were found to underestimate energy expenditure compared to DLW. Additionally, energy expenditure estimated from total steps measured by wearable devices had similar errors to the criterion-measured energy expenditure when compared to other estimates from self-report and wearable devices.[4] Steps may be frequently passed over for other outcome metrics, but with a validated tool they can be effective for assessing physical behaviors because they are more universally understood than other metrics.

Section Summary: Methods for Assessing Physical Activity and Sedentary Behavior

Although no single tool or instrument exists to comprehensively assess all components of physical behavior, practitioners are encouraged to incorporate an appropriate objective assessment method that is suited to capturing the target behaviors in free-living conditions. Important factors to consider beyond the methodological effectiveness of a tool or instrument are cost, feasibility, practicality, and patient burden. Numerous resources are available to aid in the selection process to ensure successful capture of physical behavior data for specific use cases.

Assessing Activity Spaces in Research

Activity spaces are the physical locations where people engage in physical behaviors.[66] By assessing engagement in a variety of spaces, it is possible to gain information about the context in which sedentary behavior and physical activity occur. This, in turn, sheds light on the correlates and determinants of activity levels, as well as the social and environmental factors that may influence activity levels in different groups of people. In many ways, activity-space research is an extension of the broader notion of assessing the four domains of physical behavior (domestic, occupational, transportation, and leisure time).[67,68] By adding spatial information to these domains, it becomes possible to explore how behavior is affected by the built environment and related sociopolitical factors. This is important not only for promoting health but also for advancing social justice—that is, for informing efforts to ensure that all individuals have equal access to high-quality resources for active living. Many factors warrant consideration in multiple domains. Box 8.2 provides examples of activity spaces within each physical behavior domain and factors to consider when conducting activity space–related research.

BOX 8.2

Physical Behavior Domains and Examples of Associated Activity Spaces

Domain	Associated activity spaces	Factors to consider
Domestic	Home address, both indoors (eg, cleaning) and outdoors (eg, yardwork or gardening)	Neighborhood factors such as density and lot size; climate and seasonal factors
Occupational	Industrial districts, office buildings, factories	Environmental exposures (indoor or outdoor); toxicant exposures; physiological strain (activity intensity, repetitiveness, opportunity for recovery)
Transportation	City sidewalks, greenways, bike lanes, crosswalks	Walkability, safety
Leisure time	Parks, gyms	Availability, affordability

Activity spaces can be viewed in different ways depending on the study. Some studies view them as correlates or determinants of physical behavior; others treat them as aggregation strata, independent or dependent variables, or even covariates. This range of application is important to keep in mind when conducting an assessment and selecting an appropriate measurement tool. In particular, it is important to determine whether a given instrument is designed to collect data about the environment itself or about the people interacting with it. In general, each study requires measurement tools that address the locations relevant to the research question, as well as the times when people go to those locations and how active they are while there. Few tools are effective for capturing all of these elements, so carefully designed, multi-instrument assessments are needed. The following section provides a brief overview of the types of assessment tools and how they can be applied in research settings.

Methods for Activity Space Assessments

Historically, activity space assessments have been conducted using report-based or audit-based tools.[69] Report-based tools rely on individuals to state how active they are in particular spaces. These tools include a multitude of surveys, questionnaires, and interviews.[70] Audit-based tools require researchers to directly observe an environment in order to discern its compatibility with physical activity (eg, walkability or aesthetic appeal) or to document the degree to which people are active in that space.

In recent years, global positioning system (GPS) and geographic information system (GIS) technologies have played an increasing role in activity space assessments. GPS technology uses satellite communications to log the latitude and longitude of a body-worn receiving device at regular intervals.[71,72] GIS allows those coordinates to be cross-referenced against mapping information that provides additional contextual information (eg, land use).[73]

Given the increasing influence of GPS and GIS technologies, activity space assessments are now generally categorized as report-based, audit-based, or GIS-based.[74] Hundreds of specific instruments have been developed for assessing aspects of the built environment (including activity spaces),[70] and an exhaustive listing cannot be provided here. However, we can broadly cover each category of tool and discuss its strengths and limitations, the situations in which tools of that type should be used, and prominent examples of specific instruments or techniques.

Report-Based Tools

Report-based tools represent an inexpensive and direct way to obtain information about how individuals perceive their activity levels in certain spaces.[75] While this makes the tools practical to use and scalable for a wide range of research, it also makes them susceptible to social desirability bias and related limitations of self-reported data. Thus, report-based tools are best for situations in which the goal is to measure perceptions of the physical activity environment rather than to obtain quantitative activity estimates. If quantitative estimates are needed, it is often valuable to pair the individual's self-reported perceptions with data from a separate, more objective instrument.[74] Prominent examples of report-based instruments include the Neighborhood Environment Walkability Scale[76] and the perceptions of environmental supports questionnaire.[77] The neighborhood is an activity space for which many report-based instruments are available.

Audit-Based Tools

Audit-based tools can provide activity space–related information distinct from information generated from report-based or even GIS-based methods.[70] For example, an audit-based tool might be used to collect data about the upkeep and physical dimensions of specific features in an activity space. Audits can also be used to assess how active people are while present in a certain space (eg, a park). Researcher burden is a major limitation of audit-based tools. Technicians must be trained to conduct the audits, and frequent fidelity checks are necessary to ensure data are being collected with sufficient quality. Audit-based tools should be used when exceptional detail is needed about a specific area or when observation-based assessments of group activity levels are suitable for the research question. (Notably, observation-based assessments can be logistically advantageous if specific individuals will not be identifiable, as the study will likely qualify for an expedited ethics review and waiver of informed consent requirements.) Active Living Research provides an online database (https:///activelivingresearch.org/toolsandresources/toolsandmeasures) containing references to dozens of audit-based instruments, as well as some report-based instruments. Notable audit-based examples cover a range of activity spaces, from specific parks and paths to pedestrian environments.

Geographic Information Systems–Based Tools

GIS-based tools are becoming increasingly common as technology improves.[78] Two major strengths of GIS-based tools are their ability to provide objective measures and the granularity of data they can collect. Location-based data points can typically be stored several times per minute, yielding high-resolution profiles of locations. Yet this can also become a limitation, as data sets quickly grow to sizes that are difficult to manage.[79] Additional limitations include the limited battery life of GPS receivers, their susceptibility to missing data when the satellite connection is blocked (eg, by buildings or hills), and the considerable technical expertise it can take to analyze the data.[80,81] In addition, ethical concerns require careful data anonymization to protect participant privacy.[82-84] With a sufficient team of collaborators (with expertise in health research, data science, and geography, for example), GIS-based tools are suitable for most activity space–related research. Emerging techniques include combined GIS and accelerometer methods[85,86] and other approaches that incorporate EMA with triggers based on cues from GIS-based data.[27,87] Researchers should also be aware of the robust community of researchers working with GIS-based tools, many of whom are collaborating to provide helpful tools—such as the Human Activity Behavior Identification Tool and data Unification System (HABITUS; www.habitus.eu) for merging accelerometer and GPS data—that overcome technical barriers when managing and processing complex spatial data.

Special Challenges in Geographic Information Systems–Based Assessments

A major challenge in GIS-based assessments is the operational definition of boundaries around activity spaces. It is common for operational definitions to be established with reference to existing geopolitical and municipal boundaries (eg, property and zoning lines), but the arbitrary and evolving nature of these definitions can make causal inference challenging.[88] This ultimately plays into several important concepts—namely, buffers, the modifiable areal unit problem (MAUP), the uncertain geographic context problem (UGCoP), and the selective daily mobility bias.

Buffers provide a way of defining the surrounding area, within which a person is considered to be engaged with the activity space. For example, the "home" environment may be considered any point within a 400-m (1,312-ft) radius of the home address. This common buffering approach is called a radial buffer, but there are many other approaches.[88] Buffers can be useful for establishing operational definitions of certain activity spaces, but they also have limitations. For example, the radius of a radial buffer will almost certainly be imperfect. When the radius is large, an abundance of true positive engagement (ie, correctly identifying engagement with an activity space) will be detected, but likely some false positive engagement (ie, engagement with an activity space that is identified incorrectly) as well. Conversely, when the radius is small, there will be less true positive engagement but also less false positive engagement. Therefore, the buffer setting is always a trade-off between recall and precision, and different research questions may call for different buffer settings, depending on the measurement priorities.

The MAUP and UGCoP both reference issues that arise from the subjective and fluid nature of space delineations (eg, delineations based on zoning). The MAUP acknowledges that observed differences between locations may be artifacts of how those locations were defined.[89,90] The UGCoP focuses instead on how measurements are affected at the individual level.[91] Specifically, the UGCoP acknowledges that the observed impact of an activity space on an individual may be an artifact of how the space was defined. More generally, the MAUP and UGCoP underscore the importance and difficulty of developing rigorous definitions for what constitutes an activity space.

Causal inference can also be challenging because of the selective daily mobility bias.[92] This phenomenon refers to the difficulty of discerning whether certain activity spaces (eg, parks or greenways) causally affect a person's motivation to be active or whether these spaces simply provide an outlet for existing motivation. The difference is subtle, yet it has major implications for efforts to promote active lifestyles through the built environment. New initiatives must serve not only those who already intend to be active but also those who would not otherwise become active without the initiative. The selective daily mobility bias makes it difficult to establish an evidence base that can guide policy and practice in this area of health promotion. Therefore, it is an important limitation to consider when designing new GIS-based assessments.

Section Summary: Assessing Activity Spaces in Research

Activity spaces are an important environmental contributor to physical behavior; therefore, careful assessment of these spaces is essential when evaluating a patient's physical activity and related behaviors. Assessments of activity spaces can take many forms and serve many purposes, requiring researchers to carefully consider which report-based, audit-based, or GPS- or GIS-based technique best serves the purpose of each study they design. The strengths and limitations of each method should be considered, in conjunction with how each activity space is operationally defined. In many cases, an interdisciplinary team is needed to ensure that sound decisions are made regarding what measurement techniques to use and how to implement them; this includes having team members with expertise in geospatial research when GPS- or GIS-based approaches are under consideration. Methodological choices should be clearly stated and amply justified when preparing manuscripts for publication, to ensure that nuanced interpretation and synthesis are possible as the evidence base grows across studies. Although assessing activity spaces has its difficulties, ongoing research is critical in this area for promoting active lifestyles and equitable access to them.

Assessing the Sociocultural Component of Physical Behavior

Making a complete assessment of physical behaviors goes beyond measuring and describing a person's physical behavior patterns. For example, when working on behavior change with a patient, the practitioner needs to know not only *what* the patient's current and typical physical behavior pattern is (to establish a baseline) but also *why* the patient has that pattern of physical behavior. Understanding the *why* requires evaluating both the individual-level factors and the environmental influences that have contributed to the development of the pattern over time. Contributors to physical behaviors, whether they be active or inactive (eg, sedentary) behaviors, include social, political, economic, religious, and cultural influences that are driven by a person's environment. Experts know that these influences are meaningful to the relationship an individual has with physical activity and sedentary behavior; however, it can be challenging to capture and quantify the contributions of these individual and environmental factors to habitual physical behavior and how this relates to long-term health.

Assessing Physical Behaviors With an Ecological Model

The prevailing approach to gaining a high-level understanding of a person's environment is to use an ecological model. An ecological model is a theoretical or conceptual framework that explores the interrelatedness of individual-level and environmental factors as they pertain to health. Socioecological models provide a basis for exploring correlates and determinants of physical behaviors on the microenvironmental level (within an individual) while also considering macroenvironmental factors—the larger social, political, economic, religious, and cultural influences within a community that may promote or inhibit certain aspects of physical behavior, such as engagement in physical activity.

Using an ecological model to assess physical behaviors can help the practitioner understand the complex associations and interactions that drive an individual's physical behavior while also providing a framework for developing strategies to create, execute, and evaluate methods for enacting behavior change. Because of the multidimensional relationship between physically active behavior and health, most behavior-change interventions require a multilevel approach. Developing an effective behavior-change strategy or program to achieve positive results at both the group and individual level can be challenging. For example, an individualized plan may be hindered because of specific barriers to participation, but focusing too broadly on making changes at the organizational or environmental policy level may not provide enough individualization to yield individual change across a wide range of people.

A variety of ecological models are discussed in the literature, most of which have a fair degree of overlap with but may emphasize different environmental factors from the ecological models proposed by Sallis and colleagues,[93] King and colleagues,[94] Bauman and colleagues,[95] and others. Each of these ecological models takes a slightly different approach to evaluating the determinants and correlates of physical behavior and health. Figure 8.3 provides an adapted ecological model of the determinants and correlates of physical behavior and health, specifically as they relate to sociocultural factors, that harmonizes some of the common elements and themes in the aforementioned ecological models.[94,95]

FIGURE 8.3 Adapted ecological model of the determinants of physical behaviors, illustrating how environmental influences change over the life course[94,95]

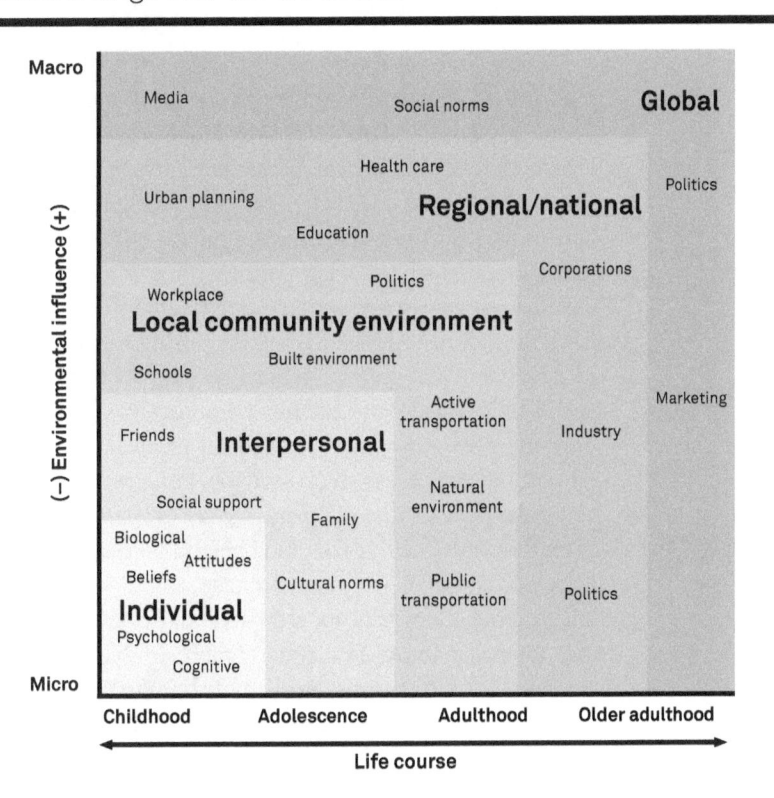

Correlates and Determinants of Sedentary Behavior and Physical Activity

Many factors at both the individual and environmental level can influence a person's relationship with physical activity and sedentary behavior. The literature refers to these factors as *correlates* and *determinants* of physical activity and sedentary behavior.[95,96] Most of the research into physical behaviors has been cross-sectional, which has introduced correlates of physical activity that are statistically associated, either positively or negatively, with participation in physical activity.[95,96] To a lesser extent, longitudinal studies describe determinants of physical behaviors, factors that have been causally linked to an individual's habitual participation in physical activity.[95,96] Research on correlates and determinants has led to the development of conceptual and theoretical frameworks for exploring the interrelatedness of individual factors and environmental variables and the interactions that influence a person's engagement in physical activity.[94-96]

Individual-Level Factors

At the individual level, several key components shape a person's perspective on and relationship with physical activity. These components include the person's beliefs, values, moods, and attitudes related to physical behaviors and health, as well as biological and genetic variables that may predispose the person to either a more active or less active lifestyle. These individual factors are influenced by family members and the individual's home life, and they begin to take shape in early childhood and continue to evolve throughout the life course. When evaluating the individual factors contributing to a patient's relationship with physical activity, it is important for the practitioner to gain an understanding of the patient's history with physical activity participation and perceived level of skill in various physical activities. Physical activity is complex and multidimensional and is known to vary across the life span, which further emphasizes the need to consider the specific individual factors that affect a person's determinants of health.[97]

Environmental Factors

People are products of their environment; therefore, it is essential to evaluate the environmental influences in a patient's life in order to understand their relationship with physical activity. A patient's workplace or school is where that person spends a lot of their wake time. This time is generally structured and drives the person's physical behavior pattern for a large portion of the waking day. For example, a school-age student's engagement with physical activity is limited to the times allotted for such activity during the school day, such as recess in primary schools and physical education courses and sporting activities in secondary schools. Similarly, an individual working in an office at a desk job has limited opportunities during the workday for physical activity compared to someone in a labor-intensive or less structured job. Policies at the organizational level can affect this balance, as some companies offer employee wellness and health promotion programs with health perks and benefits, so that employees will be more physically active during their workday. Time spent outside of school or work is considered leisure time. Generally, an individual has more autonomy during this time and is able to engage in physical activity more easily. Leisure time is a frequent target of behavioral interventions because of the flexibility. It can, however, be shaped by the resources available in the community, which is often driven by policy decisions.

Communities can promote physical activity by providing built-environment infrastructure that emphasizes activity-focused spaces, such as parks, trails, and bike lanes. The availability of these features and spaces in a community is shaped by policy and policymakers.

Methods for Assessing the Determinants of Sedentary Behavior and Physical Activity

The theoretical domains framework (TDF)[98] identifies 11 determinants of behavior change by harmonizing some of the concepts and theories from other notable behavior models, such as the health belief model[99] and the theory of planned behavior.[100] The TDF has been described as a pragmatic method that can serve as a guide for assessing current behavior and subsequently identifying avenues for intervention for the sake of behavior change.[101] Making individualized assessments of the determinants of physical activity allows for personalized and tailored interventions and treatments because potential barriers are taken into account. The Determinants of Physical Activity Questionnaire,[101] which was developed and validated using the determinants of behavior from the TDF, is a 51-item self-report questionnaire that assesses 11 different subscales representing the determinants identified in the TDF.

One aspect of health behavior determinants is the sociocultural aspect, which is important in the development of an individual's attitudes and beliefs concerning physical activity and health. These attitudes and beliefs can stem from both the microenvironment and macroenvironment.[95,102,103] The Analysis Grid for Environments Linked to Obesity (ANGELO) framework is a tool for evaluating these environments and the relevant sociocultural determinants of health as they relate to attitudes and beliefs about physical activity engagement.[103] The ANGELO framework groups sociocultural determinants into five categories: four primary microenvironments—household, educational institutions, workplace, and neighborhood—and one primary macroenvironment—city/municipality/region/country.[103] The ANGELO framework helps practitioners determine the primary environmental influences in a patient's life from a sociocultural perspective.

Barriers to Physical Activity Engagement

Individuals face many barriers, both internal and external, to engaging in sufficient physical activity. These include lack of time, the high cost of some activities, limited availability of resources, and insufficient skills. The Centers for Disease Control and Prevention developed a 21-item inventory called the Barriers to Being Active quiz to help practitioners identify a patient's perceived challenges to incorporating physical activity into daily life.[104] The quiz categorizes the barriers to physical activity into seven domains: (1) lack of time, (2) social influence, (3) lack of energy, (4) lack of willpower, (5) fear of injury, (6) lack of skill, and (7) lack of resources. For each of the seven domains, there are three related questions (for a total of 21 questions), which the patient scores on a scale of 0 (for "very unlikely") to 3 (for "very likely"). A patient's total score can range from 0 to 63 points, with a higher score indicating more perceived barriers. Practitioners can use quiz results to develop individualized strategies for their patients to help them achieve desired behavior changes. Here are a few examples[105]:

- For patients who indicate that lack of time is a barrier, map out a typical week with the patient to identify potentially available blocks of time, and then make suggestions for how that time might best be used to meet goals. This can prompt the patient to start building healthy habits by seeking ways to naturally incorporate physical activity into their lifestyle. This type of goal setting and planning can also prepare patients to approach their social support systems in order to ask for accountability partners and other adequate support as they work toward their goals.

- For patients who indicate that lack of skill is a barrier, work on skill building in the areas where the patient has indicated a feeling of inadequacy. This strategy helps build confidence and increase motivation to meet goals.
- For patients who indicate that lack of resources is a barrier, help identify available resources the community, including free or low-cost alternatives to group fitness classes and gym memberships, which may not be financially feasible.

Section Summary: Assessing the Sociocultural Component of Physical Behavior

It can be challenging to assess, quantify, and address the sociocultural component of physical behavior, but doing so can help develop an understanding of the intrapersonal characteristics and environmental factors that influence a patient's relationship with physical activity and their health. Using an ecological model to establish a high-level view of a patient's environmental influences can provide a structure that allows the practitioner to strategize and plan an effective treatment or intervention that is individualized to target behavior change. Identifying the correlates and determinants of physical activity may be challenging, but their contribution to physical behavior should not be overlooked when working toward a patient's short-term and long-term treatment goals.

Combining Assessments of Physical Activity and Sedentary Behavior in Weight Loss Trials

Weight management research often draws from the energy-balance framework, which describes the relationship between energy expenditure, energy intake, and change in body weight.[106] The energy expenditure component of energy balance is strongly influenced by both sedentary behavior and physical activity, making it crucial for researchers to account for both behaviors when examining weight loss over time. As stated previously, sedentary behavior includes both an energy expenditure component (1.5 METs or less) and a postural component (seated or lying posture, excluding sleep),[49,50] whereas physical activity is defined by movement and energy expenditure.[1] Therefore, simultaneous assessments of sedentary behavior and physical activity require attention to numerous factors that pose considerable measurement-related challenges. Fundamentally, researchers must choose appropriate instrumentation for their studies based on factors that have been described previously (refer to Figure 8.1). Additional issues to consider for combined assessments include statistical, practical, and analytical issues. Because of the overarching challenges of assessing sedentary behavior and physical activity together, successful research requires an interdisciplinary team of investigators (a biostatistician is especially important to include).

Statistical Issues

Regardless of how sedentary behavior and physical activity are assessed (eg, self-report instruments or wearable devices), appropriate statistical considerations are necessary. Historically, analyses have relied on the simple approach of fitting models with separate terms for sedentary behavior and physical activity. However, both variables are part of overall time use, meaning more time in one behavior may be compensated by less time in the other. This creates statistical dependence that undermines the validity of traditional models to examine the joint and independent effects of both variables on health.

To overcome the interdependence of sedentary behavior and physical activity, several statistical approaches may be considered. A leading example is isotemporal substitution, which seeks to model the change in a health outcome when reallocating time from one behavior to another.[107,108] For example, a model may report the predicted change in body weight associated with replacing 30 minutes of sedentary time with moderate-to-vigorous physical activity over a 6-month span. Another approach to consider is clustering-focused analyses, which places participants into categories rather than assessing sedentary behavior and physical activity on a continuous scale.[109-111] This can be as simple as creating a two-by-two table using median splits on each variable (ie, high/low sedentary behavior and high/low physical activity). This approach can work well in certain situations but may lead to imbalanced categories in others. In addition, median splits prevent comparisons across studies, as the high and low cutoffs will differ from sample to sample. Practitioners can use data mining algorithms (eg, *k*-medoid clustering) to discover richer clusters in the data, which can lead to better balance across categories when that is a priority. The cluster discovery process can also be accompanied by calibration of predictive models (eg, random forests) to determine which cluster an individual belongs to, providing an avenue for standardized assessments across studies. While the above methods offer many advantages, they can be difficult to implement and interpret, which reinforces the need for interdisciplinary teams and especially for guidance from a biostatistician.

Practical Issues

Sedentary behavior and physical activity assessments need to capture representative behavior patterns for each individual at the time of assessment. Therefore, measurements should generally be made over several days (often a week or more), and repeated measurements should be made for trials that span months or years. To avoid reactivity effects, it may also be beneficial to discard the first day or two of data collected in each assessment. Ideally, any assessment should include both weekdays and weekend days to allow for capture of normal variations in day-to-day behavior. This can also play a role in distinguishing different chronotypes of physical activity, such as "weekend warriors."[112]

The chosen assessment methods for sedentary behavior and physical activity have a profound impact on the soundness of research findings. Historically, self-report instruments have been the default method for assessing both behaviors. However, wearable devices are increasingly becoming the standard method for research assessments of sedentary behavior and physical activity, and the drawbacks (eg, higher participant burden than what occurs for self-report methods) are often offset by the advantages (eg, objective and high-resolution data capture that is not possible with self-report).

In the setting of weight loss trials, where repeat assessments will almost certainly be conducted, it is especially important that researchers select assessment tools carefully. Along with consideration of the validity, burden, cost, practicality, and feasibility of each potential method (refer to Figure 8.2), longitudinal considerations are necessary, such as responsiveness to change.[113,114] Depending on the research question, high responsiveness may be more important than criterion validity, which can dramatically change the list of assessment methods that would be appropriate for the study.

Analytical Issues

As sedentary behavior and physical activity research continues, there is increasing emphasis on analyzing data using metrics that go beyond coarse measures of overall volume (eg, total sedentary or activity time). For example, researchers are showing interest in understanding the temporal patterns of each behavior, which calls for analyzing bouts of activity. The 2008 first edition of the *Physical Activity Guidelines for Americans* recommended that moderate-to-vigorous physical activity be accumulated in bouts of at least 10 minutes.[115] However, this element was dropped from the 2018 guidelines,[34] given evidence that there are only marginal health benefits associated with continuous activity bouts.[116] For sedentary behavior, studies have shown increasing health risks as sedentary bout length increases.[117,118] Other pattern indicators have also been explored, such as usual bout duration (the bout duration below which 50% of total sedentary time occurs) and α (a statistical parameter of the bout duration distribution).

In energy-balance research (particularly focused on physical activity), researchers have become increasingly interested in not only temporal patterns but also circadian timing (ie, when behaviors occur in relation to the sleep and wake cycle).[119] This emerging area comes with unique challenges, such as the need to decide whether behavior will be assessed in terms of the time of day or relative to a specific event or circadian trigger, such as getting up in the morning.[120] Another challenge is determining how to summarize day-to-day variability within participants—for example, through a measure analogous to the sleep regularity index.[121] Currently, there are no definitive findings with respect to the influence of physical activity timing on health, and there has been very little research into circadian timing and sedentary behavior. Thus, circadian timing is an area needing further study.

Overall, it is important to consider what analytical approaches are needed to obtain a study's objectives. With the increasing sophistication of sedentary behavior and physical activity assessments, it is once again necessary to emphasize the importance of assembling an interdisciplinary research team. Experts in data science and biostatistics are crucial for completing intensive assessments at scale, which should be a prominent consideration in the planning and design stages of every study.

Section Summary: Combining Assessments of Physical Activity and Sedentary Behavior in Weight Loss Trials

Special measurement challenges arise when attempting to assess physical activity and sedentary behavior simultaneously in the context of a weight loss trial. While other considerations described remain relevant (eg, comparative strengths and limitations of self-report vs device-based methods in relation to validity, burden, cost, and practicality and feasibility), researchers must consider additional factors to address statistical, practical, and analytical issues. In general, these issues fuel the need for interdisciplinary teams that include data scientists and biostatisticians. More specifically, researchers must pay attention to the ability of potential methods to capture posture, energy expenditure, and movement (core components of sedentary behavior and physical activity), as well as the utility of potential methods for application in a longitudinal setting. With a deeper understanding of how both physical activity and sedentary behavior influence energy expenditure, energy balance, and ultimately weight management, practitioners and researchers can develop better treatments and administer them to combat the obesity epidemic and reduce its immense public health burden.

Summary

Assessing physical behavior is complex and has multiple challenges. As outlined in this chapter, practitioners and researchers should take into account several factors including the assessment method, location of the activity, and sociocultural components. This is not a comprehensive list of factors to consider, but rather a starting point.

When assessing physical activity and sedentary behavior, it is critical that researchers select the appropriate tool while factoring in practicality, feasibility, cost, and burden for both the patient and researcher. When assessing activity spaces, researchers must clearly define the activity space to be measured, as this will guide the selection of the best technique to capture the outcome of interest. Additionally, assessment of the sociocultural components that affect physical behavior is an area that is rapidly changing and needs further development. Finally, it is essential that the researchers have a clear ecological model that takes into account both the individual and environmental factors that could impact a patient's physical activity.

The field of assessing physical behavior is ever-changing with constant advancement, and there is not a one-size-fits-all approach. It is critical that practitioners have an interdisciplinary team that can work together to ensure the most appropriate assessment methods are being used. With improvements in technology and computing resources, the type of physical behavior captured, as well how it is captured, will improve over time.

References

1. Caspersen CJ, Powell KE, Christenson GM. Physical activity, exercise, and physical fitness: definitions and distinctions for health-related research. *Public Health Rep.* 1985;100(2):126-131.
2. Keadle SK, Lyden KA, Strath SJ, Staudenmayer JW, Freedson PS. A framework to evaluate devices that assess physical behavior. *Exerc Sport Sci Rev.* 2019;47(4):206-214. doi:10.1249/JES.0000000000000206
3. Sylvia LG, Bernstein EE, Hubbard JL, Keating L, Anderson EJ. Practical guide to measuring physical activity. *J Acad Nutr Diet.* 2014;114(2):199-208. doi:10.1016/j.jand.2013.09.018
4. Dowd KP, Szeklicki R, Minetto MA, et al. A systematic literature review of reviews on techniques for physical activity measurement in adults: a DEDIPAC study. *Int J Behav Nutr Phys Act.* 2018;15(1):15. doi:10.1186/s12966-017-0636-2
5. Strath SJ, Kaminsky LA, Ainsworth BE, et al. Guide to the assessment of physical activity: clinical and research applications: a scientific statement from the American Heart Association. *Circulation.* 2013;128(20):2259-2279. doi:10.1161/01.cir.0000435708.67487.da

6. Taylor HL, Jacobs DR Jr, Schucker B, Knudsen J, Leon AS, Debacker G. A questionnaire for the assessment of leisure time physical activities. *J Chronic Dis*. 1978;31(12):741-755. doi:10.1016/0021-9681(78)90058-9

7. Ainsworth BE, Haskell WL, Herrmann SD, et al. 2011 Compendium of Physical Activities: a second update of codes and MET values. *Med Sci Sports Exerc*. 2011;43(8):1575-1581.

8. Butte NF, Watson KB, Ridley K, et al. A Youth Compendium of Physical Activities: activity codes and metabolic intensities. *Med Sci Sports Exerc*. 2018;50(2):246-256. doi:10.1249/MSS.0000000000001430

9. Kozey S, Lyden K, Staudenmayer J, Freedson P. Errors in MET estimates of physical activities using 3.5 ml x kg(-1) x min(-1) as the baseline oxygen consumption. *J Phys Act Health*. 2010;7(4):508-516. doi:10.1123/jpah.7.4.508

10. Ainsworth BE, Watson KB, Ridley K, et al. Utility of the Youth Compendium of Physical Activities. *Res Q Exerc Sport*. 2018;89(3):273-281. doi:10.1080/02701367.2018.1487754

11. Pfeiffer KA, Watson KB, McMurray RG, et al. Energy cost expression for a Youth Compendium of Physical Activities: rationale for using age groups. *Pediatr Exerc Sci*. 2018;30(1):142-149. doi:10.1123/pes.2016-0249

12. Hibbing PR, Bassett DR, Coe DP, Lamunion SR, Crouter SE. Youth metabolic equivalents differ depending on operational definitions. *Med Sci Sports Exerc*. 2020;52(8):1846-1853. doi:10.1249/MSS.0000000000002299

13. American College of Sports Medicine. *ACSM's Guidelines for Exercise Testing and Prescription*. 11th ed. Lippincott Williams and Wilkins; 2021.

14. Speakman JR. The history and theory of the doubly labeled water technique. *Am J Clin Nutr*. Oct 1998;68(4):932S-938S. doi:10.1093/ajcn/68.4.932S

15. Westerterp KR. Doubly labelled water assessment of energy expenditure: principle, practice, and promise. *Eur J Appl Physiol*. 2017;117(7):1277-1285. doi:10.1007/s00421-017-3641-x

16. Gupta RD, Ramachandran R, Venkatesan P, Anoop S, Joseph M, Thomas N. Indirect calorimetry: from bench to bedside. *Indian J Endocrinol Metab*. 2017;21(4):594-599. doi:10.4103/ijem.IJEM_484_16

17. Mtaweh H, Tuira L, Floh AA, Parshuram CS. Indirect calorimetry: history, technology, and application. *Front Pediatr*. 2018;6:257. doi:10.3389/fped.2018.00257

18. Schoffelen PFM, Plasqui G. Classical experiments in whole-body metabolism: open-circuit respirometry-diluted flow chamber, hood, or facemask systems. *Eur J Appl Physiol*. 2018;118(1):33-49. doi:10.1007/s00421-017-3735-5

19. Overstreet BS, Bassett DR, Jr., Crouter SE, Rider BC, Parr BB. Portable open-circuit spirometry systems. *J Sport Med Phys Fit*. 2017;57(3):227-237. doi:10.23736/S0022-4707.16.06049-7

20. Macfarlane DJ. Open-circuit respirometry: a historical review of portable gas analysis systems. *Eur J Appl Physiol*. 2017;117(12):2369-2386. doi:10.1007/s00421-017-3716-8

21. Crouter SE, DellaValle DM, Haas JD, Frongillo EA, Bassett DR. Validity of ActiGraph 2-regression model, Matthews cut-points, and NHANES cut-points for assessing free-living physical activity. *J Phys Act Health*. 2013;10(4):504-514. doi:10.1123/jpah.10.4.504

22. Ainsworth BE, Haskell WL, Leon AS, et al. Compendium of Physical Activities: classification of energy costs of human physical activities. *Med Sci Sports Exerc*. 1993;25(1):71-80. doi:10.1249/00005768-199301000-00011

23. Ainsworth BE, Haskell WL, Whitt MC, et al. Compendium of Physical Activities: an update of activity codes and MET intensities. *Med Sci Sports Exerc*. 2000;32(9 suppl):S498-S504. doi:10.1097/00005768-200009001-00009

24. Armstrong T, Bull F. Development of the World Health Organization Global Physical Activity Questionnaire (GPAQ). *J Public Health*. 2006;14(2):66-70. doi:10.1007/s10389-006-0024-x

25. Booth M. Assessment of physical activity: an international perspective. *Res Q Exerc Sport*. 2000;71(suppl 2):114-120. doi:10.1080/02701367.2000.11082794

26. Matthews CE, Kozey Keadle S, Moore SC, et al. Measurement of active and sedentary behavior in context of large epidemiologic studies. *Med Sci Sports Exerc*. 2018;50(2):266-276. doi:10.1249/mss.0000000000001428

27. Dunton GF. Ecological momentary assessment in physical activity research. *Exerc Sport Sci Rev*. 2017;45(1):48-54. doi:10.1249/jes.0000000000000092

28. LaMunion SR, Fitzhugh EC, Crouter SE. Challenges and opportunities related to the objective assessment of physical activity within U.S. health surveys. *Ann Epidemiol*. 2020;43:1-10. doi:10.1016/j.annepidem.2020.01.011

29. Troiano RP, Berrigan D, Dodd KW, Masse LC, Tilert T, McDowell M. Physical activity in the United States measured by accelerometer. *Med Sci Sports Exerc*. 2008;40(1):181-188. doi:10.1249/mss.0b013e31815a51b3

30. Matthews CE, Chen KY, Freedson PS, et al. Amount of time spent in sedentary behaviors in the United States, 2003-2004. *Am J Epidemiol*. 2008;167(7):875-881. doi:10.1093/aje/kwm390

31. Doherty A, Jackson D, Hammerla N, et al. Large scale population assessment of physical activity using wrist worn accelerometers: the UK Biobank study. *PloS One*. 2017;12(2):e0169649. doi:10.1371/journal.pone.0169649

32. Leitzmann M, Gastell S, Hillreiner A, et al. Physical activity in the German National Cohort (NAKO): use of multiple assessment tools and initial results. Article in German. *Bundesgesundheitsblatt-Gesundheitsforschung-Gesundheitsschutz*. 2020;63(3):301-311. doi:10.1007/s00103-020-03099-7

33. Paluch AE, Bajpai S, Bassett DR, et al. Daily steps and all-cause mortality: a meta-analysis of 15 international cohorts. *Lancet Public Health*. 2022;7(3):e219-e228. doi:10.1016/S2468-2667(21)00302-9
34. US Department of Health and Human Services. *Physical Activity Guidelines for Americans*. 2nd ed. US Department of Health and Human Services; 2018. Accessed April 14, 2022. https://health.gov/sites/default/files/2019-09/Physical_Activity_Guidelines_2nd_edition.pdf
35. Piercy KL, Troiano RP, Ballard RM, et al. The *Physical Activity Guidelines for Americans*. *JAMA*. 2018;320(19):2020-2028. doi:10.1001/jama.2018.14854
36. Bull FC, Al-Ansari SS, Biddle S, et al. World Health Organization 2020 guidelines on physical activity and sedentary behaviour. *Br J Sports Med*. Dec 2020;54(24):1451-1462. doi:10.1136/bjsports-2020-102955
37. Rosenberger ME, Fulton JE, Buman MP, et al. The 24-hour activity cycle: a new paradigm for physical activity. *Med Sci Sports Exerc*. 2019;51(3):454-464. doi:10.1249/MSS.0000000000001811
38. Arvidsson D, Fridolfsson J, Börjesson M. Measurement of physical activity in clinical practice using accelerometers. *J Intern Med*. 2019;286(2):137-153. doi:10.1111/joim.12908
39. Bassett DR, Toth LP, LaMunion SR, Crouter SE. Step counting: a review of measurement considerations and health-related applications. *Sports Med*. 2016:1-13. doi:10.1007/s40279-016-0663-1
40. Crouter SE, Schneider PL, Bassett DR Jr. Spring-levered versus piezo-electric pedometer accuracy in overweight and obese adults. *Med Sci Sports Exerc*. 2005;37(10):1673-1679. doi:10.1249/01.mss.0000181677.36658.a8
41. Toth LP, Park S, Springer CM, Feyerabend MD, Steeves JA, Bassett DR. Video-recorded validation of wearable step counters under free-living conditions. *Med Sci Sports Exerc*. 2018;50(6):1315-1322. doi:10.1249/mss.0000000000001569
42. Brickwood KJ, Watson G, O'Brien J, Williams AD. Consumer-based wearable activity trackers increase physical activity participation: systematic review and meta-analysis. *JMIR Mhealth Uhealth*. 2019;7(4):e11819. doi:10.2196/11819
43. Lewis ZH, Cannon M, Rubio G, Swartz MC, Lyons EJ. Analysis of the behavioral change and utility features of electronic activity monitors. *Technologies*. 2020;8(4):75. doi:10.3390/technologies8040075
44. Castaneda D, Esparza A, Ghamari M, Soltanpur C, Nazeran H. A review on wearable photoplethysmography sensors and their potential future applications in health care. *Int J Biosens Bioelectron*. 2018;4(4):195-202. doi:10.15406/ijbsbe.2018.04.00125
45. Bent B, Goldstein BA, Kibbe WA, Dunn JP. Investigating sources of inaccuracy in wearable optical heart rate sensors. *NPJ Digit Med*. 2020;3:18. doi:10.1038/s41746-020-0226-6
46. O'Driscoll R, Turicchi J, Beaulieu K, et al. How well do activity monitors estimate energy expenditure? A systematic review and meta-analysis of the validity of current technologies. *Br J Sports Med*. 2020;54(6):332-340. doi:10.1136/bjsports-2018-099643
47. Nelson BW, Low CA, Jacobson N, Areán P, Torous J, Allen NB. Guidelines for wrist-worn consumer wearable assessment of heart rate in biobehavioral research. *NPJ Digit Med*. 2020;3:90. doi:10.1038/s41746-020-0297-4
48. Stevens ML, Gupta N, Inan Eroglu E, et al. Thigh-worn accelerometry for measuring movement and posture across the 24-hour cycle: a scoping review and expert statement. *BMJ Open Sport Exerc Med*. 2020;6(1):e000874. doi:10.1136/bmjsem-2020-000874
49. Tremblay MS, Aubert S, Barnes JD, et al. Sedentary Behavior Research Network (SBRN)—Terminology Consensus Project process and outcome. *Int J Behav Nutr Phys Act*. 2017;14(1):75. doi:10.1186/s12966-017-0525-8
50. Pate RR, O'Neill JR, Lobelo F. The evolving definition of "sedentary." *Exerc Sport Sci Rev*. 2008;36(4):173-178. doi:10.1097/JES.0b013e3181877d1a
51. Edwardson CL, Rowlands AV, Bunnewell S, et al. Accuracy of posture allocation algorithms for thigh- and waist-worn accelerometers. *Med Sci Sports Exerc*. 2016;48(6):1085-1090. doi:10.1249/MSS.0000000000000865
52. Kozey-Keadle S, Libertine A, Lyden K, Staudenmayer J, Freedson P. Validation of wearable monitors for assessing sedentary behavior. *Med Sci Sports Exerc*. 2011;43(8):1561-1567. doi:10.1249/MSS.0b013e31820ce174
53. Schneller MB, Pedersen MT, Gupta N, Aadahl M, Holtermann A. Validation of five minimally obstructive methods to estimate physical activity energy expenditure in young adults in semi-standardized settings. *Sensors (Basel)*. 2015;15(3):6133-6151. doi:10.3390/s150306133
54. Kim Y, Welk GJ. Criterion validity of competing accelerometry-based activity monitoring devices. *Med Sci Sports Exerc*. 2015;47(11):2456-2463. doi:10.1249/MSS.0000000000000691
55. Ellingson LD, Schwabacher IJ, Kim Y, Welk GJ, Cook DB. Validity of an integrative method for processing physical activity data. *Med Sci Sports Exerc*. 2016;48(8):1629-1638. doi:10.1249/MSS.0000000000000915
56. Greenwood-Hickman MA, Nakandala S, Jankowska MM, et al. The CNN Hip Accelerometer Posture (CHAP) method for classifying sitting patterns from hip accelerometers: a validation study. *Med Sci Sports Exerc*. 2021;53(11):2445-2454. doi:10.1249/MSS.0000000000002705
57. Hibbing PR, LaMunion SR, Kaplan AS, Crouter SE. Estimating energy expenditure with ActiGraph GT9X inertial measurement unit. *Med Sci Sports Exerc*. 2018;50(5):1093-1102. doi:10.1249/Mss.0000000000001532

58. Fuller D, Colwell E, Low J, et al. Reliability and validity of commercially available wearable devices for measuring steps, energy expenditure, and heart rate: systematic review. *JMIR Mhealth Uhealth*. 2020;8(9):e18694-e18694. doi:10.2196/18694
59. What is Fitabase? Fitabase. Accessed April 12, 2022. www.fitabase.com/how-it-works/faq
60. Ainsworth B, Cahalin L, Buman M, Ross R. The current state of physical activity assessment tools. *Progress in Cardiovascular Diseases*. 2015;57(4):387-395. doi:10.1016/j.pcad.2014.10.005
61. Welk G, Morrow J, Saint-Maurice P. Overview of physical activity assessment tools. In: *Measures Registry User Guide: Individual Physical Activity*. National Collaborative on Childhood Obesity Research; 2017:Section 5. www.nccor.org/tools-mruserguides/individual-physical-activity/overview-of-physical-activity-assessment-tools
62. Coravos A, Doerr M, Goldsack J, et al. Modernizing and designing evaluation frameworks for connected sensor technologies in medicine. *NPJ Digit Med*. 2020;3(1):37. doi:10.1038/s41746-020-0237-3
63. Goldsack JC, Coravos A, Bakker JP, et al. Verification, analytical validation, and clinical validation (V3): the foundation of determining fit-for-purpose for Biometric Monitoring Technologies (BioMeTs). *NPJ Digit Med*. 2020;3(1):55. doi:10.1038/s41746-020-0260-4
64. Reece JD, Bunn JA, Choi M, Navalta JW. Assessing heart rate using Consumer Technology Association standards. *Technologies*. 2021;9(3):46. doi:10.3390/technologies9030046
65. Bunn JA, Jones C, Oliviera A, Webster MJ. Assessment of step accuracy using the Consumer Technology Association standard. *J Sports Sci*. 2019;37(3):244-248. doi:10.1080/02640414.2018.1491941
66. Golledge RG, Stimson RJ. *Spatial Behavior: A Geographic Perspective*. Guilford Press; 1997.
67. Warren JM, Ekelund U, Besson H, et al. Assessment of physical activity—a review of methodologies with reference to epidemiological research: a report of the exercise physiology section of the European Association of Cardiovascular Prevention and Rehabilitation. *Eur J Prev Cardiol*. 2010;17(2):127-139. doi:10.1097/HJR.0b013e32832ed875
68. World Health Organization. *Global Action Plan on Physical Activity 2018-2030: More Active People for a Healthier World*. World Health Organization; 2019.
69. Sallis JF. Measuring physical activity environments: a brief history. *Am J Prev Med*. 2009;36(4 suppl):S86-S92. doi:10.1016/j.amepre.2009.01.002
70. Brownson RC, Hoehner CM, Day K, Forsyth A, Sallis JF. Measuring the built environment for physical activity: state of the science. *Am J Prev Med*. 2009;36(4 suppl):S99-S123.e12. doi:10.1016/j.amepre.2009.01.005
71. Maddison R, Ni Mhurchu C. Global positioning system: a new opportunity in physical activity measurement. *Int J Behav Nutr Phys Act*. 2009;6:73. doi:10.1186/1479-5868-6-73
72. Loveday A, Sherar LB, Sanders JP, Sanderson PW, Esliger DW. Technologies that assess the location of physical activity and sedentary behavior: a systematic review. *J Med Internet Res*. 2015;17(8):e192. doi:10.2196/jmir.4761
73. Butler EN, Ambs AM, Reedy J, Bowles HR. Identifying GIS measures of the physical activity built environment through a review of the literature. *J Phys Act Health*. 2011;8 (suppl 1):S91-S97. doi:10.1123/jpah.8.s1.s91
74. Carlson J, Dean K, Sallis JF. *Measures Registry User Guide: Physical Activity Environment*. National Collaborative on Childhood Obesity Research; January 2017. http://nccororgms.wpengine.com/tools-mruserguides/wp-content/uploads/sites/2/2017/NCCOR_MR_User_Guide_Physical_Activity-FINAL.pdf
75. Nasar JL. Assessing perceptions of environments for active living. *Am J Prev Med*. 2008;34(4):357-363. doi:10.1016/j.amepre.2008.01.013
76. Saelens BE, Sallis JF, Black JB, Chen D. Neighborhood-based differences in physical activity: an environment scale evaluation. *Am J Public Health*. 2003;93(9):1552-1558. doi:10.2105/ajph.93.9.1552
77. Kirtland KA, Porter DE, Addy CL, et al. Environmental measures of physical activity supports: perception versus reality. *Am J Prev Med*. 2003;24(4):323-331. doi:10.1016/s0749-3797(03)00021-7
78. Jankowska M, Schipperijn J, Kerr J, Altintas I. Applied CyberGIS in the age of complex spatial health data. *International Conference on GIScience Short Paper Proceedings* 2016;1(1). doi:10.21433/B3111jr9168v
79. Jankowska MM, Schipperijn J, Kerr J. A framework for using GPS data in physical activity and sedentary behavior studies. *Exerc Sport Sci Rev*. 2015;43(1):48-56. doi:10.1249/JES.0000000000000035
80. Kerr J, Duncan S, Schipperijn J. Using global positioning systems in health research: a practical approach to data collection and processing. *Am J Prev Med*. 2011;41(5):532-540. doi:10.1016/j.amepre.2011.07.017
81. Yi L, Wilson JP, Mason TB, Habre R, Wang S, Dunton GF. Methodologies for assessing contextual exposure to the built environment in physical activity studies: a systematic review. *Health Place*. 2019;60:102226. doi:10.1016/j.healthplace.2019.102226
82. Fuller D, Shareck M, Stanley K. Ethical implications of location and accelerometer measurement in health research studies with mobile sensing devices. *Soc Sci Med*. 2017;191:84-88. doi:10.1016/j.socscimed.2017.08.043
83. Nebeker C, Harlow J, Espinoza Giacinto R, Orozco-Linares R, Bloss CS, Weibel N. Ethical and regulatory challenges of research using pervasive sensing and other emerging technologies: IRB perspectives. *AJOB Empir Bioeth*. 2017;8(4):266-276. doi:10.1080/23294515.2017.1403980

84. Nebeker C, Linares-Orozco R, Crist K. A multi-case study of research using mobile imaging, sensing and tracking technologies to objectively measure behavior: ethical issues and insights to guide responsible research practice. *J Research Administration*. 2015;46(1):118-137.
85. Oliver M, Badland H, Mavoa S, Duncan MJ, Duncan S. Combining GPS, GIS, and accelerometry: methodological issues in the assessment of location and intensity of travel behaviors. *J Phys Act Health*. 2010;7(1):102-108. doi:10.1123/jpah.7.1.102
86. Procter DS, Page AS, Cooper AR, et al. An open-source tool to identify active travel from hip-worn accelerometer, GPS and GIS data. *Int J Behav Nutr Phys Act*. 2018;15(1):91. doi:10.1186/s12966-018-0724-y
87. Mennis J, Mason M, Ambrus A. Urban greenspace is associated with reduced psychological stress among adolescents: a Geographic Ecological Momentary Assessment (GEMA) analysis of activity space. *Landsc Urban Plan*. 2018;174:1-9. doi:10.1016/j.landurbplan.2018.02.008
88. Smith L, Foley L, Panter J. Activity spaces in studies of the environment and physical activity: a review and synthesis of implications for causality. *Health Place*. 2019;58:102113. doi:10.1016/j.healthplace.2019.04.003
89. Houston D. Implications of the modifiable areal unit problem for assessing built environment correlates of moderate and vigorous physical activity. *Applied Geography*. 2014;50:40-47. doi:10.1016/j.apgeog.2014.02.008
90. Openshaw S. *The Modifiable Areal Unit Problem*. Geo Books; 1983. *Concepts and Techniques in Modern Geography*, vol 38.
91. Kwan MP. The uncertain geographic context problem. *Ann Assoc Am Geogr*. 2012;102(5):958-968. doi:10.1080/00045608.2012.687349
92. Chaix B, Meline J, Duncan S, et al. GPS tracking in neighborhood and health studies: a step forward for environmental exposure assessment, a step backward for causal inference? *Health Place*. 2013;21:46-51. doi:10.1016/j.healthplace.2013.01.003
93. Sallis JF, Cervero RB, Ascher W, Henderson KA, Kraft MK, Kerr J. An ecological approach to creating active living communities. *Annu Rev Public Health*. 2006;27(1):297-322. doi:10.1146/annurev.publhealth.27.021405.102100
94. King KM, Gonzalez GB. Increasing physical activity using an ecological model. *ACSM's Health Fit*. 2018;22(4):29-32. doi:10.1249/fit.0000000000000397
95. Bauman AE, Reis RS, Sallis JF, Wells JC, Loos RJF, Martin BW. Correlates of physical activity: why are some people physically active and others not? *Lancet*. 2012;380(9838):258-271. doi:10.1016/S0140-6736(12)60735-1
96. Bauman AE, Sallis JF, Dzewaltowski DA, Owen N. Toward a better understanding of the influences on physical activity: the role of determinants, correlates, causal variables, mediators, moderators, and confounders. *Am J Prev Med*. 2002;23(2 suppl):5-14. doi:10.1016/s0749-3797(02)00469-5
97. Sherwood NE, Jeffery RW. The behavioral determinants of exercise: implications for physical activity interventions. *Annu Rev Nutr*. 2000;20:21-44. doi:10.1146/annurev.nutr.20.1.21
98. Michie S, Johnston M, Francis J, Hardeman W, Eccles M. From theory to intervention: mapping theoretically derived behavioural determinants to behaviour change techniques. *Appl Psychol*. 2008;57(4):660-680. doi:10.1111/j.1464-0597.2008.00341.x
99. Rosenstock IM. Historical origins of the health belief model. *Health Educ Monogr*. 1974;2(4):328-335. doi:10.1177/109019817400200403
100. Ajzen I. The theory of planned behavior. *Organ Behav Hum Decis Process*. 1991;50(2):179-211. doi:10.1016/0749-5978(91)90020-T
101. Taylor N, Lawton R, Conner M. Development and initial validation of the determinants of physical activity questionnaire. *Int J Behav Nutr Phys Act*. 2013;10(1):1-11. doi:10.1186/1479-5868-10-74
102. Jaeschke L, Steinbrecher A, Luzak A, et al. Sociocultural determinants of physical activity across the life course: a 'Determinants of Diet and Physical Activity'(DEDIPAC) umbrella systematic literature review. *Int J Behav Nutr Phys Act*. 2017;14(1):173. doi:10.1186/s12966-017-0627-3
103. Swinburn B, Egger G, Raza F. Dissecting obesogenic environments: the development and application of a framework for identifying and prioritizing environmental interventions for obesity. *Prev Med*. 1999;29(6):563-570. doi:10.1006/pmed.1999.0585
104. Barriers to Being Active Quiz. Centers for Disease Control and Prevention. Accessed December 1, 2021. www.cdc.gov/diabetes/professional-info/pdfs/toolkits/Road-to-Health-Barriers-Activity-Quiz-p.pdf
105. Overcoming barriers to physical activity. Centers for Disease Control and Prevention. Accessed December 1, 2021. www.cdc.gov/physicalactivity/basics/adding-pa/barriers.html
106. Hall KD, Heymsfield SB, Kemnitz JW, Klein S, Schoeller DA, Speakman JR. Energy balance and its components: implications for body weight regulation. *Am J Clin Nutr*. 2012;95(4):989-994. doi:10.3945/ajcn.112.036350
107. Dumuid D, Pedisic Z, Palarea-Albaladejo J, Martin-Fernandez JA, Hron K, Olds T. Compositional data analysis in time-use epidemiology: what, why, how. *Int J Environ Res Public Health*. 2020;17(7):2220. doi:10.3390/ijerph17072220
108. Mekary RA, Willett WC, Hu FB, Ding EL. Isotemporal substitution paradigm for physical activity epidemiology and weight change. *Am J Epidemiol*. 2009;170(4):519-527. doi:10.1093/aje/kwp163
109. Chinapaw MJ, de Niet M, Verloigne M, De Bourdeaudhuij I, Brug J, Altenburg TM. From sedentary time to sedentary patterns: accelerometer data reduction decisions in youth. *PloS One*. 2014;9(11):e111205. doi:10.1371/journal.pone.0111205

110. Hibbing PR, Bellettiere J, Carlson JA. Sedentary profiles: a new perspective on accumulation patterns in sedentary behavior. *Med Sci Sports Exerc*. 2022;54(4):696-706. doi:10.1249/MSS.0000000000002830

111. Aqeel M, Guo J, Lin L, et al. Temporal physical activity patterns are associated with obesity in U.S. adults. *Prev Med*. 2021;148:106538. doi:10.1016/j.ypmed.2021.106538

112. Lee IM, Sesso HD, Oguma Y, Paffenbarger RS Jr. The "weekend warrior" and risk of mortality. *Am J Epidemiol*. 2004;160(7):636-641. doi:10.1093/aje/kwh274

113. Guyatt G, Walter S, Norman G. Measuring change over time: assessing the usefulness of evaluative instruments. *J Chronic Dis*. 1987;40(2):171-178. doi:10.1016/0021-9681(87)90069-5

114. Hays RD, Hadorn D. Responsiveness to change: an aspect of validity, not a separate dimension. *Qual Life Res*. 1992;1(1):73-75. doi:10.1007/BF00435438

115. *2008 Physical Activity Guidelines for Americans*. US Department of Health and Human Services. 2008. Accessed February 28, 2023. https://health.gov/sites/default/files/2019-09/paguide.pdf

116. Saint-Maurice PF, Troiano RP, Matthews CE, Kraus WE. Moderate-to-vigorous physical activity and all-cause mortality: do bouts matter? *J Am Heart Assoc*. 2018;7(6)e007678. doi:10.1161/JAHA.117.007678

117. Diaz KM, Goldsmith J, Greenlee H, et al. Prolonged, uninterrupted sedentary behavior and glycemic biomarkers among US hispanic/latino adults: the HCHS/SOL (Hispanic Community Health Study/Study of Latinos). *Circulation*. 2017;136(15):1362-1373. doi:10.1161/circulationaha.116.026858

118. Diaz KM, Howard VJ, Hutto B, et al. Patterns of sedentary behavior and mortality in U.S. middle-aged and older adults: a national cohort study. *Ann Intern Med*. 2017;167(7):465-475. doi:10.7326/M17-0212

119. Veronda AC, Kline CE, Irish LA. The impact of circadian timing on energy balance: an extension of the energy balance model. *Health Psychol Rev*. 2022;16(2):161-203. doi:10.1080/17437199.2021.1968310

120. Blankenship JM, Rosenberg RC, Rynders CA, Melanson EL, Catenacci VA, Creasy SA. Examining the role of exercise timing in weight management: a review. *Int J Sports Med*. 2021;42(11):967-978. doi:10.1055/a-1485-1293

121. Phillips AJK, Clerx WM, O'Brien CS, et al. Irregular sleep/wake patterns are associated with poorer academic performance and delayed circadian and sleep/wake timing. *Sci Rep*. 2017;7(1):3216. doi:10.1038/s41598-017-03171-4

CHAPTER 9

Behavioral Health Assessment

Alyssa M. Minnick, PhD
Christina M. Hopkins, PhD
Kelly C. Allison, PhD
Courtney McCuen-Wurst, PsyD, LCSW

CHAPTER OBJECTIVES

- Review methods for assessing behavioral health.
- Identify psychological constructs and health behaviors affecting weight management.
- Review sociocultural factors that may influence behavioral health.
- Describe factors to consider in determining what methods of behavioral health assessment to use in outpatient settings.

Introduction

Weight management, mental health, and health behavior are fundamentally interconnected, with many psychological and behavioral factors having a bidirectional relationship with weight.[1-4] Therefore, an assessment of a patient's psychological constructs and health behaviors can help the health care practitioner choose an appropriate and effective weight-management intervention for the patient. This chapter reviews the various methods of behavioral health assessment that practitioners can use in clinical practice. The measurements reviewed can be used separately to assess specific constructs of importance to an individual patient, or a standardized battery of measures can be constructed to fit a specific clinical setting. Factors to consider when determining which assessments are appropriate are covered, as well as how behavioral health parameters can be brought together within an obesity-focused history. The importance of balancing time and patient burden of the assessment against clinical utility is also considered.

Behavioral Health Factors Within Weight Management

Mood disorders, such as depression and anxiety, have been associated with emotional eating, or eating in response to negative emotions.[5,6] As such, research has suggested that emotional eating is one mechanism linking depression to the development of overweight and obesity, and studies have shown it to be a mediating link between the two.[7,8] Research also suggests that depression and obesity are bidirectionally associated and often occur together.[9,10] Epidemiological studies indicate that clinical depression in adolescence or early adulthood often precedes the development of obesity in adulthood.[11] Additional research indicates that individuals with obesity have 55% higher odds of developing depression, and persons with depression have 58% higher odds of developing obesity; the connection between the two appears to be stronger in women than in men.[†,9,12] When people are depressed,

---

† Study participants were described as women and men. Gender was not further specified.

they may eat foods that are high in energy, sugar, fat, and carbohydrates in an attempt to improve their depressive symptoms, leading to weight gain. Their food choices tend to be energy dense and highly palatable.[7] In one study conducted in France over 2 years, emotional eating was not related to a change in BMI; however, in similar studies conducted in other countries, including the United States, South Korea, and the Netherlands, higher emotional eating at baseline led to weight gain over time.[13-16] Furthermore, a review article found that depression and emotional eating were positively associated; they were both predictors of increased BMI over 7 years.[7] Additional research suggests that emotional eating is more prevalent in women than in men.[†,17] Other lifestyle factors often associated with depression such as social isolation and fatigue may lead to a decrease in physical activity, which can also lead to weight gain. Additional mechanisms linking depression and obesity include adverse effects of antidepressant drugs or other psychotropic drugs, such as mood stabilizers and antipsychotic medications. These drugs may affect eating by causing lack of satiety and overconsumption of high-energy foods, leading to weight gain over time.[11]

In addition to mood disorders, stress has been associated with weight gain. Stress is accompanied by physiological and biological changes, and research suggests that some forms of stress can lead to depression, which as previously noted, can also lead to weight gain.[18] The accumulation of adiposity that can occur with chronic stress has been associated with activation of the hypothalamic-pituitary-adrenal axis.[19] Research seems to indicate that consuming highly palatable foods in response to stress tends to activate the reward centers of the brain, which increases the tendency to consume these foods in response to subsequent stress.[20,21] Observational studies have revealed clear associations between stress and abdominal adiposity.[22] Stress and mood disorders can also negatively impact other health behaviors, such as sleep quality, which can contribute to weight gain. Research suggests that adults with a combination of shorter sleep duration and higher frequency of eating in response to negative emotions may be more prone to overweight and obesity.[7] Short sleep duration tends to be associated with irregular eating patterns, with short-sleepers eating fewer main meals and more small, energy-dense foods and snacks more frequently throughout the day than people with longer sleep durations do. In a study conducted with Dutch employees over a 2-year period, investigators found that women[†] with both shorter sleep duration and higher levels of emotional eating experienced the greatest increase in BMI.[7] Other health behaviors, such as substance use, as well as motivations and readiness for changes in eating behaviors and physical activity levels, can also affect weight management efforts.[23,24] Consequently, it is important to assess both psychological constructs and health behaviors together, as they often influence each other, which in turn can affect weight management.

Psychological Constructs Affecting Weight Management

The most common psychological factors to consider in a behavioral health assessment for weight management are listed in Box 9.1 and expanded upon in this section.

Most of the assessment tools discussed in this chapter are self-report questionnaires, as these are easily administered in a clinical setting for the purpose of screening for important factors and to assist with the diagnosis of any comorbid conditions that may need to be incorporated into treatment planning.

---

† Study participants were described as women and men. Gender was not further specified.

> **BOX 9.1**
>
> **Common Psychological Factors to Consider in a Behavioral Health Assessment for Weight Management**
>
> Mood
> Anxiety
> Weight history and eating behaviors
> Trauma history
> Stress
> Weight-related stigma and internalization
> Quality of life

These measures can also be used to track progress and improvements during a weight-management intervention.

Mood

Mood is a primary factor to consider in weight management, given that research has consistently shown that people with depression are at a higher risk for developing obesity than those who have not experienced depression.[25] Depressed mood may be an antecedent to obesity if individuals eat in response to emotions, perhaps for distraction or comfort from negative experiences.[5,6,26] People may also feel more down or depressed because of their weight management difficulties, which may further perpetuate mood disturbances.[27] The most widely used and validated self-report measure to assess for depressed mood is the Beck Depression Inventory-II (BDI-II).[28] The BDI-II is a 21-item questionnaire that assesses for symptoms and attitudes associated with depression over the preceding 2 weeks. Each item is rated on a scale of 0 to 3 points, and a total score is calculated by summing the ratings for all items. Higher scores indicate higher levels of depressed mood. The BDI-II provides cutoff scores to help the provider determine if the patient is experiencing no-to-minimal, mild, moderate, or severe symptoms of depression.

Another well-known clinical tool for assessing depressed mood is the Patient Health Questionnaire-9 (PHQ-9).[29,30] This nine-item questionnaire also asks the patient to rate their symptoms over the preceding 2 weeks but focuses only on the criteria used for diagnosing clinical depression. Each item (symptom) is rated on a scale of 0 to 3 points, with 0 points indicating that the symptom occurred *not at all* and 3 points indicating that it occurred *nearly every day*. A final item asks patients to rate the degree to which any or all of the symptoms reported as present interfere with their ability to do their daily tasks, with 0 points indicating *not at all* and 3 points indicating that the symptoms make it *extremely difficult* to do daily tasks. There is also a shortened two-item version (PHQ-2) that can be used for quick screening to determine if additional assessment is required.[31] In addition, providers may consider using the Geriatric Depression Scale–Short Form (GDS-SF) with patients aged 65 years and older, given that some symptoms of depression may be experienced as a normal part of the aging process (eg, lower energy, changes in sleep and appetite).[32] Patients indicate whether each of the 15 items is either present or absent with a *yes* or *no* answer, and there are cutoff scores (total sum score) for normal, mild, moderate, and severely depressed mood.

Finally, suicidality can be assessed with items in the BDI-II (item 9) and the PHQ-9 (item 9), which ask something like, "Over the past 2 weeks, how often have you had thoughts that you would be better off dead or of hurting yourself?" The six-item, interview-based Columbia-Suicide Severity Rating Scale (C-SSRS) also evaluates suicide risk.[33] It is widely used for research and in clinical settings. The authors have provided an internet-based training for its administration (https://cssrs.columbia.edu/training/training-options).

Anxiety

Anxiety can be defined as excessive worry or fear that is intense and persistent in a way that interferes with daily functioning. Anxiety includes both thoughts of these worries or fears and physical sensations that may be associated with the worry or fear (eg, being fidgety or restless, sweating, increased heart rate, stomach ache).[34] Previous research has shown that individuals with overweight or obesity are more likely than individuals within a healthy weight status to have anxiety.[35] A common self-report questionnaire used to assess patients for anxiety is the Generalized Anxiety Disorder-7 (GAD-7).[36] This seven-item tool asks patients how frequently they have experienced certain symptoms of anxiety over the preceding 2 weeks, with frequency ratings ranging from *not at all* to *nearly every day*. A final question assesses for the impact that the symptoms experienced have on daily functioning. The 21-item Beck Anxiety Inventory (BAI) is another option. The BAI examines symptoms and attitudes associated with anxiety over the previous 2 weeks.[37] BAI has been shown to distinguish between anxiety and depression, which is important given the high comorbidity between these psychological disorders and because these disorders can differently influence one's choices to overeat or restrict food.[37] Higher scores on both of these questionnaires indicate higher levels of anxiety, and both measurement tools include cutoff scores to help providers determine the severity of symptoms.

Weight History and Eating Behavior

Eating behavior is one of the most important aspects of weight-management assessment and encompasses general eating behaviors and attitudes, as well as disordered eating behaviors such as binge eating, night eating, and compensatory behaviors used after eating to avoid weight gain. General assessments of weight history, eating behavior, and attitudes about eating may assist with determining developmental and maintenance factors associated with overweight and obesity, which is helpful in determining potential targets of treatment. Providers may first ask patients to detail their weight history, including their weight status at each developmental stage (childhood, adolescence, and adulthood), the age when their weight first becomes a noticeable concern, and the factors they believe contributed to their weight gain over time. These contributing factors may be biological in nature or behavioral. Examples of biological factors include genetics, family weight history, or contribution of medications (eg, steroids, some psychotropic medications). Examples of behavioral factors include specific eating behaviors, food choices, and levels of physical activity at different times in their lives.

Other assessment measures can then be used to determine additional, more current, contributing factors to weight. The Eating Inventory (formerly known as the Three-Factor Eating Questionnaire) is a 51-item instrument that assesses cognitive control over eating, disinhibition, and hunger.[38] There are also 18-item and 21-item versions of the Eating Inventory that may be more practical for clinical outpatient settings.[39,40] In addition, several questionnaires are available to assess for specific types of food experiences, including appetite management, cravings, and even "food addiction" that may influence eating behavior and subsequent weight gain. For example, the Power of Food Scale is a 21-item scale that measures a person's appetite for (but not necessarily consumption of) highly palatable foods at three different food proximities (food available, food present, and food tasted).[41] The Food Craving Inventory uses 28 items to assess a person's motivational drive for food in general, as well as the motivational drive (or craving) for specific foods, such as high-fat foods, sweets, carbohydrates or starches, and fast foods.[42] The Yale Food Addiction Scale, Version 2, proposes that individuals may have signs and symptoms of addiction to highly palatable foods that are similar to those exhibited by individuals with a substance use disorder.[43,44] This 25-item measure determines the number of food addiction symptoms a patient has; this score is then used to determine whether the patient can be considered to have food addiction. It also evaluates for the presence of substantial distress or interference with daily functioning.

Ideally, the assessment of eating behaviors should also look for potential eating pathology. The Eating Disorder Examination (EDE), a semistructured interview examining eating-disordered behaviors and attitudes, is the most widely used and best validated assessment for eating disorders.[45] It must be administered by a trained clinician and is effective for the diagnosis of anorexia nervosa, bulimia nervosa, binge eating disorder, and otherwise specified or unspecified eating disorders. The interview focuses on symptoms present within the previous 28 days and also extends to the preceding 2 months to gather diagnostic data for a full 3 months, which is required to make a diagnosis. Eating pathologies assessed by the EDE include fasting or restricting food intake, grazing (ie, picking and nibbling on small amounts of food throughout the day, between planned meals and snacks), binge eating, loss-of-control eating, and compensatory behaviors after eating to avoid gaining weight (eg, self-induced vomiting, use of laxatives or diuretics, excessive exercising). Four subscales can also be derived from the individual's responses regarding restraint, eating concerns, shape concerns, and weight concerns, as well as a global score.

Clinics that do not have a trained clinician to administer the EDE or the time to do so can use self-report questionnaires to assess eating disorder constructs. The Eating Disorder Examination-Questionnaire (EDE-Q) focuses on the previous 28 days, like the interview version, and it examines symptoms and attitudes using 28 items.[46] The EDE-Q also provides scores for the same four subscales as well as a global score. The Questionnaire on Eating and Weight Patterns-5 (QEWP-5) is a face-valid, 26-item measure that assesses patients for the symptoms listed in the fifth edition of the *Diagnostic and Statistical Manual of Mental Disorders* associated with binge eating disorder and bulimia nervosa, including loss-of-control eating and compensatory behaviors; it also collects information about weight history and family weight history.[47] The Binge Eating Scale is a 16-item self-report questionnaire designed to capture both the behavioral features of objective binge episodes (eg, consuming a large amount of food) and the cognitive and emotional features (eg, feeling out of control while eating, preoccupation with food and eating).[48] The Night Eating Questionnaire includes 14 items and assesses for the psychological and behavioral symptoms consistent with night eating syndrome.[49] In particular, it assesses for the presence of nocturnal eating episodes or consuming a large portion of one's daily energy intake after dinnertime, as well as associated symptoms of morning anorexia, mood and sleep issues, and thoughts that one must eat to resume sleep. A score of 25 or greater suggests night eating syndrome. All of these self-report questionnaires help identify the presence of disordered eating behavior and assist in making a clinical diagnosis, but they should be used in combination with a clinical interview to make a diagnosis.

Trauma

Trauma, broadly defined as the emotional reaction to a substantially disruptive or dangerous life event, has several downstream negative effects on health and health behaviors. Trauma can contribute to maladaptive thoughts about oneself and the world, which may affect one's ability or willingness to care for oneself. In adults with obesity, childhood trauma or adverse events is of particular clinical interest. A 2020 meta-analysis identified a 46% increase in the odds of having obesity in adulthood if an individual experienced multiple adverse events in childhood (odds ratio, 1.46; 95% CI, 1.28–1.64).[50] Several potential mechanisms may explain this increased risk. Systematic reviews have linked adverse childhood experiences to the development of binge eating disorder, a known contributor to obesity.[51] Furthermore, trauma can contribute to considerable neurobiological changes that can, in turn, contribute to increased inflammation in the body, poorer sleep, and increased reactivity of the hypothalamic-pituitary-adrenal axis.[52,53] Generally speaking, trauma can disrupt an individual's physiology, psychology, social connections, and ability to engage in healthy behaviors.

Childhood trauma is traditionally assessed using the Childhood Trauma Questionnaire.[54] This self-report measure is a 28-item retrospective assessment of childhood adverse experiences spanning abuse, maltreatment, and neglect. In using this assessment, clinicians can identify patterns in five subscales: emotional abuse, physical abuse, sexual abuse, emotional neglect, and physical neglect. Not all who report childhood adverse experiences have a traumatic reaction; therefore, it is imperative to pair this assessment with thoughtful and open clinical discussion of how these experiences may have affected the individual's development and the effects on health behaviors in the present day.

Stress

Stress may also play an important role in weight management. It can cause reduced appetite in some individuals, whereas in others it can induce eating or overeating.[22] The Perceived Stress Scale is a 10-item measure of the frequency of specific stressful events in a person's life over the preceding 2 weeks, as well as any thoughts and feelings associated with those events.[55] Clinicians can also assess for stress using the 21-item Depression, Anxiety, and Stress Scale, which also evaluates for depression and anxiety symptoms.[56] Each subscale score is totaled, and cutoff scores determine the severity of symptoms, ranging from *normal* to *extremely severe*. These measures may also help identify barriers and challenges to weight-management efforts, which can then be targeted by interventions.

Weight Stigma and Internalization

Individuals with obesity are commonly stereotyped, ostracized, shamed, and discriminated against. The stigma for a person who is overweight or has obesity may have a substantial impact on a person's health, health behaviors, engagement with health care services, and outcomes in weight loss interventions.[57] Weight stigma can also be internalized, causing individuals to self-stigmatize, meaning they apply these negative beliefs and stereotypes to themselves. Research suggests that the internalization of weight stigma has a considerable deleterious effect on health, over and above the health risks of obesity alone.[58] A person with a high level of internalized weight bias might avoid healthy behaviors such as engaging in physical activity or keeping their medical appointments more than someone who has a healthy weight status, and they may experience more disordered eating behaviors.[57] Furthermore, internalized weight stigma is conceptualized as a chronic discriminatory stressor; therefore, the stress associated with weight stigma may dysregulate the nervous system and contribute to obesity on a physiological level.[53]

Weight bias, both experienced and internalized, is another important psychological domain to assess for as part of weight-management interventions. Individuals should be asked whether they have experienced any of the three main forms of weight stigma: teasing, unfair treatment, or discrimination based on weight. If so, the practitioner should determine the degree to which they have internalized these experiences. Two measures are commonly used to assess the degree of self-directed weight stigma: the Weight Bias Internalization Scale (WBIS) and the Weight Self-Stigma Questionnaire (WSSQ).[58,59] The WBIS is a 10-item self-report assessment in which individuals rate their agreement with statements such as, *My weight is the major way that I value myself as a person*. The current modified version of this tool is recommended, as it has been validated for use across weight classes, whether or not the individual identifies with the label of "obesity." The WSSQ is a 12-item self-report measure with two subscales (fear of enacted stigma and self-devaluation) and may have more clinical utility than the WBIS. The WSSQ asks individuals to rate their agreement with statements such as, *I became overweight because I am a weak person*. These two instruments yield objective scores that clinicians can compare to population norms. Furthermore, the clinician should elucidate the strength of these beliefs and determine impact on day-to-day functioning, expectations about weight loss, and effects on health behaviors as they relate to weight management. In having these conversations, providers should use person-first language to prevent the occurrence of stigmazing interactions within the health care field.

Quality of Life

It is also important to assess for quality of life (QOL) when considering weight-management interventions in order to determine how a person's weight and co-occurring conditions or experiences are affecting their overall well-being. QOL assessments can be used to track a patient's progress during the course of treatment as a complement to the tracking of symptom frequency and actual weight gain or loss. The 36-item Short Form Health Survey (SF-36) is a questionnaire that assesses eight subscales: vitality, physical functioning, bodily pain, general health perceptions, physical role functioning, emotional role functioning, social role functioning, and mental health.[60] Scores on this measure range from 0 to 100, with higher scores indicating less disability and higher QOL and well-being. Another option is the Impact of Weight on Quality of Life–Lite (IWQOL-Lite).[61] It is a 31-item questionnaire that yields a total score for QOL, as well as individual scores for five domains: physical function, self-esteem, sexual life, public distress, and work.

Health Behaviors Affecting Weight Management

Health behaviors, including but not limited to substance use, sleep, physical activity, and motivation and readiness to change, are important to weight management. These factors may have direct effects on weight—for example, weight loss due to increased energy expenditure through physical activity—as well as indirect effects, including weight loss or gain due to changes in hormones associated with appetite and satiety as a result of disrupted sleep. The assessment of health behaviors may help providers determine the development and maintenance of overweight and obesity in their patients, as well as identify additional targets for a more holistic treatment plan.

Substance Use

A 2018 meta-analysis found an inverse relationship between substance use (alcohol and drug use) and overweight and obesity, such that low weight was associated with higher risk for substance use; however, substance use, including alcohol, drug, and tobacco use, may influence appetite and daily energy consumption.[23] Providers may do a simple assessment of a patient's history of substance use, including lifetime and current use, years of use, and frequency and amount of use for each substance. The Tobacco, Alcohol, Prescription medication, and other Substance use (TAPS) Tool screens for all aspects of substance use by first administering a four-item questionnaire to screen for each category of substance use, and if positive, additional questions provide further evaluation.[62] Other questionnaires, such as the Alcohol Use Disorder Identification Test (AUDIT), target specific substances.[63] AUDIT uses 10 items to assess a patient's alcohol consumption, drinking behaviors, and alcohol-related problems, and it has a cutoff score of 8 to indicate harmful alcohol use. A short version, the AUDIT-C (*C* for "concise") uses three items to help screen for problematic drinking behaviors.[64]

Sleep

Sleep disturbances are common in those with obesity. Sleep is an essential regulatory process that contributes to metabolism, mood, cognition, and health behaviors. Poorer sleep quality may result in increased impulsivity, increased disordered eating (eg, binge episodes), barriers to engaging in health behaviors, and worsening depression or anxiety. In addition to these psychological and behavioral outcomes of poor sleep, insufficient sleep can lead to disruptions in markers of appetite regulation, such as leptin or glucose. Sleep can be assessed in many ways. A thorough sleep assessment should include self-monitoring of wake times, sleep times, onset of sleep, and frequency of awakenings each night. Generally, sleeping 6 hours or less during the night is considered insufficient.[65] Self-report measures can also be used to assess sleep quality and compare against population norms. One such measure is the Pittsburgh Sleep Quality Index, which surveys several domains, such as sleep duration, subjective sleep quality, sleep latency, sleep efficiency, sleep disturbances, sleep medicine use, and daytime dysfunction due to sleep issues.[66] Finally, with the wide availability of wearable devices, several electronic watches and activity-monitoring devices can also be used to estimate sleep, although commercially available wearables are not typically as accurate as research-based wrist actigraphs.

Of note, persons with higher weight are more prone to having obstructive sleep apnea, and many individuals do not realize that they have it. The Apnea Risk Evaluation System uses 32 items to determine for risk of sleep apnea by assessing gender, age, height, weight, medical status, and domains of symptoms (eg, snoring, gasping for air).[67] The Epworth Sleepiness Scale is embedded within the Apnea Risk Evaluation System and provides cutoff scores for *low*, *high*, and *very high* risk for having sleep apnea.[68] The Epworth Sleepiness Scale is comprised of eight items and can also be used as a standalone measurement of daytime sleepiness. If indicated, patients may be referred for a sleep study to determine if sleep apnea or another sleep disorder is present and the appropriate treatment.

Physical Activity and Sedentary Behaviors

Physical activity is an important part of the energy balance equation that helps to regulate weight, and there are both self-report and objective methods for assessment. Refer to Chapter 8 for an in-depth discussion of how to assess patients for physical activity and sedentary behaviors.

Motivation and Readiness to Change

People seeking to change their behavior in any domain demonstrate varying levels of motivation and readiness to change. The transtheoretical model, also referred to as the stages of change model, proposes that individuals seeking to change a behavior move through five stages of change: precontemplation, contemplation, preparation, action, and maintenance.[69] Individuals begin in precontemplation, characterized by lack of awareness about a problem behavior and little to no intention to change it. They may then move on to the contemplation stage, at which point they may begin gathering information about the pros and cons of the behavior, considering its impact on their lives and developing intent to change the behavior. Once they voice readiness to change the behavior, they are likely in the preparation stage and will take small steps toward changing the behavior. The action stage is when concrete behavior changes are made and individuals demonstrate intent to continue to change this behavior. Finally, individuals enter the maintenance stage, which occurs after sustained behavior change and is accompanied by behaviors that provide ongoing relapse prevention.

Many people move through these stages linearly, but not all do. It is not uncommon for life events or other factors to cause a person to revert from the action stage to the contemplation stage, for instance. Some people may experience a relapse in problematic behavior and revert from maintenance to action. A person's stage of change is determined by many factors, including the history of the problematic behavior, intention to change the behavior, and knowledge of the behavior and its consequences. The University of Rhode Island Change Assessment Scale is a 32-item, validated, and widely used self-report measure of readiness to change a variety of behaviors, such as smoking cessation or beginning psychotherapy.[70] It assesses four subscales of the transtheoretical model (precontemplation, contemplation, action, and maintenance) on a 5-point Likert scale. A total readiness-to-change score can be calculated, and there are cutoff guidelines for determining low and high readiness-to-change scores. Modified versions of this questionnaire can be used to assess readiness to change weight-related behaviors. Self-report assessments can aid in evaluating an individual's stage of change and should be paired with a thorough clinical discussion to fully determine a person's readiness for behavior change.[24,71,72]

A patient may arrive for a behavioral health assessment at any stage in the process, and a thorough clinical interview and assessment of recent behavior patterns with respect to eating, physical activity, and many other constructs described in this chapter will reveal which stage the patient is currently in. Motivational interviewing is a clinical technique specifically designed to elicit and build motivation in accordance with the stages of change.[73] It involves collaborating with the patient to identify and explore ambivalence to change (eg, in weight or behavior) and supports changes that are congruous with the patient's values or goals. In these conversations, the provider asks open-ended questions about the patient's goals and ambivalence to change (in a nonjudgmental way), affirms the difficulties of change, and uses the person's strengths, reflective statements, and summaries to demonstrate active listening. The provider helps to elicit "change talk" from the patient in which the patient states their desire, reasons, ability, and commitment to change and move closer to their weight management goal. Though other constructs described in this chapter may affect the assessment plan more urgently (eg, if someone is currently in a depressive episode), collecting information about readiness and motivation to change is an essential part of building rapport and facilitates a deeper understanding of the person's knowledge, desires, and intent to follow through on suggested weight-related health behavior changes.

Strategies for Behavioral Health Assessment

The strategy used to assess each patient varies by context. A thorough assessment of behavioral health may include all of the domains described in this chapter, or it may include only the most relevant measures to the clinical situation or patient. For instance, one could pick and choose the measures of interest based on comorbid psychopathology or select only the measures necessary to assess acute risk (ie, suicidality and depression). A common framework for the behavioral health assessment of patients seeking weight management is the Biological, Environmental, Social/Psychological, and Timing (BEST) model.[74] The clinician can select measures to fulfill each of the four named areas or can use a validated integrated assessment that covers many of these topics. One such integrated assessment is the Weight and Lifestyle Inventory (WALI).[75] The WALI is a thorough assessment that covers many of the factors described in this chapter and includes a combination of open-ended questions and validated self-report measures (eg, the QEWP-5[47] or the Night Eating Questionnaire[49]). It does not cover specific symptoms of mood, anxiety, or sleep issues, so if those areas are of particular concern, a combination of tools for assessing specific psychopathologies should be added, such as the PHQ-9 for depressed mood, the GAD-7 for anxiety, and the Pittsburgh Sleep Quality Index for sleep issues. Depressive and anxiety symptoms can keep patients trapped and unable to make meaningful changes to their routines, and insufficient sleep can make it difficult to concentrate or have the energy to be active or stick to a regular meal schedule. As such, information from these domains can identify whether mental health treatment is a priority, which is the case when severe symptoms are identified or if mental health treatment would be helpful concurrently with behavioral weight-management strategies, in order to improve a patient's ability to focus on healthy lifestyle changes. If suicidal intent or ideation are identified, the appropriate level of care should be assessed. Patients with intent should call 911 or go to the nearest emergency room; patients with ideation should be referred to a mental health care provider or their primary care physician, or both, for follow-up.

If a patient is struggling with loss-of-control eating, a combination of the QEWP-5, Power of Food Scale, and Yale Food Addiction Scale could help identify whether objective binge episodes are present, consistent with binge eating disorder, or if symptoms of addictive-like eating or hedonic eating triggered by external cues are present at a high level. This approach can help determine specific interventions, such as cognitive behavioral therapy for binge eating disorder or the Regulation of Cues program for patients struggling with food-cue responsiveness and satiety responsiveness.[76]

A summary of the questionnaires and tools described in this chapter is provided in Table 9.1, on page 156.

Finally, time and patient burden are always important considerations. When considering what tools to use for an outpatient assessment, one time-saver is to send a packet electronically to the patient to complete before the intake or first in-person session. If this is an option, the initial patient contact (via telephone or otherwise), prior to the first in-person session, could include a checklist of concerns to review with the patient. As the provider goes through the checklist, the patient can identify any relevant concerns, and this way the provider can include targeted surveys in the electronic packet. To generate data on patient demographics and outcomes for clinical programs, providers can administer specific batteries or a combination of surveys and interviews at intake and then again at time intervals that match the length of the program (if predetermined) or at time points such as 3 months and 6 months.

Sociocultural Considerations

Sociocultural factors are an essential component of behavioral health assessment for weight management. A range of factors at the individual, family, community, and society levels, as well as the physical environment, can influence a person's eating behavior and physical activity in various ways. For instance, a person's socioeconomic status can affect eating behavior and food choices, given that fresh fruits and vegetables and lean proteins may be more expensive than fast foods and other higher-energy foods.[77] Race, ethnicity, and religious affiliation may also influence food choices and behaviors. For example, soul food is prominent among some Black populations, and rice is a staple of Latino and Asian cultures; and religious fasting practices, such as Ramadan for Muslims and Daniel Fast for some Christians, can affect eating schedules.[78,79] Many of these factors are not assessed on the surveys described in this chapter but should be taken into account as they can affect recommendations for dietary interventions.

Physical activity—whether through planned activities, at gyms or recreation facilities, at home on exercise equipment, or by some other means—can be too costly for some, and still others may not have the option to engage in activities within their neighborhood due to community safety concerns.[80] Thus, asking patients about their access to outdoor activities or gym memberships, as well as internet access for free online workout videos (such as those found on YouTube) is essential.

Educational level and income are also important considerations. Research has shown that poor health literacy or having limited knowledge about healthy food choices and physical activity and their impacts on health outcomes are related to poorer dietary choices, less physical activity, and higher weight status.[81] For example, individuals with lower health literacy have more difficulty reading nutrition labels, may be less likely to have resources to cook or prepare meals with healthier ingredients, and may be more likely to follow fad diets, such as juicing, which they may believe are beneficial for weight control. Health literacy can be measured in a variety of ways; one instrument, the Newest Vital Sign, is a brief (6-item) questionnaire that can be administered in about 3 minutes.[82] Food insecurity is also a concern, as people with insufficient income tend to shop once a month in large quantities. This is linked to binge eating and overeating in the first part of the month, followed by periods of low-quality dietary intake (eg, refined-carbohydrate meals such as white bread with peanut butter and jelly) or skipped meals. The most commonly used assessment of food insecurity is the US Household Food Security Survey Module, which consists of 10 items, and a 6-item version can also be used.[83] A more in-depth discussion of food insecurity assessment can be found in Chapter 7.

TABLE 9.1 Summary of Behavioral Health Assessment Questionnaires[a]

Behavioral health area	Questionnaire	Number of items	Subscales, if applicable	Clinical considerations
Mood				
	Beck Depression Inventory-II (BDI-II)	21	Item 9 assesses suicidality	The most widely used and validated depression measure
	Patient Health Questionnaire-9 (PHQ-9)	9	Item 9 assesses suicidality	Quick assessment of diagnostic criteria Shorter versions available (eg, PHQ-2)
	Geriatric Depression Scale–Short Form (GDS-SF)	15		
Suicidality				
	Columbia-Suicide Severity Rating Scale (C-SSRS)	6		Interview-based with a training module (https://cssrs.columbia.edu/training/training-options)
Anxiety				
	Generalized Anxiety Disorder-7 (GAD-7)	7		
	Beck Anxiety Inventory (BAI)	21		
Eating behavior				
	Weight and Lifestyle Inventory (WALI)	Approximately 100	Weight history Weight loss history Family weight history Substance use Eating habits Disordered eating behaviors Food recall Physical activity Mental health history Psychosocial factors Medical history	
	Questionnaire on Eating and Weight Patterns-5 (QEWP-5)	26	Binge eating Compensatory behaviors Loss-of-control eating Parental weight history	

TABLE 9.1 Summary of Behavioral Health Assessment Questionnaires[a] (continued)

Behavioral health area	Questionnaire	Number of items	Subscales, if applicable	Clinical considerations
Eating behavior (continued)				
	Eating Disorder Examination (EDE, version 17.0D)		Binge eating Compensatory behaviors Restraint Eating concerns Weight concerns Shape concerns Global score	Semistructured clinical interview that requires training to administer
	Eating Disorder Examination Questionnaire (EDE-Q)	28	Binge eating Compensatory behaviors Restraint Eating concerns Weight concerns Shape concerns Global score	
	Binge Eating Scale	16	Behavioral features Cognitive and emotional features	
	Eating Inventory	51	Cognitive restraint Disinhibition Hunger	Shorter versions available (eg, 18 and 21 items)
	Night Eating Questionnaire	14	Nocturnal ingestions Evening hyperphagia Morning anorexia Mood and sleep Total score	
	Yale Food Addiction Scale, Version 2	25	Number of food addiction symptoms Threshold for "addiction"	Based on the *Diagnostic and Statistical Manual of Mental Disorders*, 5th ed., criteria for substance use disorder, as applied to food
	Power of Food Scale	15	Appetite for highly palatable foods at three different food proximities (food available, food present, and food tasted)	
	Food Craving Inventory	28	General motivational drive for foods Motivational drive for specific foods	

Table continues

TABLE 9.1 Summary of Behavioral Health Assessment Questionnaires[a] (continued)

Behavioral health area	Questionnaire	Number of items	Subscales, if applicable	Clinical considerations
Trauma				
	Childhood Trauma Questionnaire	28	Emotional abuse Physical abuse Sexual abuse Emotional neglect Physical neglect	
Stress				
	Perceived Stress Scale	10		
	Depression, Anxiety, and Stress Scale	21		
Weight stigma and internalization				
	Weight Bias Internalization Scale	10		
	Weight Self-Stigma Questionnaire	12		
Quality of life				
	Short Form Health Survey (SF-36)	36		
	Impact of Weight on Quality of Life–Lite (IWQOL-Lite)	31		
Substance use				
	Tobacco, Alcohol, Prescription medication, and other Substance use (TAPS) Tool	4 initial items		Follow-up items administered if the patient screens positive on any of the initial items
	Alcohol Use Disorder Identification Test (AUDIT)	10		Shorter version available (three-item AUDIT-C)
Motivation and readiness to change				
	University of Rhode Island Change Assessment Scale	32		
Health literacy				
	Newest Vital Sign	6		

TABLE 9.1 Summary of Behavioral Health Assessment Questionnaires[a] (continued)

Behavioral health area	Questionnaire	Number of items	Subscales, if applicable	Clinical considerations
Sleep				
	Pittsburgh Sleep Quality Index	Approximately 25	Sleep duration Subjective sleep quality Sleep latency Sleep efficiency Sleep disturbances Sleep medicine use Daytime dysfunction due to sleep	
	Apnea Risk Evaluation System	32	Medical history related to sleep Daytime sleepiness Sleep-disordered breathing (snoring, gasping, breathing stops)	
	Epworth Sleepiness Scale	8	Daytime sleepiness	
Food insecurity				
	US Household Food Security Survey Module	Two versions available: 10 or 6 items		Most widely used assessment of food insecurity

[a] Before using any of these questionnaires, practitioners should check the copyright and correct process for using each tool in research, clinical, or for-profit settings.

Of note, the measures discussed in this chapter have been validated for adults. Adolescents have different needs, and treatment of adolescents is often tailored to a family-based approach. Also, adolescent-specific assessment measures should be used whenever possible. Older adults may also have specific needs to maintain safety and health that should be considered. These include a focus on maintaining lean mass during weight loss, so an assessment of their access to safe strength-training activities is important. In addition, their primary care physician and other health care providers should be made aware of their weight loss efforts.[84]

In summary, it is not sufficient to assess only the psychological constructs and health behaviors discussed earlier in the chapter; providers must also consider the sociocultural context in which a patient lives to better understand the factors that contribute to the eating and physical activity behaviors that regulate weight-management efforts.

Summary

Many factors influence a person's body mass and weight-related health. Behavioral health factors, including psychological constructs, health behaviors, and sociocultural considerations, often play important roles in weight gain and patients' efforts to manage their weight over the long term. The assessment of these domains can help identify treatment targets that patients may not think to report in an initial interview and also provides an important starting point for intervention as well as a measure of progress and response to treatment.

References

1. Hahn SL, Borton KA, Sonneville KR. Cross-sectional associations between weight-related health behaviors and weight misperception among U.S. adolescents with overweight/obesity. *BMC Public Health*. 2018;18(1):514. doi:10.1186//s12889-018-5394-9
2. Swencionis C, Wylie-Rosett J, Lent MR, et al. Weight change, psychological well-being, and vitality in adults participating in a cognitive-behavioral weight loss program. *Health Psychol*. 2013;32(4):439-446. doi:10.1037/a0029186
3. Pan A, Sun Q, Czernichow S, et al. Bidirectional association between depression and obesity in middle-aged and older women. *Int J Obes*. 2012;36(4):595-602. doi:10.1038/ijo.2011.111
4. Bremner JD, Moazzami K, Wittbrodt MT, et al. Diet, stress and mental health. *Nutrients*. 2020;12(8):2428. doi:10.3390/nu12082428
5. Hawkins RC II, Clement PF. Binge eating: measurement problems and a conceptual model. In: Hawkins RC II, Fremouw WJ, and Clement PF, eds. *The Binge Purge Syndrome: Diagnosis, Treatment, and Research.* Springer; 1984:229-251.
6. McCarthy M. The thin ideal, depression and eating disorders in women. *Behav Res Ther*. 1990;28(3):205-214. doi:10.1016/0005-7967(90)90003-2
7. Konttinen H. Emotional eating and obesity in adults: the role of depression, sleep and genes. *Proc Nutr Soc*. 2020;79(3):283-289. doi:10.1017/S0029665120000166
8. Konttinen H, Männistö S, Sarlio-Lähteenkorva S, Silventoinen K, Haukkala A. Emotional eating, depressive symptoms and self-reported food consumption: a population-based study. *Appetite*. 2010;54(3):473-479. doi:10.1016/j.appet.2010.01.014
9. Luppino FS, de Wit LM, Bouvy PF, et al. Overweight, obesity, and depression: a systematic review and meta-analysis of longitudinal studies. *Arch Gen Psychiatry*. 2010;67(3):220-229. doi:10.1001/archgenpsychiatry.2010.2
10. Rooke SE, Thorsteinsson EB. Examining the temporal relationship between depression and obesity: meta-analyses of prospective research. *Health Psychol Rev*. 2008;2(1):94-109. doi:10.1080/17437190802295689
11. Wurtman J, Wurtman R. The trajectory from mood to obesity. *Curr Obes Rep*. 2018;7(1):1-5. doi:10.1007/s13679-017-0291-6
12. Vittengl JR. Mediation of the bidirectional relations between obesity and depression among women. *Psychiatry Res*. 2018;264:254-259. doi:10.1016/j.psychres.2018.03.023
13. de Lauzon-Guillain B, Basdevant A, Romon M, et al. Is restrained eating a risk factor for weight gain in a general population? *Am J Clin Nutr*. 2006;83(1):132-138. doi:10.1093/ajcn/83.1.132
14. Koenders PG, van Strien T. Emotional eating, rather than lifestyle behavior, drives weight gain in a prospective study in 1562 employees. *J Occup Environ Med*. 2011;53(11):1287-1293. doi:10.1097/JOM.0b013e31823078a2
15. Vittengl JR. Mediation of the bidirectional relations between obesity and depression among women. *Psychiatry Res*. 2018;264:254-259. doi:10.1016/j.psychres.2018.03.023
16. Song YM, Lee K, Sung J, Yang Y. Changes in eating behaviors and body weight in Koreans: The Healthy Twin Study. *Nutrition*. 2013;29(1):66–70. doi:10.1016/j.nut2012.03.014

17. Péneau S, Ménard E, Méjean C, Bellisle F, Hercberg S. Sex and dieting modify the association between emotional eating and weight status. *Am J Clin Nutr*. 2013;97(6):1307-1313. doi:10.3945/ajcn.112.054916
18. Geiker NRW, Astrup A, Hjorth MF, Sjödin A, Pijls L, Markus CR. Does stress influence sleep patterns, food intake, weight gain, abdominal obesity and weight loss interventions and vice versa? *Obes Rev*. 2018;19(1):81-97. doi:10.1111/obr.12603
19. Björntorp P. Do stress reactions cause abdominal obesity and comorbidities? *Obes Rev*. 2001;2(2):73-86. doi:10.1046/j.1467-789x.2001.00027.x
20. Adam TC, Epel ES. Stress, eating and the reward system. *Physiol Behav*. 2007;91(4):449-458. doi:10.1016/j.physbeh.2007.04.011
21. Ulrich-Lai YM, Fulton S, Wilson M, Petrovich G, Rinaman L. Stress exposure, food intake and emotional state. *Stress*. 2015;18(4):381-399. doi:10.3109/10253890.2015.1062981
22. Wardle J, Chida Y, Gibson EL, Whitaker KL, Steptoe A. Stress and adiposity: a meta-analysis of longitudinal studies. *Obesity*. 2011;19(4):771-778. doi:10.1038/oby.2010.241
23. Amiri S, Behnezhad S. Obesity and substance use: a systematic review and meta-analysis. *Obes Med*. 2018;11:31-41. doi:10.1016/j.obmed.2018.06.002
24. Spiller V, Scaglia M, Meneghini S, Vanzo A. Assessing motivation for change toward healthy nutrition and regular physical activity: validation of two sets of instruments. *Mediterr J Nutr Metab*. 2009;2(1):41-47. doi:10.1007/s12349-009-0044-5
25. Blaine B. Does depression cause obesity? A meta-analysis of longitudinal studies of depression and weight control. *J Health Psychol*. 2008;13(8):1190-1197. doi:10.1177/1359105308095977
26. van Strien T. Causes of emotional eating and matched treatment of obesity. *Curr Diab Rep*. 2018;18(6):35. doi:10.1007/s11892-018-1000-x
27. Dixon JB, Dixon ME, O'Brien PE. Depression in association with severe obesity: changes with weight loss. *Arch Intern Med*. 2003;163(17):2058-2065. doi:10.1001/archinte.163.17.2058
28. Beck AT, Steer RA, Brown GK. *Beck Depression Inventory (BDI-II)*. Vol 10. Pearson; 1996.
29. Kroenke K, Spitzer RL, Williams JBW. The PHQ-9: validity of a brief depression severity measure. *J Gen Intern Med*. 2001;16(9):606-613. doi:10.1046/j.1525-1497.2001.016009606.x
30. Spitzer RL, Kroenke K, Williams JBW; Patient Health Questionnaire Primary Care Study Group. Validation and utility of a self-report version of PRIME-MD: the PHQ primary care study. *JAMA*. 1999;282(18):1737-1744. doi:10.1001/jama.282.18.1737
31. Kroenke K, Spitzer RL, Williams JBW. The Patient Health Questionnaire-2: validity of a two-item depression screener. *Med Care*. 2003;41(11):1284-1292. doi:10.1097/01.MLR.0000093487.78664.3C
32. Sheikh JI, Yesavage JA. Geriatric Depression Scale (GDS): recent evidence and development of a shorter version. *Clin Gerontol*. 1986;5(1-2):165-173. doi:10.1300/J018v05n01_09
33. Posner K, Brown GK, Stanley B, et al. The Columbia–Suicide Severity Rating Scale: initial validity and internal consistency findings from three multisite studies with adolescents and adults. *Am J Psychiatry*. 2011;168(12):1266-1277. doi:10.1176/appi.ajp.2011.10111704
34. American Psychiatric Association. *Diagnostic and Statistical Manual of Mental Disorders*. 5th ed. American Psychiatric Association; 2013.
35. Amiri S, Behnezhad S. Obesity and anxiety symptoms: a systematic review and meta-analysis. *Neuropsychiatr*. 2019;33(2):72-89. doi:10.1007/s40211-019-0302-9
36. Spitzer RL, Kroenke K, Williams JBW. A brief measure for assessing generalized anxiety disorder: the GAD-7. *Arch Intern Med*. 2006;166(10):1092-1097. doi:10.1001/archinte.166.10.1092
37. Beck AT, Epstein N, Brown G, Steer RA. An inventory for measuring clinical anxiety: psychometric properties. *J Consult Clin Psychol*. 1988;56(6):893. doi:10.1037/0022-006X.56.6.893
38. Stunkard AJ, Messick S. The three-factor eating questionnaire to measure dietary restraint, disinhibition and hunger. *J Psychosom Res*. 1985;29(1):71-83. doi:10.1016/0022-3999(85)90010-8
39. Karlsson J, Persson LO, Sjöström L, Sullivan M. Psychometric properties and factor structure of the Three-Factor Eating Questionnaire (TFEQ) in obese men and women: results from the Swedish Obese Subjects (SOS) study. *Int J Obes Relat Metab Disord*. 2000;24(12):1715-1725. doi:10.1038/sj.ijo.0801442
40. Tholin S, Rasmussen F, Tynelius P, Karlsson J. Genetic and environmental influences on eating behavior: the Swedish Young Male Twins Study. *Am J Clin Nutr*. 2005;81(3):564-569. doi:10.1093/ajcn/81.3.564
41. Lowe MR, Butryn ML, Didie ER, et al. The Power of Food Scale: a new measure of the psychological influence of the food environment. *Appetite*. 2009;53(1):114-118. doi:10.1016/j.appet.2009.05.016
42. White MA, Whisenhunt BL, Williamson DA, Greenway FL, Netemeyer RG. Development and validation of the food-craving inventory. *Obes Res*. 2002;10(2):107-114. doi:10.1038/oby.2002.17
43. Gearhardt AN, Corbin WR, Brownell KD. Preliminary validation of the Yale Food Addiction Scale. *Appetite*. 2009;52(2):430-436. doi:10.1016/j.appet.2008.12.003
44. Gearhardt AN, Corbin WR, Brownell KD. Development of the Yale Food Addiction Scale version 2.0. *Psychol Addict Behav*. 2016;30(1):113-121. doi:10.1037/adb0000136
45. Cooper Z, Fairburn C. The eating disorder examination: a semi-structured interview for the assessment of the specific psychopathology of eating disorders. *Int J Eat Disord*. 1987;6(1):1-8. doi:10.1002/1098-108X(198701)6:1<1::AID-EAT2260060102>3.0.CO;2-9
46. Fairburn CG, Beglin SJ. Assessment of eating disorders: interview or self-report questionnaire? *Int J Eat Disord*. 1994;16(4):363-370. doi:10.1002/1098-108X(199412)16:4<363::AID-EAT2260160405>3.0.CO;2-#

47. Yanovski SZ, Marcus MD, Wadden TA, Walsh BT. The Questionnaire on Eating and Weight Patterns-5 (QEWP-5): an updated screening instrument for binge eating disorder. *Int J Eat Disord*. 2015;48(3):259-261. doi:10.1002/eat.22372
48. Gormally J, Black S, Daston S, Rardin D. The assessment of binge eating severity among obese persons. *Addict Behav*. 1982;7(1):47-55. doi:10.1016/0306-4603(82)90024-7
49. Allison KC, Lundgren JD, O'Reardon JP, et al. The Night Eating Questionnaire (NEQ): psychometric properties of a measure of severity of the Night Eating Syndrome. *Eat Behav*. 2008;9(1):62-72. doi:10.1016/j.eatbeh.2007.03.007
50. Wiss DA, Brewerton TD. Adverse childhood experiences and adult obesity: a systematic review of plausible mechanisms and meta-analysis of cross-sectional studies. *Physiol Behav*. 2020;223:112964. doi:10.1016/j.physbeh.2020.112964
51. Palmisano GL, Innamorati M, Vanderlinden J. Life adverse experiences in relation with obesity and binge eating disorder: a systematic review. *J Behav Addict*. 2016;5(1):11-31. doi:10.1556/2006.5.2016.018
52. Hemmingsson E, Johansson K, Reynisdottir S. Effects of childhood abuse on adult obesity: a systematic review and meta-analysis. *Obes Rev*. 2014;15(11):882-893. doi:10.1111/obr.12216
53. Tomiyama AJ. Stress and obesity. *Annu Rev Psychol*. 2019;70(1):703-718. doi:10.1146/annurev-psych-010418-102936
54. Bernstein DP, Stein JA, Newcomb MD, et al. Development and validation of a brief screening version of the Childhood Trauma Questionnaire. *Child Abuse Negl*. 2003;27(2):169-190. doi:10.1016/S0145-2134(02)00541-0
55. Cohen S. Perceived stress in a probability sample of the United States. In: Spacapan S, Oskamp S, eds. *The Social Psychology of Health: The Claremont Symposium on Applied Social Psychology*. Sage Publications; 1988:31-67.
56. Lovibond PF, Lovibond SH. The structure of negative emotional states: comparison of the Depression Anxiety Stress Scales (DASS) with the Beck Depression and Anxiety Inventories. *Behav Res Ther*. 1995;33(3):335-343. doi:10.1016/0005-7967(94)00075-U
57. Puhl R, Suh Y. Health consequences of weight stigma: implications for obesity prevention and treatment. *Curr Obes Rep*. 2015;4(2):182-190. doi:10.1007/s13679-015-0153-z
58. Pearl RL, Puhl RM. Measuring internalized weight attitudes across body weight categories: validation of the modified Weight Bias Internalization Scale. *Body Image*. 2014;11(1):89-92. doi:10.1016/j.bodyim.2013.09.005
59. Lillis J, Luoma JB, Levin ME, Hayes SC. Measuring weight self-stigma: the Weight Self-Stigma Questionnaire. *Obesity*. 2010;18(5):971-976. doi:10.1038/oby.2009.353
60. Ware JE, Sherbourne CD. The MOS 36-item short-form health survey (SF-36): conceptual framework and item selection. *Med Care*. 1992;30(6):473-483. Accessed December 16, 2021. www.jstor.org/stable/3765916
61. Kolotkin RL, Crosby RD, Kosloski KD, Williams GR. Development of a brief measure to assess quality of life in obesity. *Obes Res*. 2001;9(2):102-111. doi:10.1038/oby.2001.13
62. McNeely J, Wu LT, Subramaniam G, et al. Performance of the Tobacco, Alcohol, Prescription medication, and other Substance use (TAPS) Tool for substance use screening in primary care patients. *Ann Intern Med*. 2016;165(10):690-699. doi:10.7326/M16-0317
63. Bohn MJ, Babor TF, Kranzler HR. The Alcohol Use Disorders Identification Test (AUDIT): validation of a screening instrument for use in medical settings. *J Stud Alcohol*. 1995;56(4):423-432. doi:10.15288/jsa.1995.56.423
64. Bush K, Kivlahan DR, McDonell MB, Fihn SD, Bradley KA; for the Ambulatory Care Quality Improvement Project (ACQUIP). The AUDIT alcohol consumption questions (AUDIT-C): an effective brief screening test for problem drinking. *Arch Intern Med*. 1998;158(16):1789-1795. doi:10.1001/archinte.158.16.1789
65. Hirshkowitz M, Whiton K, Albert SM, et al. National Sleep Foundation's updated sleep duration recommendations: final report. *Sleep Health*. 2015;1(4):233-243. doi:10.1016/j.sleh.2015.10.004
66. Buysse DJ, Reynolds CF, Monk TH, Berman SR, Kupfer DJ. The Pittsburgh Sleep Quality Index: a new instrument for psychiatric practice and research. *Psychiatry Res*. 1989;28(2):193-213. doi:10.1016/0165-1781(89)90047-4
67. Levendowski D, Olmstead R, Popovic D, Carper D, Berka C, Westbrook P. Assessment of obstructive sleep apnoea risk and severity in truck drivers: validation of a screening questionnaire. *Sleep Diagnosis and Therapy*. 2007;2:20-26.
68. Johns MW. A new method for measuring daytime sleepiness: the Epworth Sleepiness Scale. *Sleep*. 1991;14(6):540-545. doi:10.1093/sleep/14.6.540
69. Velicer WF, Rossi JS, Prochaska JO, Diclemente CC. A criterion measurement model for health behavior change. *Addict Behav*. 1996;21(5):555-584. doi:10.1016/0306-4603(95)00083-6
70. Hasler G, Klaghofer R, Buddeberg C. The University of Rhode Island Change Assessment Scale (URICA). *Psychother Psychosom Med Psychol*. 2003;53(9-10):406-411. doi:10.1055/s-2003-42172
71. Ceccarini M, Borrello M, Pietrabissa G, Manzoni GM, Castelnuovo G. Assessing motivation and readiness to change for weight management and control: an in-depth evaluation of three sets of instruments. *Front Psychol*. 2015;6:511. doi:10.3389/fpsyg.2015.00511
72. Sarkin JA, Johnson SS, Prochaska JO, Prochaska JM. Applying the transtheoretical model to regular moderate exercise in an overweight population: validation of a stages of change measure. *Prev Med*. 2001;33(5):462-469. doi:10.1006/pmed.2001.0916

73. Miller WR. Motivational interviewing with problem drinkers. *Behav Cogn Psychother*. 1983;11(2):147-172. doi:10.1017/S0141347300006583
74. Wadden TA, Phelan S. Behavioral assessment of the obese patient. In: Wadden TA, Stunkard AJ, eds. *Handbook of Obesity Treatment*. Guilford; 2002:186-208.
75. Wadden TA, Foster GD. Weight and Lifestyle Inventory (WALI). *Obes (Silver Spring)*. 2006;14(suppl 2):99S-118S. doi:10.1038/oby.2006.289
76. Boutelle KN, Manzano MA, Eichen DM. Appetitive traits as targets for weight loss: the role of food cue responsiveness and satiety responsiveness. *Physiol Behav*. 2020;224:113018. doi:10.1016/j.physbeh.2020.113018
77. Rao M, Afshin A, Singh G, Mozaffarian D. Do healthier foods and diet patterns cost more than less healthy options? A systematic review and meta-analysis. *BMJ Open*. 2013;3(12):e004277. doi:10.1136/bmjopen-2013-004277
78. Devine CM, Sobal J, Bisogni CA, Connors M. Food choices in three ethnic groups: interactions of ideals, identities, and roles. *J Nutr Educ*. 1999;31(2):86-93. doi:10.1016/S0022-3182(99)70400-0
79. James D. Factors influencing food choices, dietary intake, and nutrition-related attitudes among African Americans: application of a culturally sensitive model. *Ethn Health*. 2004;9(4):349-367. doi:10.1080/1355785042000285375
80. Rees-Punia E, Hathaway ED, Gay JL. Crime, perceived safety, and physical activity: a meta-analysis. *Prev Med*. 2018;111:307-313. doi:10.1016/j.ypmed.2017.11.017
81. Zoellner J, You W, Connell C, et al. Health literacy is associated with healthy eating index scores and sugar-sweetened beverage intake: findings from the rural lower Mississippi Delta. *J Am Diet Assoc*. 2011;111(7):1012-1020. doi:10.1016/j.jada.2011.04.010
82. Weiss BD, Mays MZ, Martz W, et al. Quick assessment of literacy in primary care: the Newest Vital Sign. *Ann Fam Med*. 2005;3(6):514-522. doi:10.1370/afm.405
83. Bickel G, Nord M, Price C, Hamilton W, Cook J. *Guide to Measuring Household Food Security, Revised 2000*. U.S. Department of Agriculture, Food and Nutrition Service; 2000.
84. Villareal DT, Aguirre L, Gurney AB, et al. Aerobic or resistance exercise, or both, in dieting obese older adults. *N Engl J Med*. 2017;376(20):1943-1955. doi:10.1056/NEJMoa1616338

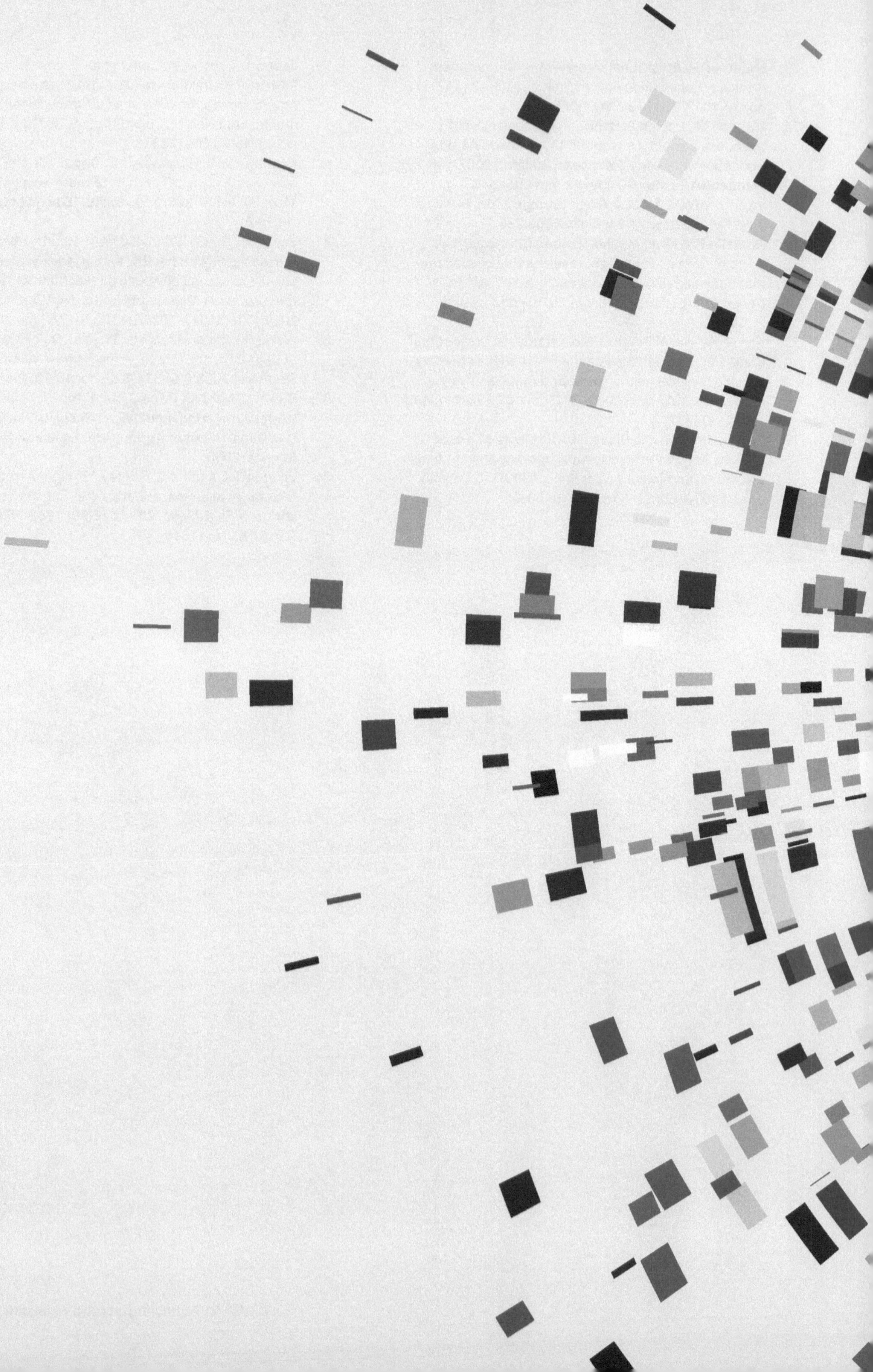

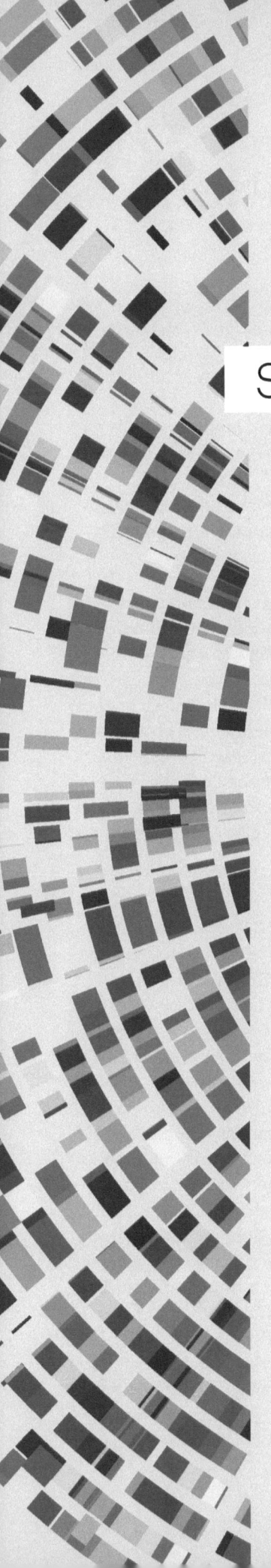

SECTION 3

Interventions for the Treatment of Overweight and Obesity

CHAPTER 10 Multicomponent Lifestyle Interventions | 166

CHAPTER 11 Dietary Interventions | 182

CHAPTER 12 Physical Activity Interventions | 195

CHAPTER 13 Counseling Approaches for Health Behavior Change | 220

CHAPTER 14 Medical and Surgical Interventions | 253

CHAPTER 15 Obesity as a Chronic Disease and Its Lifelong Management | 270

CHAPTER 16 Treatment of Obesity and Eating Disorders | 286

CHAPTER 17 The Use of Technology in the Treatment of Obesity | 316

CHAPTER 10

Multicomponent Lifestyle Interventions

Bonnie Tamis Jortberg, PhD, RDN, CDCES

CHAPTER OBJECTIVES

- Identify components of multidisciplinary lifestyle interventions for the treatment of overweight and obesity.
- Discuss the integration of lifestyle components in landmark intervention studies, including the Diabetes Prevention Program and the Look AHEAD study.
- Describe the impact that multidisciplinary intervention studies have had on the development of interventions for overweight and obesity.

Introduction

Obesity is a complex and chronic disease, and as such, it requires a multidimensional approach to treatment. This chapter discusses the rationale for and definitions of lifestyle interventions for weight management, highlighting two landmark studies for weight management and the prevention and treatment of type 2 diabetes: the Diabetes Prevention Program (DPP) and the Action for Health in Diabetes (Look AHEAD) study. This chapter elaborates on the details of these studies because they demonstrate the benefits of a comprehensive, multidimensional lifestyle approach for weight loss and maintenance. These studies had a profound positive effect on diabetes prevention and improvements in diabetes and cardiovascular outcomes for people with diabetes, and they helped to establish guidelines and policies for weight loss and maintenance.

Rationale for and Definition of Multidisciplinary Lifestyle Interventions for Weight Management

According to the US Preventive Services Task Force (USPSTF), there is strong evidence that an intensive, multicomponent behavioral intervention is the most successful method for weight management.[1] In 2018, the USPSTF upgraded their 2012 recommendations for screening for obesity in adults to a grade B.[1] (The USPSTF B recommendation means "recommend this service." There is a high certainty that the net benefit is moderate, or there is moderate certainty that the net benefit is moderate to substantial.)

The USPSTF found adequate evidence that intensive, multicomponent behavioral interventions in adults with obesity can lead to clinically significant improvements in weight status and reduce the incidence of type 2 diabetes among adults with obesity, and that there are few to no harms of intensive multicomponent behavioral interventions. These recommendations apply to adults 18 years of age or older with a BMI of 30 or higher. The "intensive behavioral weight loss interventions" considered by the USPSTF had a duration of 1 to 2 years, encouraged self-monitoring of weight, provided tools to support weight loss or weight loss maintenance (such as pedometers, food scales, or exercise videos), and often had 12 or more sessions in the first year.

The most recent (2013) guidelines from the American Heart Association (AHA), American College of Cardiology (ACC), and The Obesity Society (TOS) for the management of overweight and obesity in adults also recommend a comprehensive lifestyle intervention, alone or with adjunctive therapies (obesity pharmacotherapy) for patients with a BMI of 30 or higher or a BMI of 27 or higher in patients with comorbidities.[2] The guidelines recommend that all patients for whom weight loss is recommended should be offered or referred for comprehensive lifestyle intervention, preferably with a trained interventionist or nutrition professional, which is foundational regardless of augmentation by medications or bariatric surgery. The guidelines state that in the studies forming the evidence base for this recommendation, the nutrition professional (often a registered dietitian nutritionist, RDN) usually delivers the dietary guidance and that most interventions were delivered in a university nutrition department or in a hospital medical care setting with access to nutrition professionals. Trained interventionists included mostly health professionals (eg, RDNs, psychologists, exercise specialists, health counselors, or professionals in training) who adhered to formal protocols in weight management.

According to the 2013 AHA/ACC/TOS guidelines, the most effective behavioral treatment for weight loss is an in-person, high-intensity (14 or more sessions over 6 months), comprehensive intervention provided in individual or group sessions by a trained interventionist (an RDN). The main components of an effective, high-intensity, comprehensive lifestyle intervention include (1) the prescription of a diet that is moderately reduced in energy intake, (2) a program of increased physical activity, and (3) the use of behavioral strategies to facilitate adherence to diet and activity recommendations.

The USPSTF recommendations and the AHA/ACC/TOS guidelines are based on evidence gleaned from the DPP and the Look AHEAD study, as described in the following sections.

The Diabetes Prevention Program

The landmark study DPP (www.niddk.nih.gov/about-niddk/research-areas/diabetes/diabetes-prevention-program-dpp) changed the way people approach the prevention of type 2 diabetes worldwide. This study demonstrated that people who are at high risk for type 2 diabetes can prevent or delay the disease by losing a modest amount of weight through lifestyle changes (dietary changes and increased physical activity). The DPP, funded by the National Institute of Diabetes and Digestive and Kidney Diseases (NIDDK), was a randomized controlled trial conducted at 27 clinical centers around the United States from 1996 to 2001. The trial enrolled 3,234 participants; 55% were White, and 45% were from US minority groups at high risk for type 2 diabetes, including Black, Alaska Native, Indigenous American, Asian, Hispanic or Latino, or Pacific Islander participants.[3]

The primary DPP outcome was progression from prediabetes to diabetes; secondary outcomes related to reducing the risk of cardiovascular disease (CVD) events and risk factors. DPP participants were asked to participate for 3 to 5 years and were randomly assigned to one of three groups as shown in Box 10.1 on page 168.[3]

Why was weight loss a cornerstone of the DPP lifestyle intervention? The risk of developing diabetes increases as BMI increases; thus, researchers anticipated any decrease in BMI decreased the risk of developing diabetes.[4,5] Weight gain and obesity increase diabetes risk threefold for people who are overweight, sevenfold for people who have obesity, and 60-fold for those with severe obesity.[6] Before the launch of the DPP, several studies had reported that individuals who were overweight and then lost between 3.7 kg and 6.8 kg (8 to 15 lb) decreased their risk of diabetes by 33% compared to individuals whose weight remained stable.[7] Results from behavioral weight loss studies showed that an average weight loss of 9% of body weight at the end of a 6-month intensive program and weight maintenance of 6% of weight loss at 18 months was achievable for the majority of participants.[8,9] Given these data, a 7% weight loss goal was selected for the DPP because it appeared feasible to achieve and maintain in a multicenter trial and would likely reduce participants' risk of developing diabetes.

BOX 10.1

Diabetes Prevention Program Study Interventions[3]

Randomization group	Study intervention
Metformin group n=1,073	Metformin, 850 mg twice a day Standard advice about diet and physical activity
Lifestyle change group n=1,079	Intensive training on diet and physical activity by a trained lifestyle coach, usually a registered dietitian nutritionist Lifestyle goals: 1. A weight loss of 7% of body weight 2. A decrease in dietary fat intake to <30% of total energy intake 3. A decrease in total energy intake to promote weight loss 4. At least 150 minutes of physical activity per week Meetings with lifestyle coaches: at least 16 meetings in the first 24 weeks, and then one meeting every 2 months with at least one telephone call between visits
Placebo group n=1,082	Placebo twice a day Standard advice about diet and physical activity

Intensive Lifestyle Intervention

Individual Case Managers, or Lifestyle Coaches

At the time of their assignment to the lifestyle change group, each participant was assigned to a case manager, called a lifestyle coach. Across the 27 clinical centers, most lifestyle coaches were RDNs; a few were exercise physiologists or behavioral health specialists. The lifestyle intervention was designed to be an individual, rather than a group, intervention. The individualized approach was chosen because of the randomization process, which limited the number of participants randomly assigned each month, making it challenging to enroll enough participants for a group-based intervention. The lifestyle coach had primary responsibility for delivering the core curriculum, conducting post–core curriculum maintenance sessions, eliciting motivation from the participant to achieve lifestyle goals, and ensuring the completion of required data collection.

The DPP core curriculum included 16 sessions to be completed within the first 24 months after randomization. Content included dietary and physical activity guidance, stress management, and problem-solving skills.

Weight Loss Goal

Studies conducted prior to the DPP suggested that most individuals achieve their maximum weight loss within the first 20 to 24 weeks of intervention.[10] As a result, participants in the lifestyle change group were encouraged to achieve the 7% weight loss in the first 6 months of the DPP lifestyle intervention. The recommended pace of weight loss was 0.5 to 0.9 kg (1 to 2 lb) per week. Participants who wanted to lose more than 7% of their baseline weight were encouraged to do so as long as they continued to have a BMI of more than 21. Weight loss medications were not used as part of this trial.

Dietary Intervention

The initial focus of the dietary intervention was on reducing total fat intake rather than total energy intake. The goals were for participants to reduce their energy intake while also eating an overall healthy diet and to streamline the self-monitoring requirements. After several weeks, participants were introduced to the concept of energy balance and the need to restrict energy as well as fat intake. Energy goals were calculated by estimating the daily kilocalories needed to maintain the participant's starting weight and subtracting 500 to 1,000 kcal/d (depending on initial body weight) to achieve a weight loss of 0.5 to 0.9 kg (1 to 2 lb) per week. Fat intake goals (in grams) were based on getting 25% of energy from fat. The fat and energy goals were used as means to achieve the weight loss goal rather than as goals in themselves.

Physical Activity Goal

The goal for physical activity was selected to approximate an expenditure of at least 700 kcal/wk on physical activities. This goal was described to participants as the equivalent of at least 150 minutes of moderate physical activity, similar in intensity to brisk walking, per week. The goal was adopted for the DPP because it was determined, based on previous studies, to be achievable and likely beneficial in preventing diabetes. In addition, 150 minutes per week was chosen because it was similar to the newest public health recommendations and the Surgeon General's latest report on physical activity and health.[11]

The DPP lifestyle intervention emphasized brisk walking as the means of achieving the activity goal, but participants were given examples of other activities that are usually equivalent in intensity to brisk walking, such as aerobic dance, bicycle riding, skating, and swimming. Participants were encouraged to distribute their activity throughout the week, with a minimum frequency of three sessions weekly and at least 10 minutes per session. A maximum of 75 minutes of strength training could be applied toward the total 150-minute weekly goal. The importance of lifestyle activities such as using the stairs, stretching, and gardening were also emphasized, but these were not applied toward the 150-minute physical activity goal.

The study protocol required that each clinical center offer supervised physical activity sessions at least twice a week throughout the trial, though participant attendance was voluntary. The types of supervised activity sessions varied across centers and included activities such as neighborhood walks, cardiac rehabilitation programs affiliated with DPP clinical centers, and community aerobics classes.

Self-Monitoring of Fat and Energy Intake and Physical Activity

All participants were instructed to self-monitor their fat and energy intake daily throughout the first 24 weeks of the study and to record their minutes of physical activity. Self-monitoring was stressed as one of the most, if not the most, important strategies for changing diet and exercise behaviors. At the beginning of the lifestyle intervention, participants were given a food scale, measuring cups and spoons, and a pocket-size booklet to record food intake and track fat and energy intake levels, as well as physical activity.

Self-monitoring skills were taught gradually over the first few weeks of the core curriculum. The lifestyle coach briefly reviewed the self-monitoring booklets with the participants during each session. Between sessions, the coach provided written, constructive comments.

Adherence and Maintenance Intervention

The maintenance program used in the DPP was more intensive than that of previous clinical trials, and it employed both group and individual contacts. After completing the 16-session core curriculum, participants had to be seen in person by their lifestyle coaches at least once every 2 months for the remainder of the trial and be contacted by telephone at least once between in-person visits. The in-person contacts could occur in a group setting, as long as the lifestyle coach was able to weigh the participant and assist with solving any problems of adherence. The adherence and maintenance phase was less structured than the core curriculum, although a lifestyle intervention manual for post–core curriculum contacts was available to lifestyle coaches and provided guidelines for implementing the maintenance phase of the intervention.

Strategies for Addressing the Needs of an Ethnically Diverse Population

The DPP recruited 45% of its participants from ethnic minority groups who are disproportionately affected by type 2 diabetes, including Black, Hispanic, Indigenous, and Asian Americans. Core curriculum materials were available in Spanish and English and were designed to permit flexibility to accommodate ethnic differences.

Overall Study Results

The DPP included 3,234 persons with prediabetes who were randomly assigned across the 27 clinical centers. The average follow-up time was 2.8 years. Patient retention remained high throughout the 3-year study. Close to 100% of the study cohort was alive at the end of the study; 93% of participants completed the study, and 93% of annual visits were completed.[12] The DPP was terminated approximately a year earlier than expected because the lifestyle intervention was so effective in preventing the incidence of diabetes. The key results included the following[12]:

- The lifestyle intervention reduced the incidence of diabetes by 58% compared with the placebo; metformin reduced the incidence of diabetes by 31% compared with placebo. Refer to Figure 10.1.[12]
- The lifestyle intervention was almost twice as effective at reducing the incidence of diabetes than was metformin.

It is important to note that the intensive lifestyle intervention and the metformin intervention were effective across all ethnicities enrolled in the study, as shown in Figure 10.2.[12]

FIGURE 10.1 Cumulative incidence of diabetes according to study group[12]

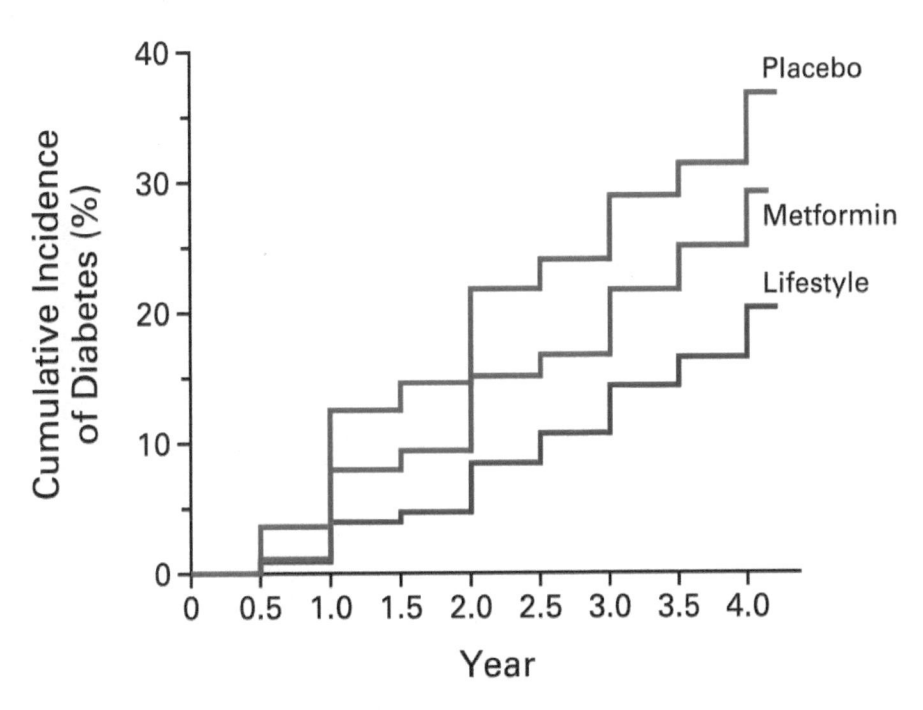

Reproduced with permission from Knowler WC, Barrett-Connor E, Fowler SE, et al. Reduction in the incidence of type 2 diabetes with lifestyle intervention or metformin. *N Engl J Med*. 2002;346(6):393-403. doi:10.1056/NEJMoa012512.[12]

FIGURE 10.2 Diabetes incidence rates by ethnicity[12]

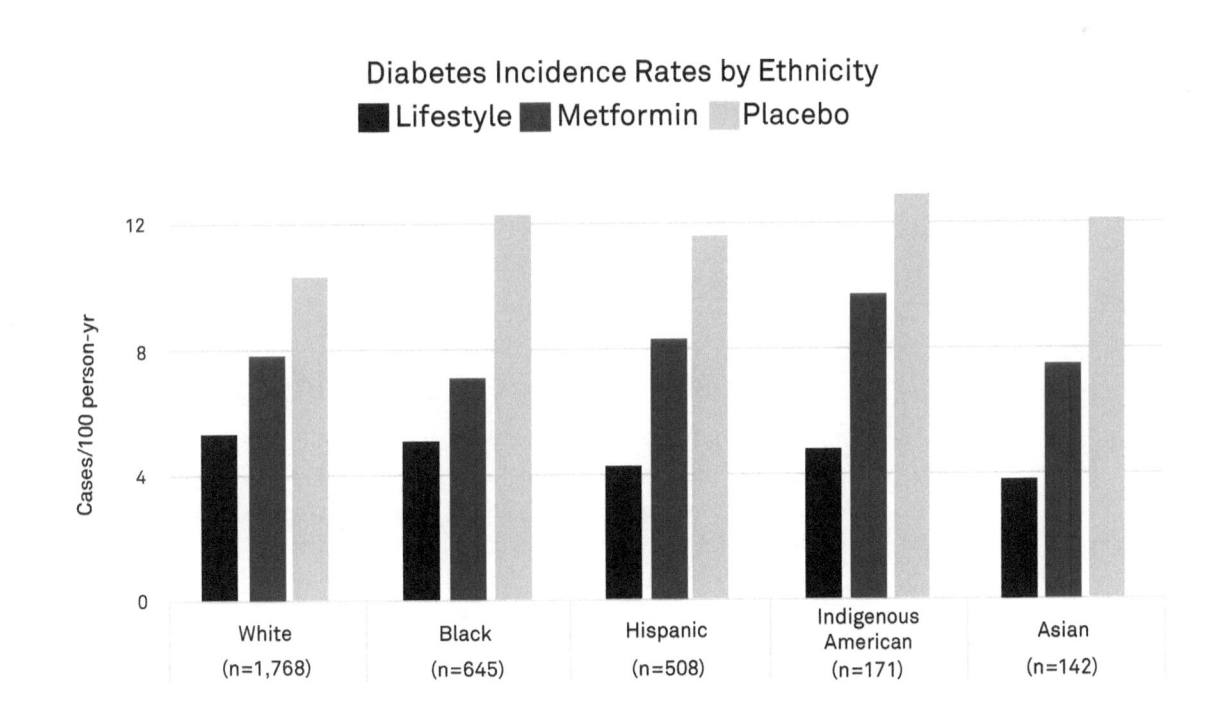

CHAPTER 10: Multicomponent Lifestyle Interventions **171**

Lifestyle Intervention Results

As previously stated, the lifestyle intervention was highly effective in the prevention of progression to diabetes. The key results for the lifestyle intervention group include the following[12]:

- By the end of 24 weeks, 50% of participants had achieved the goal of losing 7% or more of their body weight; and at the time of their most recent visit, 38% of participants were still meeting this goal.
- At 24 weeks, 74% of participants had met the goal of engaging in at least 150 minutes of physical activity per week. At 1 year, participants averaged 224 minutes of exercise per week; at 2 years, the average was 190 minutes of exercise per week. At the time of their most recent visit, 58% were still meeting this goal.
- Dietary changes were assessed yearly, and daily energy intake decreased by a mean of 450 kcal/d (±26), with the average fat intake decreasing by 6.6%.

The study concluded that "lifestyle changes and treatment with metformin both reduced the incidence of diabetes in persons at high risk. The lifestyle intervention was more effective than metformin."[12]

The DPP study group further concluded that weight loss was the dominant predictor of reduced diabetes incidence and reported the following key results related to weight loss[13]:

- For every kilogram of weight loss, there was a 16% reduction in diabetes risk, adjusted for changes in diet and activity.
- Lower percentage of energy intake from fat and increased physical activity predicted weight loss.
- Increased physical activity was important to help sustain weight loss. Among the 495 lifestyle participants who did not meet the weight loss goal at 1 year, those who still achieved the physical activity goal had a 44% lower diabetes incidence.

Of importance to weight-management health professionals, the DPP researchers concluded that interventions to reduce diabetes risk should primarily target weight reduction.

Since 2002, more than 50 articles with DPP results have been published on topics ranging from cost-effectiveness to biomarkers for the prediction of diabetes onset. The DPP publications can be found on the US National Library of Medicine's ClinicalTrials.gov website (https://clinicaltrials.gov/ct2/show/NCT00004992).

Diabetes Prevention Program Outcomes Study

Once the DPP researchers determined that the lifestyle intervention was highly effective in the prevention and delay of type 2 diabetes, the study then transitioned to the DPP Outcomes Study (DPPOS), the long-term follow-up study for the DPP, with the goal of evaluating the effects of the interventions on the further development of diabetes and diabetes complications. All active DPP participants were eligible to continue; 88% of DPP participants (910 lifestyle intervention participants; 924 metformin participants; and 932 placebo participants) enrolled in the DPPOS. Because of the benefits of the lifestyle intervention, all three groups were offered group-implemented lifestyle intervention. Placebo was discontinued for those in the original placebo group, metformin treatment was continued in the original metformin group, and the original lifestyle intervention group was offered additional lifestyle support. Table 10.1 presents key findings from the DPPOS.[14,15] The DPPOS is still active—almost 20 years later.

Other key findings from the 10-year follow-up results include the following[14]:

- Participants from the DPP lifestyle intervention group and participants who continued to take metformin or took a placebo all improved their risk factors for CVD, such as high blood pressure and high cholesterol. However, the participants from the DPP lifestyle intervention group achieved these results with fewer medications for lowering blood pressure and cholesterol levels.
- The DPP lifestyle intervention group was shown to be cost-effective, and metformin was shown to be cost-saving.

TABLE 10.1 Key Findings of the Diabetes Prevention Program Outcomes Study at 10 Years and 15 Years[14,15]

Type 2 diabetes outcome	10-year follow-up	15-year follow-up
Percentage of participants who experienced delay in progression to type 2 diabetes, compared with participants who took placebo	34%	27%
Percentage of participants aged ≥60 years in the lifestyle intervention group who experienced delay in progression to type 2 diabetes	49%	18%
Percentage of participants who continued to take metformin who experienced delay in progression to type 2 diabetes, compared with participants who took placebo	18%	Not applicable

Other key findings from the 15-year follow-up results include the following[15]:

- About half (55%) of participants from the DPP lifestyle intervention group and 56% of participants who continued to take metformin developed type 2 diabetes compared with 62% of participants who took a placebo.
- There were no overall differences in problems with small blood vessels, such as those found in the eyes, nerves, and kidneys, between participants from the DPP lifestyle intervention group and participants who continued to take metformin or took a placebo. However, women† from the DPP lifestyle intervention group developed fewer small blood vessel problems than did participants who continued to take metformin or took a placebo. Participants who did not develop diabetes had a 28% lower rate of small blood vessel problems compared with participants who developed diabetes.

In 2016, the NIDDK partnered with the National Heart, Lung, and Blood Institute and the National Cancer Institute for a third phase of the DPPOS, which is proposed to last through 2022. The goal of this partnership is to examine whether

---

† Study participants were described as women. Gender was not further specified.

people who are at high risk for type 2 diabetes and take metformin have lower rates of CVD and cancer, as has been suggested by smaller studies.

In 2010, the US Congress authorized the Centers for Disease Control and Prevention (CDC) to establish the National Diabetes Prevention Program (National DPP). This was a public-private partnership initiative to offer the program in communities across the United States to prevent type 2 diabetes. Practitioners who would like to offer the National DPP must go through a special training and meet the CDC Diabetes Prevention Recognition Program standards and operating procedures. The National DPP also requires that evaluation data be submitted to the CDC every 6 months. Data required include participant demographics, weights, and physical-activity minutes. RDNs are uniquely qualified to become National DPP lifestyle coaches; in this role, they lead lifestyle change program sessions and support and encourage participants. More information on the National DPP is available on the CDC website (www.cdc.gov/diabetes/prevention).

The Finnish Diabetes Prevention Study

At about the same time that the DPP was underway in the United States, the Finnish Diabetes Prevention Study[16] was taking place across the Atlantic Ocean. The aim of the study was to investigate the association of change in body weight and waist circumference and diabetes incidence with dietary macronutrient composition and energy density. The study randomly assigned 522 men and women[†] with impaired glucose tolerance to either standard care (control) or intensive diet and exercise counseling (lifestyle intervention). This study did not have a medication group. Interestingly, the findings of the Finnish study mirrored the findings of the DPP: namely, that an intensive lifestyle intervention was highly effective in preventing the onset of type 2 diabetes.

The lifestyle intervention in the Finnish study involved making the following five recommended lifestyle changes with the help of counseling[16]:

- losing more than 5% of initial body weight
- reducing fat intake to less than 30% of total energy intake
- reducing saturated fat intake to less than 10% of total energy intake
- increasing fiber intake to more than 15 g per 1,000 kcal
- exercising more than 4 hours per week

Participants were given a success score based on how many of the five recommended lifestyle changes they were able to achieve, earning one point for each goal successfully met. So, participants who were unable to make any of the changes had a score of zero; those who achieved one of the changes had a score of 1; and so on, up to a score of 5. Figure 10.3 illustrates the success scores of study participants in both the control and intervention groups.[16] The results demonstrate that the higher the adherence to the five lifestyle changes (the higher the success score), the greater the chance of avoiding the onset of diabetes (ie, the lower the incidence of diabetes). Participants in the lifestyle group who successfully made four or five of the recommended changes with the help of intensive counseling had an almost zero incidence of type 2 diabetes. It is worth noting that those participants in the control group who made lifestyle changes were also successful in reducing their incidence of diabetes but not as effectively as those in the lifestyle intervention group. This may indicate that support from health care professionals with expertise

---

† Study participants were described as men and women. Gender was not further specified.

FIGURE 10.3 Prevention of type 2 diabetes by changing lifestyle: the Finnish study[16]

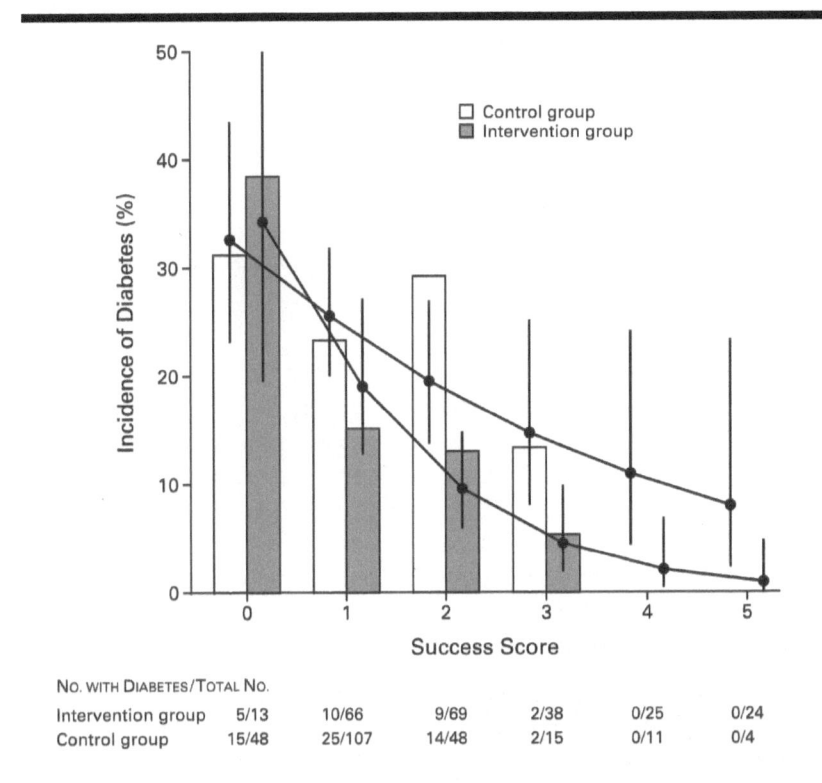

(3.2-year follow-up)

Five lifestyle changes:
Weight loss > 5%

Fat intake < 30% of energy intake

Saturated fat intake < 10% of energy intake

Fiber intake > 15 g per 1,000 kcal

Exercise > 4 h/wk

No. with Diabetes/Total No.						
Intervention group	5/13	10/66	9/69	2/38	0/25	0/24
Control group	15/48	25/107	14/48	2/15	0/11	0/4

Adapted with permission from Tuomilehto J, Lindström J, Eriksson JG, et al. Prevention of type 2 diabetes by changes in lifestyle among subjects with impaired glucose tolerance. *N Engl J Med*. 2001;344(18):1343–1350. doi:10.1056/nejm200105033441801.[16]

in lifestyle changes, such as RDNs, is crucial for making lifestyle changes that result in decreasing the incidence of diabetes.

Look AHEAD

Building on the success of the DPP, the NIDDK funded the Look AHEAD study, a 12-year, 16-center, randomized clinical trial.[17] Look AHEAD employed a group-based lifestyle modification program that included meal replacements and optional pharmacotherapy. It was designed to assess the long-term health consequences of intentional weight loss in individuals with overweight and obesity and with type 2 diabetes. More than 5,100 participants were randomly assigned to usual care (diabetes support and education, or DSE) or to an intensive lifestyle intervention (ILI), with the goal of inducing a loss of more than 7% of initial weight and increasing physical activity to more than 175 minutes per week. The groups were matched for age and sex and had a mean BMI of 36 for women and 35 for men.† The average age was 59 years, and the mean weight was approximately 94 kg (207 lb) for women and 109 kg (240 lb) for men. Approximately 63% of participants were non-Hispanic White.

Treatment Conditions

Diabetes Support and Education Group

During the first year of the study, the participants randomly assigned to the DSE group were invited to attend three 1-hour group meetings that addressed diet, physical activity, and social support. These sessions provided information but not specific behavioral strategies for adopting the diet and physical activity recommendations. Participants who wanted more support in their effort to lose weight were told to speak with their primary care providers.

Intensive Lifestyle Intervention Group

Participants in the ILI group were provided with a comprehensive intervention that was expected to induce an average weight loss of more than 7% of initial weight across all 16 centers. Individual participants were given a goal of losing more than 10% of their initial weight to increase the likelihood that they would meet the 7% study-wide goal. The weight control intervention was adopted from the DPP and was delivered to participants in groups of 10 to 20 participants. Group sessions were led by lifestyle coaches, who included RDNs, behavioral psychologists, and exercise specialists. During the first 6 months, participants attended weekly group sessions of 60 to 75 minutes each for the first 3 weeks of each month. During the fourth week of each month, participants met one-on-one with their lifestyle coaches. During months 7 through 12, participants continued to have a monthly individual meeting with their lifestyle coach, but the number of group sessions was reduced from three to two per month.

Dietary recommendations for participants in the ILI group were as follows:

- Participants weighing less than 114 kg (250 lb) were prescribed an energy goal of 1,200 to 1,500 kcal/d; those weighing more than 114 kg were prescribed an energy goal of 1,500 to 1,800 kcal/d.
- Participants were told that less than 30% of their daily energy intake should come from fat, and less than 10% should come from saturated fat.
- During weeks 3 through 19, participants were prescribed a liquid-meal-replacement plan and instructed to replace two meals with a liquid shake and one snack with a bar and to eat one meal of conventional foods. They added fruits and vegetables to their diet until they met their daily energy goal.

The physical activity goal for ILI group participants was to engage in more than 175 minutes of moderately intense activity per week. Persons who achieved this goal were encouraged to increase to more than 200 minutes of moderately intense exercise per week for months 7 through 12. Participants recorded their weekly activity in their food and activity diaries; only bouts of more than 10 minutes counted toward the weekly goal.

One-Year Results

At the 1-year mark, the average weight loss was more than 12 times greater in the ILI group than in the DSE group, as shown in Figure 10.4.[18] In addition, ILI participants reported engaging in brisk physical activity an average of 136.7 ± 110.4 minutes per week during the first year.[18]

As in the DPP study, the principal finding in the Look AHEAD study at 1 year was that the intensive lifestyle intervention induced a clinically significant weight loss in all subsets of a demographically and ethnically diverse population. Participant weight loss was related to adherence to the study's treatment recommendations. Of the three measures of adherence, physical activity most strongly correlated with weight loss. Participants in the highest quartile of self-reported physical activity lost 11.9% of their initial weight, compared with only 4.4% for those in the lowest quartile. More frequent attendance at treatment sessions and greater consumption

FIGURE 10.4 Look AHEAD results: weight loss at 1 year[18]

% Weight loss at 1 year

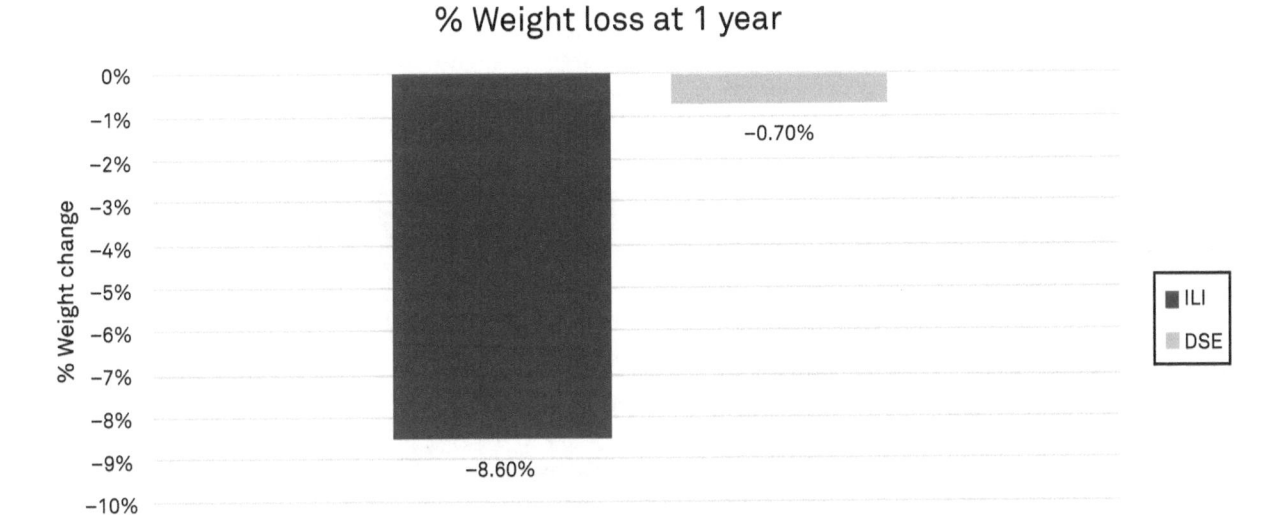

[Bar chart showing % Weight change: ILI = −8.60%, DSE = −0.70%]

Reduction in weight and cardiovascular disease risk factors in individuals with type 2 diabetes.

Abbreviations: DSE, diabetes support and education; ILI, intensive lifestyle intervention.

of meal replacements also were associated with greater weight loss, although to a lesser degree than was physical activity. In addition, participants in the ILI group saw statistically significant improvements in meeting the American Diabetes Association goals for risk factors related to hemoglobin A1c, blood pressure, and low-density lipoprotein cholesterol, and those meeting all three goals, compared to participants in the DSE group.[19]

Four-Year Results

The 4-year data from the Look AHEAD study have importance for health practitioners. The ILI group continued to demonstrate statistically significant results for weight loss, fitness improvements, glycemic control, and CVD risk factors in individuals with type 2 diabetes, compared to the DSE group.[19] The trial represented the most extensive test of long-term multidisciplinary lifestyle intervention to date and presented a unique opportunity to examine the long-term viability of lifestyle intervention. Key results at 4 years for the ILI group and the DSE group are summarized in Table 10.2 on page 178.[19] The DSE group showed greater reductions in low-density lipoprotein cholesterol levels; however, this was due to the greater use of medications to lower lipid levels in the DSE group.

Other key findings from the study at year 4 included the following[19]:

- The ILI group had a decrease in all CVD risk factors. Typically, medications target and affect only one CVD risk factor. The intensive lifestyle intervention produced positive changes in glycemic control, blood pressure, and lipid levels simultaneously.
- The data on the long-term changes in fitness were unique, as no other studies have reported fitness changes beyond 1 year for individuals with type 2 diabetes.

TABLE 10.2 Look AHEAD: Key Results at 4 Years[19]

Type 2 diabetes clinical outcomes	Intensive lifestyle intervention	Diabetes support and education
Weight loss, % initial body weight	−6.15%	−0.88%[a]
Improvements in treadmill fitness	+12.74%	+1.96%[a]
Improvements in HbA1c	−0.36%	−0.09%[a]
Improvements in systolic BP	−5.33 mm Hg	−2.97 mm Hg[a]
Improvements in diastolic BP	−2.92 mm Hg	−2.48 mm Hg[b]
Improvements in HDL cholesterol	+3.67 mg/dL	+1.97 mg/dL[a]
Triglycerides	−25.56 mg/dL	−19.75 mg/dL[a]

[a] $P = .001$.
[b] $P = .01$.
Abbreviations: BP, blood pressure; HbA1c, hemoglobin A1c; HDL, high-density lipoprotein.

- Relative to the DSE group, the ILI group demonstrated sustained benefits for high-density lipoprotein cholesterol levels. Other studies have shown a strong association between increases in high-density lipoprotein cholesterol levels and reduced heart disease.
- The intensive lifestyle intervention was shown to produce sustained weight loss and improvements in treadmill fitness, glycemic control, and CVD risk factors.

A further analysis of the 4-year weight losses in the Look AHEAD study identified factors associated with long-term success.[20] The analysis showed that a 5% or 10% weight loss in the first year by participants in the ILI group was strongly associated with maintaining this weight loss at 4 years. In addition, participants who maintained the weight loss (compared to those who did not) attended more treatment sessions and reported substantially greater physical activity and substantially lower energy intake.

Eight-Year Results

All participants in the Look AHEAD study had the opportunity to complete 8 years of intervention before the trial was halted in September 2012. Key findings at 8 years included the following[21]:

- Eighty-eight percent of both groups completed the 8-year outcomes assessment.
- ILI participants lost a mean of 4.7% of their initial weight at 8 years, compared with a loss of 2.1% for the DSE group; this difference is statistically significant ($P < .001$).
- Over the 8 years, ILI participants, compared with DSE participants, reported greater practice of several key weight-control behaviors, including:

- high levels of physical activity (the ILI group reported expending a mean of 1,040 kcal/wk, which was statistically significantly more than what the DSE group reported [P <.001])
- reduced energy intake
- frequent monitoring of body weight

The researchers summarized, "Look AHEAD advances the management of obesity by showing that a comprehensive, long-term lifestyle intervention produced ≥5% weight loss at 8 years in 50% of participants. While efforts clearly are needed to translate the current treatment approach into clinical practice, Look AHEAD provides new optimism for the long-term management of obesity and its many comorbid conditions that are ameliorated by weight loss."[21]

Additional Results

The Look AHEAD researchers published numerous articles on the results of this landmark study, a list of which can be found on the US National Library of Medicine's ClinicalTrials.gov website (https://clinicaltrials.gov/ct2/show/NCT00017953). One article addressed how to translate the results of Look AHEAD into clinical practice. According to the authors, the data indicate that supporting patients with type 2 diabetes who also have overweight or obesity in their efforts to improve their dietary intake, increase their physical activity, and engage with health care providers and community groups yields positive outcomes, including improvements in lipid levels and blood pressure, sleep apnea, renal disease, fitness, and depression. Look AHEAD also provided a comprehensive lifestyle intervention based on frequent, in-depth sessions in groups and one-on-one, several elements of which can inform clinical practice for health care providers. The ILI group sessions also fostered cohesion and a sense of community among study participants. The study also focused on using advanced behavioral strategies, such as motivational interviewing, development of problem-solving skills among participants, and increased contact with study staff to help study participants achieve weight loss goals.[22]

Another article from the Look AHEAD researchers examined the cost-effectiveness of the intensive lifestyle intervention compared with the standard approach of support and education.[23] Results from this analysis showed that the lifestyle intervention was more expensive than the standard approach ($6,666 more per person); however, the researchers concluded that the cost-effectiveness was unclear because different health-utility measures led to different conclusions. Another article looked at the weight loss experiences of Black, Hispanic, and non-Hispanic White men and women† in Look AHEAD.[24] Results showed that all subgroups averaged weight losses of 5% or more at 1 year but did experience weight regain, although losses of 5% or more were sustained at 8 years by non-Hispanic White participants and minority women (but not men). Session attendance was high (86% or more) in the first year and exceeded protocol-specific minimum levels into year 8.

A study completed in 2020 examined the translation of Look AHEAD into the primary care setting. The Reach Ahead for Lifestyle and Health–Diabetes (REAL HEALTH–Diabetes) randomized clinical trial compared the effectiveness and costs of two types of group-based, intensive lifestyle interventions for weight loss—in-person groups and group telephone conference calls—to the effectiveness and

---

† Study participants were described as men and women. Gender was not further specified.

costs of medical nutrition therapy for weight loss in primary care patients with type 2 diabetes. The results showed that both of the lifestyle intervention groups had statistically significant weight loss at 6 and 12 months compared with the group receiving medical nutrition therapy.[25]

Additional Studies

Other studies have shown that a multidisciplinary approach to weight management is effective. The US Department of Veterans Affairs has offered a multidisciplinary weight loss program for veterans, called MOVE!, since 2006. MOVE! is a standardized weight-management program with nutrition classes led by an RDN. Program results for veterans in Los Angeles showed that veterans who enrolled in the program lost an average of 2.2 kg (4.9 lb) at 1 year, compared with a weight gain of 1.4 kg (3.1 lb) at 1 year for veterans who did not enroll in the program ($P < .001$).[26]

Another study conducted in the United Kingdom found that patients with severe obesity (BMI of 40 or higher) who participated in a multidisciplinary weight-management service offered through primary care achieved a 5% weight loss at 1 year and had substantial improvements in their fruit and vegetable intake, activity level, and quality of life.[27]

Summary

A multidisciplinary team approach is highly effective for weight loss, weight maintenance, the prevention of diabetes, and improving outcomes for people with diabetes. The landmark DPP and Look AHEAD trials clearly demonstrated the positive impact of a multidisciplinary, intensive lifestyle intervention on the prevention and management of type 2 diabetes. The results from the DPP and Look AHEAD studies established the benefits of weight loss and maintenance, as these were the dominant predictors of reduced diabetes incidence and improved diabetes control. The results of these two studies changed the way health care practitioners think about weight loss and diabetes prevention, diabetes management, and the prevention and treatment of CVD risk factors. The results of these studies have been translated into community and primary care through the National DPP and REAL HEALTH–Diabetes programs.

References

1. Curry SJ, Krist AH, Owens DK, et al. Behavioral weight loss interventions to prevent obesity-related morbidity and mortality in adults: US Preventive Services Task Force recommendation statement. *JAMA*. 2018;320(11):1163-1171. doi:10.1001/jama.2018.13022
2. Jensen MD, Ryan DH, Apovian CM, et al. 2013 AHA/ACC/TOS guideline for the management of overweight and obesity in adults: a report of the American College of Cardiology/American Heart Association Task Force on Practice Guidelines and The Obesity Society. *J Am Coll Cardiol*. 2014;63(25 pt B):2985-3023. doi:10.1016/j.jacc.2013.11.004
3. Diabetes Prevention Program (DPP). National Institute of Diabetes and Digestive and Kidney Diseases. Last reviewed May 2022. Accessed February 23, 2023. www.niddk.nih.gov/about-niddk/research-areas/diabetes/diabetes-prevention-program-dpp
4. Colditz GA, Willett WC, Stampfer MJ, et al. Weight as a risk factor for clinical diabetes in women. *Am J Epidemiol*. 1990;132(3):501-513. doi:10.1093/oxfordjournals.aje.a115686
5. Knowler WC, Pettitt DJ, Savage PJ, Bennett PH. Diabetes incidence in Pima Indians: contributions of obesity and parental diabetes. *Am J Epidemiol*. 1981;113(2):144-156. doi:10.1093/oxfordjournals.aje.a113079

6. Foster D, Sanchez-Collins S, Cheskin LJ. Multidisciplinary team-based obesity treatment in patients with diabetes: current practices and the state of the science. *Diabetes Spectr*. 2017;30(4):244-249. doi:10.2337/ds17-0045
7. Moore LL, Visioni AJ, Wilson PW, D'Agostino RB, Finkle WD, Ellison RC. Can sustained weight loss in overweight individuals reduce the risk of diabetes mellitus? *Epidemiology*. 2000;11(3):269-273. doi:10.1097/00001648-200005000-00007
8. Wadden TA. The treatment of obesity: an overview. In Stunkard AJ and Wadden TA, eds. *Obesity: Theory and Therapy*. 2nd ed. Raven Press; 1993:197-218.
9. Wing RR. Behavioral approaches to the treatment of obesity. In: Bray GA, Bouchard C, and James P, eds. *Handbook of Obesity*. Marcel Dekker; 1993:855-873.
10. Jeffery RW, Wing RR, Mayer RR. Are smaller weight losses or more achievable weight loss goals better in the long term for obese patients? *J Consult Clin Psychol*. 1998;66(4):641-645. doi:10.1037//0022-006x.66.4.641
11. US Department of Health and Human Services. *Physical Activity and Health: A Report of the Surgeon General*. US Department of Health and Human Services, Centers for Disease Control and Prevention, National Center for Chronic Disease Prevention and Health Promotion; 1996.
12. Knowler WC, Barrett-Connor E, Fowler SE, et al. Reduction in the incidence of type 2 diabetes with lifestyle intervention or metformin. *N Engl J Med*. 2002;346(6):393-403. doi:10.1056/NEJMoa012512
13. Hamman RF, Wing RR, Edelstein SL, et al. Effect of weight loss with lifestyle intervention on risk of diabetes. *Diabetes Care*. 2006;29(9):2102-2107. doi:10.2337/dc06-0560
14. Knowler WC, Fowler SE, Hamman RF, et al. 10-year follow-up of diabetes incidence and weight loss in the Diabetes Prevention Program Outcomes Study. *Lancet*. 2009;374(9702):1677-1686. doi:10.1016/s0140-6736(09)61457-4
15. Diabetes Prevention Program Research Group. Long-term effects of lifestyle intervention or metformin on diabetes development and microvascular complications over 15-year follow-up: the Diabetes Prevention Program Outcomes Study. *Lancet Diabetes Endocrinol*. 2015;3(11):866-875. doi:10.1016/s2213-8587(15)00291-0
16. Tuomilehto J, Lindström J, Eriksson JG, et al. Prevention of type 2 diabetes mellitus by changes in lifestyle among subjects with impaired glucose tolerance. *N Engl J Med*. 2001;344(18):1343-1350. doi:10.1056/nejm200105033441801
17. Wadden TA, West DS, Neiberg RH, et al. One-year weight losses in the Look AHEAD study: factors associated with success. *Obesity (Silver Spring)*. 2009;17(4):713-722. doi:10.1038/oby.2008.637
18. Look AHEAD Research Group, Pi-Sunyer X, Blackburn G, Brancati FL, et al. Reduction in weight and cardiovascular disease risk factors in individuals with type 2 diabetes: one-year results of the look AHEAD trial. *Diabetes Care*. 2007;30(6):1374-1383. doi:10.2337/dc07-0048
19. Wing RR. Long-term effects of a lifestyle intervention on weight and cardiovascular risk factors in individuals with type 2 diabetes mellitus: four-year results of the Look AHEAD trial. *Arch Intern Med*. 2010;170(17):1566-1575. doi:10.1001/archinternmed.2010.334
20. Wadden TA, Neiberg RH, Wing RR, et al. Four-year weight losses in the Look AHEAD study: factors associated with long-term success. *Obesity (Silver Spring)*. 2011;19(10):1987-1998. doi:10.1038/oby.2011.230
21. Look AHEAD Research Group. Eight-year weight losses with an intensive lifestyle intervention: the look AHEAD study. *Obesity (Silver Spring)*. 2014;22(1):5-13. doi:10.1002/oby.20662
22. Salvia MG. The Look AHEAD trial: translating lessons learned into clinical practice and further study. *Diabetes Spectr*. 2017;30(3):166-170. doi:10.2337/ds17-0016
23. Zhang P, Atkinson KM, Bray GA, et al. Within-trial cost-effectiveness of a structured lifestyle intervention in adults with overweight/obesity and type 2 diabetes: results from the action for health in diabetes (Look AHEAD) study. *Diabetes Care*. 2021;44(1):67-74. doi:10.2337/dc20-0358
24. West DS, Dutton G, Delahanty LM, et al. Weight loss experiences of African American, Hispanic, and non-Hispanic White men and women with type 2 diabetes: the Look AHEAD trial. *Obesity (Silver Spring)*. 2019;27(8):1275-1284. doi:10.1002/oby.22522
25. Delahanty LM, Levy DE, Chang Y, et al. Effectiveness of lifestyle intervention for type 2 diabetes in primary care: the REAL HEALTH-Diabetes randomized clinical trial. *J Gen Intern Med*. 2020;35(9):2637-2646. doi:10.1007/s11606-019-05629-9
26. Romanova M, Liang LJ, Deng ML, Li Z, Heber D. Effectiveness of the MOVE! multidisciplinary weight loss program for veterans in Los Angeles. *Prev Chronic Dis*. 2013;10:e112. doi:10.5888/pcd10.120325
27. Jennings A, Hughes CA, Kumaravel B, et al. Evaluation of a multidisciplinary Tier 3 weight management service for adults with morbid obesity, or obesity and comorbidities, based in primary care. *Clin Obes*. 2014;4(5):254-266. doi:10.1111/cob.12066

CHAPTER 11

Dietary Interventions

Shannon M. Robson, PhD, MPH, RD

CHAPTER OBJECTIVES

- Explain the importance of negative energy balance in the treatment of obesity.
- Describe evidence-based nutrition and dietary interventions for weight management.
- Outline a critical-thinking process for analyzing fad diets, dietary supplements, and product claims.

Introduction

Energy Balance

Energy intake, energy expenditure, and energy storage are the basic components of energy balance in the human body, and this balance is governed by a complex physiological control system that is likely influenced by environmental conditions.[1,2] In accordance with the first law of thermodynamics, the amount of energy stored in the body is equal to the amount of energy taken in (energy intake) minus the amount of energy expended (energy expenditure), and this simple equation can help us understand the concept of energy balance,[3] which, in turn, can help us understand how overweight and obesity can be addressed.[4,5] Body weight cannot change when energy intake and energy expenditure are equal. When energy intake exceeds energy expenditure over a period of time, more energy is stored in the body, resulting in weight gain. When this occurs, the body is said to be in a state of *positive energy balance*. When energy expenditure exceeds energy intake over a period of time, the amount of energy stored is depleted, resulting in weight loss. In this case, the body is considered to have a *negative energy balance*. In most cases, body weight is ideally managed by changing modifiable behaviors that influence energy intake (eg, eating) and that influence energy expenditure (eg, physical activity).[4,6,7] Thus, to achieve and maintain weight loss, individuals are advised to change their energy intake through dietary approaches while at the same time increasing their energy expenditure through physical activity.

To facilitate weight loss, an energy (kilocalorie) deficit is needed.[8,9] When an energy deficit occurs over a period of time, negative energy balance results and weight loss occurs. The larger the energy deficit, the greater the weight loss. Frequently, a weight loss of 0.45 kg (1 lb) is equated to a 3,500-kcal deficit achieved through a deficit of 500 kcal/d over a period of 1 week; however, this oversimplification does not account for physiological adaptations that occur with weight loss. More precise estimates of body weight over time can be simulated using mathematical models that account for the adaptations to energy expenditure (refer to Box 11.1). The Weight Loss Predictor Calculator,[10] developed at the Pennington Biomedical Research Center, uses a predictive equation to plot weight change over time based on an identified energy deficit.[11,12] The Body Weight Planner,[13] available from the National Institute of Diabetes and Digestive and Kidney Diseases, can identify the amount of energy intake needed to maintain current weight, reach an identified goal weight, and maintain the identified goal weight.[14] Health care

> **BOX 11.1**
>
> **Calculators for Weight Loss Planning**
>
> **Weight Loss Predictor Calculator** (Pennington Biomedical Research Center): www.pbrc.edu/research-and-faculty/calculators/weight-loss-predictor
>
> **Body Weight Planner** (National Institute of Diabetes and Digestive and Kidney Diseases): www.niddk.nih.gov/bwp

practitioners can use both tools with patients or clients to demonstrate the connection between the degree of energy deficit and weight loss over a period of time.

Dietary Interventions to Achieve an Energy Deficit: An Overview

Many evidence-based dietary interventions are available to help patients or clients achieve the energy deficit needed to facilitate weight loss.[7,8,15-17] The 2013 guidelines for the management of overweight and obesity in adults issued by the American College of Cardiology (ACC), American Heart Association (AHA) Task Force on Practice Guidelines, and The Obesity Society (TOS) identified a total of 18 specific dietary approaches associated with weight loss when an energy deficit was achieved, all of which were supported by high-grade evidence (indicating high certainty of a treatment effect).[8] Across these approaches, weight loss ranged from 4 to 12 kg (9 to 26 lb) at 6 months for those that reduced energy intake by at least 500 kcal/d.[8] Dietary intervention is just one component of the recommended multicomponent behavioral intervention approach for weight loss.[18] Intensive multicomponent behavioral interventions that include a dietary approach that facilitates an energy deficit of at least 500 kcal/d can help patients or clients achieve at least a 5% weight loss.[18] Understanding the best available scientific evidence for each of the different dietary interventions that can achieve an energy deficit is essential for evidence-based practice.[19,20] When a client is interested in implementing a dietary intervention, the practitioner should review the best available evidence (preferably graded evidence) for each dietary strategy with the client, to allow the client to make an informed decision based on the their preferences and values.[19] If graded evidence is not available, such as for emerging dietary interventions, the empirical literature may be the best available evidence to present to the client. This chapter describes the various dietary approaches for weight management, including energy restriction (with an explicit energy prescription), macronutrient modifications, dietary patterns, and intermittent fasting. For each dietary approach, graded evidence from the 2013 AHA/ACC/TOS guidelines will be provided if available. If graded evidence is not available for the approach, this is also stated.

Energy-Restricted Dietary Approaches

While all dietary approaches need to produce an energy deficit to facilitate weight loss,[7,8,15-17] several energy-restricted dietary approaches provide an explicit energy prescription for the amount of amount of energy to be consumed (in kilocalories) and/or the provision of foods (eg, the number of portion-controlled meals to be eaten). The 2013 AHA/ACC/TOS guidelines identified that dietary interventions with energy goals that provide less energy intake than what is required for energy balance, such as low-calorie diets, very low-calorie diets (VCLD), and ad libitum approaches that involve portion control, have highly graded evidence.[8]

Low-Calorie Diets

Continuous (or daily) energy restriction is the most common dietary intervention for creating an energy deficit for weight loss. Low-calorie diets typically prescribe an energy intake in the range of 1,200 to 1,500 kcal/d for females[†] and 1,500 to 1,800 kcal/d for males.[8] However, a more individualized approach, based on the calculated energy expenditure of the client, may be used to establish a deficit of 500 to 750 kcal/d.[21] Regardless of the prescription, an energy-restricted diet should follow recommendations for a healthy dietary pattern from the *Dietary Guidelines for Americans, 2020–2025* (the DGA), which advise eating a variety of nutritious foods and beverages across and within food groups to enhance diet quality.[6]

Very Low-Calorie Diets

In limited cases and often out of medical necessity, such as in preparation for bariatric surgery, greater energy restriction can be achieved with a VLCD, defined as fewer than 800 kcal/d.[8] A VLCD requires medical supervision and typically prescribes high-protein meal replacement shakes with vitamin and mineral supplementation to promote weight loss with minimal loss of lean tissue. VLCDs are designed for short-term use (12 weeks or less) due to the very low energy intake. Given that a VLCD has greater energy restriction, these diets result in greater short-term weight loss than do low-energy diets, but over time the weight loss outcomes are similar.[8,22,23]

Portion-Controlled Diets

Portion-controlled diets are typically used to improve adherence to energy-restricted diets by increasing dietary structure and reducing the number of food decisions an individual has to make.[24-29] Patients or clients following these diets replace one, two, or three meals a day with portion-controlled conventional foods (eg, prepackaged, single-serving meals) or meal replacements (eg, soups, formulated shakes, bars). Research has shown that a partial meal-replacement strategy, in which patients or clients consume meal replacements for two meals and eat conventional foods for a third meal, produces significantly greater weight loss when compared to diets without meal replacements.[23,30]

Macronutrient Modification Dietary Approaches

Several dietary approaches for the treatment of obesity emphasize modifying the proportion of macronutrients (fat, carbohydrate, and protein) consumed. With these approaches, any increase or decrease in the proportion of one macronutrient necessitates an increase or decrease in another macronutrient. The name of the dietary approach—*low-fat*, *low-carbohydrate*, or *high-protein*—generally indicates the macronutrient targeted for modification, and the proportions of one or both of the other macronutrients are then modified on the basis of the dietary decisions made to meet the targeted macronutrient goal.

Low-Fat Diets

The 2013 AHA/ACC/TOS guidelines rate the evidence in support of using a low-fat diet with a realized energy deficit for the treatment of obesity as high-grade.[8] A

[†] Data for transgender people was not provided.

low-fat dietary approach is one in which not more than 30% of daily energy intake comes from fat, and a very low-fat diet is one in which not more than 10% of daily energy intake comes from fat.[8] An explicit energy-restriction goal is common in low-fat diets in order to produce the required energy deficit needed for weight loss.[31-33]

Low-Carbohydrate Diets

Definitions for low-carbohydrate diets vary and can be worded in terms of absolute grams of carbohydrate or the proportion of energy consumed that comes from carbohydrates. For weight loss, low-carbohydrate diets are usually based on the Atkins diet[34] and are defined by an initial carbohydrate intake of less than 20 g/d,[8,35,36] followed by a gradual increase to a maximum of 120 g/d for weight loss maintenance.[37] Unlike other macronutrient-based dietary interventions for weight loss, low-carbohydrate diets *do not* include explicit energy-restriction goals. Despite the lack of explicit energy restriction, low-carbohydrate diets were identified by the 2013 AHA/ACC/TOS guidelines as having high-grade evidence for obesity treatment.[8]

Ketogenic Diets

When carbohydrate intake is restricted (to less than 20–50 g/d or 10% of total energy intake) *and* fat intake is increased, with moderate protein intake, ketones become the main source of energy in the body.[38] A low-carbohydrate dietary intervention that facilitates ketosis is called a low-carbohydrate ketogenic diet, or simply a ketogenic diet. The ketogenic diet was not included in the 2013 AHA/ACC/TOS guidelines.[8] However, research shows that, like a low-carbohydrate diet, when a ketogenic diet is compared to an energy-restricted, low-fat diet, it results in an equivalent weight loss at 24 months.[39] Given the corresponding increase in fat intake, a ketogenic diet may increase satiation and decrease hunger.[40]

Recently, very low-calorie ketogenic diets have been proposed as an effective strategy for producing weight loss in a short period of time.[41,42] Very low-calorie ketogenic diets combine a VLCD (<800 kcal/d) with a low-carbohydrate ketogenic diet. Like a VLCD, this diet can be a safe approach under medical supervision. Very low-calorie ketogenic diets have shown reductions in weight over time and produce significantly greater weight loss when compared to other dietary interventions, such as low-calorie diets in the short term (≤6 months) and long term (12–24 months).[43]

High-Protein Diets

A high-protein diet is typically defined as a diet in which at least 25% of energy intake comes from protein.[8,44] High-protein, energy-restricted diets (a 500–750 kcal/d deficit) may increase satiety and energy expenditure.[45-47] According to the 2013 AHA/ACC/TOS guidelines, a high-protein diet that achieves a realized energy deficit has high-grade evidence for use in the treatment of obesity.[8]

Research on macronutrient modifications indicates that if negative energy balance is achieved, the macronutrient proportion is less relevant,[48] given that weight loss is the result of the energy deficit over a period of time.[7-9] However, given that macronutrient composition of the diet may be important for addressing other health conditions that commonly occur with overweight or obesity, the health implications of specific micronutrient modifications should be considered when choosing to implement a particular approach.

Dietary Pattern Approaches

Dietary patterns are the various combinations in which people consume nutrients, foods, and beverages; a person's dietary pattern constitutes their complete dietary intake over time. Dietary patterns provide a framework for overall eating to be achieved within energy-intake levels based on an individual's age, sex, and physical activity level. The DGA suggest three dietary patterns for the promotion of health and prevention of disease: the Healthy US-Style Dietary Pattern, the Healthy Mediterranean-Style Dietary Pattern, and the Healthy Vegetarian Dietary Pattern. The DGA are not intended to be clinical guidance for treating chronic diseases such as obesity; however, they can be used as a reference to develop clinical guidance and are viewed as the main guidance for diet quality.[6] Indeed, two of the dietary patterns suggested by the DGA (healthy Mediterranean-style and vegetarian-style) have been investigated as dietary interventions for weight management. Two additional dietary patterns, Dietary Approaches to Stop Hypertension (DASH) and the low-energy-density pattern, will also be reviewed with regard to weight outcomes.

Mediterranean-Style Dietary Pattern

The "Mediterranean diet"—so named for the dietary habits observed in the Mediterranean region in the 1960s—was initially defined as a diet low in saturated fat and high in vegetable oils.[49,50] Given the observations of lower mortality from cardiovascular disease among people in Mediterranean countries, this dietary pattern gained in popularity.[51-53] Over time, definitions have varied.[54] A Mediterranean-style dietary pattern is generally characterized by a high intake of monounsaturated fats (eg, olive oil, tree nuts), a high intake of plant-based foods (including fruits, vegetables, legumes, and whole grains), low to moderate consumption of red wine, low consumption of meat and meat products, increased consumption of fish, and moderate consumption of milk and dairy products.[55] The evidence in support of using a Mediterranean-style dietary pattern with energy restriction (a 500–750 kcal/d deficit) for weight loss is highly graded by the 2013 AHA/ACC/TOS guidelines.[8,37]

Vegetarian-Style Dietary Pattern

A vegetarian-style dietary pattern falls under the larger umbrella of plant-based diets that emphasize eating more foods derived from plant sources such as fruits, vegetables, whole grains, and legumes or beans, with no or limited animal food sources.[56,57] In general, a vegetarian diet excludes the consumption of flesh foods (meat, poultry, fish) but can include egg (ovo) or dairy (lacto). A vegan diet typically excludes all animal-derived food products.[58] Plant-based dietary patterns are widely promoted for the prevention of chronic disease (eg, cardiovascular disease).[59] The 2013 AHA/ACC/TOS guidelines identified a lacto-ovo-vegetarian–style dietary approach with energy restriction (a 500–750 kcal/d deficit) and a low-fat vegan-style diet (10%–25% of energy from fat) with a realized energy deficit as having a high-grade evidence for weight loss.[8]

The DASH Dietary Pattern

The Dietary Approaches to Stop Hypertension (DASH) dietary pattern was developed as a treatment for hypertension.[60] The original DASH dietary pattern was rich in fruits, vegetables, and low-fat dairy foods, with reduced amounts of saturated fat, total fat, and cholesterol.[61] Today, a DASH dietary pattern is supported by the

National Heart, Lung, and Blood Institute; it is characterized by the consumption of fruits, vegetables, whole grains, nonfat or low-fat dairy products, fish, poultry, beans, nuts, and vegetable oils, and by limited consumption of foods high in saturated fat, sugar-sweetened beverages, and sweets.[62] Standard characterizations of a DASH dietary pattern do not include an explicit energy restriction; however, weight loss occurred within a multicomponent behavioral intervention in which reduced total energy intake was emphasized (without an explicit prescription) within a DASH dietary pattern.[63,64] The 2013 AHA/ACC/TOS guidelines do not specifically include the DASH dietary pattern as an approach to reducing energy intake.[8]

Low-Energy-Density Dietary Pattern

Energy density is the amount of energy in a given weight of food and is presented as kilocalories per gram. Energy density can range from 0 to 9 kcal/g, depending on the macronutrient composition of the food or beverage in question. Fat and water have the greatest influence on energy density. Thus, a low-energy-density dietary pattern is one that contains foods higher in water content and lower in fat content (eg, fruits and vegetables). Because of their high water content, beverages have a low energy density and are often not included in energy-density calculations, as they would have a disproportionate impact on overall dietary energy density. No standard definition of a low-energy-density dietary pattern exists, but several cutoff values to define a food as having a low energy density have been proposed, and they range from 0.6 to 2.25 kcal/g.[65-67] Consistent evidence from laboratory studies has shown that a low-energy-density dietary pattern is associated with lower energy intake,[68-70] and consistent evidence from observational studies has shown that a low-energy-density pattern is associated with lower weight.[71-73] Several intervention trials have shown this dietary pattern to be an effective strategy for weight loss.[74,75] Despite the need for better-quality studies of longer duration, a low-energy-dense dietary pattern has been promoted as an effective approach for weight management,[76-79] but it is not an approach included in the 2013 AHA/ACC/TOS guidelines.[8]

As a dietary strategy, dietary patterns offer the opportunity to optimize diet quality, and in combination with energy restriction, they can result in weight loss.[80] Two dietary patterns, the Mediterranean-style and vegetarian-style, are supported by high-grade evidence for weight loss according to the 2013 AHA/ACC/TOS guidelines.[8]

Intermittent Fasting Dietary Approaches

While traditional dietary approaches have focused on *what* to eat, more recent dietary approaches have focused on *when* to eat. These new approaches are grouped into a category called intermittent fasting.[81] The two most-investigated intermittent fasting approaches focus on the number and pattern of days of energy restriction (periodic fasting) and when to eat during a 24-hour cycle (time-restricted eating).[81] As this is a newer area of research, there are no graded recommendations for these dietary approaches.

Periodic Fasting

Periodic fasting was initially proposed as a strategy for increasing adherence to energy restriction.[82,83] Although standardized definitions are lacking, periodic-fasting diets are generally defined by their periods of energy restriction and periods of typical energy intake.[83,84] Examples include the 5:2 diet and alternate-day fasting. The 5:2 diet involves 5 days a week of unrestricted intake and 2 days of energy restriction (typically at 60%–70% of estimated energy requirements).[85] Alternate-day fasting involves alternating a 24-hour day of typical ad libitum intake ("feast day") with a 24-hour day of either reduced energy intake (25% of usual intake or approximately 500 kcal) or no energy intake ("fast day").[86,87]

Comparable reductions in body weight have been shown between periodic-fasting diets and continuous energy-restricted diets (with the degree of restriction differing between studies), indicating that both are feasible dietary approaches for weight loss.[82-84,87-91]

Time-Restricted Eating

Time-restricted eating involves consistent ad libitum eating periods, often with no overt energy restriction, and fasting periods (of 4 to 12 hours) within a 24-hour cycle.[92-94] Thus, without energy restriction, time-restricted eating allows individuals to consume a typical diet within a certain eating period. There are many proposed advantages to time-restricted eating, including increased dietary adherence, but the literature on this dietary approach is in its infancy, and no best window of time for eating has been identified yet, neither in terms of the length of the window or when during the day the window should occur.[93] In several small studies in humans, time-restricted eating resulted in reduced energy intake and associated decreases in body weight.[95-97] A larger, randomized, clinical trial comparing time-restricted eating (8-hour window for eating) without energy restriction vs consistent meal timing without energy restriction found weight loss outcomes to be the same between the two strategies.[94] A meta-analysis determined that time-restricted eating without intentional energy restriction resulted in greater weight loss than the use of unrestricted time regimens, but the authors attributed the weight loss to changes in lean tissue.[98] Findings from a study that combined time restricted-eating (8-hour window for eating) with energy restriction (1,500–1,800 kcal/d for men; 1,200–1,500 kcal/d for women[†]) and compared it to continuous (daily) energy restriction found similar effects on weight loss.[99]

Evaluating Popular Diets and Weight Loss Products

Practitioners and scientists working in weight management should be familiar with the evidence-based literature on dietary interventions for weight loss. Consumers, on the other hand, often have little access to the scientific literature and instead are inundated with promotions for popular diets and weight loss products. Promoters of these diets and products often make unfounded health claims. Thus, the ability to work with a client to critically evaluate a popular diet or weight loss product is essential. A critical evaluation requires the practitioner to weigh and interpret the available evidence (refer to Box 11.2).

Sources such as the Academy of Nutrition and Dietetics Evidence Analysis Library (www.andeal.org) can help with synthesizing and evaluating available evidence. Unfortunately, many popular diets and weight loss products are not sufficiently evaluated, and there may be no scientific evidence available. In this case, practitioners may need to consult alternative reputable sources, particularly for products such as dietary supplements. The Office of Dietary Supplements and

---

† Study participants were described as men and women. Gender was not further specified.

BOX 11.2

Questions to Help Weigh and Interpret the Evidence for Popular Diets or Weight Loss Products

When weighing the purported evidence for a popular diet or product, practitioners should ask themselves the following questions:

- What was the stated purpose of the study?
- How long was the study?
- Does the dietary intervention create an energy deficit?
- Was the approach compared to another approach?
- What are the side effects (or harms)?
- Are the study's results statistically significant?
- Are the study's results clinically significant?
- Was the study done in animals or human beings?
- Are recommendations based on a single study?

the National Center for Complementary and Integrative Health, both of which are within the National Institutes of Health, and the US Department of Agriculture all provide online information on dietary supplements and can serve as important resources. Seeking answers to questions about a popular diet or product is also an important step in the critical evaluation of the diet or product (refer to Box 11.3). In addition, understanding what the client perceives about a specific popular diet or weight loss product is important. Gathering information on why a client is interested in trying a popular diet or weight loss product is essential given this interest has been one of the most reported factors that influences the decision to follow a popular diet.[100]

BOX 11.3

Questions to Answer About Popular Diets and Weight Loss Products

When investigating a popular diet or weight loss product, practitioners should seek answers to the following questions:

- Has research been done to evaluate the diet or weight loss product?
- Does it promise a quick fix?
- How much weight loss is expected and in what time frame?
- Does the diet or weight loss product require the client to change eating or activity behaviors? If yes, how so?
- What are the associated risks?
- Are additional health outcomes being promised beyond weight loss? If so, what are they?
- What is the cost?
- What are the credentials of the individuals or organizations promoting or selling the product?

Despite the availability of numerous effective, evidence-based dietary interventions for weight loss, popular diets and products create a competitive market and constitute a $70-billion-plus industry. The ever-changing landscape in this area makes it essential for practitioners in the field of weight management to stay educated and up to date on the latest popular diets and weight loss products.

Implications for Practice

When considering dietary interventions for weight management, the practitioner needs to understand the most relevant evidence in support of the intervention, utilize clinical expertise, and consider the characteristics of the client.[19] In addition to individual-level characteristics, various social and environmental factors may also influence a client's ability to implement a specific dietary intervention; practitioners should take this information into account. In order to effectively translate dietary interventions for weight management into practice, practitioners should keep the following points in mind:

- Weight management is ideally implemented by a multidisciplinary team.[8] Because diet is a fundamental aspect of weight management, the team should include a nutrition expert, such as a registered dietitian nutritionist with appropriate training.[7]
- An energy deficit over a given period of time results in weight loss. An energy deficit can be achieved through various dietary intervention approaches.[7,8,16,17] There is no one optimal approach.
- Helping a client make an informed decision about what dietary intervention to implement requires considering all potential individual, social, and environmental influences.
  - *Individual-level influences*: These include the client's health conditions and any opportunities for additional health benefits, as well as the client's preferences, values, medications, nutrition knowledge, and food skills (skills needed to purchase, prepare, and cook food to produce nutritious meals).
  - *Social influences*: These may include the client's socioeconomic status, cultural norms, and family or peer networks, including who is responsible for acquiring, preparing, and cooking food.
  - *Environmental influences*: These may include the client's access to food or health care services, including transportation options, and the availability of food in the home and community environment.
- The ability of a client to adhere to a dietary intervention is essential for successful weight management.[101,102] Thus, patients or clients should be encouraged to choose a dietary approach that they anticipate being able to follow.[103]

Summary

To date, an optimal dietary intervention has not been identified for weight loss; we do know, however, that adherence to a dietary intervention is essential for long-term success.[101-103] Fundamental to weight loss is the ability of the dietary intervention to create an energy deficit.[8,9] An energy deficit over a period of time results in negative energy balance and weight loss.

This energy deficit can be achieved through several dietary approaches supported by high-grade evidence,[8] but newer approaches are continually being developed to enhance outcomes. Popular diets and weight loss products can offer additional options, but they need to be critically evaluated by the health care practitioner before implementation.

References

1. Hill J, Levine J, Saris W. Energy expenditure and physical activity. In: Bray G, Bouchard C, eds. *Handbook of Obesity*. 2nd ed. Marcel Dekker; 2003:631-654.
2. Schwartz MW, Seeley RJ, Zeltser LM, et al. Obesity pathogenesis: an Endocrine Society scientific statement. *Endocr Rev.* 2017;38(4):267-296. doi:10.1210/er.2017-00111

3. Heymsfield SB, Waki M, Kehayias J, et al. Chemical and elemental analysis of humans in vivo using improved body composition models. *Am J Physiol.* 1991;261(2 pt 1):e190-198. doi:10.1152/ajpendo.1991.261.2.E190
4. Hill JO, Wyatt HR, Peters JC. Energy balance and obesity. *Circulation.* 2012;126(1):126-132. doi:10.1161/CIRCULATIONAHA.111.087213
5. Hill JO. Understanding and addressing the epidemic of obesity: an energy balance perspective. *Endocr Rev.* 2006;27(7):750-761. doi:10.1210/er.2006-0032
6. US Department of Agriculture, US Department of Health and Human Services. *Dietary Guidelines for Americans, 2020-2025.* 9th ed. US Department of Agriculture and US Department of Health and Human Services; 2020. Accessed July 11, 2022. www.dietaryguidelines.gov/resources/2020-2025-dietary-guidelines-online-materials
7. Raynor HA, Champagne CM. Position of the Academy of Nutrition and Dietetics: interventions for the treatment of overweight and obesity in adults. *J Acad Nutr Diet.* 2016;116(1):129-147. doi:10.1016/j.jand.2015.10.031
8. Jensen MD, Ryan DH, Apovian CM, et al. 2013 AHA/ACC/TOS guideline for the management of overweight and obesity in adults: a report of the American College of Cardiology/American Heart Association Task Force on Practice Guidelines and The Obesity Society. *Circulation.* 2014;129(25 suppl 2):S102-138. doi:10.1161/01.cir.0000437739.71477.ee
9. Hall KD, Guo J. Obesity energetics: body weight regulation and the effects of diet composition. *Gastroenterology.* 2017;152(7):1718-1727.e3. doi:10.1053/j.gastro.2017.01.052
10. Weight Loss Predictor Calculator. Pennington Biomedical Research Center. Accessed July 11, 2022. www.pbrc.edu/research-and-faculty/calculators/weight-loss-predictor
11. Thomas DM, Martin CK, Redman LM, et al. Effect of dietary adherence on the body weight plateau: a mathematical model incorporating intermittent compliance with energy intake prescription. *Am J Clin Nutr.* 2014;100(3):787-795. doi:10.3945/ajcn.113.079822
12. Thomas DM, Gonzalez MC, Pereira AZ, Redman LM, Heymsfield SB. Time to correctly predict the amount of weight loss with dieting. *J Acad Nutr Diet.* 2014;114(6):857-861. doi:10.1016/j.jand.2014.02.003
13. Body Weight Planner. National Institutes of Diabetes and Digestive and Kidney Diseases. Accessed July 11, 2022. www.niddk.nih.gov/bwp
14. Hall KD, Sacks G, Chandramohan D, et al. Quantification of the effect of energy imbalance on bodyweight. *Lancet.* 2011;378(9793):826-837. doi:10.1016/S0140-6736(11)60812-X
15. Looney SM, Raynor HA. Behavioral lifestyle intervention in the treatment of obesity. *Health Serv Insights.* 2013;6:15-31. doi:10.4137/HSI.S10474
16. Makris AP, Foster GD. Dietary approaches to the treatment of obesity. *Psychiatr Clin North Am.* 2005;28(1):117-139,viii-ix. doi:10.1016/j.psc.2004.11.001
17. Makris A, Foster GD. Dietary approaches to the treatment of obesity. *Psychiatr Clin North Am.* 2011;34(4):813-827. doi:10.1016/j.psc.2011.08.004
18. US Preventive Services Task Force; Curry SJ, Krist AH, et al. Behavioral weight loss interventions to prevent obesity-related morbidity and mortality in adults: US Preventive Services Task Force recommendation statement. *JAMA.* 2018;320(11):1163-1171. doi:10.1001/jama.2018.13022
19. Raynor HA, Beto JA, Zoellner J. Achieving evidence-based practice in dietetics by using evidence-based practice guidelines. *J Acad Nutr Diet.* 2020;120(5):751-756. doi:10.1016/j.jand.2019.10.011
20. Hand RK, Davis AM, Thompson KL, Knol LL, Thomas A, Proano GV. Updates to the definition of evidence-based (dietetics) practice: providing clarity for practice. *J Acad Nutr Diet.* 2021;121(8):1565-1573.e4. doi:10.1016/j.jand.2020.05.01
21. Lin PH, Proschan MA, Bray GA, et al. Estimation of energy requirements in a controlled feeding trial. *Am J Clin Nutr.* 2003;77(3):639-645. doi:10.1093/ajcn/77.3.639
22. Tsai AG, Wadden TA. The evolution of very-low-calorie diets: an update and meta-analysis. *Obesity (Silver Spring).* 2006;14(8):1283-1293. doi:10.1038/oby.2006.146
23. Astbury NM, Piernas C, Hartmann-Boyce J, Lapworth S, Aveyard P, Jebb SA. A systematic review and meta-analysis of the effectiveness of meal replacements for weight loss. *Obes Rev.* 2019;20(4):569-587. doi:10.1111/obr.12816
24. Rolls BJ. What is the role of portion control in weight management? *Int J Obes (Lond).* 2014;38 suppl 1:S1-S8. doi:10.1038/ijo.2014.82
25. Hannum SM, Carson L, Evans EM, et al. Use of portion-controlled entrees enhances weight loss in women. *Obes Res.* 2004;12(3):538-546. doi:10.1038/oby.2004.61
26. Hannum SM, Carson LA, Evans EM, et al. Use of packaged entrees as part of a weight-loss diet in overweight men: an 8-week randomized clinical trial. *Diabetes Obes Metab.* 2006;8(2):146-155. doi:10.1111/j.1463-1326.2005.00493.x
27. Cheskin LJ, Mitchell AM, Jhaveri AD, et al. Efficacy of meal replacements versus a standard food-based diet for weight loss in type 2 diabetes: a controlled clinical trial. *Diabetes Educ.* 2008;34(1):118-127. doi:10.1177/0145721707312463
28. Rolls BJ, Roe LS, James BL, Sanchez CE. Does the incorporation of portion-control strategies in a behavioral program improve weight loss in a 1-year randomized controlled trial? *Int J Obes (Lond).* 2017;41(3):434-442. doi:10.1038/ijo.2016.217
29. Ditschuneit HH, Flechtner-Mors M. Value of structured meals for weight management: risk factors and long-term weight maintenance. *Obes Res.* 2001;9 suppl 4:284S-289S. doi:10.1038/oby.2001.132
30. Heymsfield S, van Mierlo C, van der Knapp H, Heo M, Frier H. Weight management using a meal replacement strategy: meta and pooling analysis from six studies. *Int J Obes Relat Metab Disord.* 2003;27(5):537-549. doi:10.1038/sj.ijo.0802258

31. Knowler WC, Barrett-Connor E, Fowler SE, et al. Reduction in the incidence of type 2 diabetes with lifestyle intervention or metformin. *N Engl J Med*. 2002;346(6):393-403. doi:10.1056/NEJMoa012512
32. Look AHEAD Research Group; Pi-Sunyer XB, G, Brancati F, et al. Reduction in weight and cardiovascular disease risk factors in individuals with type 2 diabetes: one-year results of the look AHEAD trial. *Diabetes Care*. 2007;30(6):1374-1383. doi:10.2337/dc07-0048
33. Look AHEAD Research Group. Long-term effects of an lifestyle intervention on weight and cardiovascular risk factors in individuals with type 2 diabetes mellitus. *Arch Intern Med*. 2010;170(17):1566-1575. doi:10.1001/archinternmed.2010.334
34. Atkins R. *Dr. Atkins' New Diet Revolution*. Avon; 2002.
35. Foster GD, Wyatt HR, Hill J, et al. A randomized trial of a low-carbohydrate diet for obesity. *N Engl J Med*. 2003;348(21):2082-2090. doi:10.1056/NEJMoa022207
36. Foster GD, Wyatt HR, Hill JO, et al. Weight and metabolic outcomes after 2 years on a low-carbohydrate versus low-fat diet: a randomized trial. *Ann Intern Med*. 2010;153(3):147-157. doi:10.7326/0003-4819-153-3-201008030-00005
37. Shai I, Schwarzfuchs D, Henkin Y, et al. Weight loss in low-carbohydrate, Mediterranean, or low-fat diet. *N Engl J Med*. 2008;359(3):229-237. doi:10.1056/NEJMoa0708681
38. Kirkpatrick CF, Bolick JP, Kris-Etherton PM, et al. Review of current evidence and clinical recommendations on the effects of low-carbohydrate and very-low-carbohydrate (including ketogenic) diets for the management of body weight and other cardiometabolic risk factors: a scientific statement from the National Lipid Association Nutrition and Lifestyle Task Force. *J Clin Lipidol*. 2019;13(5):689-711.e1. doi:10.1016/j.jacl.2019.08.003
39. Bueno NB, de Melo IS, de Oliveira SL, da Rocha Ataide T. Very-low-carbohydrate ketogenic diet v. low-fat diet for long-term weight loss: a meta-analysis of randomised controlled trials. *Br J Nutr*. 2013;110(7):1178-1187. doi:10.1017/S0007114513000548
40. Gibson AA, Seimon RV, Lee CM, et al. Do ketogenic diets really suppress appetite? A systematic review and meta-analysis. *Obes Rev*. 2015;16(1):64-76. doi:10.1111/obr.12230
41. Castellana M, Conte E, Cignarelli A, et al. Efficacy and safety of very low calorie ketogenic diet (VLCKD) in patients with overweight and obesity: a systematic review and meta-analysis. *Rev Endocr Metab Disord*. 2020;21(1):5-16. doi:10.1007/s11154-019-09514-y
42. Castellana M, Biacchi E, Procino F, Casanueva FF, Trimboli P. Very-low-calorie ketogenic diet for the management of obesity, overweight and related disorders. *Minerva Endocrinol (Torino)*. 2021;46(2):161-167. doi:10.23736/S2724-6507.20.03356-8
43. Muscogiuri G, El Ghoch M, Colao A, et al. European guidelines for obesity management in adults with a very low-calorie ketogenic diet: a systematic review and meta-analysis. *Obes Facts*. 2021;14(2):222-245. doi:10.1159/000515381
44. Eisenstein J, Roberts SB, Dallal G, Saltzman E. High-protein weight-loss diets: are they safe and do they work? A review of the experimental and epidemiologic data. *Nutr Rev*. 2002;60:189-200. doi:10.1301/00296640260184264
45. Westerterp-Plantenga M, Lemmens S, Westerterp K. Dietary protein—its role in satiety, energetics, weight loss and health. *Br J Nutr*. 2012;108(suppl 2):S105-S112. doi:10.1017/S0007114512002589
46. Halton T, Hu F. The effects of high protein diets on thermogenesis, satiety and weight loss: a critical review. *J Am Coll Nutr*. 2004;23(5):373-385. doi:10.1080/07315724.2004.10719381
47. Moon J, Koh G. Clinical evidence and mechanisms of high-protein diet-induced weight loss. *J Obes Metab Syndr*. 2020;29(3):166-173. doi:10.7570/jomes20028
48. Academy of Nutrition and Dietetics. Adult weight management: executive summary of recommendations (2014): nutrition intervention: dietary approaches for caloric reduction in weight loss. Evidence Analysis Library. Accessed July 22, 2022. www.andeal.org/topic.cfm?menu=5276&cat=4690
49. Keys A, Menotti A, Karvonen MJ, et al. The diet and 15-year death rate in the seven countries study. *Am J Epidemiol*. 1986;124(6):903-915. doi:10.1093/oxfordjournals.aje.a114480
50. Kromhout D, Keys A, Aravanis C, et al. Food consumption patterns in the 1960s in seven countries. *Am J Clin Nutr*. 1989;49(5):889-894. doi:10.1093/ajcn/49.5.889
51. Kromhout D, Menotti A, Bloemberg B, et al. Dietary saturated and *trans* fatty acids and cholesterol and 25-year mortality from coronary heart disease: the Seven Countries Study. *Prev Med*. 1995;24(3):308-315. doi:10.1006/pmed.1995.1049
52. Menotti A, Kromhout D, Blackburn H, Fidanza F, Buzina R, Nissinen A. Food intake patterns and 25-year mortality from coronary heart disease: cross-cultural correlations in the Seven Countries Study. The Seven Countries Study Research Group. *Eur J Epidemiol*. 1999;15(6):507-515. doi:10.1023/a:1007529206050
53. Delarue J. Mediterranean Diet and cardiovascular health: an historical perspective. *Br J Nutr*. 2021:1-14. doi:10.1017/S0007114521002105
54. Davis C, Bryan J, Hodgson J, Murphy K. Definition of the Mediterranean diet; a literature review. *Nutrients*. 2015;7(11):9139-9153. doi:10.3390/nu7115459
55. Rees K, Takeda A, Martin N, et al. Mediterranean-style diet for the primary and secondary prevention of cardiovascular disease. *Cochrane Database Syst Rev*. 2019;3:CD009825.
56. Satija A, Hu FB. Plant-based diets and cardiovascular health. *Trends Cardiovasc Med*. 2018;28(7):437-441. doi:10.1016/j.tcm.2018.02.004

57. Hemler EC, Hu FB. Plant-based diets for cardiovascular disease prevention: all plant foods are not created equal. *Curr Atheroscler Rep.* 2019;21(5):18. doi:10.1007/s11883-019-0779-5
58. Academy of Nutrition and Dietetics. Vegetarian nutrition guideline: introduction. Evidence Analysis Library. Accessed July 11 2022. www.andeal.org/topic.cfm?menu=5271&pcat=4023&cat=5450
59. Qian F, Liu G, Hu FB, Bhupathiraju SN, Sun Q. Association between plant-based dietary patterns and risk of type 2 diabetes: a systematic review and meta-analysis. *JAMA Intern Med.* 2019;179(10):1335-1344. doi:10.1001/jamainternmed.2019.2195
60. Sacks FM, Obarzanek E, Windhauser MM, et al. Rationale and design of the Dietary Approaches to Stop Hypertension trial (DASH): a multicenter controlled-feeding study of dietary patterns to lower blood pressure. *Ann Epidemiol.* 1995;5(2):108-118. doi:10.1016/1047-2797(94)00055-x
61. Appel LJ, Moore T, Obarzanek E, et al. A clinical trial of the effects of dietary patterns on blood pressure. DASH Collaborative Research Group. *N Engl J Med.* 1997;336(16):1117-1124. doi:10.1056/NEJM199704173361601
62. DASH eating plan. National Heart, Lung, and Blood Institute. Updated December 29, 2021. Accessed July 22, 2022. www.nhlbi.nih.gov/education/dash-eating-plan
63. Appel LJ, Champagne CM, Harsha DW, et al. Effects of comprehensive lifestyle modification on blood pressure control: main results of the PREMIER clinical trial. *JAMA.* 2003;289(16):2083-2093. doi:10.1001/jama.289.16.2083
64. Blumenthal J, Babyak M, Hinderliter A, et al. Effect of the DASH diet alone and in combination with exercise and weight loss on blood pressure and cardiovascular biomarkers in men and women with high blood pressure. *JAMA.* 2010;170(2):126-135. doi:10.1001/archinternmed.2009.470
65. Rolls B, Hermann M. *The Ultimate Volumetric Diet.* HarperCollins; 2012.
66. Raynor HA, Looney SM, Steeves EA, Spence M, Gorin AA. The effects of an energy density prescription on diety quality and weight loss: a pilot randomized controlled trial. *J Acad Nutr Diet.* 2012;112(9):1397-1402. doi:10.1016/j.jand.2012.02.020
67. World Cancer Research Fund, American Institute for Cancer Research. *Diet, Nutrition, Physical Activity and Cancer: A Global Perspective.* Continuous Update Project Expert Report, 2018. Accessed July 22, 2022. www.wcrf.org/diet-activity-and-cancer/global-cancer-update-programme/about-the-third-expert-report
68. Bell EA, Rolls BJ. Energy density of foods affects energy intake across multiple levels of fat content in lean and obese women. *Am J Clin Nutr.* 2001;73(6):1010-1018. doi:10.1093/ajcn/73.6.1010
69. Kral TV, Rolls BJ. Energy density and portion size: their independent and combined effects on energy intake. *Physiol Behav.* 2004;82(1):131-138. doi:10.1016/j.physbeh.2004.04.063
70. Williams RA, Roe LS, Rolls BJ. Comparison of three methods to reduce energy density. Effects on daily energy intake. *Appetite.* 2013;66:75-83. doi:10.1016/j.appet.2013.03.004
71. Ledikwe J, Rolls B, Smiciklas-Wright H, et al. Reduction in dietary energy density are associated with weight loss in overweight and obese participants in the PREMIER trial. *Am J Clin Nutr.* 2007;85:1212-1221. doi:10.1093/ajcn/85.5.1212
72. Vernarelli JA, Mitchell DC, Rolls BJ, Hartman TJ. Dietary energy density and obesity: how consumption patterns differ by body weight status. *Eur J Nutr.* 2018;57(1):351-361. doi:10.1007/s00394-016-1324-8
73. Bes-Rastrollo M, van Dam RM, Martinez-Gonzalez MA, Li TY, Sampson LL, Hu FB. Prospective study of dietary energy density and weight gain in women. *Am J Clin Nutr.* 2008;88(3):769-777. doi:10.1093/ajcn/88.3.769
74. Ello-Martin JA, Roe LS, Ledikwe JH, Beach AM, Rolls BJ. Dietary energy-density in the treatment of obesity: a year-long trial comparing 2 weight-loss diets. *Am J Clin Nutr.* 2007;85(6):1465-1477. doi:10.1093/ajcn/85.6.1465
75. Perez-Escamilla R, Obbagy JE, Altman JM, et al. Dietary energy density a body weight in adults and children: a systematic review. *J Acad Nutr Diet.* 2012;112:671-684. doi:10.1016/j.jand.2012.01.020
76. Smethers AD, Rolls BJ. Dietary management of obesity: cornerstones of healthy eating patterns. *Med Clin North Am.* 2018;102(1):107-124. doi:10.1016/j.mcna.2017.08.009
77. National Center for Chronic Disease Prevention and Health Promotion, Division of Nutrition, Physical Activity and Obesity. *Low-Energy-Dense Foods and Weight Management: Cutting Calories While Controlling Hunger.* Research to Practice Series, no. 5. Accessed July 11, 2022. www.cdc.gov/nccdphp/dnpa/nutrition/pdf/r2p_energy_density.pdf
78. US Department of Agriculture, US Department of Health and Human Services. *Dietary Guidelines for Americans, 2010.* 7th ed. US Government Printing Office; 2010. Accessed July 11, 2022. https://health.gov/sites/default/files/2020-01/DietaryGuidelines2010.pdf
79. Rolls B, Drewnowski A, Ledikwe J. Changing the energy density of the diet as a strategy for weight management. *J Am Diet Assoc.* 2005;105(5 suppl 1):S98-S103. doi:10.1016/j.jada.2005.02.033
80. Anderson CAM. Dietary patterns to reduce weight and optimize cardiovascular health: persuasive evidence for promoting multiple, healthful approaches. *Circulation.* 2018;137(11):1114-1116. doi:10.1161/CIRCULATIONAHA.117.031429
81. Santos HO, Genario R, Tinsley GM, et al. A scoping review of intermittent fasting, chronobiology, and metabolism. *Am J Clin Nutr.* 2022;115(4):991-1004. doi:10.1093/ajcn/nqab433
82. Sundfor TM, Svendsen M, Tonstad S. Intermittent calorie restriction—a more effective approach to weight loss? *Am J Clin Nutr.* 2018;108(5):909-910. doi:10.1093/ajcn/nqy288

83. Harvie M, Howell A. Potential benefits and harms of intermittent energy restriction and intermittent fasting amongst obese, overweight and normal weight subjects—a narrative review of human and animal evidence. *Behav Sci (Basel)*. 2017;7(1):4. doi:10.3390/bs7010004

84. Rynders CA, Thomas EA, Zaman A, Pan Z, Catenacci VA, Melanson EL. Effectiveness of intermittent fasting and time-restricted feeding compared to continuous energy restriction for weight loss. *Nutrients*. 2019;11(10):2442. doi:10.3390/nu11102442

85. Schubel R, Nattenmuller J, Sookthai D, et al. Effects of intermittent and continuous calorie restriction on body weight and metabolism over 50 wk: a randomized controlled trial. *Am J Clin Nutr*. 2018;108(5):933-945. doi:10.1093/ajcn/nqy196

86. Varady KA, Hellerstein MK. Alternate-day fasting and chronic disease prevention: a review of human and animal trials. *Am J Clin Nutr*. 2007;86(1):7-13. doi:10.1093/ajcn/86.1.7

87. Trepanowski JF, Kroeger CM, Barnosky A, et al. Effect of alternate-day fasting on weight loss, weight maintenance, and cardioprotection among metabolically healthy obese adults: a randomized clinical trial. *JAMA Intern Med*. 2017;177(7):930-938. doi:10.1001/jamainternmed.2017.0936

88. Sundfor TM, Svendsen M, Tonstad S. Effect of intermittent versus continuous energy restriction on weight loss, maintenance and cardiometabolic risk: a randomized 1-year trial. *Nutr Metab Cardiovasc Dis*. 2018;28(7):698-706. doi:10.1016/j.numecd.2018.03.009

89. Sundfor TM, Tonstad S, Svendsen M. Effects of intermittent versus continuous energy restriction for weight loss on diet quality and eating behavior: a randomized trial. *Eur J Clin Nutr*. 2019;73(7):1006-1014. doi:10.1038/s41430-018-0370-0

90. Steger FL, Donnelly JE, Hull HR, Li X, Hu J, Sullivan DK. Intermittent and continuous energy restriction result in similar weight loss, weight loss maintenance, and body composition changes in a 6 month randomized pilot study. *Clin Obes*. 2021;11(2):e12430. doi:10.1111/cob.12430

91. Pannen ST, Maldonado SG, Nonnenmacher T, et al. Adherence and dietary composition during intermittent vs. continuous calorie restriction: follow-up data from a randomized controlled trial in adults with overweight or obesity. *Nutrients*. 2021;13(4):1195. doi:10.3390/nu13041195

92. Chaix A, Manoogian ENC, Melkani GC, Panda S. Time-restricted eating to prevent and manage chronic metabolic diseases. *Annu Rev Nutr*. 2019;39:291-315. doi:10.1146/annurev-nutr-082018-124320

93. O'Connor SG, Boyd P, Bailey CP, et al. Perspective: time-restricted eating compared with caloric restriction: potential facilitators and barriers of long-term weight loss maintenance. *Adv Nutr*. 2021;12(2):325-333. doi:10.1093/advances/nmaa168

94. Lowe DA, Wu N, Rohdin-Bibby L, et al. Effects of time-restricted eating on weight loss and other metabolic parameters in women and men with overweight and obesity: the TREAT randomized clinical trial. *JAMA Intern Med*. 2020;180(11):1491-1499. doi:10.1001/jamainternmed.2020.4153

95. Hutchison AT, Regmi P, Manoogian ENC, et al. Time-restricted feeding improves glucose tolerance in men at risk for type 2 diabetes: a randomized crossover trial. *Obesity (Silver Spring)*. 2019;27(5):724-732. doi:10.1002/oby.22449

96. Anton SD, Lee SA, Donahoo WT, et al. The effects of time restricted feeding on overweight, older adults: a pilot study. *Nutrients*. 2019;11(7):1500. doi:10.3390/nu11071500

97. Wilkinson MJ, Manoogian ENC, Zadourian A, et al. Ten-hour time-restricted eating reduces weight, blood pressure, and atherogenic lipids in patients with metabolic syndrome. *Cell Metab*. 2020;31(1):92-104.e5. doi:10.1016/j.cmet.2019.11.004

98. Chen JH, Lu LW, Ge Q, et al. Missing puzzle pieces of time-restricted-eating (TRE) as a long-term weight-loss strategy in overweight and obese people? A systematic review and meta-analysis of randomized controlled trials. *Crit Rev Food Sci Nutr*. Published online September 23, 2021. doi:10.1080/10408398.2021.1974335

99. Liu D, Huang Y, Huang C, et al. Calorie restriction with or without time-restricted eating in weight loss. *N Engl J Med*. 2022;386(16):1495-1504. doi:10.1056/NEJMoa2114833

100. Spadine M, Patterson M. Social influence on fad diet use: a systematic literature review. *Nutr Health*. 2022;28(3):369-388. doi:10.1177/02601060211072370

101. Gibson AA, Sainsbury A. Strategies to improve adherence to dietary weight loss interventions in research and real-world settings. *Behav Sci (Basel)*. 2017;7(3):44. doi:10.3390/bs7030044

102. Chao AM, Quigley KM, Wadden TA. Dietary interventions for obesity: clinical and mechanistic findings. *J Clin Invest*. 2021;131(1):e140065. doi:10.1172/JCI140065

103. Koliaki C, Spinos T, Spinou M, Brinia ME, Mitsopoulou D, Katsilambros N. Defining the optimal dietary approach for safe, effective and sustainable weight loss in overweight and obese adults. *Healthcare (Basel)*. 2018;6(3):73. doi:10.3390/healthcare6030073

CHAPTER 12

Physical Activity Interventions

Brenda Davy, PhD, RDN
Kristen Howard, MSN, ARNP, CBN
Kevin P. Davy, PhD

CHAPTER OBJECTIVES

- Contrast the roles of physical activity in weight-gain prevention, weight loss, weight maintenance, and cardiometabolic health.
- Delineate approaches to physical activity for patients or clients with overweight or obesity.
- Discuss practice points to consider when personalizing physical activity interventions.
- List physical activity resources for health professionals.

Introduction

Regular engagement in physical activity is recommended by both national and international guidelines for weight loss, maintenance of weight loss, and prevention of weight gain. The second edition of the *Physical Activity Guidelines for Americans*[1] and the *WHO Guidelines on Physical Activity and Sedentary Behaviour*[2] recommend reducing sedentary time and engaging in muscle strengthening activity at least 2 days per week for additional weight management and health benefits. Although the importance of *physical activity* and *exercise* (which are defined in the next section) for inducing weight loss has been debated, systematic reviews and meta-analyses have concluded that regular physical activity or exercise participation produces modest weight loss (1–3 kg) when used as a singular strategy[3-6] or in combination with a hypocaloric diet,[3,5,7] including after bariatric surgery.[8] Regular engagement in physical activity and exercise is generally associated with successful long-term maintenance of weight loss,[9-12] although uncertainties exist in findings from randomized controlled trials, likely because of suboptimal adherence to physical activity in these trials.[5,11] Physical activity, either alone or as part of a multicomponent lifestyle intervention, is effective for preventing weight gain (ie, maintaining a stable weight over time, which is distinct from weight loss maintenance, which refers to maintaining a weight loss following a weight loss intervention), particularly among individuals with normal body weight or who are overweight,[6] and when a specific exercise prescription is provided (one that includes targets or goals).[13,14]

This chapter addresses the benefits of engaging in physical activity and reducing sedentary behavior for weight management, body composition, and cardiometabolic health; it presents the current physical activity guidelines for weight-gain prevention, weight loss, and weight loss maintenance (summarized in Box 12.1 on page 196[2,6,15-17]); and it discusses the effectiveness of different physical activity approaches, including reducing sedentary behavior, for weight management. Lastly, practical applications for health professionals to consider when prescribing physical activity and exercise to patients are included.

BOX 12.1

Guidelines and Position Stands: Physical Activity, Exercise, and Weight Management[1,2,6,15-17]

Physical Activity Guidelines for Americans (2018)[1]

Weight-gain prevention
Achieve 150 to 300 min/wk moderate-intensity[a] aerobic activity or 75 to 150 min/wk vigorous-intensity[b] aerobic activity. Achieve minimum recommendations, but 300 or more minutes per week of moderate-intensity aerobic activity may be needed to prevent weight gain.

Engage in muscle-strengthening activity[c] involving all major muscle groups 2 or more days per week.

Reduce sedentary time.

Weight loss
Achieve 150 to 300 min/wk moderate-intensity aerobic activity or 75 to 150 min/wk vigorous-intensity aerobic activity. Achieve minimum recommendations, but 300 or more minutes per week of wk moderate-intensity aerobic activity may be needed for weight loss of greater than 5% body weight.

Engage in muscle-strengthening activity involving all major muscle groups 2 or more days per week.

Reduce sedentary time.

Weight loss maintenance
Achieve 150 to 300 min/wk moderate-intensity aerobic activity or 75 to 150 min/wk vigorous-intensity aerobic activity. Achieve minimum recommendations, but 300 or more minutes per week of moderate-intensity aerobic activity may be needed to maintain weight loss.

Engage in muscle-strengthening activity involving all major muscle groups 2 or more days per week.

Reduce sedentary time.

Academy of Nutrition and Dietetics Adult Weight Management Guideline (2014)[15]

Weight-gain prevention
Not addressed

Weight loss
Achieve 150 to 420 min/wk or more of physical activity, depending on intensity.

Weight loss maintenance
Achieve 200 to 300 min/wk or more of physical activity, depending on intensity.

2013 AHA/ACC/TOS Guideline for the Management of Overweight and Obesity in Adults (2014)[16]

Weight-gain prevention
Not addressed

Weight loss
Increase aerobic activity to more than 150 min/wk (30 min/d, most days of the week).

Weight loss maintenance
Achieve 200 to 300 min/wk aerobic activity.

Box continues

BOX 12.1 (CONTINUED)

American College of Sports Medicine Position Stand: Appropriate Physical Activity Intervention Strategies for Weight Loss and Prevention of Weight Regain for Adults (2009)[17]

Weight-gain prevention	Achieve 150 to 250 min/wk moderate-intensity physical activity.
Weight loss	Achieve 150 to 250 min/wk moderate-intensity physical activity for modest weight loss and more than 250 min/wk for clinically significant weight loss.
Weight loss maintenance	Achieve more than 250 min/wk moderate-intensity physical activity.

European Association for the Study of Obesity Physical Activity Working Group recommendations (2021)[6]

Weight-gain prevention	Not addressed
Weight loss	Achieve 150 to 200 min/wk aerobic exercise of at least moderate intensity. Engage in supervised high-intensity interval training (HIIT)[d] after a thorough assessment of cardiovascular risk. Engage in resistance training at moderate-to-high intensity (60% of the one-repetition maximum) to preserve lean mass during weight loss.
Weight loss maintenance	Achieve 200 to 300 min/wk moderate-intensity aerobic exercise.

World Health Organization Guidelines on Physical Activity and Sedentary Behaviour (2020)[2]

Weight-gain prevention	Achieve at least 150 to 300 min/wk moderate-intensity aerobic activity or at least 75 to 150 min/wk vigorous-intensity aerobic activity.
	Increase aerobic activity to more than 300 min/wk moderate-intensity activity or more than 150 min/wk vigorous activity for additional health benefits.
	Engage in muscle-strengthening activities of moderate or higher intensity that involve all major muscle groups 2 or more days per week.
	Limit sedentary time. Replace sedentary time with physical activity of any intensity.
Weight loss	Recommendations only address adiposity in general.[e]
Weight loss maintenance	Recommendations only address adiposity in general.[e]

[a] Moderate-intensity aerobic activity is aerobic activity that uses 3.0 to 5.9 metabolic equivalents (METs; 1 MET=energy expended at rest). Examples include brisk walking and doubles tennis.
[b] Vigorous-intensity aerobic activity is aerobic activity that uses 6.0 or more METs. Examples include running, jogging, or a strenuous fitness class.
[c] Examples of muscle-strengthening activity include resistance training, weight lifting, training with elastic bands, and calisthenics such as push-ups.
[d] HIIT consists of short periods (ie, <1 min) of high-intensity anaerobic exercise alternated with short periods of recovery.
[e] Recommendations are associated with health benefits; measures of adiposity "may also improve." Adiposity includes all weight outcomes: weight gain, weight change, weight control, weight stability, weight status, and weight maintenance.

Defining Physical Activity, Exercise, and Sedentary Behavior

The term *exercise* refers to planned, structured physical activity that is undertaken to promote health or fitness, whereas *physical activity* denotes "any bodily movement produced by the contraction of skeletal muscle that increases energy expenditure" above resting levels,[1] including participation in household activities, such as gardening, and occupational and leisure activities, such as walking. *Sedentary behavior* is defined as "any waking behavior characterized by a low level of energy expenditure (less than or equal to 1.5 METs [metabolic equivalents; rest = .0 MET]) while sitting, reclining, or lying."[1]

Benefits of Physical Activity for Weight-Gain Prevention, Weight Loss, and Weight Loss Maintenance

Strong evidence links exercise and physical activity with numerous cardiometabolic benefits,[6] although the role of exercise and physical activity in weight management, particularly for weight loss, has been questioned.[18] Exercise alone is effective for preventing weight gain[13] and as a strategy for weight loss, albeit with modest reductions in body weight and body fat.[3-6] Interventions that combine exercise and diet produce greater long-term weight loss (ie, 12 months) than diet-only interventions.[7] Engaging in 250 minutes or more per week of moderate-intensity physical activity or exercise is associated with successful maintenance of weight loss.[6] The limited weight loss induced by exercise suggests that some behavioral or metabolic compensation may occur to limit the degree of negative energy balance produced by exercise. Yet collectively, the effectiveness of exercise as a weight-management strategy suggests that exercise may improve energy intake regulation or increase daily energy expenditure, or both. This section reviews these areas, as well as the benefits of engaging in physical activity and reducing sedentary behaviors on body composition and cardiometabolic health.

Improved Appetite Control and Regulation of Energy Intake

Relative energy intake is reduced for 24 hours after an acute bout of exercise, and this effect is not moderated by BMI or exercise mode.[19] Over a period of several days (eg, 2–14 days), regular exercise may produce a short-term energy deficit, as energy intake is not increased to match the energy expended in exercise.[20,21] Among adults with overweight or obesity who begin regular exercise training, neither daily hunger nor energy intake is generally reported to increase compared to their baseline pretraining state or nonexercising controls.[6,21] Although individual responses may vary, the effect of exercise on energy intake does not appear to differ by sex, exercise dose, or training duration.[19-21] The impact of exercise intensity, timing, and training mode (eg, aerobic, resistance, or high-intensity interval training [HIIT]) on appetite control in individuals with overweight and obesity is not yet clear,[6,21] although some research suggests that morning exercise may be more effective at reducing energy intake than exercise later in the day.[22]

Exercise training may affect the regulation of energy intake in adults with overweight or obesity in several ways. Regular exercisers who meet or exceed current physical activity recommendations can better match their daily energy intake to their energy expenditure than insufficiently active individuals, and this could promote weight stability over time.[23] Exercise training increases dietary restraint and decreases disinhibition or uncontrolled eating in individuals with overweight or obesity, an effect that is possibly related to reduced neural activation to food cues.[20] Compared to sedentary individuals, active individuals report a lower overall liking for foods (ie, regardless of a food's fat or sugar content) and a lower liking for high-fat, energy-dense sweet and savory foods.[24] Thus, regular exercise may have a favorable impact on food preference and food reward systems. Importantly, adults with overweight or obesity who participate in exercise training demonstrate a reduced susceptibility to overconsumption.[6]

In addition to the beneficial effects of exercise on hedonic systems that regulate appetite and energy intake, physiological systems such as the gastrointestinal (GI) tract are affected. High-intensity exercise acutely reduces the gastric emptying rate,[25] which in turn may affect GI-derived appetite hormones. Exercise acutely reduces the orexigenic hormone ghrelin and increases the anorexigenic hormones peptide YY, glucagon-like peptide 1, and pancreatic polypeptide[26]; longer-term effects are uncertain. These potential benefits of regular exercise on hedonic and homeostatic energy-intake regulation systems may support behavioral change strategies aimed at facilitating weight management.[27]

Existing research shows that regular exercise helps to control appetite and regulate energy intake for weight-gain prevention, weight loss, and weight loss maintenance, although there is considerable variability among individuals. In an environment where energy-dense foods are readily available and the need to expend energy is low, daily physical activity that includes planned, structured exercise may allow individuals to maintain a higher state of energy flux, whereby intake is more accurately matched with expenditure.[28]

Increasing Energy Expenditure

The impact of physical activity on total daily energy expenditure (TDEE) is a complex and unsettled matter. TDEE consists of three main components: resting energy expenditure (REE, also called basal energy expenditure or basal metabolic rate), the thermic effect of food (TEF), and physical activity energy expenditure (PAEE). REE reflects the energy required to maintain vital organ function at rest and is determined primarily by fat-free mass. TEF is the energy required for digestion, absorption, and assimilation of nutrients after a meal. PAEE, the most variable component, is the energy expended with all physical activity and encompasses exercise as well as nonexercise activity thermogenesis such as fidgeting. How and under what circumstances physical activity increases TDEE is not entirely clear, but multiple models have been proposed. A more complete understanding of this issue is needed to determine the impact of prescribing exercise and physical activity for weight management.

Much of the confusion regarding the impact of physical activity on weight loss assumes that REE and PAEE are independent and not correlated. The *additive model* predicts that any increase in PAEE results in an equivalent increase in TDEE. In contrast, the *performance model* predicts that an increase in TDEE with physical activity will be greater than just the increase in PAEE because of the additional cost of recovery and maintenance associated with the support of this greater "metabolic machinery."[29] However, there may be a compensatory reduction in other components of TDEE in response to an increase in physical activity. That is, the *constrained model* proposes that energy expenditure is "constrained" and that an increase in physical activity is accompanied by behavioral or metabolic compensation; thus, the increase in TDEE is smaller than predicted by the energy cost of physical activity. Figure 12.1 compares the additive, performance, and constrained models of energy expenditure.[29,30] Figure 12.2 displays energy balance predictions in the additive vs constrained models.

Recent research utilizing doubly labeled water[29] supports the constrained model. On average, higher physical activity was accompanied by a reduction of REE amounting to 28% of the increased energy expended in physical activity. This compensation was as high as 50% among individuals with obesity. Both increases in energy intake[31,32] and reductions in energy expenditure associated with nonstructured physical activity have been reported following exercise interventions.[33-35] Interestingly, the results of a study of middle-aged and older adults published in 2022 suggested that during negative energy balance the constrained model was supported, whereas in positive energy balance the additive model was supported.[36] The latter observation may have important implications for understanding the impact of physical activity on the prevention of weight gain.

Benefits of Physical Activity on Body Composition, Cardiometabolic Health, Fitness, and Well-Being

Improvements in Body Composition and Regional Fat Distribution

Exercise training is an efficacious strategy for reducing total body and visceral fat in individuals with obesity.[5] In addition, reductions in liver and skeletal-muscle fat have been observed.[37,38] The latter could translate into clinically significant reductions in cardiometabolic disease risk, given the deleterious impact of these depots on cardiometabolic health.[39] The magnitude of reduction in visceral fat appears to be influenced largely by the amount of total-body fat mass that is lost.[40] In addition, total-body and visceral fat mass change in parallel, independent of the weight loss method (eg, diet, exercise, bariatric surgery). However, exercise may reduce visceral fat more than pharmacological[41,42] or diet-induced[43] weight loss interventions do, with similar amounts of total fat loss. Importantly, increasing the intensity or volume of exercise may be a means for increasing the number of individuals who achieve a clinically meaningful reduction in visceral fat.[43]

Evidence linking sedentary time with adiposity and weight status is limited, and it is not clear if associations between sedentary time and adiposity are modified by the level of moderate or vigorous physical activity.[2] However, sedentary behavior is associated with increased risk of cardiovascular disease and other health outcomes (eg, cancer), and this risk is mitigated with higher levels of moderate and vigorous physical activity.[2]

Cardiometabolic and Other Health Benefits

Blood Pressure

Elevated blood pressure (BP), defined as systolic blood pressure greater than 120 mm Hg and/or diastolic blood pressure greater than 80 mm Hg, is a major risk factor for cardiovascular disease (CVD) morbidity and mortality.[44,45] The association between obesity and hypertension is well documented, and although not all individuals with obesity have hypertension, weight gain is invariably associated with increased BP.[46] Though weight loss plays a critical role in the management of hypertension and the accompanying target organ damage associated with obesity, exercise independent of weight loss is an effective means for lowering BP.[47]

The incidence of elevated BP is lowest in lean, physically active people and highest in sedentary people with obesity.[48] The risk of developing hypertension

FIGURE 12.1 Comparative models of energy expenditure[29,30]

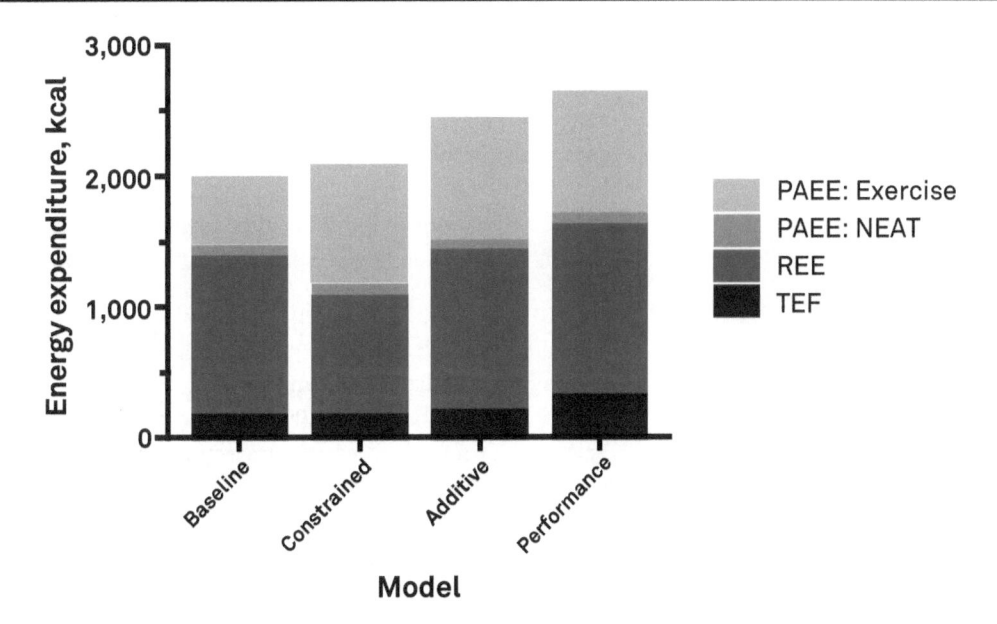

Abbreviations: PAEE, physical activity energy expenditure; NEAT, non-exercise thermogenesis; REE, resting energy expenditure; TEF, thermic effect of food.

The constrained model predicts that as energy expended in physical activity increases, total energy expenditure rises to a lesser degree. This is explained by compensation shown here resulting from a decrease in resting energy expenditure. In contrast, the additive model predicts no compensation and an increase in total energy expenditure equivalent to the additional kilocalories expended in physical activity. The performance model predicts an increase in both resting energy expenditure and physical activity energy expenditure as a result of increased physical activity.

FIGURE 12.2 Energy balance predictions in constrained vs additive models of energy expenditure

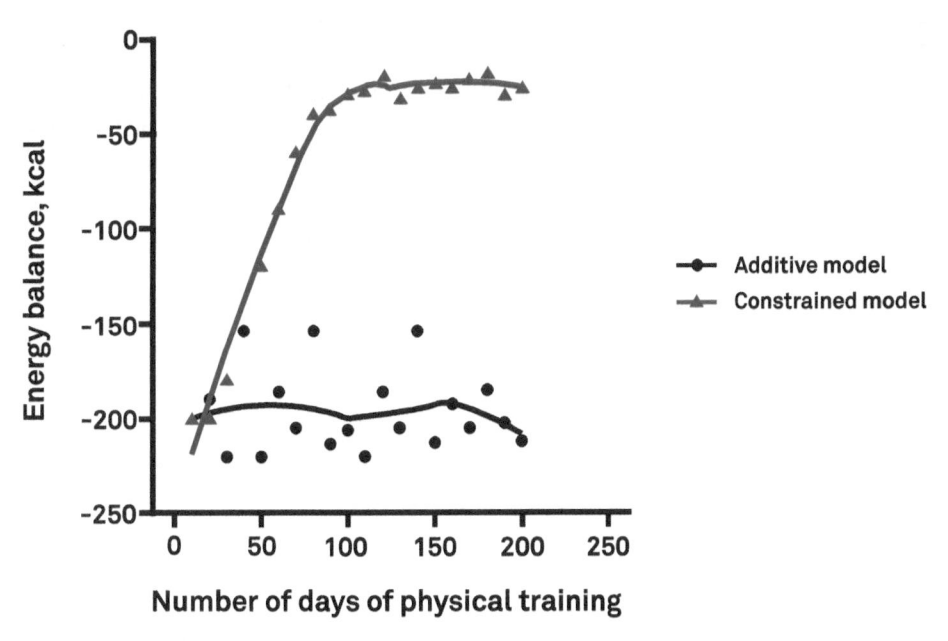

The additive model of energy expenditure predicts a constant negative energy balance following increased physical activity assuming the elevated physical activity remains constant and there is no change in dietary intake. The constrained model predicts an energy deficit that is constrained within limits due to a compensatory decrease in resting energy expenditure.

CHAPTER 12: Physical Activity Interventions

is reduced in physically active individuals compared with sedentary individuals. In addition, physical activity reduces the risk of hypertension with weight gain. As such, regular aerobic exercise is recommended for patients with elevated BP.[49] Meta-analyses indicate that regular aerobic exercise produces clinically significant reductions in systolic and diastolic BP; the effect is largest in those with hypertension.[50] Importantly, the systolic BP–lowering effect of exercise appears similar to some commonly used antihypertensive medications.[51] Resistance exercise may also be effective for lowering BP.[52] The reduction in BP with regular exercise appears to be independent of baseline adiposity and changes in body composition[53,54]; the impact of reduction in visceral fat on BP is less clear.

Lipid and Lipoprotein Concentrations

Dyslipidemia, particularly an elevated level of low-density lipoprotein (LDL) cholesterol, has been causally linked to the development of atherosclerosis.[55,56] Perhaps the most successful strategy in the prevention and treatment of CVD has been through the use of statins.[55] However, CVD remains the leading cause of death in the United States, and substantial residual risk attributable to lipid and lipoprotein concentrations remains.[57] Obesity is associated with an adverse lipid and lipoprotein profile. Elevated levels of small, dense LDL particles (and apolipoprotein B) and triglycerides and reduced levels of high-density lipoprotein (HDL) cholesterol occur more frequently in patients with an accumulation of abdominal visceral fat.[58] Weight loss, regardless of the mode used to achieve it, is associated with reductions in most lipid and lipoprotein levels with the exception of HDL cholesterol,[59] but diet composition can have a profound impact on the direction and magnitude of change in lipid and lipoprotein concentrations.[60] A high intake of saturated fatty acids and dietary fiber are associated with increases and decreases in LDL concentrations, respectively.[61,62]

Regular aerobic exercise has a positive impact on fasting lipid and lipoprotein concentrations, independent of weight loss.[63] The effect of exercise on levels of lipoprotein subclasses is beyond the scope of this chapter but, in general, exercise reduces triglyceride concentrations and results in a distribution of LDL and HDL particles toward larger species.[64] Importantly, exercise reduces the number of more atherogenic, small, dense LDL particles. Reductions in total body fat, and particularly visceral fat, with exercise training are associated with more favorable changes in lipid and lipoprotein levels than is exercise without changes in body composition and regional fat distribution.[63]

Insulin Resistance and Type 2 Diabetes

Impaired insulin-stimulated glucose disposal (ie, insulin resistance) is common in individuals with obesity,[65] particularly those with abdominal obesity.[66] Obesity and insulin resistance are associated with a high risk of developing type 2 diabetes, as well as CVD.[67] Skeletal-muscle insulin resistance has been implicated as a key defect in the development of type 2 diabetes.[68] Fortunately, insulin resistance in skeletal muscle can be improved even after a single bout of exercise.[69,70] However, repeated bouts are needed to ensure durability of the effect. Exercise training improves insulin sensitivity in individuals with obesity with and without type 2 diabetes.[71] Exercise does not have to be prolonged or of high intensity to favorably affect insulin sensitivity,[72] although recent findings suggest that low-volume HIIT improved insulin sensitivity in individuals with obesity.[73] Importantly, daily exercise does not have to be completed in a single session (eg, 30 minutes) to improve insulin sensitivity but can be accumulated throughout the day.[74]

There is a strong inverse relationship between physical activity and type 2 diabetes, although this may be mediated, in part, by reduced adiposity.[75,76] Most types of physical activity that have been studied, including leisure-time activity, walking, low-intensity activity, moderate-intensity activity, high-intensity activity, and occupational activity, are associated with reductions in the risk of developing type 2 diabetes. Sedentary behavior (eg, sitting time, time spent watching television, total time sedentary) is associated with increased risk for type 2 diabetes.[2] Some evidence suggests that larger reductions in risk can be achieved with lower levels of leisure time and higher levels of vigorous physical activity, thus interventions targeting individuals with low levels of physical activity may be particularly important from a public health viewpoint.[75,76]

Cardiorespiratory Fitness and Muscular Strength

Cardiorespiratory fitness and muscular strength are well-defined health-related components of physical fitness. Cardiorespiratory fitness is a sensitive measure of physical activity and is defined as the maximal ability of the cardiovascular and respiratory systems to supply exercising skeletal muscle with oxygen during large-muscle, dynamic exercise. Low cardiorespiratory fitness is as strong an independent risk factor for all-cause mortality as are type 2 diabetes, hypertension, smoking, and dyslipidemia.[77] While the relative contribution of cardiorespiratory fitness and adiposity to mortality risk continue to be debated, it is important to emphasize that the association between cardiorespiratory fitness and mortality is independent of BMI.[78] As such, moderate-to-vigorous physical activity should be encouraged in all individuals, regardless of BMI and weight loss goals. Importantly, the availability of valid and reliable tools for estimating cardiorespiratory fitness provide a cost-effective substitute for monitoring this important health metric without the need for the expensive equipment required for measurement in laboratory settings.[79]

Muscular strength is another health-related component of physical fitness and is defined as the maximal force that a muscle or muscle group can generate. Muscular strength is inversely associated with incidence of type 2 diabetes, as well as CVD, cancers, and all-cause mortality risk in healthy individuals and those with chronic diseases, including obesity.[80,81] Resistance exercise is particularly effective for increasing muscle strength and mass.[82] The latter may be particularly important in the setting of sarcopenic obesity, the age-related loss of skeletal muscle mass in the presence of obesity in older adults.[83] In addition, resistance exercise may be effective in minimizing the loss of muscle mass with weight loss in individuals with obesity.[84] As such, resistance exercise should be recommended for all patients with obesity unless otherwise contraindicated.

Mental Health and Quality of Life

Obesity is associated not only with an increased risk of poor physical health but also with poor mental health. Individuals with obesity are susceptible to weight bias, stigma, and discrimination.[85,86] The internalization of weight bias may be, at least indirectly, associated with physical inactivity and weight gain.[87,88] Physical activity is associated with reduced risk of anxiety[89] and depression[90] and with improved sleep and health-related quality of life[91,92] in adults. Regular exercise has been reported to reduce anxiety symptoms in healthy individuals and in those with chronic disease.[93] Regular aerobic exercise improves depressive symptoms, as a singular therapy or as an adjuvant or combination therapy.[94] However, a systematic review and meta-analysis published in 2021 concluded that regular exercise did not consistently reduce depression or anxiety in individuals with overweight or obesity.[95] Whether the internalization of weight stigma and weight bias moderates the impact of exercise on these outcomes is unclear. However, regular aerobic exercise improves quality of life in healthy individuals and among those with chronic diseases,[96] including overweight and obesity.[95]

Current Physical Activity Guidelines

Recommendations and guidelines related to physical activity and weight management are provided in Box 12.1.[1,2,6,15-17] For the prevention of weight gain, 150 minutes per week or more of moderate-intensity aerobic activity (eg, brisk walking) is recommended, along with muscle-strengthening activity two or more times per week. This weekly volume and intensity of aerobic activity is also recommended for weight loss. Higher volumes of aerobic activity (200–250 minutes or more per week) are generally recommended for maintaining weight loss.

Experts recommend reducing sedentary behavior (eg, sitting time) for preventing weight gain, weight loss, and maintaining weight loss in the *Physical Activity Guidelines for Americans*,[1] but it is not specifically addressed in other guidelines for weight management. WHO recommends limiting sedentary time and replacing sedentary time with physical activity of any intensity. Currently, however, there is insufficient evidence of associations between sedentary behaviors and adiposity or weight status; additional research is needed. It is also uncertain how these relationships may vary with moderate and vigorous physical activity.[2] Evidence is not yet available to support time-based recommendations for sedentary behavior or the frequency and duration of breaks in sedentary behavior. This has been identified as an area in need of additional research.[2,6] People who successfully maintain weight loss report spending less time sitting (approximately 3 hours less per day) than weight-stable individuals with obesity,[97] but experts do not know if reducing sitting time is an effective strategy for weight loss or the maintenance of weight loss maintenance.[6]

There is inadequate research to support guidelines related to exercise timing and weight management,[6] although consistent timing (particularly morning exercise) is suggested as a strategy for promoting exercise adherence through habit formation and improved self-regulation.[19] According to recommendations made by the European Association for the Study of Obesity, the effectiveness of HIIT as a weight loss strategy is comparable to that of aerobic activity, but more research is needed to address its feasibility and acceptability in individuals with overweight or obesity.[6]

Physical Activity Approaches for Weight-Gain Prevention, Weight Loss, and Weight Loss Maintenance

Box 12.2 on page 206 summarizes the effectiveness of various physical activity approaches for weight management among individuals with overweight or obesity.[4,5,12,13,97-102]

Weight-Gain Prevention

It is unclear whether targeting sedentary behavior alone (ie, without also targeting an increase in physical activity) can prevent weight gain or promote weight loss.[2,12] Aerobic exercise (at a level of 2,000 kcal expended per week) prevents long-term weight gain in women† in the absence of other lifestyle changes.[13] Prescriptive programs—that is, programs conducted in controlled settings (eg, gym, classes,

---

† Study participants were described as women. Gender was not further specified.

research facilities) or that provide specific energy-expenditure targets, or both—are substantially more effective in preventing weight gain than nonprescriptive programs (a weight change of −0.8 kg vs 1.6 kg, respectively).[14] Though research is limited, practicing yoga may prevent weight gain.[103,104]

Weight Loss and Maintenance

Compared to no change in activity level, participating in moderate-intensity aerobic exercise (eg, brisk walking, jogging, or cycling over a period of more than 12 weeks) without other lifestyle interventions leads to modest weight loss (1.6–2.0 kg).[4,99,100] Greater weight losses may occur with moderate-intensity exercise in men compared to women.[†,99] Longer duration of participation (eg, 6–12 months) does not appear to increase the magnitude of weight loss.[4] A comparison of aerobic vs resistance vs combined (aerobic plus resistance) training programs for weight loss ranked combined programs as the most effective, followed by aerobic training alone. Higher-intensity programs were more effective than low-to-moderate-intensity programs.[3,98] Although resistance training may not be effective for weight loss,[98,100] it is effective for preserving lean body mass during weight loss efforts[5,6] and for improving body composition.[100]

Among patients with overweight and obesity, continuous moderate-intensity exercise produces greater weight loss than HIIT does, unless the energy expended within sessions is matched. When isocaloric, HIIT may lead to slightly greater weight loss (−0.41 kg) than continuous moderate-intensity exercise.[5,101] Protocols using running (vs cycling) and employing higher exercise intensities (achieving greater than 90% peak heart rate) result in a greater loss of body fat than do cycling or lower-intensity protocols.[105] The efficiency and safety of isocaloric HIIT and moderate-intensity continuous exercise appear to be similar; thus, individual preference and enjoyment of physical activity should be considered when prescribing HIIT or continuous exercise.[101]

Few controlled trials have examined yoga as a singular or adjunct component to behavioral interventions for weight management.[106] Depending on the style practiced, yoga could be considered light or moderate physical activity, or a muscle-strengthening activity.[1] A randomized trial compared two forms of yoga (Vinyasa vs Hatha; 5 d/wk) as part of a standard 6-month behavioral weight loss intervention.[107] Session duration progressed from 20 to 60 minutes over the course of the study. Participants completed an average of 2.5 to 3 yoga sessions per week, with each session lasting an average of 30 to 35 minutes. Mean weight loss at 6 months was approximately 3.6 kg, which did not differ by yoga form. Long session duration (ie, 60 minutes) was cited as a barrier to participation, but a majority of participants reported that they planned to continue yoga after the study. In another study, reductions in body weight were similar (approximately 2–3 kg) following an 8-week intervention in which women† were randomly assigned to either a hypocaloric diet or to yoga (5 d/wk, 60 min/session) with a less energy-restricted diet.[108] A study of Asian Indian adults with obesity found that those who practiced yoga reported a higher quality of life, greater physical activity enjoyment, and better self-esteem compared to those who did not practice yoga.[109]

For long-term weight loss (12–18 months), behavioral weight-management programs that combine diet and physical activity approaches are more effective than those that focus on a single component (ie, diet only or physical activity only).[7] However, weight loss in response to exercise varies widely among individuals.[5] To successfully maintain long-term weight loss, patients need to sustain high levels of weekly moderate-to-vigorous physical activity (refer to Box 12.1).[6,9]

Working With Patients

Prescribing Exercise and Physical Activity

After assessing a patient's usual physical activity level (refer to Chapter 8) and comparing the results to existing recommendations, the practitioner can then develop an exercise or physical activity prescription based on the patient's weight-management goal. Physical activity guidelines for weight-gain prevention, weight loss, and weight loss maintenance are provided in Box 12.1. The recommended minimum amount of physical activity per week for weight-gain prevention or modest weight loss (ie, 1–3 kg) is 150 minutes of moderate-intensity aerobic activity (eg, brisk walking) or 75 minutes of vigorous-intensity activity (eg, jogging). If patients desire a more substantial weight loss, higher levels of physical activity (250–300 minutes or more of moderate-intensity activity) may be needed. This increase in activity may also be needed for successful weight loss maintenance. For all weight-management goals, reducing sedentary time and engaging in muscle strengthening activity, such as resistance training, 2 days or more per week are recommended. A physical activity prescription may include replacing sedentary time (eg, time spent sitting) with physical activity of any intensity, including light-intensity activity.[1,2] There is insufficient evidence to support a specific recommendation for the timing, frequency, or duration of breaks in sedentary time.[2]

A prescription that includes both aerobic activity and resistance training is more effective for promoting weight loss than one that includes aerobic activity or resistance training alone.[6,98] Both continuous physical activity (ie, a single bout) and intermittent physical activity consisting of multiple short bouts (more than 10 minutes per bout) are effective in promoting weight loss, provided the minimum weekly goal of 150 minutes is achieved (refer to Box 12.2).[102] Depending on patient preference, a prescription for high-intensity exercise (eg, HIIT) may be appropriate, but the total energy expended by the patient should be comparable to that expended in continuous exercise.[5,101] The timing of exercise-program initiation (ie, at the onset of a combined diet and exercise intervention or following a period of dietary intervention alone) can also be determined by patient preference.[110] An exercise prescription can incorporate patient-specific strategies that support success, such as a clear and structured physical activity plan, a regular physical activity schedule, personalized physical activity goals, and the use of self-monitoring tools.[111] A plan that includes consistent morning exercise sessions may facilitate habit formation, simplify daily planning, and lead to greater weight loss.[19,112]

BOX 12.2

Physical Activity Approaches for Weight Management in Individuals With Overweight or Obesity[4,5,12,13,97-102]

Reducing sedentary time

Weight-gain prevention	Uncertain[12]
Weight loss	Uncertain[12]
Weight loss maintenance	Not addressed

BOX 12.2 (CONTINUED)

Aerobic exercise

Weight-gain prevention	Moderate-intensity aerobic exercise (expending 2,000 kcal/wk for 16 months) prevents weight gain in women.[13]
Weight loss	Moderate-intensity aerobic exercise (for >12 weeks) alone reduces body weight by approximately 1 to 2 kg.[4,98,99]
Weight loss maintenance	Moderate-intensity aerobic exercise (>250 min/wk) is associated with successful weight loss maintenance.

Resistance/strength training (RT)

Weight-gain prevention	Not addressed
Weight loss	RT alone may not reduce body weight.[97,100]
Weight loss maintenance	Not addressed

Combined aerobic exercise and RT

Weight-gain prevention	Not addressed
Weight loss	High-intensity combined programs reduce body weight more than low-to-moderate–intensity combined programs; both are superior to aerobic alone and RT alone.[5,98]
Weight loss maintenance	Not addressed

High-intensity interval training (HIIT)

Weight-gain prevention	Not addressed
Weight loss	HIIT (3–4 sessions/wk) can reduce body weight but is not superior to continuous exercise unless energy expended is matched.[5,101]
Weight loss maintenance	Not addressed

Continuous vs accumulated short bouts of exercise

Weight-gain prevention	Not addressed
Weight loss	Accumulated short bouts reduce body weight. Greater effects are seen with a total weekly exercise time of 150 or more per week (bout duration >10 minutes).[102]
Weight loss maintenance	Not addressed

Yoga

Weight-gain prevention	Uncertain
Weight loss	Uncertain
Weight loss maintenance	Uncertain

Health professionals specializing in weight management can provide patients or clients who are in good health with general guidance on physical activity recommendations using credible sources such as the *Physical Activity Guidelines for Americans*[1] and the *WHO Guidelines on Physical Activity and Sedentary Behaviour*.[2] For patients without contraindications,[113] preexercise medical clearance is generally not necessary when prescribing light-intensity and moderate-intensity physical activity (eg, brisk walking).[2] More detailed, individualized physical activity prescriptions can be provided based on the client's health status and the practitioner's knowledge, competence, and scope of practice. The *Physical Activity Toolkit for RDNs* (refer to Box 12.3 on page 210) was collaboratively developed by the American College of Sports Medicine and the Academy of Nutrition and Dietetics. This no-cost tool kit provides details on scope of practice; a link to a scope-of-practice decision algorithm; tips for incorporating physical activity assessment, diagnosis, and intervention in the Nutrition Care Process; and information about referral to qualified exercise professionals when appropriate. For additional physical activity tool kits and patient resources, refer to Box 12.3.

Personalizing Physical Activity Recommendations

Addressing Expectations

Although the benefits of physical activity and exercise for cardiometabolic health and body composition are clear, its role in weight loss has been debated. Exercise-induced increases in energy expenditure may allow individuals to more accurately regulate their energy intake and avoid future weight gain,[13] which is an important achievement in itself. Exercise intervention alone (ie, without energy-intake restriction) may induce a weight loss of 1 to 3 kg,[3,6] which may be far less than what many individuals expect to achieve. Combining increased physical activity with energy restriction may result in a weight loss of approximately 5 to 6 kg, which exceeds typical weight loss through the use of either strategy alone. However, these results may occur over a long period of time: several months to a year or more.[7] Weight-management practitioners should discuss expectations for weight loss with their patients to ensure that their expectations are realistic for the exercise program being prescribed.

Patient Perspectives and Motivation

Patients report that health care providers support their weight-management efforts in several ways.[111] Provider feedback, interest, and support in making lifestyle changes are important external motivators for patients. Discussing provider-defined goals and providing accountability are also beneficial. Practitioners can also acknowledge and address the challenges commonly encountered by patients as they adopt and endeavor to maintain a regular physical activity program, including lack of time, stress, stigma, navigating holidays and major life events, and prioritizing goals.[111]

Patients may vary in their degree of motivation for engaging in physical activity during an intervention. Individuals with a high degree of intrinsic motivation to engage in exercise—for example, those who value its benefits and report enjoying exercise—are more likely to sustain a regular pattern of physical activity over the long term without supervision or external support.[114] Others may benefit from external supports, such as supervised exercise programs or coaching.[113]

Older Adults

The weekly physical activity recommendations for the general adult population also apply to older adults (aged 65 years and older), including the recommendations for muscle strengthening and reducing sedentary time.[1,2] To reduce the risk of falling and to preserve functional capacity, older adults may also include multicomponent activity programs that incorporate balance, strength, gait, and endurance-training components (eg, dancing, yoga, tai chi).[1,2] However, older adults may be managing chronic health conditions that affect their physical capabilities. If older adults cannot achieve recommendations for physical activity because of chronic health conditions, practitioners should encourage them to be as active as possible and reduce their sedentary time.[1,2] When prescribing physical activity to older adults, providers may find that gradual increases in physical activity are helpful for reducing the risk of injury.

Orthopedic Limitations

Individuals with obesity may experience single and widespread joint, knee, and foot pain.[115] Among those with knee and hip osteoarthritis, it is unclear whether high-intensity exercise poses a greater risk for adverse events compared to low-intensity exercise.[116] In this population, weight-management programs that include an exercise component may improve objective and self-reported measures of physical function. Physical activity delays the progression of disability from osteoarthritis, the leading cause of orthopedic-related disability. Walking, cycling, and swimming are joint-friendly options. Cardiorespiratory fitness develops more quickly than joints are able to adapt, so gradually increasing activity is important for patients with joint limitations. Breaking up exercise into two or more small sessions per day may be helpful—for example, beginning with 5 minutes of walking twice daily. Strategies also include parking one's car a distance away from one's destination and progressively increasing this distance to help to incorporate small amounts of exercise into a daily routine. Aerobic activity is important, but resistance, flexibility, and balance exercises are also essential. Finally, safety is an important consideration. Individuals with orthopedic conditions may find that recruiting friends to exercise with or attending group exercise classes can make for a safer exercise experience. Although 150 minutes of moderate-intensity activity per week is the goal, some exercise is better than none.[117]

Physical Activity and Pharmacotherapy

For weight-management interventions that include pharmacotherapy, the addition of an exercise program may increase long-term weight and body-fat loss compared to interventions without an exercise component.[118] A randomized controlled trial placed patients on an 8-week, low-calorie diet and divided them into four groups:

- those who received liraglutide with moderate-to-vigorous exercise
- those who received liraglutide without moderate-to-vigorous exercise
- those who received placebo with exercise
- those who received placebo with usual activity

After 1 year, the liraglutide-plus-exercise group demonstrated the greatest weight and body-fat loss (9.5 kg; 3.9% of body fat) compared to either treatment alone (liraglutide alone, 6.8 kg; exercise alone, 4.1 kg).[118,119] The additive effects of pharmacotherapy and physical training after weight loss surgery remains unexplored.

BOX 12.3

Physical Activity Resources for Health Professionals

Tool kits

Physical Activity Toolkit for RDNs (2021), American College of Sports Medicine and the Academy of Nutrition and Dietetics

Description	Reviews physical activity (PA) guidelines, how to incorporate PA into the Nutrition Care Process, scope of practice, referrals, certifications
	Provides links to client-appropriate exercise handouts for various medical conditions, examples of how to add PA into counseling, case studies
Where to access online	www.exerciseismedicine.org/a-physical-activity-toolkit-for-registered-dietitians-a-collaborative-effort-between-eim-and
	www.eatrightpro.org/practice/dietetics-resources/chronic-disease-sports-wellness-and-behavioral-health/a-physical-activity-toolkit-for-rdns-exercise-is-medicine

Move Your Way campaign, US Department of Health and Human Services

Description	Promotional campaign for the *Physical Activity Guidelines for Americans*
	Includes tools, fact sheets, posters, videos, graphics, sample social media messages, community playbook
	Provides information for consumers, including fact sheets, interactive weekly planner, videos, infographics
	Spanish-language materials available
Where to access online	https://health.gov/our-work/nutrition-physical-activity/move-your-way-community-resources
	https://health.gov/moveyourway#adults

Active People, Healthy Nation initiative, Centers for Disease Control and Prevention

Description	Provides infographics, fact sheets, resource library, sample social media messages, statewide programs
Where to access online	www.cdc.gov/physicalactivity/activepeoplehealthynation

National Center on Health, Physical Activity and Disability (NCHPAD)

Description	Provides tool kits for public health professionals, health care providers, educators, and fitness professionals to help build inclusivity in health and fitness for those living with disabilities
Where to access online	www.nchpad.org

BOX 12.3 (CONTINUED)

Patient resources

SilverSneakers

Description	A health and fitness program for seniors included with many Medicare plans
	Includes online fitness classes
Where to access online	https://tools.silversneakers.com

14 Weeks to a Healthier You, NCHPAD

Description	A personalized health and fitness program for people living with disabilities
Where to access online	www.nchpad.org/14weeks

YMCA: Health, Well-Being and Fitness

Description	Provides group exercise programs, personal training, programs for older adults
	Search for programs by state or region
Where to access online	www.ymca.org/what-we-do/healthy-living/fitness

Cooperative Extension System physical activity programs (vary by state)

Description	Programs offered by cooperative extensions through the states' designated land-grant universities in partnership with the National Institute of Food and Agriculture of the US Department of Agriculture
	Provides statewide physical activity programs, handouts
Where to access online	www.nifa.usda.gov/about-nifa/how-we-work/extension/cooperative-extension-system
	Example from Virginia:
	https://ext.vt.edu/food-health/physical-activity.html

SNAP-Ed physical activity programs, US Department of Agriculture

Description	Provides physical activity programs and resources offered by various states
	Spanish-language materials available
Where to access online	https://snaped.fns.usda.gov/nutrition-education/nutrition-education-materials/physical-activity

There is little evidence in the literature regarding the interaction of obesogenic pharmacologic agents (eg, psychotropics, including antipsychotics and antidepressants; and hypoglycemics, including insulin, sulfonylureas, and meglitinides) and physical activity. However, patients prescribed one or more obesogenic medications who participate in a behavioral intervention that includes physical activity may experience less weight loss than those not prescribed these medications[120,121]; this includes patients who have undergone bariatric surgery.[122]

Physical Activity and Bariatric Surgery

There are no physical activity or exercise guidelines specific to patients who have undergone bariatric surgery; thus, current recommendations are based on those for the general population.[123] Consensus guidelines recommend 30 minutes of exercise daily following bariatric surgery. Individuals with class 3 obesity (BMI >40) might have unique considerations for physical activity prescription, such as orthopedic limitations, limited aerobic capacity, mechanical difficulties, and other comorbidities and psychosocial considerations.

Although physical activity is important for maintaining weight loss in patients in the general population, high-level evidence regarding its role in weight maintenance following bariatric surgery is limited. Observational studies using objective measures have reported an association between postoperative, moderately vigorous physical activity and sedentary behavior and weight loss outcomes following bariatric surgery at 6 and 18 months[124] and at 3 years.[125] Behavioral interventions initiated preoperatively to increase physical activity may increase moderately vigorous physical activity postoperatively,[126,127] but evidence from objective data and long-term follow-up are limited. Preoperative exercise training may mitigate surgical risk associated with venous thromboembolism and cardiorespiratory capacity[128] and can improve short-term and long-term fitness postoperatively.[129] Nonetheless, evidence to confirm that presurgery exercise training results in improved weight loss outcomes is lacking.[129] In contrast, postoperative exercise training for more than 1 year after bariatric surgery may increase weight loss.[8] Those who undergo exercise training after bariatric surgery demonstrate greater reductions in body weight and fat mass but no differences in fat-free mass, compared to nonexercise controls.[126] Moreover, postoperative exercise training improves cardiorespiratory fitness and reduces insulin resistance following weight loss in this population.[130,131]

Loss of fat-free mass is significant postoperatively, and loss of lean mass is a potential mechanism for metabolic adaptation after weight loss surgery. Resistance training can minimize loss of lean mass and bone mass in this population.[132,133] Exercise intervention can also reverse loss of fat-free mass after gastric bypass surgery.[134] The extent to which resistance training interacts with protein-intake adequacy to preserve bone and muscle mass following weight loss surgery (a postsurgery concern) is not clear.[135]

Physical Activity Resources for Health Professionals

A variety of freely accessible tool kits and resources for physical activity are available for health professionals and patients; they are listed in Box 12.3. Several organizations and agencies, including the American College of Sports Medicine, the Academy of Nutrition and Dietetics, the US Department of Health and Human Services, the Centers for Disease Control and Prevention, and the National Center on Health, Physical Activity and Disability, provide infographics, fact sheets, and tool kits for health professionals and patients. Information about exercise programs available to patients, such as SilverSneakers and the YMCA, is also included in Box 12.3.

Summary

A large body of evidence links engagement in exercise and physical activity with cardiometabolic and other health benefits, although the role of exercise and physical activity in weight management, particularly for weight loss, has been questioned. Exercise alone is effective for preventing weight gain and as a weight loss strategy, promoting modest reductions in body weight and body fat. Engaging in moderately intense physical activity for at least 250 minutes per week is associated with successful maintenance of weight loss. The limited weight loss induced by exercise suggests that some behavioral or metabolic compensation may occur to limit the degree of negative energy balance produced by exercise. Regular exercise may improve energy intake regulation or increase daily energy expenditure, or both; however, the limited degree of weight loss induced by exercise has led to the investigation of new models for total daily energy expenditure. The constrained model of energy expenditure suggests that metabolic compensation may occur to limit the degree of negative energy balance produced by exercise; thus, the increase in total energy expenditure is smaller than predicted by the energy cost of physical activity. Current physical activity guidelines also recommend reducing sedentary behavior, but at this time it is unclear whether targeting sedentary behavior alone can prevent weight gain or promote weight loss.

When developing personalized exercise prescriptions, health care providers should discuss expectations with their patients to ensure that they are realistic and should also address strategies for overcoming challenges to adoption and maintenance. The individual's age, degree of motivation, and any medical issues that may affect physical activity capabilities should also be considered. With the provider's support, the individual's efforts to engage in lifestyle change can be facilitated.

References

1. US Department of Health and Human Services. *Physical Activity Guidelines for Americans*. 2nd ed. US Department of Health and Human Services; 2018. Accessed December 21, 2021. https://health.gov/paguidelines/second-edition/pdf/Physical_Activity_Guidelines_2nd_edition.pdf
2. World Health Organization. *WHO Guidelines on Physical Activity and Sedentary Behaviour*. World Health Organization; 2020. Accessed March 24, 2022. https:::/apps.who.int/iris/handle/10665/336656
3. Shaw K, Gennat H, O'Rourke P, Del Mar C. Exercise for overweight or obesity. *Cochrane Database Syst Rev*. 2006;(4):CD003817. doi:10.1002/14651858.CD003817.pub3
4. Thorogood A, Mottillo S, Shimony A, et al. Isolated aerobic exercise and weight loss: a systematic review and meta-analysis of randomized controlled trials. *Am J Med*. 2011;124(8):747-755. doi:10.1016/j.amjmed.2011.02.037
5. Bellicha A, van Baak MA, Battista F, et al. Effect of exercise training on weight loss, body composition changes, and weight maintenance in adults with overweight or obesity: an overview of 12 systematic reviews and 149 studies. *Obes Rev*. 2021;22 suppl 4(suppl 4):e13256. doi:10.1111/obr.13256
6. Oppert JM, Bellicha A, van Baak MA, et al. Exercise training in the management of overweight and obesity in adults: synthesis of the evidence and recommendations from the European Association for the Study of Obesity Physical Activity Working Group. *Obes Rev*. 2021;22 suppl 4(suppl 4):e13273. doi:10.1111/obr.13273

7. Johns DJ, Hartmann-Boyce J, Jebb SA, Aveyard P; Behavioural Weight Management Review Group. Diet or exercise interventions vs combined behavioral weight management programs: a systematic review and meta-analysis of direct comparisons. *J Acad Nutr Diet*. 2014;114(10):1557-1568. doi:10.1016/j.jand.2014.07.005

8. Ren ZQ, Lu GD, Zhang TZ, Xu Q. Effect of physical exercise on weight loss and physical function following bariatric surgery: a meta-analysis of randomised controlled trials. *BMJ Open*. 2018;8(10):e023208. doi:10.1136/bmjopen-2018-023208

9. Unick JL, Gaussoin SA, Hill JO, et al. Objectively assessed physical activity and weight loss maintenance among individuals enrolled in a lifestyle intervention. *Obesity (Silver Spring)*. 2017;25(11):1903-1909. doi:10.1002/oby.21971

10. Paixao C, Dias CM, Jorge R, et al. Successful weight loss maintenance: a systematic review of weight control registries. *Obes Rev*. 2020;21(5):e13003. doi:10.1111/obr.13003

11. Foright RM, Presby DM, Sherk VD, et al. Is regular exercise an effective strategy for weight loss maintenance? *Physiol Behav*. 2018;188:86-93. doi:10.1016/j.physbeh.2018.01.025

12. Jakicic JM, Rogers RJ, Davis KK, Collins KA. Role of physical activity and exercise in treating patients with overweight and obesity. *Clin Chem*. 2018;64(1):99-107. doi:10.1373/clinchem.2017.272443

13. Donnelly JE, Hill JO, Jacobsen DJ, et al. Effects of a 16-month randomized controlled exercise trial on body weight and composition in young, overweight men and women: the Midwest Exercise Trial. *Arch Intern Med*. 2003;163(11):1343-1350. doi:10.1001/archinte.163.11.1343

14. Martin JC, Awoke MA, Misso ML, Moran LJ, Harrison CL. Preventing weight gain in adults: a systematic review and meta-analysis of randomized controlled trials. *Obes Rev*. 2021;22(10):e13280. doi:10.1111/obr.13280

15. Academy of Nutrition and Dietetics. Adult weight management (AWM) guideline (2014). Evidence Analysis Library. Accessed December, 21, 2021. www.andeal.org/topic.cfm?menu=5276&cat=4688

16. Jensen MD, Ryan DH, Apovian CM, et al. 2013 AHA/ACC/TOS guideline for the management of overweight and obesity in adults: a report of the American College of Cardiology/American Heart Association Task Force on Practice Guidelines and The Obesity Society. *Circulation*. 2014;129(25 suppl 2):S102-S138. doi:10.1161/01.cir.0000437739.71477.ee

17. Donnelly JE, Blair SN, Jakicic JM, et al. American College of Sports Medicine Position Stand: appropriate physical activity intervention strategies for weight loss and prevention of weight regain for adults. *Med Sci Sports Exerc*. 2009;41(2):459-471. doi:10.1249/MSS.0b013e3181949333

18. Malhotra A, Noakes T, Phinney S. It is time to bust the myth of physical inactivity and obesity: you cannot outrun a bad diet. *Br J Sports Med*. 2015;49(15):967-968. doi:10.1136/bjsports-2015-094911

19. Schubert MM, Desbrow B, Sabapathy S, Leveritt M. Acute exercise and subsequent energy intake: a meta-analysis. *Appetite*. 2013;63:92-104. doi:10.1016/j.appet.2012.12.010

20. Beaulieu K, Blundell JE, van Baak MA, et al. Effect of exercise training interventions on energy intake and appetite control in adults with overweight or obesity: a systematic review and meta-analysis. *Obes Rev*. 2021;22 suppl 4(suppl 4):e13251. doi:10.1111/obr.13251

21. Donnelly JE, Herrmann SD, Lambourne K, Szabo AN, Honas JJ, Washburn RA. Does increased exercise or physical activity alter ad-libitum daily energy intake or macronutrient composition in healthy adults? A systematic review. *PLoS One*. 2014;9(1):e83498. doi:10.1371/journal.pone.0083498

22. Schumacher LM, Thomas JG, Raynor HA, Rhodes RE, Bond DS. Consistent morning exercise may be beneficial for individuals with obesity. *Exerc Sport Sci Rev*. 2020;48(4):201-208. doi:10.1249/JES.0000000000000226

23. Van Walleghen EL, Orr JS, Gentile CL, Davy KP, Davy BM. Habitual physical activity differentially affects acute and short-term energy intake regulation in young and older adults. *Int J Obes (Lond)*. 2007;31(8):1277-1285. doi:10.1038/sj.ijo.0803579

24. Horner KM, Finlayson G, Byrne NM, King NA. Food reward in active compared to inactive men: roles for gastric emptying and body fat. *Physiol Behav*. 2016;160:43-49. doi:10.1016/j.physbeh.2016.04.009

25. Horner KM, Schubert MM, Desbrow B, Byrne NM, King NA. Acute exercise and gastric emptying: a meta-analysis and implications for appetite control. *Sports Med*. 2015;45(5):659-678. doi:10.1007/s40279-014-0285-4

26. Schubert MM, Sabapathy S, Leveritt M, Desbrow B. Acute exercise and hormones related to appetite regulation: a meta-analysis. *Sports Med*. 2014;44(3):387-403. doi:10.1007/s40279-013-0120-3

27. Anton S, Das SK, McLaren C, Roberts SB. Application of social cognitive theory in weight management: time for a biological component? *Obesity (Silver Spring)*. 2021;29(12):1982-1986. doi:10.1002/oby.23257

28. Melby CL, Paris HL, Sayer RD, Bell C, Hill JO. Increasing energy flux to maintain diet-induced weight loss. *Nutrients*. 2019;11(10):2533. doi:10.3390/nu11102533

29. Careau V, Halsey LG, Pontzer H, et al. Energy compensation and adiposity in humans. *Curr Biol*. 2021;31(20):4659-4666.e2. doi:10.1016/j.cub.2021.08.016

30. Pontzer H. Constrained total energy expenditure and the evolutionary biology of energy balance. *Exerc Sport Sci Rev*. 2015;43(3):110-116. doi:10.1249/JES.0000000000000048

31. Martin CK, Johnson WD, Myers CA, et al. Effect of different doses of supervised exercise on food intake, metabolism, and non-exercise physical activity: the E-MECHANIC randomized controlled trial. *Am J Clin Nutr*. 2019;110(3):583-592. doi:10.1093/ajcn/nqz054

32. Thomas DM, Ivanescu AE, Martin CK, et al. Predicting successful long-term weight loss from short-term weight-loss outcomes: new insights from a dynamic energy balance model (the POUNDS Lost study). *Am J Clin Nutr*. 2015;101(3):449-454. doi:10.3945/ajcn.114.091520

33. Hand GA, Shook RP, O'Connor DP, et al. The effect of exercise training on total daily energy expenditure and body composition in weight-stable adults: a randomized, controlled trial. *J Phys Act Health*. 2020;17(4):456-463. doi:10.1123/jpah.2019-0415

34. Flack KD, Ufholz K, Johnson L, Fitzgerald JS, Roemmich JN. Energy compensation in response to aerobic exercise training in overweight adults. *Am J Physiol Regul Integr Comp Physiol*. 2018;315(4):R619-R626. doi:10.1152/ajpregu.00071.2018

35. Riou ME, Jomphe-Tremblay S, Lamothe G, et al. Energy compensation following a supervised exercise intervention in women living with overweight/obesity is accompanied by an early and sustained decrease in non-structured physical activity. *Front Physiol*. 2019;10:1048. doi:10.3389/fphys.2019.01048

36. Willis EA, Creasy SA, Saint-Maurice PF, et al. Physical activity and total daily energy expenditure in older US adults: constrained versus additive models. *Med Sci Sports Exerc*. 2022;54(1):98-105. doi:10.1249/MSS.0000000000002759

37. Brouwers B, Hesselink MK, Schrauwen P, Schrauwen-Hinderling VB. Effects of exercise training on intrahepatic lipid content in humans. *Diabetologia*. 2016;59(10):2068-2079. doi:10.1007/s00125-016-4037-x

38. Bruce CR, Thrush AB, Mertz VA, et al. Endurance training in obese humans improves glucose tolerance and mitochondrial fatty acid oxidation and alters muscle lipid content. *Am J Physiol Endocrinol Metab*. 2006;291(1):E99-E107. doi:10.1152/ajpendo.00587.2005

39. Goossens GH. The metabolic phenotype in obesity: fat mass, body fat distribution, and adipose tissue function. *Obes Facts*. 2017;10(3):207-215. doi:10.1159/000471488

40. Hallgreen CE, Hall KD. Allometric relationship between changes of visceral fat and total fat mass. *Int J Obes (Lond)*. 2008;32(5):845-852. doi:10.1038/sj.ijo.0803783

41. Rao S, Pandey A, Garg S, et al. Effect of exercise and pharmacological interventions on visceral adiposity: a systematic review and meta-analysis of long-term randomized controlled trials. *Mayo Clin Proc*. 2019;94(2):211-224. doi:10.1016/j.mayocp.2018.09.019

42. Abe T, Song JS, Bell ZW, et al. Comparisons of calorie restriction and structured exercise on reductions in visceral and abdominal subcutaneous adipose tissue: a systematic review. *Eur J Clin Nutr*. 2022;76(2):184-195. doi:10.1038/s41430-021-00942-1

43. Brennan AM, Day AG, Cowan TE, Clarke GJ, Lamarche B, Ross R. Individual response to standardized exercise: total and abdominal adipose tissue. *Med Sci Sports Exerc*. 2020;52(2):490-497. doi:10.1249/MSS.0000000000002140

44. Olsen MH, Angell SY, Asma S, et al. A call to action and a lifecourse strategy to address the global burden of raised blood pressure on current and future generations: the Lancet Commission on hypertension. *Lancet*. 2016;388(10060):2665-2712. doi:10.1016/S0140-6736(16)31134-5

45. Zhou B, Perel P, Mensah GA, Ezzati M. Global epidemiology, health burden and effective interventions for elevated blood pressure and hypertension. *Nat Rev Cardiol*. 2021;18(11):785-802. doi:10.1038/s41569-021-00559-8

46. Davy KP, Hall JE. Obesity and hypertension: two epidemics or one? *Am J Physiol Regul Integr Comp Physiol*. 2004;286(5):R803-R813. doi:10.1152/ajpregu.00707.2003

47. Cifu AS, Davis AM. Prevention, detection, evaluation, and management of high blood pressure in adults. *JAMA*. 2017;318(21):2132-2134. doi:10.1001/jama.2017.18706

48. Paffenbarger RS, Jr., Wing AL, Hyde RT, Jung DL. Physical activity and incidence of hypertension in college alumni. *Am J Epidemiol*. 1983;117(3):245-257. doi:10.1093/oxfordjournals.aje.a113537

49. Whelton PK, Carey RM. The 2017 clinical practice guideline for high blood pressure. *JAMA*. 2017;318(21):2073-2074. doi:10.1001/jama.2017.18209

50. Cornelissen VA, Smart NA. Exercise training for blood pressure: a systematic review and meta-analysis. *J Am Heart Assoc*. 2013;2(1):e004473. doi:10.1161/JAHA.112.004473

51. Naci H, Salcher-Konrad M, Dias S, et al. How does exercise treatment compare with antihypertensive medications? A network meta-analysis of 391 randomised controlled trials assessing exercise and medication effects on systolic blood pressure. *Br J Sports Med*. 2019;53(14):859-869. doi:10.1136/bjsports-2018-099921

52. Abrahin O, Moraes-Ferreira R, Cortinhas-Alves EA, Guerreiro JF. Is resistance training alone an antihypertensive therapy? A meta-analysis. *J Hum Hypertens*. 2021;35(9):769-775. doi:10.1038/s41371-021-00582-9

53. Hagberg JM, Park JJ, Brown MD. The role of exercise training in the treatment of hypertension: an update. *Sports Med*. 2000;30(3):193-206. doi:10.2165/00007256-200030030-00004

54. Carroll JF, Kyser CK. Exercise training in obesity lowers blood pressure independent of weight change. *Med Sci Sports Exerc*. 2002;34(4):596-601. doi:10.1097/00005768-200204000-00006

55. Boren J, Chapman MJ, Krauss RM, et al. Low-density lipoproteins cause atherosclerotic cardiovascular disease: pathophysiological, genetic, and therapeutic insights: a consensus statement from the European Atherosclerosis Society Consensus Panel. *Eur Heart J*. 2020;41(24):2313-2330. doi:10.1093/eurheartj/ehz962

56. Ference BA, Ginsberg HN, Graham I, et al. Low-density lipoproteins cause atherosclerotic cardiovascular disease: 1. Evidence from genetic, epidemiologic, and clinical studies. A consensus statement from the European Atherosclerosis Society Consensus Panel. *Eur Heart J*. 2017;38(32):2459-2472. doi:10.1093/eurheartj/ehx144

57. Sampson UK, Fazio S, Linton MF. Residual cardiovascular risk despite optimal LDL cholesterol reduction with statins: the evidence, etiology, and therapeutic challenges. *Curr Atheroscler Rep*. 2012;14(1):1-10. doi:10.1007/s11883-011-0219-7

58. Despres JP. Dyslipidaemia and obesity. *Baillieres Clin Endocrinol Metab*. 1994;8(3):629-660. doi:10.1016/s0950-351x(05)80289-7

59. Hasan B, Nayfeh T, Alzuabi M, et al. Weight loss and serum lipids in overweight and obese adults: a systematic review and meta-analysis. *J Clin Endocrinol Metab*. 2020;105(12):dgaa673. doi:10.1210/clinem/dgaa673

60. Chawla S, Tessarolo Silva F, Amaral Medeiros S, Mekary RA, Radenkovic D. The effect of low-fat and low-carbohydrate diets on weight loss and lipid levels: a systematic review and meta-analysis. *Nutrients*. 2020;12(12):3774. doi:10.3390/nu12123774

61. Fechner E, Smeets E, Schrauwen P, Mensink RP. The effects of different degrees of carbohydrate restriction and carbohydrate replacement on cardiometabolic risk markers in humans—a systematic review and meta-analysis. *Nutrients*. 2020;12(4):991. doi:10.3390/nu12040991

62. Whitehead A, Beck EJ, Tosh S, Wolever TM. Cholesterol-lowering effects of oat β-glucan: a meta-analysis of randomized controlled trials. *Am J Clin Nutr*. 2014;100(6):1413-1421. doi:10.3945/ajcn.114.086108

63. Gordon B, Chen S, Durstine JL. The effects of exercise training on the traditional lipid profile and beyond. *Curr Sports Med Rep*. 2014;13(4):253-259. doi:10.1249/JSR.0000000000000073

64. Sarzynski MA, Burton J, Rankinen T, et al. The effects of exercise on the lipoprotein subclass profile: a meta-analysis of 10 interventions. *Atherosclerosis*. 2015;243(2):364-372. doi:10.1016/j.atherosclerosis.2015.10.018

65. Hoddy KK, Axelrod CL, Mey JT, et al. Insulin resistance persists despite a metabolically healthy obesity phenotype. *Obesity (Silver Spring)*. 2022;30(1):39-44. doi:10.1002/oby.23312

66. Tchernof A, Despres JP. Pathophysiology of human visceral obesity: an update. *Physiol Rev*. 2013;93(1):359-404. doi:10.1152/physrev.00033.2011

67. Powell-Wiley TM, Poirier P, Burke LE, et al. Obesity and cardiovascular disease: a scientific statement from the American Heart Association. *Circulation*. 2021;143(21):e984-e1010. doi:10.1161/CIR.0000000000000973

68. DeFronzo RA, Tripathy D. Skeletal muscle insulin resistance is the primary defect in type 2 diabetes. *Diabetes Care*. 2009;32 suppl 2:S157-S163. doi:10.2337/dc09-S302

69. Heath GW, Gavin JR III, Hinderliter JM, Hagberg JM, Bloomfield SA, Holloszy JO. Effects of exercise and lack of exercise on glucose tolerance and insulin sensitivity. *J Appl Physiol Respir Environ Exerc Physiol*. 1983;55(2):512-517. doi:10.1152/jappl.1983.55.2.512

70. Perseghin G, Price TB, Petersen KF, et al. Increased glucose transport-phosphorylation and muscle glycogen synthesis after exercise training in insulin-resistant subjects. *N Engl J Med*. 1996;335(18):1357-1362. doi:10.1056/NEJM199610313351804

71. Battista F, Ermolao A, van Baak MA, et al. Effect of exercise on cardiometabolic health of adults with overweight or obesity: focus on blood pressure, insulin resistance, and intrahepatic fat-a systematic review and meta-analysis. *Obes Rev*. 2021;22 suppl 4:e13269. doi:10.1111/obr.13269

72. Houmard JA, Tanner CJ, Slentz CA, Duscha BD, McCartney JS, Kraus WE. Effect of the volume and intensity of exercise training on insulin sensitivity. *J Appl Physiol (1985)*. 2004;96(1):101-106. doi:10.1152/japplphysiol.00707.2003

73. Ryan BJ, Schleh MW, Ahn C, et al. Moderate-intensity exercise and high-intensity interval training affect insulin sensitivity similarly in obese adults. *J Clin Endocrinol Metab*. 2020;105(8):e2941-e2959. doi:10.1210/clinem/dgaa345

74. Balkau B, Mhamdi L, Oppert JM, et al. Physical activity and insulin sensitivity: the RISC study. *Diabetes*. 2008;57(10):2613-2618. doi:10.2337/db07-1605

75. Aune D, Norat T, Leitzmann M, Tonstad S, Vatten LJ. Physical activity and the risk of type 2 diabetes: a systematic review and dose-response meta-analysis. *Eur J Epidemiol*. 2015;30(7):529-542. doi:10.1007/s10654-015-0056-z

76. Smith AD, Crippa A, Woodcock J, Brage S. Physical activity and incident type 2 diabetes mellitus: a systematic review and dose-response meta-analysis of prospective cohort studies. *Diabetologia*. 2016;59(12):2527-2545. doi:10.1007/s00125-016-4079-0

77. Ross R, Blair SN, Arena R, et al. Importance of assessing cardiorespiratory fitness in clinical practice: a case for fitness as a clinical vital sign: a scientific statement from the American Heart Association. *Circulation*. 2016;134(24):e653-e699. doi:10.1161/CIR.0000000000000461

78. Wei M, Kampert JB, Barlow CE, et al. Relationship between low cardiorespiratory fitness and mortality in normal-weight, overweight, and obese men. *JAMA*. 1999;282(16):1547-1553. doi:10.1001/jama.282.16.1547

79. Qiu S, Cai X, Sun Z, Wu T, Schumann U. Is estimated cardiorespiratory fitness an effective predictor for cardiovascular and all-cause mortality? A meta-analysis. *Atherosclerosis*. 2021;330:22-28. doi:10.1016/j.atherosclerosis.2021.06.904

80. Stenholm S, Mehta NK, Elo IT, Heliovaara M, Koskinen S, Aromaa A. Obesity and muscle strength as long-term determinants of all-cause mortality—a 33-year follow-up of the Mini-Finland Health Examination Survey. *Int J Obes (Lond)*. 2014;38(8):1126-1132. doi:10.1038/ijo.2013.214

81. Xie Y, Wu Z, Sun L, et al. The effects and mechanisms of exercise on the treatment of depression. *Front Psychiatry*. 2021;12:705559. doi:10.3389/fpsyt.2021.705559
82. Grgic J, Schoenfeld BJ, Orazem J, Sabol F. Effects of resistance training performed to repetition failure or non-failure on muscular strength and hypertrophy: a systematic review and meta-analysis. *J Sport Health Sci*. 2022;11(2):202-211. doi:10.1016/j.jshs.2021.01.007
83. Batsis JA, Haudenschild C, Roth RM, et al. Incident impaired cognitive function in sarcopenic obesity: data from the national health and aging trends survey. *J Am Med Dir Assoc*. 2021;22(4):865-872.e5. doi:10.1016/j.jamda.2020.09.008
84. Cava E, Yeat NC, Mittendorfer B. Preserving healthy muscle during weight loss. *Adv Nutr*. 2017;8(3):511-519. doi:10.3945/an.116.014506
85. Gariepy G, Nitka D, Schmitz N. The association between obesity and anxiety disorders in the population: a systematic review and meta-analysis. *Int J Obes (Lond)*. 2010;34(3):407-419. doi:10.1038/ijo.2009.252
86. Pereira-Miranda E, Costa PRF, Queiroz VAO, Pereira-Santos M, Santana MLP. Overweight and obesity associated with higher depression prevalence in adults: a systematic review and meta-analysis. *J Am Coll Nutr*. 2017;36(3):223-233. doi:10.1080/07315724.2016.1261053
87. Pearl RL, Puhl RM. Weight bias internalization and health: a systematic review. *Obes Rev*. 2018;19(8):1141-1163. doi:10.1111/obr.12701
88. Pearl RL, Puhl RM, Lessard LM, Himmelstein MS, Foster GD. Prevalence and correlates of weight bias internalization in weight management: a multinational study. *SSM Popul Health*. 2021;13:100755. doi:10.1016/j.ssmph.2021.100755
89. McDowell CP, Dishman RK, Gordon BR, Herring MP. Physical activity and anxiety: a systematic review and meta-analysis of prospective cohort studies. *Am J Prev Med*. 2019;57(4):545-556. doi:10.1016/j.amepre.2019.05.012
90. Dishman RK, McDowell CP, Herring MP. Customary physical activity and odds of depression: a systematic review and meta-analysis of 111 prospective cohort studies. *Br J Sports Med*. 2021;55(16):926-934. doi:10.1136/bjsports-2020-103140
91. Ul-Haq Z, Mackay DF, Fenwick E, Pell JP. Meta-analysis of the association between body mass index and health-related quality of life among adults, assessed by the SF-36. *Obesity (Silver Spring)*. 2013;21(3):e322-e327. doi:10.1002/oby.20107
92. Posadzki P, Pieper D, Bajpai R, et al. Exercise/physical activity and health outcomes: an overview of Cochrane systematic reviews. *BMC Public Health*. 2020;20(1):1724. doi:10.1186/s12889-020-09855-3
93. Kandola A, Stubbs B. Exercise and anxiety. *Adv Exp Med Biol*. 2020;1228:345-352. doi:10.1007/978-981-15-1792-1_23
94. McLeod JC, Stokes T, Phillips SM. Resistance exercise training as a primary countermeasure to age-related chronic disease. *Front Physiol*. 2019;10:645. doi:10.3389/fphys.2019.00645
95. Carraca EV, Encantado J, Battista F, et al. Effect of exercise training on psychological outcomes in adults with overweight or obesity: a systematic review and meta-analysis. *Obes Rev*. 2021;22 suppl 4:e13261. doi:10.1111/obr.13261
96. Marquez DX, Aguinaga S, Vasquez PM, et al. A systematic review of physical activity and quality of life and well-being. *Transl Behav Med*. 2020;10(5):1098-1109. doi:10.1093/tbm/ibz198
97. Roake J, Phelan S, Alarcon N, Keadle SK, Rethorst CD, Foster GD. Sitting time, type, and context among long-term weight-loss maintainers. *Obesity (Silver Spring)*. 2021;29(6):1067-1073. doi:10.1002/oby.23148
98. O'Donoghue G, Blake C, Cunningham C, Lennon O, Perrotta C. What exercise prescription is optimal to improve body composition and cardiorespiratory fitness in adults living with obesity? A network meta-analysis. *Obesity Reviews*. 2021;22(2):e13137. doi:10.1111/obr.13137
99. Mabire L, Mani R, Liu L, Mulligan H, Baxter D. The influence of age, sex and body mass index on the effectiveness of brisk walking for obesity management in adults: a systematic review and meta-analysis. *J Phys Act Health*. 2017;14(5):389-407. doi:10.1123/jpah.2016-0064
100. Morze J, Rucker G, Danielewicz A, et al. Impact of different training modalities on anthropometric outcomes in patients with obesity: a systematic review and network meta-analysis. *Obes Rev*. 2021;22(7):e13218. doi:10.1111/obr.13218
101. Andreato LV, Esteves JV, Coimbra DR, Moraes AJP, de Carvalho T. The influence of high-intensity interval training on anthropometric variables of adults with overweight or obesity: a systematic review and network meta-analysis. *Obes Rev*. 2019;20(1):142-155. doi:10.1111/obr.12766
102. Kim H, Reece J, Kang M. Effects of accumulated short bouts of exercise on weight and obesity indices in adults: a meta-analysis. *Am J Health Promot*. 2020;34(1):96-104. doi:10.1177/0890117119872863
103. Neumark-Sztainer D, MacLehose RF, Watts AW, Eisenberg ME, Laska MN, Larson N. How is the practice of yoga related to weight status? Population-based findings from Project EAT-IV. *J Phys Act Health*. 2017;14(12):905-912. doi:10.1123/jpah.2016-0608
104. Kristal AR, Littman AJ, Benitez D, White E. Yoga practice is associated with attenuated weight gain in healthy, middle-aged men and women. *Altern Ther Health Med*. 2005;11(4):28-33.
105. Maillard F, Pereira B, Boisseau N. Effect of high-intensity interval training on total, abdominal and visceral fat mass: a meta-analysis. *Sports Med*. 2018;48(2):269-288. doi:10.1007/s40279-017-0807-y

106. Rioux JG, Ritenbaugh C. Narrative review of yoga intervention clinical trials including weight-related outcomes. *Altern Ther Health Med*. 2013;19(3):32-46.

107. Jakicic JM, Davis KK, Rogers RJ, et al. Feasibility of integration of yoga in a behavioral weight-loss intervention: a randomized trial. *Obesity (Silver Spring)*. 2021;29(3):512-520. doi:10.1002/oby.23089

108. Yazdanparast F, Jafarirad S, Borazjani F, Haghighizadeh MH, Jahanshahi A. Comparing between the effect of energy-restricted diet and yoga on the resting metabolic rate, anthropometric indices, and serum adipokine levels in overweight and obese staff women. *J Res Med Sci*. 2020;25:37. doi:10.4103/jrms.JRMS_787_19

109. Telles S, Sharma SK, Singh A, et al. Quality of life in yoga experienced and yoga naive Asian Indian adults with obesity. *J Obes*. 2019;2019:9895074. doi:10.1155/2019/9895074

110. Catenacci VA, Ostendorf DM, Pan Z, et al. The impact of timing of exercise initiation on weight loss: an 18-month randomized clinical trial. *Obesity (Silver Spring)*. 2019;27(11):1828-1838. doi:10.1002/oby.22624

111. Spreckley M, Seidell J, Halberstadt J. Perspectives into the experience of successful, substantial long-term weight-loss maintenance: a systematic review. *Int J Qual Stud Health Well-being*. 2021;16(1):1862481. doi:10.1080/17482631.2020.1862481

112. Willis EA, Creasy SA, Honas JJ, Melanson EL, Donnelly JE. The effects of exercise session timing on weight loss and components of energy balance: midwest exercise trial 2. *Int J Obes (Lond)*. 2020;44(1):114-124. doi:10.1038/s41366-019-0409-x

113. Liguori G, Magal M, Riebe D. ACSM's new exercise preparticipation screening: removing barriers to initiating exercise. American College of Sports Medicine blog. February 1, 2018. Accessed March 27, 2022. www.acsm.org/blog-detail/acsm-certified-blog/2018/02/01/exercise-preparticipation-screening-removing-barriers-initiating-exercise

114. Ostendorf DM, Schmiege SJ, Conroy DE, Phelan S, Bryan AD, Catenacci VA. Motivational profiles and change in physical activity during a weight loss intervention: a secondary data analysis. *Int J Behav Nutr Phys Act*. 2021;18(1):158. doi:10.1186/s12966-021-01225-5

115. Walsh TP, Arnold JB, Evans AM, Yaxley A, Damarell RA, Shanahan EM. The association between body fat and musculoskeletal pain: a systematic review and meta-analysis. *BMC Musculoskelet Disord*. 2018;19(1):233. doi:10.1186/s12891-018-2137-0

116. Regnaux JP, Lefevre-Colau MM, Trinquart L, et al. High-intensity versus low-intensity physical activity or exercise in people with hip or knee osteoarthritis. *Cochrane Database Syst Rev*. 2015;(10):CD010203. doi:10.1002/14651858.CD010203.pub2

117. Increasing physical activity among adults with disabilities. Centers for Disease Control and Prevention. Updated August 5, 2021. Accessed December 15, 2021. www.cdc.gov/ncbddd/disabilityandhealth/pa.html

118. Sarma S, Lipscombe LL. In persons with obesity, exercise plus liraglutide improved weight-loss maintenance vs. exercise or placebo. *Ann Intern Med*. 2021;174(9):JC102. doi:10.7326/ACPJ202109210-102

119. Lundgren JR, Janus C, Jensen SBK, et al. Healthy weight loss maintenance with exercise, liraglutide, or both combined. *N Engl J Med*. 2021;384(18):1719-1730. doi:10.1056/NEJMoa2028198

120. Desalermos A, Russell B, Leggett C, et al. Effect of obesogenic medications on weight-loss outcomes in a behavioral weight-management program. *Obesity (Silver Spring)*. 2019;27(5):716-723. doi:10.1002/oby.22444

121. Moon RC, Almuwaqqat Z. Effect of obesogenic medication on weight- and fitness-change outcomes: evidence from the Look AHEAD study. *Obesity (Silver Spring)*. 2020;28(11):2003-2009. doi:10.1002/oby.22997

122. Leggett CB, Desalermos A, Brown SD, et al. The effects of provider-prescribed obesogenic drugs on post-laparoscopic sleeve gastrectomy outcomes: a retrospective cohort study. *Int J Obes (Lond)*. 2019;43(6):1154-1163. doi:10.1038/s41366-018-0207-x

123. Adil MT, Jain V, Rashid F, et al. Meta-analysis of the effect of bariatric surgery on physical activity. *Surg Obes Relat Dis*. 2019;15(9):1620-1631. doi:10.1016/j.soard.2019.06.014

124. Nielsen MS, Alsaoodi H, Hjorth MF, Sjodin A. Physical activity, sedentary behavior, and sleep before and after bariatric surgery and associations with weight loss outcome. *Obes Surg*. 2021;31(1):250-259. doi:10.1007/s11695-020-04908-3

125. King WC, Hinerman AS, White GE, Courcoulas AP, Saad MAB, Belle SH. Associations between physical activity and changes in weight across 7 years after Roux-en-Y gastric bypass surgery: a multicenter prospective cohort study. *Ann Surg*. 2022;275(4):718-726. doi:10.1097/SLA.0000000000004456

126. Bond DS, Vithiananthan S, Thomas JG, et al. Bari-Active: a randomized controlled trial of a preoperative intervention to increase physical activity in bariatric surgery patients. *Surg Obes Relat Dis*. 2015;11(1):169-177. doi:10.1016/j.soard.2014.07.010

127. Bond DS, Thomas JG, Vithiananthan S, et al. Intervention-related increases in preoperative physical activity are maintained 6-months after bariatric surgery: results from the Bari-Active trial. *Int J Obes (Lond)*. 2017;41(3):467-470. doi:10.1038/ijo.2016.237

128. Bellicha A, Ciangura C, Poitou C, Portero P, Oppert JM. Effectiveness of exercise training after bariatric surgery—a systematic literature review and meta-analysis. *Obes Rev*. 2018;19(11):1544-1556. doi:10.1111/obr.12740

129. Durey BJ, Fritche D, Martin DS, Best LMJ. The effect of pre-operative exercise intervention on patient outcomes following bariatric surgery: a systematic review and meta-analysis. *Obesity Surg*. 2022;32(1):160-169. doi:10.1007/s11695-021-05743-w

130. da Silva ALG, Sardeli AV, André LD, et al. Exercise training does improve cardiorespiratory fitness in post-bariatric surgery patients. *Obes Surg*. 2019;29(4):1416-1419. doi:10.1007/s11695-019-03731-9

131. Cohen RV, Cummings DE. Weight regain after bariatric/metabolic surgery: a wake-up call. *Obesity (Silver Spring)*. 2020;28(6):1004. doi:10.1002/oby.22822

132. Carnero EA, Dubis GS, Hames KC, et al. Randomized trial reveals that physical activity and energy expenditure are associated with weight and body composition after RYGB. *Obesity (Silver Spring)*. 2017;25(7):1206-1216. doi:10.1002/oby.21864

133. Scibora LM. Skeletal effects of bariatric surgery: examining bone loss, potential mechanisms and clinical relevance. *Diabetes Obes Metab*. 2014;16(12):1204-1213. doi:10.1111/dom.12363

134. Marchesi F, De Sario G, Reggiani V, et al. Road running after gastric bypass for morbid obesity: rationale and results of a new protocol. *Obes Surg*. 2015;25(7):1162-1170. doi:10.1007/s11695-014-1517-2

135. Morales-Marroquin E, Kohl HW III, Knell G, de la Cruz-Muñoz N, Messiah SE. Resistance training in post-metabolic and bariatric surgery patients: a systematic review. *Obes Surg*. 2020;30(10):4071-4080. doi:10.1007/s11695-020-04837-1

CHAPTER 13

Counseling Approaches for Health Behavior Change

Gareth R. Dutton, PhD
Alena C. Borgatti, MA
Kathryn P. King, MA
Andrea L. Davis, MA

CHAPTER OBJECTIVES

- Define and discuss the evidence-based counseling approaches to changing health behaviors.
- Define and discuss alternative, "nondiet" counseling approaches to changing health behaviors.
- Discuss tips and other factors to consider when determining which counseling approach to use with a patient or client.

Introduction

Multicomponent lifestyle interventions for weight management that target dietary change and promote physical activity require the use of evidence-based counseling techniques and behavioral strategies to help patients or clients adhere to these lifestyle changes. Cognitive-behavioral counseling has been part of multicomponent lifestyle interventions since its inception, and there is robust empirical support for this approach and the behavioral techniques it encompasses. More recently, another evidence-based counseling approach—acceptance and commitment therapy—has been successfully applied in weight-management programs, and although it shares many components with traditional cognitive-behavioral therapy, the two approaches differ in important and meaningful ways. Finally, several other counseling strategies, including mindful eating, intuitive eating, and the Health at Every Size approach, have gained popularity for their applicability to healthy lifestyle promotion among individuals with overweight and obesity. Some of these alternative approaches, however, are less focused on weight loss as a treatment goal; therefore, there is less empirical support for them as successful weight-management tools. This chapter reviews the theoretical frameworks, primary components, and evidence supporting each of these counseling approaches as they apply to weight management and health promotion. Considerations for the selection and application of these approaches with patients or clients are also discussed.

Cognitive-Behavioral Approaches

Cognitive-behavioral therapy (CBT) is well established and has ample empirical support for its use in addressing a number of psychological conditions and facilitating adherence to treatment regimens for acute and chronic medical conditions (eg, type 2 diabetes and cardiac rehabilitation).[1-3] For weight management, CBT principles and techniques have been key elements of lifestyle interventions for decades and have robust empirical support for promoting weight loss and improving other metabolic, behavioral, and psychological outcomes.

Theoretical Frameworks

Cognitive-behavioral interventions for weight management are focused primarily on the principles of three theoretical frameworks: classical conditioning, operant conditioning, and social cognitive theory.[4-9] In the classical conditioning paradigm, eating behaviors become associated with stimuli such as situations, routines, activities, locations, or other people. These associations develop through the repeated pairing of eating with these stimuli, such that the nonfood stimuli become potent triggers for weight-altering behaviors. The goals of CBT are to learn to identify these triggers and disrupt the associations by either avoiding the triggers when possible or modifying one's learned responses to them (ie, replacing them with healthier responses that can lead to weight reduction).[1,7,9,10] Individuals can also learn to develop new associations for stimuli that promote healthier eating and activity behaviors.

Operant conditioning posits that behaviors are more or less likely to occur based on their consequences.[11] Positive consequences, such as the gratification of eating a savory food, are reinforced and make a behavior more likely to occur in the future, whereas negative consequences, such as the dislike of and discomfort associated with exercise, make a behavior less likely to occur. Because the short-term consequences of many behaviors associated with weight gain (eg, eating palatable, energy-dense foods) are positive and the negative effects of these behaviors (eg, development of chronic medical conditions, impaired mobility) take longer to manifest, operant conditioning illustrates why behavior change can be so challenging. Thus, CBT for weight management works to raise one's awareness of the positive and negative consequences of one's eating and activity behaviors while also bolstering the short-term, positive consequences of behavioral changes associated with weight reduction.[5,7,8,10]

Social cognitive theory recognizes the importance of social support and social context in adopting and maintaining behavior change. It also emphasizes an individual's motivation and perceived ability (ie, self-efficacy) to make specific behavioral changes. Finally, social cognitive theory recognizes the internal (cognitive) factors that influence behaviors and the need to modify cognitions when they are irrational or maladaptive and subsequently undermine behavior change.[6]

In applying the principles of these frameworks to weight management, CBT focuses on developing, practicing, and maintaining cognitive and behavioral skills that support behavioral changes in eating and activity routines. CBT practitioners help patients or clients identify salient internal and external cues for weight-altering behaviors, as well as the consequences of these behaviors, and encourage patients or clients to consistently practice and maintain new skills to modify these associations and patterns.

Specific Tools and Strategies

Self-Monitoring

Self-monitoring is a foundational element of CBT for weight management. Practitioners typically make recommendations for a patient or client's daily self-monitoring of food intake (including timing, servings, and energy content of meals and snacks) and physical activity (type and duration). CBT providers may also address other factors associated with eating or activity, which may include external (locations, social settings) and internal experiences (emotions and cognitions). Such information can be particularly helpful in identifying salient triggers for eating or activity behaviors.[12] In addition, self-weighing between intervention visits is encouraged and constitutes another key element of self-monitoring.[13] Of note, patients or clients can self-monitor using traditional methods ("paper and pencil") or via electronic means (smartphone applications to track food intake and wearable devices to monitor physical activity). Self-monitoring provides the crucial feedback needed to evaluate a patient or client's progression toward stated goals and modify strategies to better align current behaviors with goals.

Goal Setting

Specific and measurable goals for eating, activity, and weight loss are provided by the CBT practitioner in collaboration with the patient or client. Consistent with evidence-based lifestyle interventions, such as those delivered in the Diabetes Prevention Program and the Action for Health in Diabetes (Look AHEAD) trial, CBT interventions often involve an overall weight loss goal of 7% to 10% of initial body weight, restriction of energy intake to 1,200 to 1,800 kcal/d, and a physical activity goal of at least 150 minutes of moderate-intensity physical activity per week.[14,15] Dietary goals can vary by program and in accordance with relevant patient or client characteristics, such as the patient or client's starting weight, current activity level, age, and sex.[14,15] Physical activity goals are provided with an understanding that higher levels of activity are associated with greater benefits.[14,15] Lifestyle-based activity goals in the form of monitoring step counts and increasing them over time are also encouraged. In addition to goals related to weight, eating habits, and physical activity, CBT promotes setting goals specific to other behaviors targeted in the program (eg, identifying effective sources of social support), as established during treatment sessions. Throughout treatment, the practitioner monitors the patient or client's goals, making adjustments as needed, and works to connect progress made toward these goals with specific behavioral strategies employed by the patient or client.

Problem-Solving

Patients or clients may encounter obstacles and setbacks when trying to initiate and maintain cognitive and behavioral strategies for weight management. These challenges can be related to internal barriers (eg, diminished motivation or irrational cognitions), environmental factors (eg, unsupportive family and friends, stigma experienced in physical activity settings), or deficits in behavior-monitoring skills (eg, inconsistent or incorrect weighing and measuring of foods). In CBT, problem-solving involves five iterative steps: (1) problem orientation, (2) problem definition, (3) generation of potential solutions, (4) decision-making to identify the most viable solution, and (5) implementation and evaluation of the selected solution.[16,17] The practitioner initially guides the patient or client in the effective use of this model, with a goal of having the patient or client gradually develop skills and learn to independently address challenges and setbacks over time.

Stimulus Control

Stimulus control involves modifying one's environment in order to promote behaviors conducive to weight loss and diminish behaviors associated with overeating or sedentary time.[18] For example, practitioners may encourage patients or clients to remove energy-dense, highly palatable snacks from the pantry or make such foods less accessible in the home. Alternatively, patients or clients may be encouraged to keep healthy snacks (eg, fresh fruits and vegetables) washed, packaged, and ready for consumption. Thus, key elements of stimulus control include the availability, visibility, and accessibility of cues that promote healthy choices and restrict less healthy options. Patients or clients are encouraged to apply stimulus control in any setting where diet and activity behaviors may be affected, including at home, work, or school, and in transportation environments.

Cognitive Restructuring

In the CBT paradigm, thoughts are considered important precursors to the experience of emotions and subsequent behavioral responses. In particular, irrational thoughts can lead to negative emotions and behaviors that are inconsistent with weight-management goals.[8,18] For example, a patient or client may think "I've blown it!" after eating an energy-dense meal and exceeding their energy goal for the day. Such thoughts may lead to feelings of disappointment and frustration, which may cause that person to go home and eat even more energy-dense foods that evening. Thus, modifying irrational thought processes is an important step in promoting healthy behaviors. CBT practitioners can advise patients or clients on how to monitor their thoughts and emotions during and between sessions in order to identify irrational thoughts that may be interfering with their weight-management progress. Once irrational thoughts are identified, practitioners can help patients or clients modify or replace such thoughts with more rational ones that are more supportive of behavior change. For example, instead of thinking, "I've blown it!" in response to having eaten one unhealthy meal, a patient or client may identify an alternative thought, such as "No meal or food choice has to derail my efforts. I can make my next meal a healthy one." Through cognitive restructuring, patients or clients may become better equipped to avoid negative mood states and unhealthy behavioral responses.

Social Support

Drawing on social cognitive theory, CBT recognizes the importance of an individual's interactions with others in behavior-change efforts.[19,20] Social support can come from the practitioner and, in the case of group-based interventions, from other program participants. In addition, CBT providers can help patients or clients identify and seek out the support of important people in their everyday environments, such as family, friends, and coworkers. Support may include emotional support or encouragement, or it may come in the form of instrumental support, such as time or resources (eg, a partner could offer to do the laundry or other chores so that the patient or client can go for a walk). Also, providers should describe and offer opportunities in sessions for patients or clients to practice effective and assertive communication strategies to use in enlisting support from others and effectively dealing with difficult people or situations.

Relapse Prevention

CBT distinguishes between behavioral lapses and relapses. A lapse is a temporary movement away from one's behavioral or weight loss goals. A relapse is a more substantial and prolonged departure from one's goals.[21] The aim of relapse prevention is to develop cognitive and behavioral strategies to prevent a lapse from progressing to a full-blown relapse. Other CBT strategies previously discussed, such as cognitive restructuring, problem-solving, and stimulus control, are useful in relapse prevention. For example, part of the cognitive restructuring work entails reframing a slip as a temporary setback caused by insufficient planning and as a learning opportunity rather than as a lack of motivation or a personal failure.[5]

Other Techniques

Additional strategies may be incorporated in a CBT-based curriculum for weight management. Stress management and addressing body image concerns,[15] for example, may facilitate a patient or client's adherence to the other behavioral strategies fundamental to successful weight loss. High levels of stress can interfere with treatment adherence, and practitioners can introduce patients or clients to various techniques for better handling stress, such as diaphragmatic breathing, progressive muscle relaxation, guided imagery, and time management. Targeting body image dissatisfaction uses cognitive restructuring to help patients or clients identify and modify maladaptive thoughts, attitudes, and emotional reactions to their body shape or size. This may be particularly useful for patients or clients whose negative thoughts about their bodies interfere with program engagement and success.[22]

Treatment Format and Structure

CBT for weight management typically involves weekly visits for the first 4 to 6 months of treatment. This often transitions to visits every 2 weeks or monthly.[5,7,8] Visits can be one-on-one, group-based, or some combination of the two. Group sessions typically last 60 to 90 minutes, whereas individual sessions commonly last 30 minutes or less. Regardless of the format, the session usually begins with a private weigh-in, during which time the practitioner can review the patient or client's progress, reinforce behavioral changes adopted or maintained, and problem-solve if the patient or client has not achieved weight loss goals or has encountered barriers to progress. During the private weigh-in, the practitioner can also review the patient or client's self-monitoring records (ie, food logs, activity trackers) and provide feedback, and can help the patient or client identify connections between any weight change and behavioral changes adopted since the previous visit. The weigh-in is followed by an interactive discussion and the provision of educational content on a prespecified topic (eg, making healthy selections when dining out). Finally, the practitioner and patient or client (or patients or clients) engage in goal setting for the period between the current visit and the next.[7,23]

Empirical Support

The efficacy of CBT for weight loss is well-documented. Data from a multitude of efficacy trials show that statistically and clinically significant reductions in weight among study subjects participating in intensive, multicomponent programs grounded in CBT range from 8% to 10%.[5,7,16,24] This result is typically achieved after 4 to 6 months of treatment, which equates to a weight loss rate of approximately 0.5 to 1 kg/wk during this period of initial treatment.[18] This level of weight loss is associated with clinically meaningful improvements in a variety of health indicators, including blood pressure, cholesterol levels, and blood glucose levels.[25-29]

After the initial, maximal weight reductions achieved during the first 6 months of treatment, gradual and consistent weight regain is common. Within the first year following initial treatment, patients or clients often regain about half of the weight they lost; at 5 years from the time treatment is terminated, most patients or clients have regained all of the weight lost.[23,30,31] However, there are some encouraging signs in terms of long-term outcomes. First, the benefits of continued contacts and practitioner support are clear for improving weight loss maintenance.[32,33] Extended-care contacts designed to support the maintenance of health behaviors associated with weight management (eg, continued dietary self-monitoring, regular physical activity) can substantially reduce the amount of weight regained. In fact, current clinical guidelines for the treatment of obesity recommend ongoing extended-care contacts following initial treatment in order to improve long-term outcomes.[34] Several large-scale trials of weight loss and weight loss maintenance have demonstrated clinically meaningful weight loss maintenance up to 8 years after treatment initiation, particularly when continued long-term support is provided.[35] Although it is blunted, weight regain still occurs. Thus, weight loss maintenance remains one of the most substantial challenges and limitations of weight-management programs, including CBT-based interventions.

Given the weight loss values observed with treatment, it is not surprising that CBT-based interventions effectively improve patients or clients' reduction in energy intake, increases in physical activity levels, and engagement in self-monitoring behaviors.[36] However, adherence to self-monitoring and other behavioral strategies tends to decline over the course of treatment,[37,38] which corresponds to the gradual weight regain commonly observed. Other benefits achieved with CBT have been observed, including improvements in a variety of psychosocial outcomes. For instance, CBT-based interventions have been shown to improve patients or clients' depressive symptoms, quality of life, mobility, and physical functioning.[39-41]

Population Considerations

Although CBT for weight management has been used in a variety of populations with encouraging results, some issues warrant consideration. In most efficacy trials, individuals with more severe levels of obesity (BMI >40–50) are often excluded. Thus, some of this research may not generalize to this group. If individuals with a higher BMI or significant medical comorbidities (eg, uncontrolled type 2 diabetes, congestive heart failure) participate in treatment, medical clearance and close supervision may be indicated. CBT-based interventions tend to heavily promote physical activity, so medical clearance and ongoing monitoring may be necessary for patients or clients with multiple or medically complex conditions as they engage in increased activity. Also, some of the techniques integral to CBT (eg, self-monitoring of dietary intake, interpreting food labels) require a reasonable amount of health literacy and numeracy to implement. Thus, some of these strategies may be challenging for groups with limitations in these domains. Additional training or adaptations to these treatment techniques (eg, simplified self-monitoring instructions and records) may be appropriate. Similarly, individuals with impaired executive functioning—the higher-order cognitive processes necessary for planning and self-regulation—may experience less benefit from CBT, although research results in this area are mixed.

Acceptance and Commitment–Based Approaches

Acceptance and commitment therapy (ACT) is considered the next generation therapy following CBT. ACT builds on CBT's philosophies augmented by patient or client-centered therapy and several evidence-based theories, including functional contextualism, applied behavior analysis, and relational frame theory.[42,43] ACT is a type of contextual CBT that emphasizes behavioral engagement, psychological openness, and flexibility. Psychological flexibility is the primary target of this type of therapy, and this flexibility is increased through various strategies in order to encourage patients or clients to behaviorally engage in increasingly meaningful ways, despite psychological, social, and environmental barriers.[42,44] Notably, ACT relies on experiential exercises based in metaphor and imagery far more than other evidence-based therapies do.[42] It has been adapted and applied to a number of conditions, including weight management.[44] In the context of behavioral weight management, ACT has been termed *acceptance-based behavioral therapy*. Before one can understand ACT's fine-tuned approach for weight management, however, it is helpful to understand its foundations and basic tenants.

Theoretical Frameworks

Functional Contextualism

Functional contextualism holds that the functions of concepts, as well as objects, are dependent on their context. For example, a broken chair may be (or function as) a useless hazard in the context of an office space, but in the context of a play portraying a fight scene, it may be (or function as) a useful prop. In ACT, patients or clients are taught to observe and evaluate the function of their own behaviors and thoughts in multiple contexts, particularly in the context of their value system (ie, the things they value, such as family).[43] For example, in weight-management counseling, a patient or client may be asked to evaluate the function of their emotional eating in the context of their family. Although the short-term function of emotional eating may be to provide the patient or client with brief relief from negative emotions, when asked to evaluate it in the context of family, the patient or client may come to see that it is functioning as a model for coping that they do not want their children to follow. Alternatively, emotional eating may be viewed in the context of family as functioning to decrease their chances of living a long life and thus reduce the time they will have to spend with their family. The hope is that the patient or client will realize that emotional eating is drawing them farther away from a value-congruent life. Teaching the principles of functional contextualism helps patients or clients observe, predict, and influence their behavior to better align with their values and goals.

Applied Behavior Analysis

Applied behavior analysis grew out of the school of radical behaviorism. Radical behaviorists consider *everything* an organism does as behavior; even thinking, feeling, and remembering are considered behaviors. In this school of thought, behaviors are classified as either private or public.[45] The scientific contributions of radical behaviorists have led to many effective techniques for shaping behavior, including classical and operant conditioning using something called applied behavior analysis. Applied behavior analysis involves examining a target behavior (by asking questions such as "What behavior are we interested in?" and "Is it a public or private behavior?") and the antecedents and consequences of that behavior. A behavior's antecedents are what happens immediately before the behavior and can include thoughts, feelings, or actions of both a private and public nature. A behavior's consequences are the effects of the behavior on the self, others, or the environment. Like antecedents, consequences can also be thoughts, feelings, or actions. It is important to identify both the short-term and long-term consequences of the behavior. Applied behavior analysis develops increased awareness of behavioral patterns and identifies opportunities to increase or decrease target behaviors.

Relational Frame Theory

Relational frame theory emphasizes the connections of one's thoughts and feelings to an interconnected network of words and learned responses to these words. For example, the word *comfort* typically leads to thoughts and feelings of relaxation or relief from stress. If this word is used in conjunction with the word *food* in reference to a particular food, then the thoughts and feelings associated with comfort become applied to that comfort food, and one may seek out that food when feeling stressed or having difficulty relaxing. This idea is called *transfer of stimulus functions* in relational frame theory, and this kind of transfer can either steer people away from valued paths or be harnessed as a powerful tool for achieving value-congruent living.[43] For example, if the given comfort food is viewed in the context of values, it can be associated with the term *value-incongruent*, and the behaviors and motivation that are associated with value-incongruent concepts can more easily be applied to the comfort food to the point that comfort becomes less associated with the given food. It is not difficult to see how our ability to associate responses with words is adaptive, and it is essential to consider how these associations influence mental and physical health, as is done in ACT.

Psychological Flexibility

Psychological flexibility is at the core of ACT, and the model of psychological flexibility is derived from the three theoretical frameworks just described. Psychological flexibility involves six components: (1) acceptance, (2) contact with the present moment, (3) self as context, (4) committed action, (5) values, and (6) defusion.[43] These six constructs constitute the six primary strategies of traditional ACT. As previously mentioned, when ACT is applied to weight management, it is called acceptance-based behavioral therapy, or ABT. ABT has a similar focus on psychological flexibility, which is defined as the ability to take value-congruent action rather than acting on short-term feelings, impulses, or thoughts. However, in ABT, the six components of psychological flexibility from traditional ACT are organized into three primary categories: (1) value-congruent action, (2) mindful decision-making, and (3) acceptance.[44] We review each of these next in the context of ABT, with references to the six traditional components or strategies of ACT throughout.

Specific Tools and Strategies

Value-Congruent Action

Value-congruent action (also called values-driven action) is emphasized in ABT. Values are defined as "the ideas, principles, and domains of our lives that are most important to us."[44] Practitioners using ABT must take care to explain this definition to patients or clients and help them distinguish it from any preconceived notions they may have about what values are. For example, it is helpful to clarify that values are not goals or achievements; nor are they aptitudes or talents beyond one's control (eg, intelligence) or particular feelings (eg, the feeling of happiness).[43] It may also be useful for practitioners to distinguish values from goals by describing values as cardinal directions and goals as destinations. In this therapeutical approach, practitioners guide patients or clients in identifying and clarifying their values. For example, the practitioner might ask, "Why do you go to work?"[44] Aside from the need for money, a patient or client's answer to this question may reveal certain underlying values.[44]

ABT's emphasis on value-congruent action likewise emphasizes making a commitment to one's values in the context of one's actions. This increases the patient or client's focus on living according to their identified values, even if it causes pain and discomfort. Patients or clients learn that their commitment to difficult goals—especially goals that involve prolonged exposure to unpleasant stimuli—is more easily sustained when those goals are connected to their core values.[44] Interestingly, this component of ABT incorporates some traditional, evidence-based behavioral intervention techniques found in CBT, such as goal setting, planning, and stimulus control. Incorporated in the approach is a discussion of potential barriers to success and the patient or client's willingness to experience these barriers. Patients or clients are also taught strategies for increasing awareness of their behavioral choices in order to increase the likelihood that they will take value-congruent actions.[44]

Mindful Decision-Making

This component of ABT focuses on increasing the patient or client's awareness of the present moment through mindfulness. Patients or clients are taught how to observe perceptual, affective, and cognitive aspects of their food intake and physical activity to facilitate present-moment decision-making regarding these behaviors and to reduce the tendency to make mindless decisions regarding eating and activity.[44] Patients or clients practice monitoring their body sensations before, during, and after a physical activity, exercise, or eating. The primary goal is to consciously engage oneself in the present moment in order to disrupt automatic responses, such as sedentary behavior or overeating.[44] Mindfulness creates opportunities for the individual to plan for value-congruent action. Examples of mindful decision-making encouraged in ABT include mindfully deciding what foods to purchase and eat, mindfully deciding when to start eating or engaging in physical activity and when to stop, and mindfully deciding how to structure one's environment, including the food and physical activity cues in that environment.[44]

Acceptance

The acceptance component of ABT focuses on the patient or client's ability to make room for painful or unpleasant feelings, sensations, urges, and emotions. It helps patients or clients recognize that distress may accompany their efforts to eat healthily and engage in physical activity, and that avoiding these feelings of distress is not useful and can be counterproductive.[44] The concept of willingness is taught along with acceptance, as willingness promotes engagement in valued activities (while accepting the discomfort they may bring) and deciding that the value-congruent behavior is worth the associated distress.[43] Willingness strategies are also discussed in ABT. Patients or clients are taught urge surfing as a tool for tolerating feelings of distress. *Urge surfing* involves picturing oneself riding atop a wave of discomfort.[44] This visual helps patients or clients realize that distressing internal experiences will pass on their own, thus decreasing the urge to act on feelings of distress.

Cognitive defusion is also taught in conjunction with acceptance and willingness. This technique is the distancing of oneself from one's thoughts, feelings, or sensations, rather than identifying oneself with these thoughts, feelings, or sensations or considering them to be absolute truths.[44] The process of defusion can also be thought of as looking *at* one's thoughts rather than *from* one's thoughts—noticing rather than getting caught up in thoughts, or letting thoughts come and go rather than holding onto them.[42,43] This strategy helps prevent behaviors such as overeating or sedentary behavior, which can occur when people identify themselves with their distressing thoughts, feelings, or sensations and act on them. To practice defusion, patients or clients are guided in several experiential activities to help them notice their thought content and their own "fusion" with their thoughts (ie, how much they buy into or get caught up in their own thoughts). These activities help patients or clients recognize that they are not their minds and their thoughts are not necessarily themselves speaking so that they are better able to freely choose value-congruent behavior.[44]

"Control What You Can, Accept What You Can't"

ABT for weight management provides a useful mantra that sums up the approaches just described. The mantra "Control what you can, accept what you can't" is taught to patients or clients to help them distinguish between the facets of weight management that are within their control (eg, one's personal food environment) and those that are outside of their control (eg, food environment on a societal level). It is also a useful tool for identifying what type of strategy to use in which situation. When patients or clients encounter distressing situations that are outside of their control (eg, a coworker brings a lot of sweets to a work party and the patient or client has the urge to try them all), acceptance-based psychological strategies such as defusion and urge surfing are useful. When patients or clients encounter distressing situations that are within their control (eg, the patient or client sees the candy bowl on their own dinner table and has an urge to eat several candies), behavioral strategies such as stimulus control, portion control, or planning are more appropriate.[44]

Treatment Format and Structure

ABT is generally delivered in a group setting over the course of 1 year but can be adapted to an individual format. Over the year, 25 sessions are offered: 16 weekly sessions followed by six biweekly sessions, and finally three sessions offered monthly or bimonthly. As in CBT, each session begins with a weigh-in and a check-in, when patients or clients are prompted to report their activity (ie, exercise in minutes), behavior goal progress, daily energy intake, number of days they recorded food intake, and experiential exercise practice. *Experiential exercise* refers to activities introduced in session and assigned as homework to illustrate and develop psychological strategies, such as acceptance, willingness, defusion, and urge surfing.[44]

At the beginning of treatment, patients or clients are introduced to behavioral strategies for weight management and relevant psychoeducation; starting with the fifth session, psychological strategies are introduced. Early in treatment, patients or clients set attainable goals for weight loss, with guidance from the practitioner; a goal of 10% weight loss is recommended. Patients or clients switch to a weight-maintenance goal once they have met their initial weight loss goal, when their weight loss has plateaued, or when the end of the treatment is near (to allow for time to practice weight maintenance).[44]

Of note, some research has examined 1-day, acceptance-based workshops as a way to address specific aspects of weight management, such as emotional eating or physical activity; this format shows some promise in terms of acceptability, feasibility, and efficacy in behavior change.[46,47] However, given the limited research in this area and the smaller scope of behavior change being addressed, more studies are needed to evaluate the feasibility and utility of delivering the full ABT for weight management in a workshop-based format.

Empirical Support

Researchers have examined the efficacy of ACT and ABT over the past several decades, and several studies from the pioneers of ACTs demonstrate its application to weight management. In an initial study of feasibility and preliminary test of effectiveness, participants engaging in a 12-week ABT weight-management intervention lost 8.1% of their initial body weight on average, and an additional 2.2% on average during the maintenance phase.[48] Another pilot study found clinically significant decreases in energy intake, weight, and intake of sodium and saturated fats, as well as increased physical activity, among patients or clients with cardiac conditions.[49] Another trial enrolled individuals classified as overweight with disinhibited eating found that after 24 sessions of ABT the mean weight loss was 12 kg, which was much higher than expected, and this weight loss was maintained at 3-month follow-up visits.[50] A randomized controlled trial of a 40-session, yearlong program compared ABT with CBT and demonstrated significantly greater weight loss with ABT at 18 months. Furthermore, individuals with greater responsivity to food cues, a greater degree of emotional eating, and symptoms of depression all demonstrated a particular advantage in increased weight loss when assigned to ABT vs CBT.[51] Long-term follow-up data from the same clinical trial indicated that at 36 months, differences in weight loss between participants assigned to CBT vs those assigned to ABT were attenuated. However, significantly more treatment "completers" maintained at least a 10% weight loss in the ABT vs CBT group when assessed at 36 months. Furthermore, quality of life was higher at 36 months in the ABT group than in the CBT group.[52]

Researchers have also examined ABT in unique populations. One study investigated the effect of ABT vs CBT on weight management in individuals with high disinhibition. They found no significant difference in percentage of weight lost at 24 months, but secondary analyses showed that those in the ABT group regained significantly less weight from the time of treatment's end to the final follow-up visit than did individuals in the CBT group. Similarly, a greater percentage of participants in the ABT group achieved 5% weight loss at 24 months.[53] Another study compared the effects of behavioral treatment as usual (BT), behavioral treatment plus skills for coping with the obesogenic food environment (BT+E), and a behavioral treatment utilizing both environmental strategies and acceptance-based strategies (BT+EA).[54] Findings showed no differences in weight change among the treatment groups throughout the 12-month program but did show that race moderated the response to the intervention, such that disparities in weight loss between Black participants and non-Hispanic White participants, apparent in both the BT and BT+E groups, were significantly reduced in the BT+EA group.[54]

Population Considerations

As just noted, research demonstrates that ABT has advantages over CBT among individuals with greater disinhibition, greater food-cue responsivity, a greater degree of emotional eating, and symptoms of depression. However, for patients or clients who do not exhibit these traits or symptoms, CBT may be equally or even more effective for weight loss than ABT.[44] ABT may also have advantages for Black patients or clients, given the results of aforementioned study that observed diminished racial disparities in weight loss when an acceptance-based approach was used vs other treatments. However, additional studies are needed to support this potential recommendation.

Given ABT's similarities to CBT in terms of behavioral strategies in particular, the same populations should be treated with caution in both CBT and ABT. As previously described, this includes individuals with multiple or medically complex conditions who may need medical clearance or individually tailored dietary and physical activity plans. In addition, ABT has not been evaluated in people with a BMI higher than 50. ABT could be of benefit in this population, but such individuals are also more likely to experience medical complications that could limit their response to ABT.[44]

Certain psychological conditions should be considered with caution. If a psychiatric condition is severe enough to compromise the patient or client's ability to engage in behavior changes, it may be necessary to treat that condition before initiating ABT.[44] Similarly, people with night eating syndrome and binge eating disorder may benefit from pursuing treatment for the eating disorder alongside ABT, as they may show less weight loss in response to ABT because of their eating disorder.[44]

Motivational Interviewing Approaches

Motivational interviewing is an empathic approach to behavior-change counseling that has demonstrated positive effects on patient or client-provider interactions, patient or client attrition and adherence, and clinical outcomes.[55,56] It employs a goal-oriented, collaborative communication style that particularly attends to and elicits "change talk," language that alludes to one's consideration of a behavior change. Practitioners of motivational interviewing are guided by four principles: (1) express empathy by reflectively listening to the patient or client's concerns, (2) develop the discrepancy between the patient or client's current behaviors and their values, (3) sidestep resistance to change through empathy rather than confrontation, and (4) develop patient or client self-efficacy by building the patient or client's confidence in their ability to change.[57]

Motivational interviewing is predicated on several key assumptions, many of which relate to theories that have been linked to the approach (see next section).[58] First, it is *patient* or *client-centered* rather than provider-centered. Similarly, it emphasizes *collaboration* between patient or client and practitioner such that the interaction is not prescriptive, as in traditional clinical settings, but rather dependent on the patient or client's goals, values, and preferences. Likewise, patients or clients are considered *autonomous* individuals, and it is important for them to recognize their autonomy in choosing to change their behavior. Relatedly, this approach holds that *motivation* is essential to behavior change, exists within the patient or client, can be dynamic, and can be influenced by social interaction or the clinician's style. Finally, the patient or client's *environment* must be conducive to behavior change or made conducive to behavior change.

Theoretical Framework

Motivational interviewing was first developed by clinicians who working with patients or clients with alcohol use disorders and noticed that confrontational styles of clinical interviewing led to resistance on the part of the patient or client.[56] Initial clinical anecdotes eventually fostered research into techniques used in motivational interviewing, which has become associated with several evidence-based theories and therapies. It has been linked to Carl Rogers's work on patient or client-centered therapy.[59] Patient or client-centered therapy emphasizes nondirective, reflective listening, with the provider serving as a mirror to the patient or client. Rogers posited several key characteristics of a provider-patient or client relationship that are required for the patient or client to make changes, including: the relationship must be genuine; it must be characterized by empathy; and the provider must have unconditional positive regard for the patient or client.[59] Motivational interviewing also operates on these patient or client-centered principles to create the necessary environment between patient or client and provider in which to discuss behavior change.

A second theory linked to motivational interviewing is the theory of cognitive dissonance. The concept of cognitive dissonance derives from the work of Leon Festinger, who proposed that human beings possess an inner drive to have their cognitions (thoughts, attitudes, beliefs, and the like) be in agreement—that is, to be consistent with one another.[60] When an individual experiences conflict or tension among their cognitions, discomfort arises; the person's inner drive motivates them to resolve the dissonance, which they can do either through behavior change or, alternatively, through denial and resistance. Motivational interviewing can elicit cognitive dissonance in patients or clients because it guides patients or clients to consider the agreements or disagreements between their thoughts, beliefs, and actions in a nonjudgmental way, which can facilitate behavior change.

A third theory that has been related to motivational interviewing is self-perception theory. Developed by Daryl Bem, self-perception theory holds that people develop beliefs and attitudes about themselves based on their behavior, just as they would develop beliefs and attitudes about other people based on the behavior of those people.[61] This theory could help explain why motivational interviewing is effective, because if an individual spends time talking about making a change (which is a behavior in itself), that talking can then contribute to the individual's own belief or attitude about the importance of making that change.

The final and perhaps best-known theory linked with motivational interviewing is the transtheoretical model of behavior change (refer to Chapter 9). This model posits that a person seeking to change a behavior moves through several stages of change: precontemplation, contemplation, preparation, action, maintenance, and termination. Motivational interviewing's focus on change talk can clarify for both the patient or client and the interviewer (provider) the stage of change that the patient or client is in and how the provider can best support the patient or client accordingly. The transtheoretical model also posits several processes by which people make changes, some of which are included in CBT (eg, stimulus control, contingency management) and some of which map onto motivational interviewing's focus on change talk (eg, evaluating one's self and one's environment to ascertain the role played by the target behavior and how it affects one's self-concept or others around the individual).[62]

Specific Tools and Strategies

Supporting the generalizability and utility of motivational interviewing are its various tools and strategies, which can be employed across a variety of clinical settings and by a variety of clinical providers.

OARS

At the heart of motivational interviewing is a set of four tools known collectively by the acronym OARS, which stands for open-ended questions, affirmations, reflections, and summary statements.[58]

Open-ended questions elicit a wider range of replies than do close-ended questions and thereby facilitate a conversational interaction. In contrast, close-ended questions yield a narrower range of responses (eg, *yes* or *no* answers, brief words or phrases) and lead to an interview-style or interrogation-style interaction; they can cause patients or clients to feel defensive and make it easier for patients or clients to answer dishonestly. Open-ended questions are helpful for exploring the advantages of the desired target behavior, the disadvantages of the current (undesirable) behavior, and the patient or client's beliefs and intentions regarding making a change.

Affirmations are compliments paid to patients or clients on their efforts, strengths, abilities, and good intentions. Effective affirmations should be sincere and empathic. When done well, affirmations can boost patients or clients' confidence in their ability to change (ie, they support self-efficacy), lead to increases in praised habits, and build rapport.

Making reflections or reflectively listening to the patient or client's perspective is so important to the motivational interviewing process that training in the process encourages providers to make three reflections for every one question asked during intervention sessions. Reflections can range from simple to complex in both their content and impact. Simple reflections involve restating what the patient or client said, which shows understanding and facilitates interaction. This type of reflection does not add much meaning to the conversation, however. Complex reflections, on the other hand, can draw out emotions, direct the patient or client toward positive change statements, add substantial meaning to what the patient or client has already communicated, make a point, change the direction of the conversation, make a guess, or add more momentum to the exploration process.

Finally, summary statements are used to reprise the core points discussed during the interview, but they can also send the conversation in a new direction in order to facilitate change or even keep the conversation going. Summaries also help structure the conversation and maintain the conversation's focus while emphasizing change talk.

Box 13.1 provides weight-management–related examples of each of the OARS components.

BOX 13.1

The OARS Strategy Applied to Weight Management

OARS strategy component	Weight-management example
Open-ended questions	How would you go about planning your meals?
	What do you think about the national recommendation to get 150 minutes of moderate physical activity a week?
	Can you tell me more about your family's eating patterns?
Affirmations	You really persevered on your step goal this week by using the treadmill when the weather got in the way of outdoor walking!
	Even though you are not sure about setting aside time to work out, I can tell that being active is important to you by the way you have been taking the stairs and parking farther away from your destination—way to be creative about increasing activity!
	It sounds like you held your goal in mind when your coworker brought a cake to the office on Friday, and that helped you stick to a small portion size—great job!
Reflections	Simple: It sounds like you discussed changing your eating habits with your partner this week.
	Complex: It sounds like you were at least open to the idea of changing your eating habits and you discussed that with your partner, who also seems open to making this change with you.
Summary statements	We've discussed the pros and cons of decreasing your sugar intake—the pros being that you can reverse your prediabetes and model healthy eating for your children, and the cons being that you have several stressors in your life and would feel overwhelmed by making a drastic change in your eating patterns at the moment. You mentioned that a small change could be reasonable, though, and indicated that decreasing your consumption of soft drinks to one or two on the weekend would be a great place to start. Before we wrap up, would you mind if I share some strategies people have found useful for tracking their progress?

DARN

A second strategy in the motivational-interviewer's toolbox is represented by the acronym *DARN*, which stands for *desire*, *ability*, *reason*, and *need*. These four words represent the four types of change talk that are important to elicit from patients or clients in order to develop their motivation to change.[63] Practitioners of motivational interviewing listen for these four types of change talk and ask the patient or client open-ended questions or provide reflections to further elicit them. Box 13.2 provides examples of how an interviewer might draw out each type of change talk in a weight-management setting.

BOX 13.2

The DARN Strategy Applied to Weight Management

Type of change talk	Weight-management examples
Desire	What do you want to achieve by changing your eating and exercise habits?
	How might you want to change your diet?
Ability	What is possible for your family to eat, given your dietary restrictions?
	How can you feasibly change your physical activity given your resources?
Reason	Why would you want to make changes to your eating behavior and exercise habits?
	What benefits do you see to decreasing your sugar intake?
Need	How badly do you need to increase your physical activity?
	How important is it to you to change your eating habits?

Confidence and Importance

Motivational interviewing also employs "rulers" to elicit self-report data on the key constructs of confidence and importance. Called readiness rulers, these tools prompt practitioners to ask patients or clients to rate how ready (confident) they are for change or how important the change is to them on a scale of 1 to 10. Patients or clients' answers can be tracked over time to assess readiness, and the provider can discuss these data with the patient or client, particularly when a change or pattern is identified.

Additional Tools

Additional types of change talk that the motivational interviewer should listen for and elicit are mentions of commitment to change (including ambivalence) and steps taken toward change (both preparation and action). When a patient or client discusses commitment, the interviewer should emphasize how the patient or client can strengthen their commitment via strategies such as negotiating a plan, creating a menu of choices, enlisting social support, and identifying and addressing barriers to change.[58] Research has shown that patient or client-generated change talk at the end of a session is most predictive of future change.

Finally, providers using the motivational-interviewing approach are encouraged to "roll with resistance." Resistant behaviors from patients or clients are many and diverse. They can include arguing, interrupting, ignoring, negating, disagreeing, excusing, blaming, minimizing, reluctance, pessimism, and unwillingness to change, among others. Resistant responses are to be expected; however, if resistance is persistent, the issue likely lies with the practitioner and how that practitioner is applying the approach. To roll with patient or client resistance, interviewers must avoid the "righting reflex"—the temptation to tell patients or clients the correct solution to a problem or to fix patients or clients' problems for them, without allowing them to invite such advice or giving them the space to choose the solution for themselves.[58] Although typically well-intentioned, the righting reflex is a directive style of interaction with the patient or client that minimizes the opportunity to enhance patient or client motivation via a patient or client-centered style of interaction.

Treatment Format and Structure

Given its conversational nature, motivational interviewing can be used during almost any encounter with a patient or client, including medical, dietetic, physical therapy, and counseling appointments. Research on the efficacy of motivational interviewing for weight loss has primarily examined the approach in the context of counseling appointments; therefore, the treatment format and structure details discussed here pertain mainly to counseling encounters.

The patient or client-centered nature of motivational interviewing and its focus on behavior-related change talk lends the approach to a format that is guided by change talk and patient or client priorities and desires rather than to one that is practitioner-generated and agenda-based. Motivational interviewing is traditionally delivered in person, but it can also be delivered via telehealth (ie, via telephone coaching or videoconferencing). Limited research has investigated delivery by eHealth (ie, via email, internet, social media, or smartphone applications); some efficacy has been demonstrated for this, but additional research is needed.[64] Recommended length of appointment varies considerably in the literature, with randomized controlled trials using appointment durations ranging from 20 to 60 minutes.[65] The optimum number of sessions is also variable; three to 11 sessions is the typical range studied in randomized controlled trials, although one trial indicated that sessions continued indefinitely until weight loss goals were achieved.[65] The data on frequency of sessions and treatment duration are also highly variable; a meta-analysis published in 2011 indicated that studies with a treatment duration of 6 months or longer demonstrated significantly greater weight loss among participants than did studies with treatment durations of less than 6 months.[65] Of the studies that lasted longer than 6 months, the number of sessions was typically four to six, and the sessions were typically spread out over 12 to 18 months. Lastly, research indicates that motivational interviewing is more effective in an individual (one-on-one) format than in the group setting.

Empirical Support

Motivational interviewing as a tool for weight management is supported by a wealth of evidence. A systematic review and meta-analysis revealed that, across randomized controlled trials of the effect of motivational interviewing on weight management, motivational interviewing demonstrated a medium-size effect for decreasing body mass as compared to control treatments. In this same review, studies comparing patients in motivational-interviewing groups to patients in control groups receiving equivalent attention or information demonstrated that participants in the motivational-interviewing groups lost 1.47 kg of weight over and above those in control groups.[65] As for the primary care setting, more than one-third of studies included in a systematic review reported that motivational interviewing led to a clinically significant weight loss of more than 10% of body weight, and half of the included studies demonstrated a 5% weight loss on average. Weight-related variables such as food intake, physical activity, and metabolic markers were evaluated in several included studies, with one-third of these studies reporting significant improvements in the motivational-interviewing group compared with controls.[66] The authors indicated that variability in findings may have been due to a lack of monitoring of treatment fidelity (the degree to which practitioners adhered to the treatment protocol) in most studies.

As for long-term outcomes, a randomized controlled feasibility trial examined the effect of motivational interviewing on participants who lost at least 5% of their body weight in the preceding year. Those receiving intensive motivational interviewing demonstrated additional weight loss maintenance compared to controls.[67] However, in another study that compared an online motivational-interviewing intervention to an online nutrition and psychoeducation intervention, no significant differences were seen between the intervention groups in terms of weight loss maintained. This finding, in light of other literature, suggests that motivational interviewing is useful in weight loss maintenance but that delivering it online may compromise its effectiveness.[64]

Aside from its effect on weight, motivational interviewing has been shown to improve patient or client retention and engagement in treatment. It can also enhance the effects of other interventions, such as those reviewed in this chapter. Motivational interviewing as an intervention for weight loss has also been shown to decrease alcohol consumption, improve glycemic control, decrease overall energy and fat intake, increase the number of fruits and vegetables consumed, increase the number of sit-ups done per minute, and increase physical activity. It has mixed effects on decreasing sodium intake and improving blood pressure, with some studies showing a significant difference over control interventions and others showing no significant differences.[65]

Population Considerations

The patient- or client-centered nature of motivational interviewing makes it very generalizable across populations. However, it may not be effective if the patient or client's environment is not conducive to change—for example, if the patient or client has poor access to treatment, lacks transportation (thus limiting access to healthy foods or gyms), lives in a food desert, or does not live in or have access to a walking-friendly neighborhood.[58] A potential first step in such cases could be to involve social workers or other social and community resources to enhance the patient or client's environment, making it more suitable for behavior change, if such options are feasible. Of note, a conducive environment is also likely important for CBT and ACT to be successful as well. In addition, motivational interviewing is not ideal for people of a young chronological age or developmental age given their limited ability to make substantial behavior changes without the support of a caregiver. In these cases, including the caregiver in sessions, providing caregiver training, and incorporating other behavioral strategies are all indicated.

Nondiet Approaches

Mindful eating, intuitive eating, and Health at Every Size (HAES) are three similar, complementary counseling techniques for addressing health in individuals with obesity and unhealthy eating behaviors. All three are considered nondiet approaches, in that the traditional focus on dieting for weight loss is downplayed; instead, the focus is on increasing one's body awareness (to enhance the ability to recognize internal cues for fullness and satiety), improving one's attention to food and the process of eating, moving away from dieting and toward sustained lifestyle changes, and promoting an "all foods fit" mentality. This section discusses all three techniques as distinct but interrelated approaches for health promotion among individuals with obesity. Certain strategies or techniques are common to all three approaches, and distinctions or components unique to each approach are noted.

Mindful Eating

The term *mindfulness* typically refers to an intentional, nonjudgmental awareness of the present moment.[68] In the late 1990s, research emerged on the development and efficacy of mindful eating as a treatment for individuals with binge eating disorder.[69] Originally called mindfulness-based eating awareness training (MB-EAT), the approach stressed the importance of improving awareness of one's internal experiences and eating behaviors, enhancing self-efficacy and self-acceptance, interrupting unhealthy behavioral patterns through conscious food and activity choices, and decreasing reactivity to emotions and stress.[70,71] In addition, mindful eating approaches work to avoid mind*less* eating practices, or moments where the mind might be less able to concentrate on food, taste, and hunger (ie, when eating in front of a television or working through a lunch break).[72] With mindful eating, there are no restrictions on the types of food eaten as long as foods are eaten in a mindful way. These treatment strategies are thought to reduce emotional, appetite, and food-intake dysregulation.[73-75]

A core component of mindful eating is the identification of emotional and physical triggers for hunger, coupled with an increased awareness of sensory-specific satiety, a process whereby one's taste sensitivity decreases after eating small amounts of food. Together, these processes are thought to help individuals recognize taste satiety earlier, better regulate reward sensitivity in areas of the brain associated with eating and obesity, and rely more on internal physical cues to reduce overeating and food intake.[70] In contrast to similar approaches, mindfulness meditations are integral to the intervention. Mindful eating has been incorporated into a variety of treatment approaches for obesity, including ACT, intuitive eating, and HAES; however, MB-EAT and other mindfulness-based approaches are also used as standalone treatments for weight management.

Intuitive Eating

Intuitive eating is very similar to mindful eating (the two terms are often used interchangeably); however, it is a more weight-inclusive approach to health that focuses on rejecting diet culture and relying on internal as opposed to external cues in order to recognize and respond appropriately to satiety and fullness.[72,76] Like mindful eating practices, intuitive eating treatments involve improving one's awareness of hunger, fullness, and satiety cues.[72,76] However, intuitive eating also aims to give patients or clients unconditional permission to eat and to empower them to eat whatever and whenever they choose. Although this may seem counterintuitive and is different from traditional weight-management advice, giving the patient or client permission to eat is thought to reduce guilt and emotion-driven eating, thereby reducing the cycle of restriction and overeating as well as eating in the absence of hunger.[72,74] Unlike mindful eating approaches, the importance of rejecting dieting or weight loss is essential to intuitive eating, as diet culture is believed to trigger the cycle of restriction and subsequent emotional eating and binge eating. Thus, intuitive eating interventions focus on repairing a patient or client's relationship with food and with their body so that they are able to eat in a way that is more attuned to their hunger level and tastes.[77] The main tenets of intuitive eating are summarized in Box 13.3.[77]

BOX 13.3

Guiding Principles of Intuitive Eating[77]

1. Reject the diet mentality.
2. Honor your hunger.
3. Make peace with food.
4. Challenge the food police.
5. Discover the satisfaction factor.
6. Feel your fullness.
7. Cope with your emotions with kindness.
8. Respect your body.
9. Movement—feel the difference.
10. Honor your health with gentle nutrition.

Health at Every Size

The Health at Every Size (HAES) approach was popularized in research and weight-management literature in the early 2000s, although the origins of the HAES movement date back to the 1980s with the development of the National Association to Advance Fat Acceptance and the work of feminist scholars throughout this era. The movement emerged partially in response to perceived failures of traditional weight loss interventions to achieve or sustain prolonged weight loss, as well as increasing recognition of the negative impacts that weight-related stigma and sizeism can have on the health of people with obesity.[78,79] The HAES philosophy involves moving away from weight-focused strategies for health in individuals with larger body sizes and toward a health-focused paradigm that encourages body acceptance, intuitive eating, and intuitive exercise or "active embodiment."[80,81] Traditional HAES treatment programs include five key components: body acceptance, physical activity, nutrition, psychosocial support, and eating behaviors. At the initial phase of treatment, and continuing throughout, emphasis is placed on self-acceptance and self-worth, with the goal of enjoying life to the fullest, regardless of one's weight or shape.[82] Subsequently, psychoeducation on nutrition and exercise are provided through an intuitive eating lens (eg, relying on hunger, taste, and satiety cues).

Like intuitive eating, HAES is a more radical approach to healthy eating and activity, as it focuses not only on weight management but on the rejection of diet culture and the concept of health as defined by a "normal" weight.[83] The modern HAES movement also includes a focus on social justice—including the understanding of how systemic societal inequities contribute to health care inequities—as foundational to personal and societal health management.[84] Among other important distinctions, HAES requires practitioners and participants alike to reject the notions of "healthy" and "unhealthy" weights and sizes, to recognize the inherent dangers of dieting, and to promote acceptance of body diversity.[85] A key principle of HAES is the belief that any obesity intervention should, first and foremost, support and promote the development of health; thus, some weight-management techniques may be ineffective or even cause harm by strictly targeting weight loss.[82] To the extent that a healthy-lifestyle program stresses weight loss as a primary goal, even if conceived through an intuitive eating or mindful eating lens, it is incompatible with HAES.[86]

Figure 13.1 illustrates the similarities and differences between the three alternative counseling approaches to health in individuals with obesity.

Specific Tools and Strategies

Attuned Eating

The practice of attuned eating is used across HAES, mindful eating, and intuitive eating interventions, although it is perhaps best known within intuitive eating approaches. The central concept behind it is twofold: (1) regulate eating according to internal physical cues of hunger and satiety, and (2) mindfully attend to the process of consuming food.[74] The first component can be fostered through intuitive eating "check-ins" of one's level of hunger, fullness, and satiety throughout different parts of a meal. Especially in intuitive-eating approaches, this is often done by rating one's hunger and taste satisfaction on a scale of 0 to 10 throughout meals and snacks, with the intention of avoiding substantial hunger (which may lead to binge-eating behavior) and substantial fullness (which can trigger guilt, fasting, and then binge-eating behaviors).[76,87] Furthermore, individuals are challenged to distinguish between physical and emotional reasons for eating and to honor physical cues for hunger rather than psychological or environmental cues.

Perhaps one of the best-known mindful eating meditations for fostering attuned eating involves the careful observation, interaction, and eating of a single raisin.[88,89] This

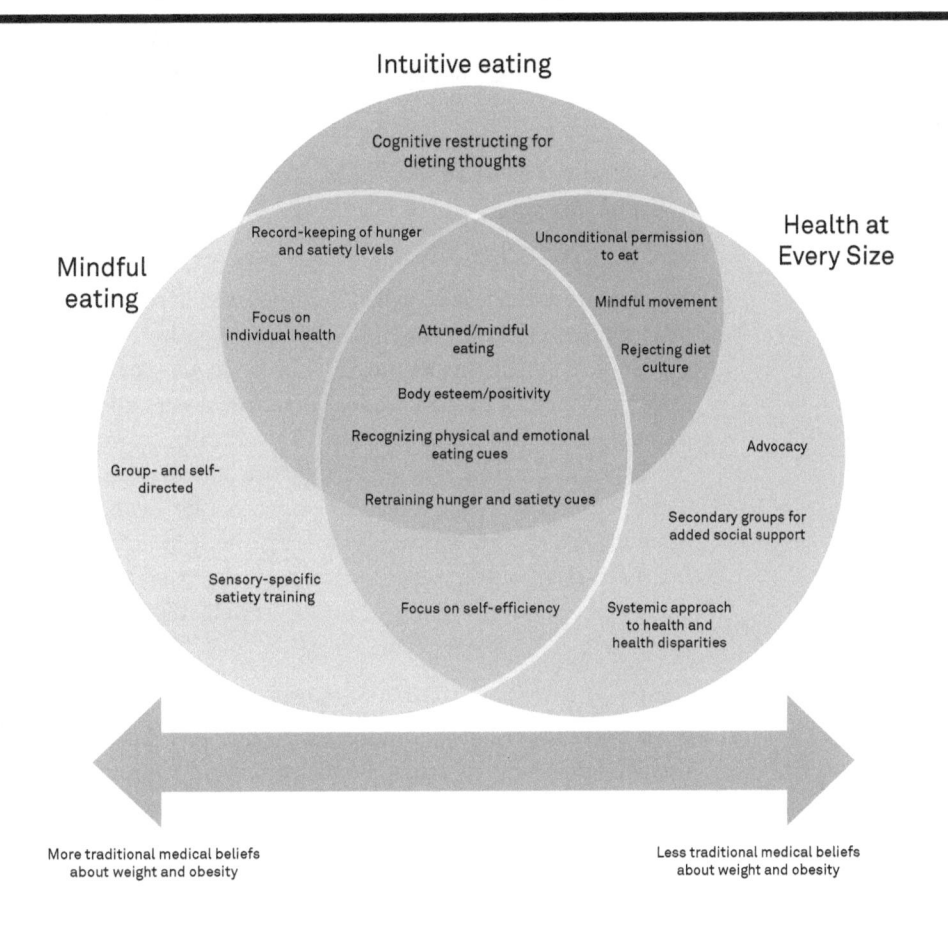

FIGURE 13.1 The overlap between the three nondiet approaches to health

meditation, which embodies the second component of attuned eating, involves attending to the sight, smell, feel, and context of a single raisin and where it came from, prior to the slow and careful consumption of that raisin. The aim of this meditation is to foster food and body awareness, reduce mindless or automatic food consumption, and promote slower, more careful eating.[88,89]

Daily Meditation

Meditation is a core component of mindful eating and has been shown to reduce emotional eating and binge eating among individuals with obesity.[90] Mindful eating interventions typically include a meditation exercise at each session, which can include breathing meditations, mindful eating meditations, and brief meditations for mealtimes and increasing mindfulness throughout the day.[71] Experts believe that frequent mindfulness meditation may increase body awareness, including the ability to better respond to hunger and satiety cues; moreover, increased mindfulness may reduce stress, negative emotions, and emotional reactivity, which are correlated with mindless eating, overeating, and binge eating.[90-94]

Unconditional Permission to Eat

Providing patients or clients with unconditional permission to eat is a core component of both the intuitive eating and HAES approaches.[77] This practice helps patients or clients feel empowered to eat wherever, whenever, and however much they want, and it aligns strongly with the goal of rejecting a diet culture that dichotomizes foods into good or bad, healthy or unhealthy.[77,85] Proponents of both HAES and intuitive eating suggest that removing such "food rules" reduces activation of the neurological reward pathway for previously forbidden foods, and that this, in turn, reduces emotional eating, binge eating, and feelings of guilt or shame following moments of eating less nutritionally dense foods.[95] To implement this strategy, providers sometimes ask patients or clients to bring their favorite foods to sessions and practice attuned eating. The intentional exposure to and consumption of previously forbidden, unhealthy, or off-limit foods help patients or clients understand and accept the idea that they have unconditional permission to eat.

Active Embodiment

Active embodiment (also called intuitive exercising or mindful movement) is the participation in movement and physical activity for the sake of enjoyment and for the physical benefits experienced in the body, as opposed to having weight loss as the objective.[82,96] This technique is practiced across all weight-neutral approaches to health and emphasizes exposure to a variety of activities and bringing attention to the physical sensations induced before and after any kind of physical activity. Some mindful eating interventions incorporate meditative activities, such as a mindful walk or yoga practice, to increase body awareness during exercise. Across most variations of these approaches, however, the intention of movement is deliberately separated from energy-burning or weight loss goals.

Rejecting Diet Culture

A central tenant of both intuitive eating and HAES is the rejection of dieting and societal constructs regarding food restriction.[77,84] From a HAES perspective, this includes the rejection of several key premises of weight loss medicine, including the beliefs that adiposity alone poses a major health risk, that weight can be used as an effective measure of health, and that weight loss is a practical and important goal for individuals with obesity.[86] Diet culture is, instead, seen as promoting poor body image, internalized weight stigma, negative emotions, disordered eating, and a drive for thinness, among other things.[77,97] These mental states are both highly unpleasant and counterproductive, as they can trigger feelings of deprivation, which are followed shortly after by craving and unhealthy eating behaviors, ultimately reducing a person's self-efficacy and causing more weight gain and poor health.[83,98] The strategy of rejecting diet culture may include having patients or clients throw away food and weight scales, uninstall calorie-counting smartphone applications, and learn about the purported dangers associated with chronic dieting.[77,99]

Body Respect and Body Positivity

A related but different technique used in interventions involving mindful eating, intuitive eating, and HAES is the promotion of positive body esteem. This can be accomplished in a variety of ways, including through body-positivity meditations, the recognition and rejection of self-perceptions caused by internalized diet culture, attuned eating, and unconditional permission to eat. From a HAES perspective, this may also involve engaging in activities or events that one previously avoided because of concerns about being viewed negatively by others; such activities may include swimming, dining out at restaurants, flying on an airplane, or going for a health check-up.[100,101] Other strategies may focus on improving body image through gratitude journaling, yoga interventions, and fostering self-compassion.[102] Finally, the HAES approach to body respect and positivity involves showing respect not only for one's own body but for the bodies of others as well.

Social Support

Although social support is a core component of all group interventions, it is especially important within the HAES framework.[82,83] Social support is often provided in the form of supplemental groups that meet separately during HAES interventions. These groups allow individuals to discuss their experiences of living in larger bodies, including their experiences of weight stigma and its impact on their physical and mental health. By providing this venue for individuals to voice these concerns, providers of HAES interventions can encourage their patients or clients to share strategies for asserting themselves or confronting stigma, for reducing feelings of internalized shame or guilt, and for making life choices based on quality of life over weight loss.[82,83]

Advocacy

Advocating for the rights and needs of individuals of all weights and sizes is a central theme in the HAES movement, which argues that the only effective approach to health is one that is systems-based and addresses systemic inequalities.[80,84,103] Advocacy in the HAES model encompasses both advocating for others and advocating for oneself. The former includes promoting size diversity by avoiding discriminating against others, supporting infrastructure that enables individuals of all sizes and abilities to participate equally, and speaking up for others when they are disregarded or stigmatized. Self-advocacy includes speaking up for oneself in the face of harmful comments made by family members, providers, and friends; refusing to weigh-in at physicians' offices; and insisting on weight-inclusive accommodations as needed.

Treatment Format and Structure

Recent reviews of the nondiet interventions—mindful eating, intuitive eating, and HAES—found that the duration of interventions was highly variable, ranging from 1.5 to 12 months, with 60- to 90-minute sessions on average.[104] However, most interventions lasted between 3 and 5 months, with some including monthly follow-up sessions or subsequent group-based opportunities to provide ongoing support for behavior change.[104,105] Interventions were almost exclusively delivered in groups, with the majority of interventions being delivered in person. Most treatment programs included weekly homework assignments that varied across approaches and interventions.[70,82,106] In all three types of nondiet interventions, didactic information on nutrition, exercise, and eating behaviors was provided, but it was given considerably less emphasis than in traditional weight-management programs.[72,94] Typically, weigh-ins, weight loss goals, and calorie-counting or food records were either secondary to intervention aims or actively discouraged as part of these treatment approaches.[74,80]

Although similar in many ways, these three interventions differ in key aspects of their treatment structure and format. Because mindful eating emphasizes meditation, a brief meditation is commonly included in each session to promote body awareness and enhance meditative practice. Intuitive eating interventions may involve having participants keep records of hunger, satiety, and fullness in order to better monitor satiety and promote intuitive eating. Finally, HAES groups traditionally include a strong element of social support and self-advocacy, with patients or clients learning techniques to assert themselves, reject stigma, and produce change to empower themselves.[82,86]

Empirical Support

Although the purpose of this chapter is to evaluate weight-management approaches for individuals with obesity, all three alternative approaches covered in this section are partially or radically opposed to weight loss as a primary health outcome for people with obesity. As one might expect, intuitive eating, mindful eating, and HAES interventions are less successful at producing short-term weight loss than traditional dieting programs.[76,83,107] In general, trials comparing HAES or intuitive eating interventions with traditional weight loss programs found that more conventional programs produced greater weight loss.[82,86,108] However, multiple reviews of all three alternative approaches concluded that these programs appear to promote weight maintenance and reduce weight gain during the intervention and through repeated follow-up.[76,105,107] Importantly, due to the nature of weight-neutral approaches, only some studies included outcomes on weight, thus limiting results and conclusions about efficacy for sustained prevention of weight gain. Moreover, most of these approaches are still relatively new, and studies evaluating longer-term weight outcomes of nondiet interventions (ie, beyond 24-month follow-up) are lacking.

Apart from weight-related outcomes, there is some support for the use of these alternative approaches in improving other indicators of health. In general, reviews suggest positive or neutral effects on physiological markers of health for all three approaches. Reviews identified generally positive improvements in blood pressure with HAES interventions, although this effect was not maintained at follow-up.[86,104,107] Additional benefits were found for glycemic control in patients or clients with obesity, particularly with HAES interventions, and positive or neutral findings were reported regarding improvements in cholesterol levels.[86,107]

Although there is limited evidence to support intuitive eating and HAES interventions as helpful for reducing overall food intake, partial support was found for using a mindful eating approach; this said, the findings were mixed with regard to improvements in diet quality and consumption of fruits and vegetables across all three approaches.[76,104,105,109] In contrast, many studies identified improvements in physical activity among mindful eating, intuitive eating, and HAES groups, and these improvements were at least partially sustained at follow-up visits.[104]

In addition to physical indicators of health, all three nondiet approaches may have benefits for mental health and general psychological well-being. Systematic reviews have identified that participants frequently score higher on measures of mindful eating, intuitive eating, self-esteem, body awareness, quality of life, and body satisfaction after these interventions.[76,86,104,107] Reduced symptoms or frequency of binge eating, disinhibited eating, emotional eating, and disordered eating have also been observed across all three approaches.[76,81,86,107] Individuals also tend to score lower on measures of dietary restraint, negative affect, drive for thinness measures, and disordered eating attitudes following treatment, and these benefits appear to be maintained at least partially at follow-up visits.[81,104,107] In addition, intuitive eating and HAES have demonstrated efficacy in reducing weight self-stigma among study participants.[81] Finally, a notable benefit of these programs is improved patient or client satisfaction and retention. Studies suggest that HAES and intuitive eating interventions may be perceived as more worthwhile or empowering relative to traditional diet interventions.[86,104] In addition, HAES and other nondiet approaches tend to have very good patient or client retention rates.[86,104]

Population Considerations

Individuals with frequent weight cycling, a history of chronic dieting, and a high degree of internalized weight stigma may be good candidates for intuitive eating, mindful eating, and HAES interventions.[83,86] In addition, all three interventions have demonstrated efficacy in reducing disordered eating behaviors as well as emotional eating, and the HAES approach specifically has been endorsed by several national and international organizations dedicated to eating disorders.[69,70,86] From a weight-management perspective, preliminary evidence suggests that these interventions may be effective for individuals who do not necessarily hope to lose weight but would like to improve their health or maintain a stable weight.[81,86] Finally, because HAES specifically addresses intersectional systems of health disparities and teaches self-advocacy within and outside of a health care system, some researchers have proposed that it may be effective at promoting healthy behaviors in individuals of color and those within lesbian, gay, bisexual, transgender, queer (or questioning), asexual (or allied), and intersex (LGBTQAI+) communities.[103] However, if the primary goal of an individual and their treatment team is weight loss, these interventions are unlikely to be very effective. Finally, for individuals with medical comorbidities with substantial dietary restrictions or who would benefit from adherence to a specific, structured dietary plan, these approaches may be contraindicated, given their emphasis on an all-foods-fit approach.

Other Treatment Considerations

Selection and Integration of Counseling Approaches

It is important that the counseling approach employed with a patient or client be consistent with the patient or client's needs, preferences, values, and treatment goals. In addition, the practitioner must be properly trained and equipped to engage in the selected counseling approach. Practitioners should have the appropriate qualifications for the selected approach, as qualifications differ by modality. For example, CBT and ABT for weight management involve a variety of techniques and often require specialized skills and training for their proper implementation. Thus, these modalities are often delivered or supervised by a clinical psychologist or other mental health practitioner. However, other specialized providers (eg, registered dietitian nutritionists) can be taught to deliver many elements of these interventions with thorough training, experience, and supervision. Because CBT is more established and widespread than ABT, more practitioners are trained in the former than in the latter. Although ABT-based interventions share many common elements with CBT, practitioners require additional formal training in ABT for these interventions to be effective. Motivational interviewing can be effectively delivered by a wide range of health care providers, many of whom participate in a full day of training (or more) in this modality prior to its implementation. Like CBT and ABT, motivational interviewing is most effective when the practitioner has sufficient "hands-on" experience in using the approach and the associated counseling techniques.

Across all counseling strategies, developing and maintaining a strong rapport and trust with the patient or client is crucial to treatment engagement and successful outcomes, and a patient or client-centered stance should be maintained throughout treatment. In some instances, this may require making adaptations to counseling strategies and specific behavior-change techniques used in treatment. For instance, if a patient or client is particularly ambivalent about behavior change, more motivational interviewing may be needed to increase treatment buy-in, bolster motivation, and facilitate change talk. A patient or client who responds to major life challenges with impulsive or mindless eating may benefit from placing greater emphasis on these topics in treatment and incorporating more attuned-eating exercises into treatment sessions.

In many respects, the different counseling approaches described in this chapter there are substantial and complementarity. Thus, integration of different approaches and techniques is appropriate and even expected in some cases. In particular, as ABT builds on CBT, it is not difficult to incorporate ABT-informed strategies into CBT interventions and vice versa. For example, a discussion of values-congruent behavior could be a valuable addition to a CBT intervention and result in better treatment adherence. Although ABT and CBT share many common features, there are important distinctions as well. Perhaps one of the biggest differences lies in the specific tools used in each (eg, distress tolerance in ABT vs cognitive restructuring in CBT). Acceptance and defusion strategies in ABT are forms of cognitive restructuring that are well suited to patients or clients with cognitive disinhibition or cognitive inflexibility. ABT and CBT also differ in their strategies for dealing with environmental stimuli. A CBT practitioner might encourage a patient or client to remove energy-dense foods from the home so that the stimulus can be avoided. In contrast, an ABT practitioner might encourage urge surfing as a tool for distress tolerance in the presence of energy-dense, highly palatable foods. However, stimulus control could be used in ABT, as long as it is value-congruent and does not foster avoidance on the patient or client's part.

Similarities between ABT, mindful eating, and intuitive eating are also apparent, and these approaches are complementary in some respects. Yet, like CBT and ABT, they differ in important ways. Both mindful eating and intuitive eating emphasize minimizing distractions while eating and paying attention to hunger and satiety cues. However, intuitive eating does not restrict the type of food eaten and gives patients or clients unconditional permission to eat. Intuitive eating may be a more appropriate strategy for patients or clients with a history of unhealthy food restriction. Some mindful eating programs share characteristics with ABT approaches as well. Both approaches emphasize value clarification and psychological flexibility. Mindful eating, however, places much more emphasis on mindfulness. Mindful eating does not necessarily involve a goal of weight loss; therefore, many of the other behavioral strategies present in ABT are not present in mindful eating approaches.

Special Populations

Older adults and young adults are two groups that are typically underrepresented in weight loss interventions. Young adults (aged 18 to 35 years) experience major life changes that can be associated with weight gain, such as leaving home, getting married, and having children. This age group demonstrates high rates of weight gain,[110] but young adults do not typically enroll in weight loss intervention programs. If they do enroll, they experience higher rates of attrition and lower rates of weight loss compared to their older counterparts.[111] When interventions are tailored to young adults, they are successful at producing weight loss.[112] Similarly, older adults also have unique risk factors to consider, such as limitations on physical activity and high rates of medical comorbidities. Existing interventions may need to be modified for older adults, specifically with regard to physical activity recommendations.

Race can also influence treatment outcomes, and practitioners may consider a patient or client's race when deciding on a treatment plan (refer to Chapter 2). Historically, participants in behavioral weight loss interventions have usually been White cisgender women. Obesity interventions are understudied in minority populations, even though non-White individuals are disproportionately affected by obesity and its comorbid conditions. Culturally sensitive interventions for diverse populations are beginning to emerge. A 2021 meta-analysis of weight loss interventions for Hispanic women† concluded that outcomes of weight loss interventions in Hispanic women are highly variable and more research is needed with adequate sample sizes to determine how effective interventions are with this population.[113] Black individuals demonstrate attenuated weight loss outcomes in response to CBT interventions compared to White individuals during the initial phase of weight loss, though this discrepancy may be less pronounced over the long term.[114-116] As previously discussed, ABT-based interventions may be more effective for Black patients or clients,[54] although additional work is needed to replicate these findings.

In general, more research on how to tailor existing interventions to improve outcomes for Black patients or clients (and patients or clients from other minority groups) is needed. Research efforts need to increase focus on recruiting diverse samples, as minority populations are disproportionately affected by obesity and comorbid conditions but are greatly underrepresented in the intervention literature. Males are also substantially underrepresented in studies of weight loss treatments. Recruitment strategies intended to increase the number of males in behavioral interventions is needed to investigate the efficacy of such approaches. HAES approaches may be well-accepted and effective for health promotion among patients or clients of color and patients or clients who are LGBTQIA+,[105] but these alternative approaches do not typically achieve substantial weight reductions.

---

† Study participants were described as women. Gender was not further specified.

Weight loss interventions can also be tailored to patients or clients with serious mental illnesses who may not be able to participate in traditionally delivered interventions. Rates of obesity are high among people with serious mental illnesses, and many medications traditionally prescribed for serious mental illnesses have weight gain as a side effect. Furthermore, cardiovascular disease, a consequence of obesity, is a leading cause of death in this population, thus highlighting the need for effective weight-management interventions for this group. Interventions can be modified for this patient or client population to accommodate cognitive deficits as well as barriers to healthy eating and physical activity.[117] Interventions that are longer in duration; that target deficits in motivation, memory, and executive function; and that include group exercise sessions have been shown to be effective for this population.[117,118]

Delivery Modality

Generally, CBT and ABT interventions are delivered in a weekly, in-person format, and there is some indication that group-based interventions may be more effective than individual treatment.[119] Alternative modalities have also been explored. In particular, technology-based weight-management interventions have garnered much attention among researchers in recent years (refer to Chapter 17). Because in-person treatment sessions can be burdensome to patients or clients in that they require time, means of transportation, and proximity to programs and centers, interventions delivered via the internet or smartphone applications (eHealth interventions) have been developed to address these barriers. The amount of interaction of patients or clients with each other (in the case of group-based interventions) and with practitioners varies in eHealth interventions. A meta-analysis published in 2019 suggests that eHealth interventions are effective at producing clinically significant weight loss, but the amount of weight lost is less than with in-person interventions.[120] High heterogeneity between eHealth intervention trials suggests that more research is needed to identify intervention components that are associated with positive outcomes. Some components of eHealth interventions that have been shown to improve outcomes are financial incentives,[121] frequent engagement with treatment materials,[122] and support from practitioners with personalized feedback.[123,124]

ABT interventions are typically delivered via in-person groups, but some researchers are investigating remotely delivered ABT. Although eHealth ABT interventions have not been extensively studied, results from one trial indicated that an online, guided, self-help, ABT-based program achieved significant improvements in healthy eating, psychological inflexibility, and weight self-stigma, but not in physical activity.[125] More research is warranted. Another intriguing alternative method for delivering ABT-based interventions is through relatively brief, in-person workshops. Some evidence suggests that these types of workshops can increase participants' level of physical activity and satisfaction with their bodies in as little as one 4-hour session, and participants also showed decreases in internalized weight stigma and food dependence. Although ABT workshop interventions have not been shown to improve weight loss outcomes, the other benefits make them a promising area of future research.[47,126]

Future Directions

Several topics warrant more research in order to better understand the most effective and feasible counseling approaches for weight management and health promotion in individuals with obesity. Currently, little is known about which interventions may be most suitable for certain individuals or groups. Identifying which treatments works best for whom and under what conditions (ie, precision medicine and nutrition) is an exciting and challenging frontier for researchers in the field of obesity and weight management. In addition, adaptive interventions, which involve modifications to the type or intensity of treatment (or both) based on an individual patient or client's characteristics or response to initial treatment, offer another opportunity to better meet the needs of patients or clients and improve treatment outcomes. With the development of mobile technology (eg, wearable devices, smartphone applications), adaptive interventions can be tailored to individuals in real time based on their current actions, situations, resources, or challenges. Called "just-in-time" adaptive interventions, these novel interventions are typically used in conjunction with mobile devices such as smartphones, digital scales, or activity tracking devices, and they prompt the patient or client to rate their mood, cravings, and other factors several times throughout the day. If a patient or client reports distress, a craving, or a negative emotional state, for instance, intervention and support can be delivered to the patient or client in real time. Although such approaches have great potential, more research is needed to determine efficacy for weight loss.[127]

Additional research is also needed into effective weight-management interventions and counseling approaches that target certain high-risk life stages for obesity. Some life stages—adolescence, young adulthood, pregnancy, and the postpartum period, for example—are associated with accelerated weight gain or increased susceptibility to developing obesity. Although some effort has been made to tailor interventions to patients or clients in these life stages,[128] these populations remain relatively understudied in terms of weight management.

Regardless of the population targeted, many weight-management interventions are intensive, require frequent provider-patient or client contact, and can thus be burdensome for providers and program participants. Research is needed to develop streamlined and potentially targeted interventions that reduce this burden and the resources required to sustain treatment yet still maintain their efficacy. Future advances in this area are particularly relevant to the ongoing effort to translate evidence-based interventions into "real-world" community and clinical settings.

Finally, one of the greatest opportunities we have to improve the impact of counseling and behavior-change strategies for weight management is to address the challenge of weight loss maintenance following treatment. Novel strategies for maintaining patient or client engagement and motivation for sustained behavior change are crucial for maximizing the public health impact of these interventions.

Summary

Several counseling approaches, including CBT, ABT, and motivational interviewing, have strong empirical support for their application in weight-management interventions. Even in the absence of substantial weight loss, a number of non-diet counseling strategies (mindful eating, intuitive eating, and HHAES) may be beneficial for improving physical and psychological health in targeted populations. Although there is some overlap among the various counseling approaches, each has its important distinguishing characteristics. These defining characteristics and areas of emphasis may make certain counseling strategies more appropriate than others for certain populations or treatment goals. The various counseling approaches can also be integrated when appropriate. Regardless of the specific approach or combination of approaches employed, evidence-based counseling strategies represent an essential component of lifestyle interventions for weight management. Effective counseling and evidence-based techniques are necessary for the initiation and maintenance of behavior change and sustained motivation for behavior change to promote successful weight management.

References

1. Nezu CM, Nezu AM, eds. *The Oxford Handbook of Cognitive and Behavioral Therapies*. Oxford University Press; 2016.
2. Hofmann SG, Asnaani A, Vonk IJJ, Sawyer AT, Fang A. The efficacy of cognitive behavioral therapy: a review of meta-analyses. *Cogn Ther Res*. 2012;36(5):427-440. doi:10.1007/s10608-012-9476-1
3. Sperry L. *Treatment of Chronic Medical Conditions Cognitive-Behavioral Therapy Strategies and Integrative Treatment Protocols*. American Psychological Association; 2009.
4. Ferster CB, Nurnberger JI, Levitt EB. The control of eating. *Obes Res*. 1996 [1962];4(4):401-410.
5. Foster GD, Makris AP, Bailer BA. Behavioral treatment of obesity. *Am J Clin Nutr*. 2005;82(1 suppl):230S-235S. doi:10.1093/ajcn/82.1.230S
6. Bandura A. *Social Foundations of Thought and Action: A Social Cognitive Theory*. Prentice-Hall; 1986:xiii, 617.
7. Dutton GR, Perri MG. Delivery, evaluation, and future directions for cognitive-behavioral treatments of obesity. In: Nezu CM, Nezu AM, eds. *The Oxford Handbook of Cognitive and Behavioral Therapies*. Oxford University Press; 2016:419-437.
8. Wadden TA, Foster GD. Behavioral treatment of obesity. *Med Clin North Am*. 2000;84(2):441-461, vii. doi:10.1016/s0025-7125(05)70230-3
9. Stuart RB. Behavioral control of overeating. *Behav Res Ther*. 1967;5(4):357-365. doi:10.1016/0005-7967(67)90027-7
10. Butryn ML, Webb V, Wadden TA. Behavioral treatment of obesity. *Psychiatr Clin North Am*. 2011;34(4):841-859. doi:10.1016/j.psc.2011.08.006
11. Skinner BF. *Science and Human Behavior*. Macmillan; 1953.
12. Burke LE, Wang J, Sevick MA. Self-monitoring in weight loss: a systematic review of the literature. *J Am Diet Assoc*. 2011;111(1):92-102. doi:10.1016/j.jada.2010.10.008
13. Zheng Y, Klem ML, Sereika SM, Danford CA, Ewing LJ, Burke LE. Self-weighing in weight management: a systematic literature review. *Obes (Silver Spring)*. 2015;23(2):256-265. doi:10.1002/oby.20946
14. Diabetes Prevention Program (DPP) Research Group. The Diabetes Prevention Program (DPP): description of lifestyle intervention. *Diabetes Care*. 2002;25(12):2165-2171. doi:10.2337/diacare.25.12.2165
15. Look AHEAD Research Group; Wadden TA, West DS, et al. The Look AHEAD study: a description of the lifestyle intervention and the evidence supporting it. *Obes (Silver Spring)*. 2006;14(5):737-752. doi:10.1038/oby.2006.84
16. Perri MG, Nezu AM, McKelvey WF, Shermer RL, Renjilian DA, Viegener BJ. Relapse prevention training and problem-solving therapy in the long-term management of obesity. *J Consult Clin Psychol*. 2001;69(4):722-726.
17. Murawski ME, Milsom VA, Ross KM, et al. Problem solving, treatment adherence, and weight-loss outcome among women participating in lifestyle treatment for obesity. *Eat Behav*. 2009;10(3):146-151. doi:10.1016/j.eatbeh.2009.03.005
18. Berkel LA, Poston WSC, Reeves RS, Foreyt JP. Behavioral interventions for obesity. *J Am Diet Assoc*. 2005;105(5 suppl 1):S35-S43. doi:10.1016/j.jada.2005.02.031

19. Gorin A, Phelan S, Tate D, Sherwood N, Jeffery R, Wing R. Involving support partners in obesity treatment. *J Consult Clin Psychol*. 2005;73(2):341-343. doi:10.1037/0022-006X.73.2.341
20. Wing RR, Jeffery RW. Benefits of recruiting participants with friends and increasing social support for weight loss and maintenance. *J Consult Clin Psychol*. 1999;67(1):132-138. doi:10.1037/0022-006X.67.1.132
21. Brownell KD, Marlatt GA, Lichtenstein E, Wilson GT. Understanding and preventing relapse. *Am Psychol*. 1986;41(7):765-782. doi:10.1037//0003-066x.41.7.765
22. Cash TF. Body-image attitudes: evaluation, investment, and affect. *Percept Mot Skills*. 1994;78(3 pt 2):1168-1170. doi:10.2466/pms.1994.78.3c.1168
23. Wadden TA, Butryn ML, Byrne KJ. Efficacy of lifestyle modification for long-term weight control. *Obes Res*. 2004;12 suppl:151S-162S. doi:10.1038/oby.2004.282
24. Wing RR. Behavioral weight control. In: Wadden TA, Stunkard AJ, eds. *Handbook of Obesity Treatment*. Guilford Press; 2002:301-316.
25. Wing RR, Lang W, Wadden TA, et al. Benefits of modest weight loss in improving cardiovascular risk factors in overweight and obese individuals with type 2 diabetes. *Diabetes Care*. 2011;34(7):1481-1486. doi:10.2337/dc10-2415
26. Cardiovascular effects of intensive lifestyle intervention in type 2 diabetes. *N Engl J Med*. 2013;369(2):145-154. doi:10.1056/NEJMoa1212914
27. Knowler WC, Barrett-Connor E, Fowler SE, et al. Reduction in the incidence of type 2 diabetes with lifestyle intervention or metformin. *N Engl J Med*. 2002;346(6):393-403. doi:10.1056/NEJMoa012512
28. Look AHEAD Research Group; Pi-Sunyer X, Blackburn G, et al. Reduction in weight and cardiovascular disease risk factors in individuals with type 2 diabetes: one-year results of the Look AHEAD trial. *Diabetes Care*. 2007;30(6):1374-1383. doi:10.2337/dc07-0048
29. Effects of weight loss and sodium reduction intervention on blood pressure and hypertension incidence in overweight people with high-normal blood pressure: the Trials of Hypertension Prevention, phase II. *Arch Intern Med*. 1997;157(6):657-667.
30. Perri MG, Corsica JA. Improving the maintenance of weight lost in behavioral treatment of obesity. In: Wadden TA, Stunkard AJ, eds. *Handbook of Obesity Treatment*. Guilford Press; 2002:357-379.
31. Kramer FM, Jeffery RW, Forster JL, Snell MK. Long-term follow-up of behavioral treatment for obesity: patterns of weight regain among men and women. *Int J Obes*. 1989;13(2):123-136.
32. Perri MG, Nezu AM, Patti ET, McCann KL. Effect of length of treatment on weight loss. *J Consult Clin Psychol*. 1989;57(3):450-452.
33. Perri MG. Effects of behavioral treatment on long-term weight loss: lessons learned from the Look AHEAD trial. *Obes (Silver Spring)*. 2014;22(1):3-4. doi:10.1002/oby.20672
34. Jensen MD, Ryan DH, Apovian CM, et al. 2013 AHA/ACC/TOS guideline for the management of overweight and obesity in adults: a report of the American College of Cardiology/American Heart Association Task Force on Practice Guidelines and The Obesity Society. *Circulation*. 2014;129(25 suppl 2):S102-S138. doi:10.1161/01.cir.0000437739.71477.ee
35. Look AHEAD Research Group. Eight-year weight losses with an intensive lifestyle intervention: the Look AHEAD study. *Obes (Silver Spring)*. 2014;22(1):5-13. doi:10.1002/oby.20662
36. Wadden TA, Neiberg RH, Wing RR, et al. Four-year weight losses in the Look AHEAD study: factors associated with long-term success. *Obes (Silver Spring)*. 2011;19(10):1987-1998. doi:10.1038/oby.2011.230
37. Burke LE, Conroy MB, Sereika SM, et al. The effect of electronic self-monitoring on weight loss and dietary intake: a randomized behavioral weight loss trial. *Obes (Silver Spring)*. 2011;19(2):338-344. doi:10.1038/oby.2010.208
38. Krukowski RA, Harvey-Berino J, Bursac Z, Ashikaga T, West DS. Patterns of success: online self-monitoring in a web-based behavioral weight control program. *Health Psychol*. 2013;32(2):164-170. doi:10.1037/a0028135
39. Williamson DA, Rejeski J, Lang W, et al. Impact of a weight management program on health-related quality of life in overweight adults with type 2 diabetes. *Arch Intern Med*. 2009;169(2):163-171. doi:10.1001/archinternmed.2008.544
40. Rubin RR, Wadden TA, Bahnson JL, et al. Impact of intensive lifestyle intervention on depression and health-related quality of life in type 2 diabetes: the Look AHEAD Trial. *Diabetes Care*. 2014;37(6):1544-1553. doi:10.2337/dc13-1928
41. Rejeski WJ, Ip EH, Bertoni AG, et al. Lifestyle change and mobility in obese adults with type 2 diabetes. *N Engl J Med*. 2012;366(13):1209-1217. doi:10.1056/NEJMoa1110294
42. Hayes SC, Strosahl KD, Wilson KG. *Acceptance and Commitment Therapy: An Experiential Approach to Behavior Change*. Guilford Press; 1999.
43. Harris R. *ACT Made Simple: An Easy-to-Read Primer on Acceptance and Commitment Therapy*. New Harbinger Publications; 2019.
44. Forman EM, Butryn ML. *Effective Weight Loss: An Acceptance-Based Behavioral Approach: Clinician Guide*. Oxford University Press; 2016.
45. Skinner BF. *About Behaviorism*. Knopf; 1974.
46. Frayn M, Khanyari S, Knäuper B. A 1-day acceptance and commitment therapy workshop leads to reductions in emotional eating in adults. *Eat Weight Disord*. 2020;25(5):1399-1411. doi:10.1007/s40519-019-00778-6
47. Lillis J, Schumacher LM, Bond DS. Preliminary evaluation of a 1-day acceptance and commitment therapy workshop for increasing moderate-to-vigorous physical activity in adults with overweight or obesity. *Int J Behav Med*. 2021;28(6):827-833. doi:10.1007/s12529-021-09965-1

48. Forman EM, Butryn ML, Hoffman KL, Herbert JD. An open trial of an acceptance-based behavioral intervention for weight loss. *Cogn Behav Pract*. 2009;16(2):223-235.

49. Goodwin CL, Forman EM, Herbert JD, Butryn ML, Ledley GS. A pilot study examining the initial effectiveness of a brief acceptance-based behavior therapy for modifying diet and physical activity among cardiac patients. *Behav Modif*. 2012;36(2):199-217. doi:10.1177/0145445511427770

50. Niemeier HM, Leahey T, Reed KP, Brown RA, Wing RR. An acceptance-based behavioral intervention for weight loss: a pilot study. *Behav Ther*. 2012;43(2):427-435. doi:10.1016/j.beth.2011.10.005

51. Forman EM, Butryn ML, Juarascio AS, et al. The mind your health project: a randomized controlled trial of an innovative behavioral treatment for obesity. *Obesity (Silver Spring)*. 2013;21(6):1119-1126. doi:10.1002/oby.20169

52. Forman EM, Manasse SM, Butryn ML, Crosby RD, Dallal DH, Crochiere RJ. Long-term follow-up of the Mind Your Health project: acceptance-based versus standard behavioral treatment for obesity. *Obesity (Silver Spring)*. 2019;27(4):565-571. doi:10.1002/oby.22412

53. Lillis J, Niemeier HM, Thomas JG, et al. A randomized trial of an acceptance-based behavioral intervention for weight loss in people with high internal disinhibition. *Obesity (Silver Spring)*. 2016;24(12):2509-2514. doi:10.1002/oby.21680

54. Butryn ML, Forman EM, Lowe MR, Gorin AA, Zhang F, Schaumberg K. Efficacy of environmental and acceptance-based enhancements to behavioral weight loss treatment: the ENACT trial. *Obesity (Silver Spring)*. 2017;25(5):866-872. doi:10.1002/oby.21813

55. Resnicow K, Davis R, Rollnick S. Motivational interviewing for pediatric obesity: conceptual issues and evidence review. *J Am Diet Assoc*. 2006;106(12):2024-2033. doi:10.1016/j.jada.2006.09.015

56. Miller WR, Rollnick S. *Motivational Interviewing: Preparing People to Change Addictive Behaviour*. Guilford Press; 1991.

57. Treasure J. Motivational interviewing. *Adv Psychiatr Treat*. 2004;10(5):331-337.

58. Miller WR, Rollnick S. *Motivational Interviewing: Helping People Change*. Guilford Press; 2012.

59. Rogers CR. *Client-Centered Therapy; Its Current Practice, Implications, and Theory*. Houghton Mifflin; 1951.

60. Festinger L. *A Theory of Cognitive Dissonance*. Stanford University Press; 1957.

61. Bem DJ. Self-perception: an alternative interpretation of cognitive dissonance phenomena. *Psychol Rev*. 1967;74(3):183.

62. Prochaska JO, Velicer WF. The transtheoretical model of health behavior change. *Am J Health Promot*. 1997;12(1):38-48.

63. Levounis P, Arnaout B, Marienfeld C, eds. *Motivational Interviewing for Clinical Practice*. American Psychiatric Association Publishing; 2017.

64. Patel ML, Wakayama LN, Bass MB, Breland JY. Motivational interviewing in eHealth and telehealth interventions for weight loss: a systematic review. *Prev Med*. 2019;126:105738.

65. Armstrong MJ, Mottershead TA, Ronksley PE, Sigal RJ, Campbell TS, Hemmelgarn BR. Motivational interviewing to improve weight loss in overweight and/or obese patients: a systematic review and meta-analysis of randomized controlled trials. *Obes Rev*. 2011;12(9):709-723.

66. Barnes RD, Ivezaj V. A systematic review of motivational interviewing for weight loss among adults in primary care. *Obes Rev*. 2015;16(4):304-318.

67. Simpson SA, McNamara R, Shaw C, et al. A feasibility randomised controlled trial of a motivational interviewing-based intervention for weight loss maintenance in adults. *Health Technol Assess*. 2015;19(50):v-vi, xix-xxv, 1-378. doi:10.3310/hta19500

68. Nelson JB. Mindful eating: the art of presence while you eat. *Diabetes Spectr*. 2017;30(3):171-174. doi:10.2337/ds17-0015

69. Kristeller JL, Hallett CB. An exploratory study of a meditation-based intervention for binge eating disorder. *J Health Psychol*. 1999;4(3):357-363. doi:10.1177/135910539900400305

70. Kristeller J, Wolever RQ, Sheets V. Mindfulness-Based Eating Awareness Training (MB-EAT) for binge eating: a randomized clinical trial. *Mindfulness*. 2014;5(3):282-297. doi:10.1007/s12671-012-0179-1

71. Kristeller JL, Wolever RQ. Mindfulness-based eating awareness training for treating binge eating disorder: the conceptual foundation. *Eat Disord*. 2011;19(1):49-61. doi:10.1080/10640266.2011.533605

72. Mathieu J. What should you know about mindful and intuitive eating? *J Am Diet Assoc*. 2009;109(12):1987. doi:10.1016/j.jada.2009.10.023

73. Pivarunas B, Conner BT. Impulsivity and emotion dysregulation as predictors of food addiction. *Eat Behav*. 2015;19:9-14. doi:10.1016/j.eatbeh.2015.06.007

74. Kerin JL, Webb HJ, Zimmer-Gembeck MJ. Intuitive, mindful, emotional, external and regulatory eating behaviours and beliefs: an investigation of the core components. *Appetite*. 2019;132:139-146. doi:10.1016/j.appet.2018.10.011

75. VanderBroek-Stice L, Stojek MK, Beach SRH, vanDellen MR, MacKillop J. Multidimensional assessment of impulsivity in relation to obesity and food addiction. *Appetite*. 2017;112:59-68. doi:10.1016/j.appet.2017.01.009

76. Warren JM, Smith N, Ashwell M. A structured literature review on the role of mindfulness, mindful eating and intuitive eating in changing eating behaviours: effectiveness and associated potential mechanisms. *Nutr Res Rev*. 2017;30(2):272-283. doi:10.1017/S0954422417000154

77. 10 principles of intuitive eating. IntuitiveEating.org. Accessed January 5, 2022. www.intuitiveeating.org/10-principles-of-intuitive-eating

78. Tomiyama AJ, Carr D, Granberg EM, et al. How and why weight stigma drives the obesity "epidemic" and harms health. *BMC Med*. 2018;16(1):123. doi:10.1186/s12916-018-1116-5

79. O'Hara L, Ahmed H, Elashie S. Evaluating the impact of a brief Health at Every Size®-informed health promotion activity on body positivity and internalized weight-based oppression. *Body Image*. 2021;37:225-237. doi:10.1016/j.bodyim.2021.02.006

80. Penney TL, Kirk SFL. The Health at Every Size paradigm and obesity: missing empirical evidence may help push the reframing obesity debate forward. *Am J Public Health*. 2015;105(5):e38-e42. doi:10.2105/AJPH.2015.302552

81. Ulian MD, Aburad L, da Silva Oliveira MS, et al. Effects of Health at Every Size® interventions on health-related outcomes of people with overweight and obesity: a systematic review. *Obes Rev*. 2018;19(12):1659-1666. doi:10.1111/obr.12749

82. Bacon L, Keim NL, Van Loan MD, et al. Evaluating a "non-diet" wellness intervention for improvement of metabolic fitness, psychological well-being and eating and activity behaviors. *Int J Obes Relat Metab Disord*. 2002;26(6):854-865. doi:10.1038/sj.ijo.0802012

83. Bacon L, Stern JS, Van Loan MD, Keim NL. Size acceptance and intuitive eating improve health for obese, female chronic dieters. *J Am Diet Assoc*. 2005;105(6):929-936. doi:10.1016/j.jada.2005.03.011

84. Health at Every Size community resources. Accessed January 5, 2022. https://haescommunity.com

85. Robison J, Putnam K, McKibbin L. Health at Every Size: a compassionate, effective approach for helping individuals with weight-related concerns—part II. *AAOHN J*. 2007;55(5):185-192. doi:10.1177/216507990705500503

86. Bacon L, Aphramor L. Weight science: evaluating the evidence for a paradigm shift. *Nutr J*. 2011;10(1):9. doi:10.1186/1475-2891-10-9

87. Hinton EC, Leary SD, Comlek L, Rogers PJ, Hamilton-Shield JP. How full am I? The effect of rating fullness during eating on food intake, eating speed and relationship with satiety responsiveness. *Appetite*. 2021;157:104998. doi:10.1016/j.appet.2020.104998

88. Mantzios M, Egan H, Asif T. A randomised experiment evaluating the mindful raisin practice as a method of reducing chocolate consumption during and after a mindless activity. *J Cogn Enhanc*. 2020;4(3):250-257. doi:10.1007/s41465-019-00159-y

89. Alber S. *Eating Mindfully*. 3rd ed. New Harbinger Publications; 2012.

90. Katterman SN, Kleinman BM, Hood MM, Nackers LM, Corsica JA. Mindfulness meditation as an intervention for binge eating, emotional eating, and weight loss: a systematic review. *Eat Behav*. 2014;15(2):197-204. doi:10.1016/j.eatbeh.2014.01.005

91. Fjorback LO, Walach H. Meditation based therapies—a systematic review and some critical observations. *Religions*. 2012;3(1):1-18. doi:10.3390/rel3010001

92. Rose MH, Nadler EP, Mackey ER. Impulse control in negative mood states, emotional eating, and food addiction are associated with lower quality of life in adolescents with severe obesity. *J Pediatr Psychol*. 2018;43(4):443-451. doi:10.1093/jpepsy/jsx127

93. Boggiano MM, Burgess EE, Turan B, et al. Motives for eating tasty foods associated with binge-eating: results from a student and a weight-loss seeking population. *Appetite*. 2014;83:160-166. doi:10.1016/j.appet.2014.08.026

94. Dalen J, Smith BW, Shelley BM, Sloan AL, Leahigh L, Begay D. Pilot study: Mindful Eating and Living (MEAL): weight, eating behavior, and psychological outcomes associated with a mindfulness-based intervention for people with obesity. *Complement Ther Med*. 2010;18(6):260-264. doi:10.1016/j.ctim.2010.09.008

95. Carbonneau E, Bégin C, Lemieux S, et al. A Health at Every Size intervention improves intuitive eating and diet quality in Canadian women. *Clin Nutr*. 2017;36(3):747-754. doi:10.1016/j.clnu.2016.06.008

96. Brevers D, Rogiers A, Defontaine A, et al. Implementation intention for initiating intuitive eating and active embodiment in obese patients using a smartphone application. *Front Psychiatry*. 2017;8:243. doi:10.3389/fpsyt.2017.00243

97. Braun TD, Unick JL, Abrantes AM, et al. Intuitive eating buffers the link between internalized weight stigma and body mass index in stressed adults. *Appetite*. 2022;169:105810. doi:10.1016/j.appet.2021.105810

98. Tomiyama AJ. Weight stigma is stressful: a review of evidence for the Cyclic Obesity/Weight-Based Stigma model. *Appetite*. 2014;82:8-15. doi:10.1016/j.appet.2014.06.108

99. Memon AN, Gowda AS, Rallabhandi B, et al. Have our attempts to curb obesity done more harm than good? *Cureus*. 12(9):e10275. doi:10.7759/cureus.10275

100. Lewis S, Thomas SL, Blood RW, Castle DJ, Hyde J, Komesaroff PA. How do obese individuals perceive and respond to the different types of obesity stigma that they encounter in their daily lives? A qualitative study. *Soc Sci Med*. 2011;73(9):1349-1356. doi:10.1016/j.socscimed.2011.08.021

101. Thedinga HK, Zehl R, Thiel A. Weight stigma experiences and self-exclusion from sport and exercise settings among people with obesity. *BMC Public Health*. 2021;21(1):565. doi:10.1186/s12889-021-10565-7

102. Guest E, Costa B, Williamson H, Meyrick J, Halliwell E, Harcourt D. The effectiveness of interventions aiming to promote positive body image in adults: a systematic review. *Body Image*. 2019;30:10-25. doi:10.1016/j.bodyim.2019.04.002

103. Rauchwerk A, Vipperman-Cohen A, Padmanabhan S, Parasram W, Burt KG. The case for a Health at Every Size approach for chronic disease risk reduction in women of color. *J Nutr Educ Behav*. 2020;52(11):1066-1072. doi:10.1016/j.jneb.2020.08.004

104. Schaefer JT, Magnuson AB. A review of interventions that promote eating by internal cues. *J Acad Nutr Diet*. 2014;114(5):734-760. doi:10.1016/j.jand.2013.12.024

105. Grider HS, Douglas SM, Raynor HA. The influence of mindful eating and/or intuitive eating approaches on dietary intake: a systematic review. *J Acad Nutr Diet.* 2021;121(4):709-727.e1. doi:10.1016/j.jand.2020.10.019

106. Beintner I, Emmerich OLM, Vollert B, Taylor CB, Jacobi C. Promoting positive body image and intuitive eating in women with overweight and obesity via an online intervention: results from a pilot feasibility study. *Eat Behav.* 2019;34:101307. doi:10.1016/j.eatbeh.2019.101307

107. Clifford D, Ozier A, Bundros J, Moore J, Kreiser A, Morris MN. Impact of non-diet approaches on attitudes, behaviors, and health outcomes: a systematic review. *J Nutr Educ Behav.* 2015;47(2):143-155.e1. doi:10.1016/j.jneb.2014.12.002

108. Mensinger JL, Calogero RM, Stranges S, Tylka TL. A weight-neutral versus weight-loss approach for health promotion in women with high BMI: a randomized-controlled trial. *Appetite.* 2016;105:364-374. doi:10.1016/j.appet.2016.06.006

109. Leblanc V, Provencher V, Bégin C, Corneau L, Tremblay A, Lemieux S. Impact of a Health-At-Every-Size intervention on changes in dietary intakes and eating patterns in premenopausal overweight women: results of a randomized trial. *Clin Nutr.* 2012;31(4):481-488. doi:10.1016/j.clnu.2011.12.013

110. Lanoye A, Gorin AA, LaRose JG. Young adults' attitudes and perceptions of obesity and weight management: implications for treatment development. *Curr Obes Rep.* 2016;5(1):14-22. doi:10.1007/s13679-016-0188-9

111. Gokee-LaRose J, Gorin AA, Raynor HA, et al. Are standard behavioral weight loss programs effective for young adults? *Int J Obes.* 2009;33(12):1374-1380. doi:10.1038/ijo.2009.185

112. Poobalan AS, Aucott LS, Precious E, Crombie IK, Smith WCS. Weight loss interventions in young people (18 to 25 year olds): a systematic review. *Obes Rev.* 2009;11(8):580-592. doi:10.1111/j.1467-789X.2009.00673.x

113. Morrill KE, Lopez-Pentecost M, Molina L, et al. Weight loss interventions for Hispanic women in the United States: a systematic review. *J Environ Public Health.* 2021;2021:1-14. doi:10.1155/2021/8714873

114. Tussing-Humphreys LM, Fitzgibbon ML, Kong A, Odoms-Young A. Weight loss maintenance in African American women: a systematic review of the behavioral lifestyle intervention literature. *J Obes.* 2013;2013:1-31. doi:10.1155/2013/437369

115. Fitzgibbon ML, Tussing-Humphreys LM, Porter JS, Martin IK, Odoms-Young A, Sharp LK. Weight loss and African-American women: a systematic review of the behavioural weight loss intervention literature. *Obes Rev.* 2012;13(3):193-213. doi:10.1111/j.1467-789X.2011.00945.x

116. Svetkey LP, Ard JD, Stevens VJ, et al. Predictors of long-term weight loss in adults with modest initial weight loss, by sex and race. *Obesity.* 2012;20(9):1820-1828. doi:10.1038/oby.2011.88

117. Cabassa LJ, Ezell JM, Lewis-Fernández R. Lifestyle interventions for adults with serious mental illness: a systematic literature review. *Psychiatr Serv.* 2010;61(8):9. doi:10.1176/ps.2010.61.8.774

118. Daumit GL, Dickerson FB, Wang NY, et al. A behavioral weight-loss intervention in persons with serious mental illness. *N Engl J Med.* 2013;368(17):1594-1602. doi:10.1056/NEJMoa1214530

119. Paul-Ebhohimhen V, Avenell A. A systematic review of the effectiveness of group versus individual treatments for adult obesity. *Obes Facts.* 2009;2(1):17-24. doi:10.1159/000186144

120. Ryan K, Dockray S, Linehan C. A systematic review of tailored eHealth interventions for weight loss. *Digit Health.* 2019;5:2055207619826685. doi:10.1177/2055207619826685

121. Leahey TM, Subak LL, Fava J, et al. Benefits of adding small financial incentives or optional group meetings to a web-based statewide obesity initiative. *Obesity.* 2015;23(1):70-76. doi:10.1002/oby.20937

122. Manzoni GM, Pagnini F, Corti S, Molinari E, Castelnuovo G. Internet-based behavioral interventions for obesity: an updated systematic review. *Clin Pract Epidemiol Ment Health.* 2011;7(1):19-28. doi:10.2174/1745017901107010019

123. Kim M, Kim Y, Go Y, et al. Multidimensional cognitive behavioral therapy for obesity applied by psychologists using a digital platform: open-label randomized controlled trial. *JMIR MHealth UHealth.* 2020;8(4):e14817. doi:10.2196/14817

124. Sherrington A, Newham JJ, Bell R, Adamson A, McColl E, Araujo-Soares V. Systematic review and meta-analysis of internet-delivered interventions providing personalized feedback for weight loss in overweight and obese adults. *Obes Rev.* 2016;17(6):541-551. doi:10.1111/obr.12396

125. Levin ME, Petersen JM, Durward C, et al. A randomized controlled trial of online acceptance and commitment therapy to improve diet and physical activity among adults who are overweight/obese. *Transl Behav Med.* 2021;11(6):1216-1225. doi:10.1093/tbm/ibaa123

126. Lillis J, Hayes SC, Bunting K, Masuda A. Teaching acceptance and mindfulness to improve the lives of the obese: a preliminary test of a theoretical model. *Ann Behav Med.* 2009;37(1):58-69. doi:10.1007/s12160-009-9083-x

127. Miller CK. Adaptive intervention designs to promote behavioral change in adults: what is the evidence? *Curr Diab Rep.* 2019;19(2):7. doi:10.1007/s11892-019-1127-4

128. Bennion KA, Tate D, Muñoz-Christian K, Phelan S. Impact of an internet-based lifestyle intervention on behavioral and psychosocial factors during postpartum weight loss. *Obesity.* 2020;28(10):1860-1867. doi:10.1002/oby.22921

CHAPTER 14

Medical and Surgical Interventions

Jessica Bartfield, MD, DABOM

CHAPTER OBJECTIVES

- Discuss the role of medical supervision during weight loss.
- Outline the criteria for medical and surgical interventions for obesity.
- Identify the antiobesity medications available and considerations for their use.
- Describe the surgical treatment of obesity and considerations for its use.

Introduction

Although the scientific study of obesity dates to at least the beginning of the 20th century, the American Medical Association only recognized it as a disease in 2013.[1] Through scientific progress and advancements, we now better understand the complexities and chronicity of the disease of obesity. Thanks to ongoing research and development, providers now have safer and more effective treatment options for obesity than at any other time in the past. Effective weight management demands multiple targeted approaches of indefinite duration. This chapter focuses on two arenas of treatment: antiobesity pharmacotherapy and surgical obesity treatment.

Choosing an Obesity Treatment Plan

Initiating a conversation on obesity treatment offers enough of a challenge to providers. Once the conversation starts, how then does one begin to select the appropriate treatment? As with other chronic diseases, the complexity of the disease (mild, moderate, or severe) dictates the intensity (low, moderate, or high) of the treatment. Currently, most obesity treatment guidelines remain weight-centric rather than disease-centric: patients meet the criteria for medical or surgical treatment when their BMI reaches a certain threshold, rather than when obesity-related health complications develop. The risks and benefits of this approach to treatment go beyond the scope of this chapter, but have been described elsewhere.[2] For example, providers could intervene earlier or be more aggressive with medical or surgical obesity treatments once weight-related complications arise—thus creating the potential for faster and more robust health improvement in their patients—instead of having to limit treatment until a patient's weight reaches a specific threshold. Providers also must appreciate that clinically meaningful weight loss of 5% to 10%, as defined by expert panels such as the World Health Organization and National Institutes of Health, translates into substantial improvement in metabolic diseases, including insulin resistance, hypertension, and dyslipidemia.[3] Although 5% weight loss is considered to be clinically effective, the average expected weight loss with more intensive pharmacotherapy or surgical treatment tends to be much higher. Understanding the expected weight response for a given treatment optimizes patient care, as providers can better manage patients' expectations and promptly change treatment if the response suggests it is not effective.

Current guidelines recommend screening patients for overweight and obesity using BMI at least annually.[4,5] The US Preventive Services Task Force recommends that providers refer patients with obesity (a BMI of 30 or higher) to intensive, multidisciplinary behavioral treatment.[4] Practice guidelines from The Obesity Society and the American College of Cardiology/American Heart Association Task Force on Practice Guidelines recommend assessing all patients with a BMI of more than 25 for risk of cardiovascular disease and all other obesity-related comorbidities.[5] Use of antiobesity pharmacotherapy should be considered for patients who have both a BMI of 27 or higher and weight-related complications, or a BMI of 30 or higher regardless of active or previous obesity-related health complications. Providers can offer surgical obesity treatment to patients who have both a BMI of 35 or higher and obesity-related complications, or to those who have a BMI of 40 or higher regardless of obesity related complications.[5] Table 14.1 provides a summary of obesity treatment options.[4,5]

TABLE 14.1 Obesity Treatment Options[4,5]

	BMI >25	BMI ≥27 with weight-related complications	BMI 30-34.9	BMI 35-39.9 with weight-related complications	BMI ≥40
Intensive behavioral modifications	Approved	Approved	Approved	Approved	Approved
Antiobesity pharmacotherapy		Approved	Approved	Approved	Approved
Endoscopic bariatric therapy or device			Approved	Approved	Approved[a]
Surgical obesity treatment				Approved	Approved

[a] Not all endoscopic bariatric therapies and devices are approved for BMI of greater than 40.

Patients with sufficient need and readiness for weight loss should be referred for comprehensive, high-intensity behavioral interventions. These are multifactorial and may include energy restriction, increased physical activity, goal setting, self-monitoring, and stimulus control. An interdisciplinary team (medical providers, dietitians, exercise specialists, behaviorists) should deliver care over at least 14 sessions within the first 6 months, with a minimum goal of 5% to 10% weight loss.[5-7] Other chapters in this book (Chapters 10 through 13) address the specifics of intensive behavior modifications for weight management. As patients transition from active weight loss to weight loss maintenance, care may drop in frequency and intensity but must remain *indefinite*.

Medical Supervision During Obesity Treatment

Medical supervision during obesity treatment focuses mainly on the management and monitoring of treatment side effects and changes in obesity-related complications. Common side effects of weight loss include constipation, fatigue, and headaches. More intensive treatment and weight loss may result in dehydration, electrolyte disturbances, hypoglycemia, or gallstones. Clinical monitoring typically includes weight trajectory, laboratory tests (electrolytes, renal function, liver function, lipid panel, glucose), blood pressure, and heart rate. As blood pressure or glycemic control improves with weight management, doses of antihypertensive and antidiabetes medications need to be lowered or discontinued. Patients with type 2 diabetes who are taking insulin or certain oral agents that increase insulin production (ie, sulfonlyureas) face a higher risk of hypoglycemia with effective obesity treatment. Thus, obesity medicine providers will recommend that patients closely monitor their blood glucose levels at home (via fingerstick or continuous glucose monitor) and often stop oral hypoglycemic medications or decrease insulin doses at the start of treatment to reduce this risk. If the patient's weight has not responded as expected, the treatment strategy should be assessed and intensity of care increased.

Medication Use in Weight Management

Antiobesity medications provide the increased intensity of care that some patients require. These medications control patients' symptoms (excessive hunger, cravings, poor satiety), strengthen behavior-change consistency, and improve weight response. Advancements in drug development and the science of obesity have expanded the number of available effective antiobesity medications. As of the printing of this book, Table 14.2 lists antiobesity medications approved by the US Food and Drug Administration (FDA).[8-19]

TABLE 14.2 Medications Approved by the US Food and Drug Administration for Obesity Treatment[8-19]

Drug (brand name) and available doses	Mechanism of action	Most common side effects	Contraindications[a]	Average weight loss[b]
Phentermine (Lomaira, Adipex-P) 8 mg (Lomaira), prescribed 1-3 times per day 15 mg (generic phentermine) prescribed 1-2 times per day 30 mg (generic phentermine) or 37.5 mg (Adipex-P) prescribed once daily	Works centrally to increase release of norepinephrine, dopamine, serotonin; sympathomimetic	Dry mouth Increased irritability, agitation Elevated heart rate and BP Insomnia	Uncontrolled hypertension Open-angle glaucoma Uncontrolled hyperthyroidism Uncontrolled anxiety History of cardiovascular disease Structural heart disease History of drug abuse MAOI use within 14 days	4.4% at 28 weeks[14]
Phendimetrazine (Bontril) 17.5-35 mg prescribed 1-2 times per day 105 mg extended-release prescribed once daily	Works centrally to increase norepinephrine and dopamine release; sympathomimetic	Dry mouth Agitation Insomnia Elevated BP and heart rate	Uncontrolled hypertension Open-angle glaucoma Uncontrolled hyperthyroidism Uncontrolled anxiety History of cardiovascular disease Structural heart disease History of drug abuse	Not well established
Diethylpropion (Tenuate) 25 mg prescribed 1-3 times per day 75 mg extended-release prescribed once daily	Works centrally to increase norepinephrine and dopamine release; sympathomimetic	Dry mouth Constipation Nausea Dyspepsia Insomnia Elevated BP or heart rate, or both	Uncontrolled hypertension Open-angle glaucoma Uncontrolled hyperthyroidism Uncontrolled anxiety History of cardiovascular disease Structural heart disease History of drug abuse Heart murmur	6.6% at 6 months[15]

Table continues

TABLE 14.2 Medications Approved by the US Food and Drug Administration for Obesity Treatment[8-19] (continued)

Drug (brand name) and available doses	Mechanism of action	Most common side effects	Contraindications[a]	Average weight loss[b]
Orlistat (Xenical, Alli[c]) 120 mg prescribed 3 times per day with meals containing fat (Xenical) 60 mg prescribed 3 times per day with meals containing fat (Alli[c])	Inhibits pancreatic and gastric lipase, reducing amount of dietary fat absorbed *Only antiobesity medication that does not work through appetite suppression*	Increased stool frequency and urgency Flatus with discharge Fatty diarrhea	Cholestasis Chronic malabsorption syndromes	3.8%[16]
Phentermine and topiramate extended-release (Qsymia) 3.75 mg phentermine/23 mg topiramate prescribed once daily 7.5 mg phentermine/46 mg topiramate prescribed once daily 11 mg phentermine/69 mg topiramate prescribed once daily 15 mg phenterimine/92 mg topiramate prescribed once daily	Works centrally to increase norepinephrine release and GABA release; inhibits carbonic anhydrase	Dry mouth Paresthesias Constipation Taste changes Insomnia Dizziness	Uncontrolled hypertension Open-angle glaucoma Uncontrolled hyperthyroidism Uncontrolled anxiety History of cardiovascular disease Structural heart disease History of drug abuse MAOI use within 14 days	8.6%[8]
Naltrexone and bupropion (Contrave) 8 mg naltrexone/90 mg bupropion prescribed as 2 tablets taken 2 times per day	Inhibits norepinephrine and dopamine reuptake; blocks opioid receptor	Nausea Vomiting Constipation Headache Insomnia Flushing	MAOI use within 14 days End-stage renal disease Uncontrolled hypertension Seizure disorder or history Bulimia Anorexia Opioid use or dependence	4.8%[9]
Liraglutide (Saxenda) 3 mg subcutaneous injection prescribed once daily	Activates GLP-1 receptor	Nausea Dyspepsia Diarrhea Constipation Fatigue	Medullary thyroid cancer history or family history of medullary thyroid cancer Multiple endocrine neoplasia type 2 Pancreatitis history Suicidal ideation or treatment	5.4%[11]
Semaglutide (Wegovy) 0.25 mg, 0.5 mg, 1 mg, 1.7 mg, or 2.4 mg subcutaneous injection once weekly	Activates GLP-1 receptor	Nausea Vomiting Dyspepsia Diarrhea Constipation Fatigue	Medullary thyroid cancer history or family history of medullary thyroid cancer Multiple endocrine neoplasia type 2 Pancreatitis history Suicidal ideation or treatment Acute gallstones	12.7%[17]
Tirzepatide (Zepbound) 2.5 mg, 5.0 mg, 10.0 mg, or 15.0 mg subcutaneous injection once weekly	Dual incretin, GLP-1 RA/GIP agonist	Nausea Vomiting Dyspepsia Diarrhea Constipation	Medullary thyroid cancer history or family history of medullary thyroid cancer Multiple endocrine neoplasia type 2 Pancreatitis	15% at 5 mg, 19.5% at 10 mg, 20.9% at 15 mg (all over 72 weeks)

TABLE 14.2 Medications Approved by the US Food and Drug Administration for Obesity Treatment[8-19] (continued)

Drug (brand name) and available doses	Mechanism of action	Most common side effects	Contraindications[a]	Average weight loss[b]
Setmelanotide (Imcivree) 2 mg subcutaneous injection prescribed once daily (ages 12 y and older) 1 mg subcutaneous injection prescribed once daily (ages 6-12 y) Can titrate up to 3 mg daily	MC4R agonist Restores MC4R activity in the brain and downstream pathways Only approved for patients with proven POMC deficiency, PCSK1 deficiency, or leptin receptor deficiency *Not approved for polygenic (common) obesity*	Hyperpigmentation Injection site reaction Nausea Vomiting Diarrhea Abdominal pain Fatigue	None	23% at 1 year for patients with POMC or PCSK1 deficiency[10] 9.7% at 1 year for patients with leptin receptor deficiency
Oral superabsorbent hydrogel (Plenity)[d] 3 capsules prescribed 20-30 min before each meal (with 500 mL water)	Particles absorb water in stomach and mix with foods Occupies about 25% of average stomach volume	Diarrhea Abdominal distension Constipation Gas Abdominal pain	Esophageal abnormalities (webs, rings), stricture, prior gastrointestinal surgery	2% at 6 months[18]

Abbreviations: BP, blood pressure; GABA, γ-aminobutyric acid; GIP, glucose-dependent insulinotropic polypeptide; GLP-1, glucagon-like peptide 1; MAOI, monoamine oxidase inhibitor; MC4R, melanocortin-4 receptor; PCSK1, proprotein convertase subtilisin/kexin type 1; POMC, pro-opiomelanocortin; RA, receptor agonist.

[a] All antiobesity medications are contraindicated in pregnancy and breastfeeding.
[b] Placebo-subtracted average weight loss with the highest dose at 1 year unless otherwise stated.
[c] Alli is the only FDA-approved over-the-counter weight loss medication.
[d] Plenity is obtained through a prescription but considered a device, not a medication, which is delivered through capsules but not systemically absorbed.

Appetite regulation involves a complex system of both central and peripheral signals, and this system is further influenced by external factors. Appetite control is not just a matter of increased self-discipline or having the willpower to "eat less." Antiobesity medications, once termed *appetite suppressants*, increase weight loss mainly by influencing the various signals involved in appetite regulation which decrease hunger, increase satiety, or reduce hedonic responses to food. Most of the medications' direct effects work centrally to reduce appetite and increase satiety. Phentermine, for example, increases norepinephrine levels. Topiramate's mechanism for weight loss remains uncertain, but its inhibition of carbonic anhydrase, antagonism of α-amino-3-hydroxy-4-isoxazole-propionic acid kainate (AMPA/KA) receptors, and activation of γ-aminobutyric acid receptors likely contribute.[8] Combination naltrexone and bupropion increases dopamine levels and activates pro-opiomelanocortin (POMC) cells found in the hypothalamus, which in turn activate the melanocortin-4 receptors (MC4R) and shut down feeding.[9,20] One of the newest medications treats patients whose obesity arises from specific genetic causes related to leptin receptor deficiency or POMC deficiency.[10] GLP-1 receptor agonists improve incretin function, both peripherally by increasing insulin release, suppressing hepatic gluconeogenesis and decreasing glucagon secretion. They also delay gastric emptying and reduce food intake.

The Academy of Nutrition and Dietetics strongly supports the inclusion of medical nutrition therapy by a registered dietitian nutritionist for all patients prescribed antiobesity medications to support healthy weight loss, minimize loss of muscle mass, and help minimize medication side effects.[21] A prospective study found that combined therapy with lifestyle modification and antiobesity medication resulted in a 12.1-kg weight loss over 1 year, compared to 5 kg lost with medication alone.[22]

A medication must prove an average weight loss of 5% to receive FDA approval for weight management. Of note, the highest velocity of weight loss occurs within the first 6 months of treatment with an antiobesity medication. Studies demonstrate that patients who have had less than 5% weight loss by 3 to 4 months of therapy are likely nonresponders to the medication and require either a dose increase or an alternative medication.[11] If patients respond appropriately to an antiobesity medication, it should be continued indefinitely; if stopped, weight gain should be expected.

Prescribers must remember that patients need not "fail" behavior therapy prior to initiating antiobesity medications. As with other chronic diseases, such as hypertension and type 2 diabetes, early disease control improves long-term disease sequelae. Few providers would hesitate to start a medication in patients with uncontrolled blood pressure or a hemoglobin A1c level greater than 7%, even if they also recommended lifestyle changes. Likewise, patients with overweight or obesity may also benefit from pharmacotherapy at the start of treatment. Furthermore, providers should view obesity treatment as a necessary component of the treatment of other diseases. For example, rather than adding another antihypertensive or antidiabetic medication to the regimen of a patient with obesity and uncontrolled blood pressure or blood glucose levels, a clinician could instead begin an antiobesity medication to promote weight loss and optimize blood pressure or glycemic control.

Selecting a Medication

Guidelines do not yet recommend an algorithm for prescribing specific antiobesity medications. Multiple factors influence the selection of antiobesity medications. Typically, providers try to match a medication to a patient's specific symptoms or challenges (eg, hyperphagia, poor satiety, depressed resting metabolic rate). Contraindications and potential side effects of each medication must be carefully reviewed and either avoided (contraindications) or minimized (adverse effects) when selecting an antiobesity medication. Insurance coverage and cost of these medications vary considerably and influence which medication may be prescribed, particularly as antiobesity medicines need to be used indefinitely when effective. For example, a nonprofit research institute investigating the coverage of obesity treatment by state insurance plans found pharmacotherapy to be the least likely obesity treatment option to be covered.[23] Currently Medicare does not cover any antiobesity medications; only 15 Medicaid programs nationwide cover antiobesity medications in fee-for-service plans, and only 16 state-employee plans offer coverage of these medications. Prescribers also need to elicit and appreciate their patients' preferences for medication use, such as opting for an oral pill rather than a subcutaneous injection or one with an easier dosing regimen. Patients may find one medication more appealing than another based on side-effect profiles. Finally, providers should consider a medication's potential ability to treat multiple conditions, such as prediabetes, type 2 diabetes, or depression, in addition to treating obesity. In addition to antiobesity medications, drugs that are associated with weight loss rather than approved for weight loss can often offer this dual benefit, as discussed next. Providers unfamiliar with pharmacotherapy for the treatment of obesity should refer patients to an obesity medicine specialist.

Additional Considerations for Medications

In order to enhance the medical treatment of obesity, providers should be aware of other medications that their patients may take (ie, medications other than those being prescribed for weight loss) that can cause weight gain. Examples include psychotropic medications, antidiabetes medications, and antiepileptics, among others. Typically, medication-induced weight gain is defined by a 5% or higher increase in body weight, although individual effects vary tremendously. The same medication may cause one person to gain a modest amount of weight (5% to 10%) over a long period of time (years), whereas another person may gain more weight very rapidly (15% or more in a matter of months). Mechanisms for weight gain include appetite stimulation or decreased inhibition through changes in neural pathways, altered glucose absorption and storage, increased fatigue, and reduced energy expenditure. Often the mechanism remains unclear. Fortunately, some classes of medications include alternatives that are either weight neutral or weight reducing, and providers should make every effort to utilize these when treating patients with obesity. Box 14.1 lists common medications that may induce weight gain and provides examples of weight-neutral alternatives.[24-26]

BOX 14.1

Medications Associated With Weight Gain and Examples of Weight-Neutral Alternatives[24-26]

Class of medication	Examples of medications that may lead to weight gain	Examples of weight-neutral alternatives
Antidiabetics	Insulin Sulfonylureas (glipizide) Thiazolidinediones (pioglitazone)	Metformin Pramlintide (adjunct to insulin) Glucagon-like peptide 1 (GLP-1) agonists (exenatide, dulaglutide, liraglutide, semaglutide) Sodium-glucose cotransporter-2 (SGLT2) inhibitors (empagliflozin, canagliflozin) Tirzepatide
β-Blockers	Metoprolol Propranolol	Carvedilol Nebivolol
Antidepressants	Selective serotonin reuptake inhibitor (SSRIs) (paroxetine) Tricyclic antidepressants (TCAs; amitriptyline) Mirtazapine Selective serotonin and norepinephrine reuptake inhibitors (desvenlafaxine, duloxetine)	Sertraline Fluoxetine Citalopram Bupropion

Box continues

BOX 14.1 (CONTINUED)

Class of medication	Examples of medications that may lead to weight gain	Examples of weight-neutral alternatives
Antipsychotics	Clozapine Olanzapine Quetiapine Risperidone	Ziprasidone Aripiprazole
Contraceptives	Injectable contraceptives (medroxyprogesterone acetate)	Oral contraceptives
Antiepileptics	Valproic acid Carbamazepine Gabapentin Pregabalin	Topiramate Zonisamide Felbamate
Steroids	Corticosteroids (prednisone)	Nonsteroidal anti-inflammatory drugs (NSAIDs; diclofenac, meloxicam) Disease-modifying antirheumatic drugs (methotrexate) Biologics
Antihistamines	First-generation antihistamines (diphenhydramine)	Second-generation antihistamines (loratadine)

Finally, providers can also consider off-label use of medications for obesity treatment, particularly when they offer a dual benefit, as previously explained. Common examples include metformin for prediabetes, polycystic ovary syndrome, or metabolic dysfunction–associated steatotic liver disease. Metformin has also been shown to mitigate psychotropic-induced weight gain, particularly weight gain that is caused by antipsychotics.[27] Topiramate and zonisamide can offer dual-benefit weight loss and migraine treatment. Topiramate has also shown benefit for weight regain following bariatric surgery, night eating syndrome, and binge eating.[28-30] Lisdexamfetamine is approved for binge eating, not for obesity treatment, but often results in a dual benefit as well. The newer antidiabetes medications are frequently used to optimize obesity treatment. Furthermore, recent trials now suggest a substantial reduction in major cardiac adverse events with semaglutide.[31] Box 14.2 lists common medications used off label for obesity treatment.

Surgical Treatment of Obesity

For patients with a BMI of 35 or higher and obesity-related comorbidities (hypertension, dyslipidemia, type 2 diabetes, obstructive sleep apnea) or patients with a BMI of 40 or higher, guidelines recommend that providers consider referral for

BOX 14.2

Common Medications Used Off Label for Weight Management

Phentermine (long-term use)

Diethylpropion (long-term use)

Metformin

Topiramate

Zonisamide

Pramlintide

Sodium-glucose cotransporter-2 inhibitors

Bupropion

Dulaglutide (4.5-mg weekly dose)

Lisdexamfetamine

Semaglutide (Ozempic)

Tirzepatide (Mounjaro)

---

bariatric surgery.[5] Surgical options include adjustable gastric banding, vertical sleeve gastrectomy, Roux-en-Y gastric bypass, biliopancreatic diversion with duodenal switch, and the single anastomosis duodeno-ileal switch endorsed in 2020 by the American Society for Metabolic and Bariatric Surgery (ASMBS).[32] Currently, the sleeve gastrectomy and the Roux-en-Y gastric bypass are the two most common procedures performed (refer to Figure 14.1 below and Figure 14.2 on page 262).[33] Refer to Table 14.3 on page 262 for a summary of current surgical options.[33-35]

FIGURE 14.1 Sleeve gastrectomy

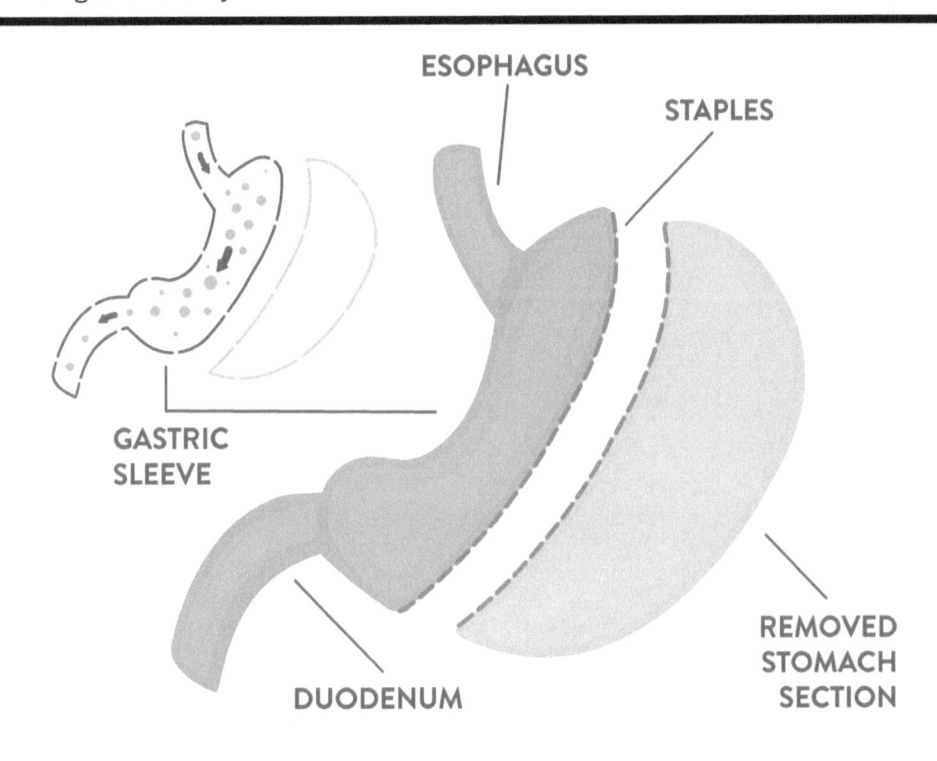

FIGURE 14.2 Roux-en-Y gastric bypass

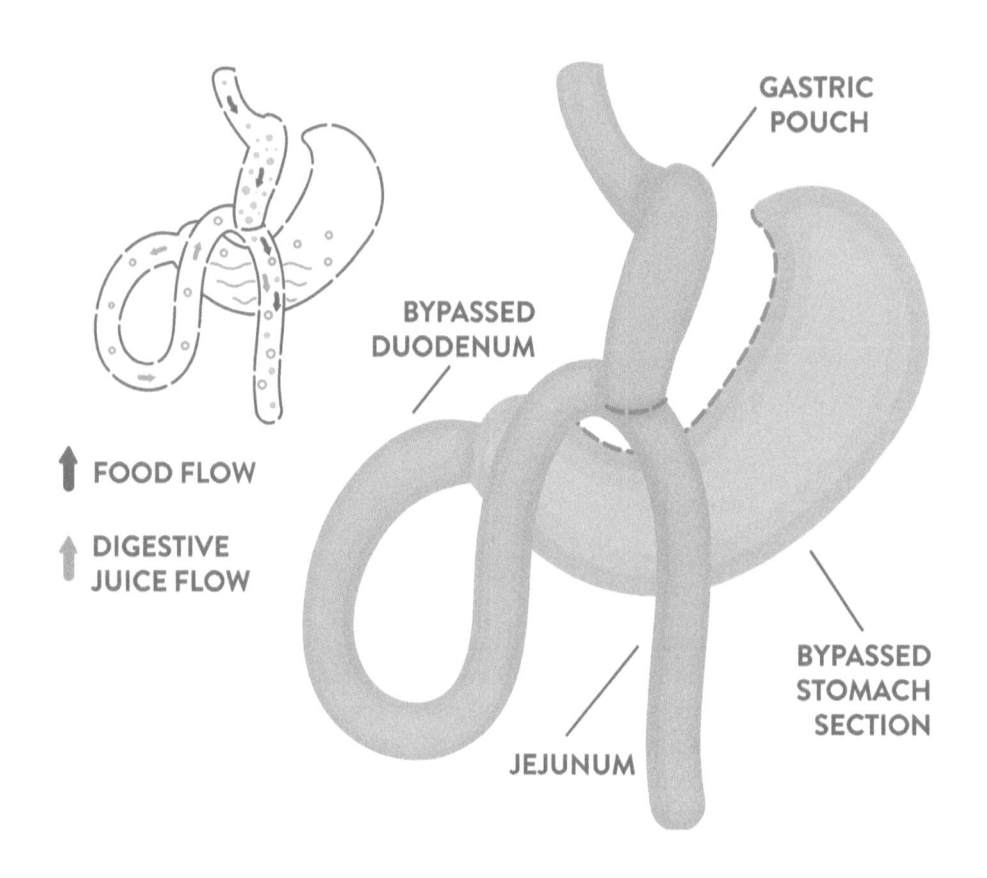

TABLE 14.3 Surgical Interventions for Obesity Treatment[33-35]

Procedure	Mechanism of action	Benefits	Potential complications	Average % of excess body weight lost[a]	Average % of total weight lost
Laparoscopic adjustable gastric banding	An adjustable inflatable band placed around the upper portion of the stomach decreases food intake.	Indicated for BMI of 30-40 Early satiety Very low risk for vitamin deficiencies Reversible, adjustable	Band slippage or erosion Foreign-body reaction Esophageal dysmotility or dilation	40-50	20-25
Vertical sleeve gastrectomy	Approximately 80% of the stomach is removed. Energy intake is reduced.	Early satiety No bypass or foreign objects involved Lower risk of complications compared with Roux-en-Y gastric bypass and BPD-DS Fewer nutrient deficiencies	Not reversible Nutrient deficiencies (vitamin B12, iron, vitamin D, calcium, folate) Potential worsening of GERD, so not recommended for patients with severe reflux or Barrett esophagus	>50	25-30

SECTION 3: Interventions for the Treatment of Overweight and Obesity

TABLE 14.3 Surgical Interventions for Obesity Treatment[33-35] (continued)

Procedure	Mechanism of action	Benefits	Potential complications	Average % of excess body weight lost[a]	Average % of total weight lost
Roux-en-Y gastric bypass	The stomach is divided to create a small pouch, and the first portion of the small intestine is divided and reattached distally. This results in both reduced energy intake and decreased energy absorption.	Early satiety Strong metabolic effects (especially type 2 diabetes improvement) independent of weight loss Favorable improvement in gut hormones (eg, GLP-1) Recommended for patients with severe GERD	Anastomotic leak or marginal ulcer, so *not* recommended for patients requiring long-term NSAID use or with high-risk tobacco use Nutrient deficiencies (fat-soluble vitamins, B vitamins, iron, calcium, zinc, copper) Early dumping—occurs within 30 minutes after eating (usually simple carbohydrates) and is characterized by diarrhea, abdominal cramping, flushing, need to lie down Late dumping—occurs at least 1 hour after eating (simple carbohydrates) and is characterized by hypoglycemia, feeling lightheaded, sweating, shaking, tachycardia, syncope; occurs in pateints at least 1 yr post operation	60	30-35
Biliopancreatic diversion with duodenal switch	A stomach pouch is created, and the first ¾ of the small intestine is bypassed via diversion. This results in reduced energy intake and >70% reduction in fat absorption.	Effective for higher BMI Greatest weight loss of all bariatric procedures Improved satiety Greatest improvement in type 2 diabetes and other metabolic diseases	Highest rate of complications and mortality of all bariatric surgeries More severe nutrient deficiencies (fat-soluble vitamins, B vitamins, iron, calcium, folate, zinc, copper) Requires the most vitamin and mineral supplementation (lifelong) Internal hernia Steatorrhea	≥70	35-45
Single anastomosis duodeno-ileal switch	The goal is to decrease long-term nutritional complications and technical difficulty of BPD-DS. The Roux-en-Y reconstruction of BPD-DS is replaced with a single duodeno-ileostomy with a longer common channel.	Improved satiety Substantial improvement in type 2 diabetes and other metabolic diseases Potentially fewer short-term and long-term complications (eg, internal hernia, marginal ulceration) than with Roux-en-Y gastric bypass or BPD-DS	Nutrient deficiencies still a substantial risk Considerable variation in small-bowel length among individuals; difficult to predict necessary common channel length Fewer long-term data available	70 (as suggested by early studies)	

Abbreviations: BPD-DS, biliopancreatic diversion with duodenal switch; GERD, gastroesophageal reflux disease; GLP-1, glucagon-like peptide 1; NSAID, nonsteroidal anti-inflammatory drug.

[a] This percentage is determined by dividing the amount of weight lost as a result of surgery by the patient's excess weight before surgery. Excess weight is calculated by subtracting the patient's ideal weight at a BMI of 25 from the patient's actual weight.

Preoperative Care

The updated 2019 clinical practice guidelines for perioperative care of patients undergoing bariatric procedures from the American Association of Clinical Endocrinologists/American College of Endocrinology, The Obesity Society, the American Society for Metabolic and Bariatric Surgery, the Obesity Medicine Association, and the American Society of Anesthesiologists include a comprehensive checklist that clinicians can follow preoperatively to appropriately prepare patients for surgery.[34] This includes routine laboratory tests, nutrition screening for active deficiencies, specialty evaluation as needed (cardiology, gastroenterology, endocrinology), pregnancy counseling for people of childbearing age, and lifestyle medicine evaluation and counseling. Although no absolute contraindications for bariatric surgery exist, relative contraindications include end-stage lung disease, active cancer treatment, portal hypertension, active substance use, and inability to tolerate general anesthesia. According to the guidelines, the type of procedure offered should be based on patient preference, weight severity, weight loss goals, presence of obesity-related comorbidities, and surgeon expertise. These considerations are highlighted in Box 14.3. Furthermore, providers should refer patients to surgical practices designated as Centers of Excellence. The ASMBS Bariatric Surgery Center of Excellence distinction is one of the most widely used distinctions by various insurance companies, including the Centers for Medicare and Medicaid Services. To receive this distinction, surgeons must demonstrate a certain level of expertise (50 cases per year, 125 lifetime cases), hospitals must meet specific surgical case volumes, and the center must utilize a multidisciplinary team for patient care.[36] Once a patient commits to having bariatric surgery, an interdisciplinary team should thoroughly evaluate and treat any existing behavioral disorders and counsel patients extensively on postoperative care and potential complications. Chapter 9 further discusses behavioral health assessments.

BOX 14.3

Preoperative Checklist for Bariatric Surgery

Routine laboratory tests (in the fasting state): blood glucose level, lipid panel, complete blood count, comprehensive metabolic panel, thyrotropin level

Nutrition screening: vitamin B12 level, 25-hydroxyvitamin D level, iron studies

Sleep apnea screening (or adherence to treatment), deep vein thrombosis risk evaluation

Helicobacter pylori evaluation; upper gastrointestinal series or esophagogastroduodenoscopy (or both)

Optimization of glycemic control in patients with type 2 diabetes: goal hemoglobin A1c level <10% prior to surgery (may be variable by surgeon recommendations)

Age-appropriate cancer screening

Nutrition evaluation by a registered dietitian nutritionist

Tobacco cessation

Perioperative Care

New clinical pathways for enhanced recovery after bariatric surgery have been researched and developed. Some of the recommendations include carbohydrate loading, sips of clear liquid up to 2 hours before surgery, deep breathing exercises, intraoperative protective ventilation strategies, leg exercises, and preemptive antiemetics and nonopioid analgesic medications. These intraoperative and perioperative steps reduce pain and pulmonary complications and speed up bowel recovery, among other benefits.

Postoperative Care

The aforementioned 2019 guidelines also advise practitioners on early and long-term postoperative care, providing specific recommendations for vitamin supplementation, diet progression, and frequency of nutritional deficiency screening and other laboratory monitoring (eg, glucose level, lipid levels, thyroid function).[34] Particularly, the guidelines contain greater detail on immediate postoperative complications (eg, deep vein thrombosis, nausea and pain management, internal hernias) and criteria for hospital admission.

The most rapid weight loss occurs within the first 6 to 12 months following surgery, and weight stabilizes around 12 to 18 months after surgery. Patients need to be counseled regarding the average pattern of weight loss postsurgery, including rate of weight loss and total expected weight loss, to help manage expectations for the selected procedure. Generally, a loss of 50% of presurgical excess body weight at 12 months postsurgery suggests an appropriate response to surgical treatment. (Excess body weight is ideal weight at a BMI of 25 minus actual weight.)

Vitamin and Mineral Supplementation

Each surgical procedure requires the patient to adhere to lifelong vitamin and mineral supplementation, but the regimen varies according to procedure type and institutional practice. In the first year after surgery, nutrition screening for deficiencies typically occurs at 3 months, 6 months, and 12 months. Key recommendations include indefinite annual screening for vitamin B12, folate, iron, and vitamin D deficiencies in all patients, and copper, zinc, selenium, and thiamine deficiencies pending clinical suspicion for deficiencies. If deficiencies occur, the patient's supplementation regimen should be adjusted and repeat screening done within 1 to 3 months to ensure resolution of the deficiency. Patients' long-term adherence to vitamin and mineral supplementation following surgical treatment for obesity tends to wane, and the risk of deficiencies remains substantial, even with appropriate recommended vitamin and mineral supplementation.[37] Therefore, providers need to consistently ensure that their patients take vitamins and minerals indefinitely after surgery. Also, providers should continue long-term assessment of lipid levels, hemoglobin A1c levels, and thyroid function. Guidelines recommend screening for osteoporosis with bone mineral density testing for patients once they are 2 years out from bariatric surgery.[34]

Medication Considerations

Finally, in addition to trying to avoid prescribing medications that may lead to weight gain in patients, providers need to consider potential changes in how the body absorbs medications following surgical treatment for obesity. For example, the use of immediate-release, rather than extended-release, formulations of medications is preferred. And patients taking medications that require therapeutic drug monitoring (eg, warfarin, levothyroxine, lithium) should have their levels checked more frequently until their weight stabilizes.

Postoperative Outcomes

Currently, surgery is the most effective treatment for obesity. A meta-analysis including 22,094 patients who underwent bariatric surgery demonstrated a mean excess-body-weight loss of 61.2%, remission of type 2 diabetes in 76.8% of patients, resolution of hypertension in 61.7% of patients, and improved or resolved obstructive sleep apnea in 83.6% of patients.[38] Again, all guidelines regard surgical obesity treatment as an *adjunct* to intensive behavioral interventions and include lifestyle interventions in both the preoperative and postoperative recommendations.[5,34] Patients must understand that weight loss responses to each type of obesity treatment can vary substantially among individuals and that any single treatment, including a surgical procedure, is typically not curative. Clinicians caring for patients undergoing bariatric surgery should carefully monitor their patients' weight changes, mood changes, sleep habits, and activity habits, and they should screen for nutritional deficiencies and substance use (particularly tobacco and alcohol). Lifelong care is needed to help sustain post–bariatric surgery lifestyle habits that promote long-term maintenance of weight loss. Refer to Box 14.4 for a summary of postoperative recommendations.

BOX 14.4

Recommendations for Postoperative Care Following Bariatric Surgery

Monitor weight changes on an annual basis (minimum) and initiate treatment if weight regain exceeds 20% of total weight loss or if the percentage of excess body weight lost is less than 50% at least 1 year postsurgery.

Provide dietary counseling, advising patients to prioritize protein intake, minimize intake of simple carbohydrates, avoid carbonated beverages, and consume adequate amounts of water. Monitor for increased alcohol intake.

Provide physical activity counseling, advising patients to avoid prolonged sedentary behaviors, progress toward 150 minutes of moderate activity per week, and engage in a minimum of 2 days of strength and resistance training per week.

Screen for alcohol and tobacco use.

Instruct patients on vitamin and mineral supplementation.

Screen for nutritional deficiencies on annual basis.

Weight Regain After Surgical Treatment

The Endocrine Society released post–bariatric surgery management guidelines in 2010.[39] Although these guidelines have been superseded by the 2019 guidelines previously discussed, these initial guidelines distinctly highlighted weight regain after bariatric surgery. Prevention and treatment of weight regain is an important consideration for clinicians when discussing surgical treatment options with their patients. An estimated 20% to 25% of patients will experience weight regain or inadequate weight loss after surgery.[40] A loss of less than 50% of one's excess body weight typically signals inadequate weight loss. Weight regain, however, remains less well defined. Multiple definitions for weight regain have been proposed, including percent weight regain from nadir weight, percent weight regain from total weight loss, or increase in BMI points from nadir BMI. Furthermore, a threshold for weight regain warranting intervention has yet to be agreed upon by experts. Depending on which definition and threshold providers use, the number of patients requiring adjunct treatment for active weight loss instead of treatment for weight loss maintenance will vary. The causes of weight regain after surgery resemble the multifactorial etiologies of obesity for the general population and include lifestyle changes (eg, changes in eating patterns, levels of activity, stress levels, and sleep patterns), hormonal changes (eg, changes in leptin, insulin, or ghrelin levels), environmental changes, and degree of clinical follow-up. Patients experiencing weight regain should undergo a comprehensive evaluation by the interdisciplinary team to identify specific causes and challenges unique to the patient. A tailored treatment plan can then be designed to include the necessary behavior interventions and, potentially, antiobesity pharmacotherapy. Surgical conversion or revision treatment for patients with severe or refractory weight regain or inadequate weight loss may be advised. Recent data analyses found that revisions constitute about 17% of all bariatric procedures.[33]

Dietary Considerations of Medical and Surgical Treatments for Obesity

Both pharmacotherapy and surgery often require dietary management beyond energy restriction. Providers need to routinely assess patients' daily dietary practices. Side effects of certain antiobesity medications may cause dry mouth, taste changes, constipation, or nausea. Symptoms management and mitigation may include increased fluids, fiber supplementation, or changing the number or timing of eating episodes. Similarly, surgery can cause nausea, increased reflux, hypoglycemia, altered bowel movements, and taste or palatability changes. Although the details are specified by individual surgeons and institutions, dietary progression usually spans the first 4 to 6 weeks after surgery. Initially, it focuses on hydration with clear liquids 1 to 2 days after surgery, followed by full liquids or pureed foods for 10 to 14 days. Soft or texture-modified foods are then introduced, and by 6 weeks patients are consuming regular textured foods. Typical dietary remedies to prevent surgical side effects include strategic diet progression in the early postoperative period from liquids to solids, waiting 30 minutes between eating and fluid intake, slowing the pace of eating, increased mastication of food, and prioritizing protein intake (minimum 60 g/d up to 2.1 g per kilogram of ideal body weight, depending on needs).[41]

Summary

Obesity treatment demands a patient-centered, targeted strategy employing multiple approaches and having an indefinite duration. Options for treatment include intensive behavioral interventions, antiobesity pharmacotherapy, endoscopic interventions, and surgical interventions. Often a combination of all four treatment options may yield the best results. Multiple guidelines exist to help providers navigate treatment. A modest weight loss of 5% to 10% can translate into substantial improvements in obesity-related comorbidities for type 2 diabetes, hypertension, and dyslipidemia. It is imperative that clinicians counsel patients on the chronic, relapsing nature of obesity. Weight loss plateaus and weight regain should be *expected* and should prompt a change in treatment rather than feelings of fear, futility, or failure. By utilizing current treatment guidelines and emphasizing long-term monitoring, clinicians can best support patients' health and weight loss goals.

References

1. AMA House of Delegates adopts policy to recognize obesity as a disease. Obesity Medicine Association. June 19, 2013. Accessed December 20, 2021. https://obesitymedicine.org/ama-adopts-policy-recognize-obesity-disease
2. Daniel S, Soleymani T, Garvey WT. A complications-based clinical staging of obesity to guide treatment modality and intensity. *Curr Opin Endocrinol Diabetes Obes*. 2013;20(5):377-388. doi:10.1097/01.med.0000433067.01671.f
3. Douketis JD, Macie C, Thabane L, Williamson DF. Systematic review of long-term weight loss studies in obese adults: clinical significance and applicability to clinical practice. *Int J Obes (Lond)*. 2005;29(10):1153-1167. doi:10.1038/sj.ijo.0802982
4. US Preventive Services Task Force; Curry SJ, Krist AH, et al. Behavioral weight loss interventions to prevent obesity-related morbidity and mortality in adults: US Preventive Services Task Force recommendation statement. *JAMA*. 2018;320(11):1163-1171. doi:10.1001/jama.2018.13022
5. Jensen MD, Ryan DH, Apovian CM, et al. 2013 AHA/ACC/TOS guideline for the management of overweight and obesity in adults: a report of the American College of Cardiology/American Heart Association Task Force on Practice Guidelines and The Obesity Society. *J Am Coll Cardiol*. 2014;63(25 pt B):2985-3023. doi:10.1016/j.jacc.2013.11.004
6. Wadden TA, Webb VL, Moran CH, Bailer BA. Lifestyle modification for obesity: new developments in diet, physical activity, and behavior therapy. *Circulation*. 2012;125:1157-1170. doi:10.1161/CIRCULATIONAHA.111.039453
7. Wadden TA, Tsai AG, Tronieri JS. A protocol to deliver intensive behavioral therapy (IBT) for obesity in primary care settings: the MODEL-IBT Program. *Obesity (Silver Spring)*. 2019;27(10):1562-1566. doi:10.1002/oby.22594
8. Shin JH, Gadde KM. Clinical utility of phentermine/topiramate (Qsymia™) combination for the treatment of obesity. *Diabetes Metab Syndr Obes*. 2013;6:131-139. doi:10.2147/DMSO.S43403
9. Sherman MM, Ungureanu S, Rey JA. Naltrexone/bupropion ER (Contrave): newly approved treatment option for chronic weight management in obese adults. *P T*. 2016;41(3):164-172.
10. Markham A. Setmelanotide: first approval. *Drugs*. 2021;81(3):397-403. doi:10.1007/s40265-021-01470-9
11. Fujioka K, O'Neil PM, Davies M, et al. Early weight loss with liraglutide 3.0 mg predicts 1-year weight loss and is associated with improvements in clinical markers. *Obesity (Silver Spring)*. 2016;24(11):2278-2288. doi:10.1002/oby.21629
12. Micromedex (database). IBM Watson Health. Accessed December 21, 2021. www.micromedexsolutions.com
13. Igel LI, Kumar RB, Saunders KH, Aronne LJ. Practical use of pharmacotherapy for obesity. *Gastroenterology*. 2017;152(7):1765-1779. doi:10.1053/j.gastro.2016.12.049
14. Kaplan LM. Pharmacologic therapies for obesity. *Gastroenterol Clin Am*. 2005;39:69-79. doi:10.1016/j.gtc.2010.01.001
15. Cercato C, Roizenblatt VA, Leança CC, et al. A randomized double-blind placebo-controlled study of the long-term efficacy and safety of diethylpropion in the treatment of obese subjects. *Int J Obes (Lond)*. 2009;33(8):857-865. doi:10.1038/ijo.2009.124
16. Foxcroft DR, Milne R. Orlistat for the treatment of obesity: rapid review and cost-effectiveness model. *Obes Rev*. 2000;1(2):121-126. doi:10.1046/j.1467-789x.2000.00011.x
17. Wadden TA, Berkowitz RI, Womble LG, et al. Randomized trial of lifestyle modification and pharmacotherapy for obesity. *N Engl J Med*. 2005;353(20):2111-2120. doi:10.1056/NEJMoa050156
18. Greenway FL, Aronne LJ, Raben A, et al. A randomized, double-blind, placebo-controlled study of Gelesis100: a novel nonsystemic oral hydrogel for weight loss. *Obesity (Silver Spring)*. 2019;27(2):205-216. doi:10.1002/oby.22347
19. Jastreboff AM, Aronne LJ, Ahmad NN et al. Tirzepatide once weekly for the treatment of obesity. *N Engl J Med* 2022;387(3):205-216. doi:10.1056/NEJMoa2206038

20. Greenway FL, Whitehouse MJ, Guttadauria M, et al. Rational design of a combination medication for the treatment of obesity. *Obesity (Sliver Spring)*. 2009;17:30-39. doi:10.1038/oby.2008.461
21. Academy of Nutrition and Dietetics. Anti-obesity medication and the role of lifestyle interventions delivered by RDNs. eatrightPRO.org website. 2024. Accessed February 22, 2024. www.eatrightpro.org/aom
22. Wadden TA, Bailey TS, Billings LK, et al. Effect of subcutaneous semaglutide vs placebo as an adjunct to intensive behavioral therapy on body weight in adults with overweight or obesity: the STEP 3 randomized clinical trial. *JAMA*. 2021;325(14):1403-1413. doi:10.1001/jama.2021.1831
23. Waidmann TA, Waxman E, Pancini V, Gupta P, Tabb LP. *Obesity Across America: Geographic Variation in Disease Prevalence and Treatment Options*. Urban Institute; February 17, 2022. Accessed April 1, 2022. www.urban.org/research/publication/obesity-across-america
24. Domecq JP, Prutsky G, Leppin A, et al. Clinical review: drugs commonly associated with weight change: a systematic review and meta-analysis. *J Clin Endocrinol Metab*. 2015;100(2):363-370. doi:10.1210/jc.2014-3421
25. Apovian CM, Aronne LJ, Bessesen DH, et al. Pharmacological management of obesity: an Endocrine Society clinical practice guideline. *J Clin Endocrinol Metab*. 2015;100(2):342-362. doi:10.1210/jc.2014-3415
26. Ferrannini E, Solini A. SGLT2 inhibition in diabetes mellitus: rationale and clinical prospects. *Nat Rev Endocrinol*. 2012;8(8):495-502. doi:10.1038/nrendo.2011.243
27. Zhou J, Massey S, Story D, Li L. Metformin: an old drug with new applications. *Int J Mol Sci*. 2018;19(10):2863. doi:10.3390/ijms19102863
28. Stanford FC, Alfaris N, Gomez G, et al. The utility of weight loss medications after bariatric surgery for weight regain or inadequate weight loss: a multi-center study. *Surg Obes Relat Dis*. 2017;13(3):491-500. doi:10.1016/j.soard.2016.10.018
29. Amodeo G, Cuomo A, Bolognesi S, et al. Pharmacotherapeutic strategies for treating binge eating disorder: evidence from clinical trials and implications for clinical practice. *Expert Opin Pharmacother*. 2019;20(6):679-690. doi:10.1080/14656566.2019.1571041
30. Kucukgoncu S, Midura M, Tek C. Optimal management of night eating syndrome: challenges and solutions. *Neuropsychiatr Dis Treat*. 2015;11:751-760. doi:10.2147/NDT.S70312
31. Lincoff AM, Brown-Frandsen K, Colhoun HM, et al. Semaglutide and Cardiovascular Outcomes in Obesity without Diabetes. *N Engl J Med*. Published online November 11, 2023. doi:10.1056/NEJMoa2307563
32. Kallies K, Rogers AM; American Society for Metabolic and Bariatric Surgery Clinical Issues Committee. American Society for Metabolic and Bariatric Surgery updated statement on single-anastomosis duodenal switch. *Surg Obes Relat Dis*. 2020;16(7):825-830. doi:10.1016/j.soard.2020.03.020
33. Estimate of bariatric surgery numbers, 2011-2019. American Society for Metabolic and Bariatric Surgery. March 2021. Accessed December 21, 2021. https://asmbs.org/resources/estimate-of-bariatric-surgery-numbers
34. Mechanick JI, Apovian C, Brethauer S, et al. Clinical practice guidelines for the perioperative nutrition, metabolic, and nonsurgical support of patients undergoing bariatric procedures—2019 update: cosponsored by American Association of Clinical Endocrinologists/American College of Endocrinology, The Obesity Society, American Society for Metabolic and Bariatric Surgery, Obesity Medicine Association, and American Society of Anesthesiologists—executive summary. *Endocr Pract*. 2019;25(12):1346-1359. doi:10.4158/GL-2019-0406
35. Arterburn DE, Courcoulas AP. Bariatric surgery for obesity and metabolic conditions in adults. *BMJ*. 2014;349:g3961. doi:10.1136/bmj.g3961
36. Pratt GM, Greer-Ullrich P. Bariatric Surgery Centers of Excellence®: Why they are important when selecting your surgeon and hospital. Obesity Action Coalition. Fall 2009. Accessed June 1, 2022. www.obesityaction.org/resources/bariatric-surgery-centers-of-excellence-why-they-are-important-when-selecting-your-surgeon-and-hospital
37. Ha J, Kwon Y, Kwon JW, et al. Micronutrient status in bariatric surgery patients receiving postoperative supplementation per guidelines: insights from a systematic review and meta-analysis of longitudinal studies. *Obes Rev*. 2021;22(7):e13249. doi:10.1111/obr.13249
38. Buchwald H, Avidor Y, Braunwald E, et al. Bariatric surgery: a systematic review and meta-analysis. *JAMA*. 2004;292(14):1724-1737. doi:10.1001/jama.292.14.1724
39. Heber D, Greenway FL, Kaplan LM, et al. Endocrine and nutritional management of the post-bariatric surgery patient: an Endocrine Society clinical practice guideline. *J Clin Endocrinol Metab*. 2010;95(11):4823-4843. doi:10.1210/jc.2009-2128
40. El Ansari W, Elhag W. Weight regain and insufficient weight loss after bariatric surgery: definitions, prevalence, mechanisms, predictors, prevention and management strategies, and knowledge gaps—a scoping review. *Obes Surg*. 2021;31(4):1755-1766. doi:10.1007/s11695-020-05160-5
41. Sherf Dagan S, Goldenshluger A, Globus I, et al. Nutritional recommendations for adult bariatric surgery patients: clinical practice. *Adv Nutr*. 2017;8(2):382-394. doi:10.3945/an.116.014258

CHAPTER 15

Obesity as a Chronic Disease and Its Lifelong Management

Chloe Panizza Lozano, PhD, MHlthProm, GradDip Dietetics
Corby K. Martin, PhD, FTOS

CHAPTER OBJECTIVES

- Discuss obesity as a chronic disease and the implications for its lifelong management.
- Describe the pathophysiology of obesity and the obesogenic environment that affects lifelong weight management.
- Discuss various interventions for the lifelong management of overweight and obesity.
- Summarize the Chronic Care Model and its application to overweight and obesity.

Introduction

Obesity is a complex, chronic disease with many factors contributing to its etiology and maintenance, including genetics, environment, metabolism, socioeconomic factors, lifestyle, and behavior.[1,2] Obesity was acknowledged as a chronic disease by the American Medical Association in 2013. This important decision was made to recognize the physiology and pathology of obesity, change the bias and stigma associated with obesity, improve the available resources for education and management of obesity, encourage further funding for obesity-related research, and improve access to evidenced-based obesity care.[3] A dominant belief in the United States is that people with obesity lack the willpower to control their weight, thus the individual is cast as being at fault for their condition.[4] This philosophy creates *weight stigma*, which leads to additional physical and psychological health problems for people with obesity (refer to Chapter 3).[5,6] The eating and activity behaviors that are needed to manage long-term weight loss are challenging due to the current obesogenic environment[7] and to physiological changes that occur in response to weight loss.[8]

The factors affecting the maintenance of weight loss are examined in this chapter, with the intention of highlighting obesity as a complex disease that requires lifelong management, with ongoing support from family, the community, health care services, and policy makers.[7]

Pathophysiology and Environment: Implications for the Lifelong Management of Obesity

The Pathophysiology of Obesity

Body weight is controlled by complex neuroendocrine and behavioral factors (detailed in Chapter 1) that, theoretically, should maintain the body at a healthy weight through homeostasis.[5] For example, the hypothalamus responds to interoceptive signals (signals from within the body) by affecting changes in dietary behaviors and energy expenditure. An example of a key producer of interoceptive signals is the hormone leptin, which is secreted from adipose tissue and assists in maintaining levels of fat stores.[9] However, the ability to translate the administration of exogenous leptin into an effective therapy is limited,[10] demonstrating the complexity of body weight regulation. Homeostasis—achieved through internal, physical, and chemical conditions—should ensure that body weight stays within preset limits to allow for optimal functioning of the human body.[11] Unfortunately, as evidenced by changes in body weight that occur throughout the life span and the increasing prevalence of obesity, these homeostatic mechanisms appear to be less effective at addressing positive energy balance and preventing obesity. Difficulties in managing body weight are likely the result of interactions between physiology, genetics, behavioral predispositions, and the obesogenic environment. Thus, homeostatic mechanisms to preserve body weight are challenged and overcome by an environment that promotes excess energy intake and reduced energy expenditure.[7]

Body weight regulation is complex, and more simplistic models fail to find broad levels of support. For example, the set point model of body weight regulation (which states that body weight has a set point that is biologically determined and defended) and the lipostatic set point model of body weight regulation (which states that body fat is regulated at a set point by feedback between adipose tissue and the brain) fail to address environmental interactions that influence weight regulation.[11] In addition, there is a wide range of factors involved in the risk of mortality, which would make it unlikely for the set point theory to evolve.[12]

Metabolic Adaptation

Shifts in body weight of 5% to 10% can be achieved through diet and lifestyle.[5] However, such weight loss can be difficult to maintain over time[13] given the difficulties of maintaining energy restriction over time, as well as the physiological changes that occur with weight loss. One such physiological change is metabolic adaptation. With weight loss there is an expected reduction in metabolism, as there is less body mass to maintain.[14] However, the decrease in energy expenditure after weight loss is variable,[14-16] and metabolic adaptation occurs when the reduction in energy expenditure is greater than what would be predicted based on the loss of body mass.[17] From a weight loss perspective, metabolic adaptation is intuitively viewed as negative because it could contribute to weight regain. From another perspective, however, metabolic adaptation is seen as a marker of improved health; specifically, it is considered an indication that a dietary intervention—namely, energy restriction with optimal nutrition—is effectively promoting health span (the length of time during one's life that one is healthy) and longevity. This view supports the rate of living hypothesis, which states that organisms with a higher metabolic rate per unit of mass have shorter life spans.[18] In this regard, a lower metabolic rate per unit of mass is associated with a longer life.[19]

Perceptions of metabolic adaptation as "good" or "bad" aside, there is no agreed-upon method for calculating metabolic adaptation. Recently, researchers assessed 13 methods for calculating metabolic adaptation and found disparate results among people who lost 4.8% of their body weight during a lifestyle intervention and a control group. Specifically, the magnitude of metabolic adaptation across the calculations varied widely, from 65 to 230 kcal/d, with all calculations detecting metabolic adaptation in the intervention group, though three calculations also detected metabolic adaptation in the control group.[14] The persistence of metabolic adaptation during weight loss maintenance and weight regain has also been questioned, as researchers recently concluded that metabolic adaptation is dependent on the presence of an energy deficit. These authors also found that metabolic adaptation did not predict weight regain after 1 year of follow-up.[20] This finding is consistent with the failure of metabolic adaptation to predict weight regain following participation in the televised weight loss competition *The Biggest Loser*, though metabolic adaptation was found to persist 6 years after the competition. Importantly, data from *The Biggest Loser* showed that metabolic adaptation persisted to a greater degree among those who maintained the most weight loss after 6 years, which supports the hypothesis that metabolic adaptation is greatest when weight reductions and energy deficits are maintained.[21]

Changes in Appetite

After a person loses weight, hormonal changes (eg, decreased leptin and increased ghrelin)[22,23] and neuronal signaling changes[22] occur that increase appetite and delay satiation. In neuroimaging studies of people with obesity, researchers found that the areas of the brain associated with food reward (eg, the orbitofrontal cortex) were more greatly stimulated when food images were shown during the weight loss maintenance phase.[22] These findings highlight biological factors that make it difficult for people to behaviorally sustain reduced energy intake during the maintenance phase,[5,24] particularly in an obesogenic environment where palatable foods are plentiful and accessible. Nonetheless, some studies that quantify changes in subjective ratings of appetite during weight loss offer paradoxical yet promising findings for those seeking to lose weight. For example, a consistent observation over the past 35 years is that people who eat less food, primarily through medically supervised very low-calorie diets (VLCD), report less hunger than people who eat relatively higher-energy balanced diets. In one study, people with obesity who were randomly assigned to a protein-sparing modified fast vs a 1,200 kcal/d balanced diet reported less hunger, despite experiencing significantly larger weight loss.[25] Other markers of appetite have been found to behave similarly. For example, food cravings decreased to a larger extent among people following a VLCD than among people eating a less restrictive balanced diet, despite the fact that those following the VLCD lost almost three times as much weight as those on the balanced diet (16.7% vs 6.6% weight loss).[26] These and other findings have contributed to the theory that measures of appetite, such as food cravings, reflect a conditioned expression of hunger.[26,27] This highlights the ways in which behavior, dietary patterns, and environment can interact to drive energy intake and how these factors affect a person's ability to maintain weight loss.

The Obesogenic Environment

The obesogenic environment is a key factor contributing to weight gain. An obesogenic environment is defined as "the sum of influences that the surroundings, opportunities, or conditions of life have on promoting obesity in individuals or populations."[28] The hedonic controls of body weight include the sensory, emotional, and cognitive pathways of the nervous system involved with "reward" and are influenced by the environment, including the taste and appearance of food. The homeostatic control of body weight, however, is more focused on maintaining energy balance.[29] There may be bidirectional communication between the hedonic and the homeostatic controls of body weight. For example, activity in the hypothalamus can be affected by exteroceptive signals (ie, signals from outside the body).[30] An example of hedonic influences on weight maintenance can be demonstrated by the consumption of ultraprocessed foods and hyperpalatable foods. Previous research has shown that ad libitum consumption of ultraprocessed foods overrides homeostatic control mechanisms and leads to increased energy intake and weight gain.[31-34] According to Monteiro et al,[35] *ultraprocessed foods* are defined as "formulations mostly of cheap industrial sources of dietary energy and nutrients plus additives, using a series of processes." The NOVA system of food classification places foods into four groups (one of which is ultraprocessed foods), as described in Box 15.1. Interestingly, in mouse models, once ultraprocessed foods are removed from the environment and the mouse's diet is returned to "normal," weight gain is reversed.[36]

BOX 15.1

NOVA Food Classification System[35]

Group 1: Unprocessed or minimally processed foods	Edible parts of plants or animals after separation from nature (eg, raw fruits and vegetables, animal muscle, milk, eggs)
Group 2: Processed culinary ingredients	Derived from Group 1 foods with a small amount of processing; designed to aid in cooking (eg, oil, butter, sugar)
Group 3: Processed foods	Preserved, cooked, or fermented versions of Group 1 or Group 2 foods (eg, canned vegetables, bread, cheese)
Group 4: Ultraprocessed foods	Man-made formulations that contain few intact Group 1 foods and often contain processed derivatives of food constituents, as well as preservatives, stabilizers, added colors, and flavor enhancers; designed to create convenient, attractive, shelf-stable products (eg, soft drinks, packaged snacks, pre-prepared frozen meals)

Recently, a method was developed to quantitatively define and categorize hyperpalatable foods,[37] and many ultraprocessed foods fall within these categories. The three main clusters of hyperpalatable foods are detailed in Box 15.2 on page 274.[37]

Subsequent research on hyperpalatable and ultraprocessed foods has demonstrated the complex processes by which food groups may or may not drive increased intake and body weight. For example, and as noted earlier, consuming a diet rich in ultraprocessed foods increases energy intake and body weight over the short-term,[37] but a 1-year longitudinal study found that only the consumption of hyperpalatable foods that were high in carbohydrates and sodium predicted weight and fat gain 1 year later, whereas the consumption of ultraprocessed foods and energy-dense foods did not predict weight or fat-mass gain.[38] Together, the results of these studies demonstrate that: (1) clinicians can use various food categorizations, like hyperpalatable foods, to try to determine what types of foods contribute to excess intake and weight gain for individual clients, and (2) more research is needed to fully understand how characteristics of foods drive intake and body weight. Lastly, and unfortunately, in the current obesogenic environment, it does not seem possible to remove access to ultraprocessed foods or hyperpalatable foods without close collaboration with the food industry or a substantial shift in the willingness of governments to regulate such products, or both. In fact, 62% of foods in the US Department of Agriculture's Food and Nutrient Database for Dietary Studies were found to be hyperpalatable.[37]

BOX 15.2

Hyperpalatable Food Clusters[37]

Fat and sodium cluster	A food falls into this cluster if greater than 25% of its kilocalorie content comes from fat and if it contains 0.3% or greater sodium by weight.
Fat and simple sugars cluster	A food falls into this cluster if greater than 20% of its kilocalorie content comes from fat and greater than 20% comes from sugar.
Carbohydrates and sodium cluster	A food falls into this cluster if greater than 40% of its kilocalorie content comes from carbohydrates and if it contains 0.2% or greater sodium by weight.

The ability of ultraprocessed foods and hyperpalatable foods to disrupt the homeostasis of weight maintenance is only one example of how the obesogenic environment influences obesity. Other environmental factors affecting weight loss maintenance will be discussed in the interventions section of this chapter.

The Importance of Lifelong Management of Obesity

It is not unusual for a client to report a history of multiple weight loss attempts followed by weight regain. A meta-analysis of 29 studies of weight loss found that 80% of weight lost was regained after 5 years.[39] Weight regain can contribute to feelings of hopelessness and failure and may not only cause a client to give up but can also contribute to a lack of urgency on the part of the health professional to address weight with a client.

Despite the many barriers to maintaining weight loss, successful long-term weight loss can be achieved. The National Weight Control Registry (NWCR) is an observational study of participants who report a weight loss of more than 13.6 kg (30 lb) and maintenance of that weight loss for more than 1 year.[40,41] Participants report that an average weight loss of 32.4 kg (71 lb) was maintained after 6 years.[42] Researchers have identified that one of the most important factors for long-term maintenance of weight loss is keeping the weight off for at least 2 years. Once weight loss has been maintained for 2 years, the risk of weight regain is lowered by approximately 50%.[40] This highlights that resources dedicated to helping people with obesity lose weight should be made available for at least 2 years to help establish more permanent healthy behavior changes.

Strong data exist to support the long-term health benefits of weight loss and interventions for maintaining weight loss. Research has established that a weight loss of 5% to 10% leads to substantial improvements in health outcomes, including lowering the risk of type 2 diabetes and heart disease.[40] Therefore, even if weight regain occurs, maintaining at least a 5% to 10% weight loss over the long term is considered a success.

A reduction in body weight to shift someone from the obese to the overweight category also positively affects mortality risk. An analysis of more than 24,000 adults monitored for more than 10 years found that weight loss from obese to overweight resulted in a 54% reduction in mortality risk compared to remaining in the obese category.[43] Also, patients undergoing bariatric surgery may not have the same life expectancy as the general population, but their mortality risk is lower compared to people with obesity who do not undergo bariatric surgery. For example, a 20-year follow-up of patients who underwent bariatric surgery found that the life expectancy of these patients was 3 years longer than that of the control group with obesity, though their life expectancy was still 5 years shorter than that of the general population.[44]

Long-term weight loss is challenging but achievable. If patients with obesity do experience some degree of weight regain, they should be encouraged and recognized for the health benefits they achieved by maintaining at least some weight loss over the long term.

Interventions for the Lifelong Management of Obesity

Planning for Long-Term Attention

Short-term diets are not a cure for overweight or obesity, and long-term lifestyle change is necessary for weight loss maintenance.[45,46] Clients with overweight or obesity benefit from ongoing support in developing the skills they need to manage a lower body weight. According to guidelines issued in 2013 by the American College of Cardiology/American Heart Association Task Force on Practice Guidelines and The Obesity Society for the management of overweight and obesity in adults (hereafter, the 2013 AHA/ACC/TOS guidelines), the graded evidence is strong for participation in a comprehensive weight loss maintenance program for 1 or more years following weight loss in these clients.[24] Interventions for weight management are of much longer duration than interventions for weight loss.

Managing Expectations

Clients may set goals to lose weight in order to reach an "ideal" weight or BMI or a weight experienced at an earlier time in life—for example, during high school or when they were first married. Such goals often far exceed the amount of weight loss needed for health benefits and, more important, the degree of lifestyle change needed to maintain that weight loss. Ideally, a conversation about realistic goals takes place before the client embarks on a weight loss program, and it is an important part of the discussion for long-term management. Clients may experience a decrease in their rate of weight loss or a weight loss plateau, causing them to become frustrated and give up, only to regain lost weight. Focusing on the health benefits of the weight loss achieved to date and other non–scale-related victories can help clients shift their focus to weight maintenance and management strategies for keeping the weight off. Because clients often feel rewarded when they see decreases in their weight on the scale, other strategies, such as the use of graphs or photographs, may be useful in helping clients restructure their thoughts and perceptions about weight.[46,47]

Addressing Metabolic Adaptation

As previously discussed, weight loss triggers metabolic adaptation, and it is essential for practitioners to understand (1) the extent to which metabolic adaptation should be a focus of treatment, (2) whether efforts are needed to mitigate metabolic adaptations, and (3) whether effective interventions exist to mitigate it. Metabolic adaptation is not a predictor of weight regain. Weight loss maintenance is largely dependent on the persistence of an energy deficit below baseline levels.[20,21] Consequently, the presence and persistence of metabolic adaptation can be an objective marker of successful weight loss maintenance.[18] It is also unclear to what extent metabolic adaptation needs to be addressed in clinical encounters given its limited clinical implications, particularly in comparison with the large effect of food intake on weight regain. Moreover, effective strategies for combating metabolic adaptation are lacking, other than increased energy intake and weight regain, though practitioners hope that pharmacotherapy will offer effective methods for reducing or eliminating metabolic adaptation in the future; exogenous leptin administration offers promise in this regard.[10]

Clients may ask about metabolic adaptation; hence, failing to address it may not be an option. Furthermore, metabolic adaptation puts a person at a daily energetic disadvantage after weight loss, and this intuitively implies that weight regain is more likely. However, by comparing the energy value of metabolic adaptation to the energy equivalent in food, clinicians can shift their clients' focus away from what is difficult, if not impossible, to change without weight regain (metabolic adaptation) to something that they can address immediately (diet modification). For example, typical metabolic adaptation over 6 months is approximately 90 kcal/d, or the equivalent of 1 tablespoon of peanut butter per day.[48] This means that a person who has lost weight will have to eat the energetic equivalent of approximately 1 tablespoon of peanut butter less each day compared to a person with similar body mass who is not weight suppressed in order to maintain their weight loss. This information is valuable to clients as it provides a clear behavioral and dietary goal while shifting attention away from metabolic adaptation, which cannot easily be manipulated, does not necessarily predict weight regain, and suggests that biology is destiny and that people have limited tools to prevent weight regain.

Self-Monitoring Lifestyle Behaviors

During periods of weight loss and weight loss maintenance, the body often experiences changes in the hormones associated with increased hunger and decreased satiation, leading to changes in appetite.[22] However, these changes in appetite may be managed through supportive diet therapy (refer to Chapter 11).[25,26] It is important for practitioners to communicate this information to clients so that they can monitor their appetite and its effect on weight loss maintenance. Also, an increased awareness of energy intake, energy expenditure, and body weight may help clients resist the urge to respond to the increased hunger and decreased satiety. Evidence from the NWCR supports that self-monitoring of weight, eating, and physical activity are associated with successful weight loss maintenance. The frequency and intensity with which patients monitor these behaviors was also positively associated with maintaining weight loss over time.[40,41] In addition, a qualitative analysis found that people who maintained their weight loss were more likely to weigh themselves regularly, use productive problem-solving skills, and practice positive self-talk.[49]

Addressing Dietary Behaviors for Weight Loss Maintenance

Just as a variety of dietary behaviors can contribute to weight loss, there is no one dietary prescription for maintaining weight loss. A client-centered counseling approach helps to reveal the dietary adjustments a client is willing to make and adhere to over the long term. These are often a continuation of the same dietary behaviors a client followed for weight loss, with an adjustment to allow for energy balance at the new weight instead of a continued energy deficit for weight loss.

Dietary behaviors associated with successful weight loss maintenance are listed in Box 15.3.[40,42,50] Approximately 78% of participants in the NWCR reported eating breakfast every day, and approximately 59% of participants reported following similar eating patterns on weekdays and weekends. Also, among NWCR participants, allowing oneself more freedom in food choices when on vacation was associated with weight regain.[40,50] This research highlights the importance of consistently following a balanced, healthy eating pattern that can be sustained in any setting. Among participants in the NWCR, weight regain was also associated with increased energy intake from total fat and decreased dietary restraint.[40] As previously discussed, eating ultraprocessed foods and hyperpalatable foods can lead to the excessive energy intake. Changing public policies to reduce the availability of ultraprocessed foods and hyperpalatable foods would require major shifts in the obesogenic environment and would likely receive pushback from industry and consumers given that ultraprocessed foods and hyperpalatable foods are relatively inexpensive, highly palatable, desirable, and lead to high profits. Therefore, interventions aimed at reducing the intake of ultraprocessed foods and hyperpalatable foods in the short term may need to rely on nutrition education and self-management.

BOX 15.3

Dietary Behaviors Associated With Weight Loss Maintenance[40,42,50]

- Eating breakfast regularly
- Following a similar dietary pattern across weekdays and weekends
- Eating a diet low in energy and fat
- Exhibiting higher levels of dietary restraint and lower levels of disinhibition

---

Planning for Physical Activity for Weight Loss Maintenance

Given the reduction in energy expenditure after weight loss, physical activity has been consistently identified as important for maintaining weight loss.[51] Increasing physical activity may help to increase energy expenditure and to counteract any additional energy intake from increased hunger and reduced satiety during the weight-maintenance phase.[52] The recommendation for prevention of weight regain from the 2013 AHA/ACC/TOS guidelines is 200 to 300 minutes of exercise per week.[24] (This is considerably higher than the guidelines' recommendation for health benefits, which is 150 minutes of moderate-intensity exercise per week.) However, many clients find it challenging to consistently add physical activity to their daily regimen. Practitioners should note that new research found that higher levels of exercise following weight loss did not result in better weight loss maintenance compared to lower levels of exercise (less than 200 min/wk). Thus, lower levels of exercise appear to assist with weight loss maintenance.[53]

One's physical environment includes the walkability, street connectivity, land-use mix, residential density, availability of public transportation, and green space where one lives, among other factors,[54] and is associated with the incidence and prevalence of obesity.[55] For example, a meta-analysis of prospective cohort studies from the United States, Australia, and Europe found that higher walkability and less urban sprawl were associated with lower obesity incidence.[55] Given that physical activity is important for maintaining weight loss, supportive physical environments are likely needed for facilitating this healthy behavior change.

Considering the Mode of Care Delivery

With advances in technology, there have been substantial changes in the way health information is collected, tracked, and communicated between health care professionals and patients.[56] Especially since COVID-19 first appeared in December 2019, providers have sought to provide health care remotely through technology-based methods to reduce the spread of the virus while maintaining much-needed care.[57] These advancements in technology include the use of the internet for self-management support (eg, through secure portals), social networking or eHealth communities, telehealth (eg, videoconferencing), mobile health (mHealth, including wearable physical activity monitors and mHealth apps), and electronic health records.[56-58] Chapter 17 provides more information on this topic.

As for the mode of delivery, some evidence suggests that various modes of delivering weight loss support—in person, in a group setting, or via the telephone—are equally effective.[5,59] The 2013 AHA/ACC/TOS guidelines reflect a high strength of evidence for comprehensive weight loss interventions delivered in person, though the strength of evidence is moderate for electronically delivered interventions and low for interventions delivered via telephone.[24] Nonetheless, research continues and more work is needed to evaluate the utility and effectiveness of interventions delivered via communication technology, such as video-based telehealth.[5,59] Telehealth may not be suitable for people with unreliable telephone service or poor internet access. Limited evidence exists regarding the delivery of interventions primarily through technology and with no human intervention (eg, through a website platform, text messages, or smartphone apps).[5,59] However, these technology-based tools are very important for supporting weight loss through the self-monitoring of diet, physical activity, and body measurements, and for providing real-time feedback to patients and their health care providers.[5,57,59] These tools facilitate a platform for remote delivery of care, which may greatly enhance the feasibility and affordability of the long-term support essential for maintaining weight loss.[57]

Managing Relapses

Given the obesogenic environment and the challenges of managing energy intake over one's lifespan, weight regain can occur even when a client follows the various strategies that have been outlined here. Earlier intervention to "get back on track" increases the likelihood of reinitiating lapsed behaviors and reversing weight gain. This highlights the value of self-weighing and other forms of self-monitoring in long-term management. Clients may find it useful to identify a weight or other threshold at which they will reengage with interventions and support. Thus, retreatment and managing lapses or relapses are crucial aspects of long-term weight management.[45]

The Chronic Care Model

The Chronic Care Model (CCM), developed in the 1990s, is an important framework for the management of chronic disease.[60-62] The model focuses on patient-centered care, which is supported by intricate partnerships between the patient, health care providers, the community, and policy makers.[63] The CCM replaces more acute and disease-focused therapies previously used in primary care, as chronic diseases are far more complex and persistent than are acute illnesses. Historically, disease-focused therapies have relied heavily on physicians and were contributing to physician burnout, patient dissatisfaction, and poor health outcomes for patients when applied to chronic diseases.[62]

The CCM includes six components: (1) the health system or health organization; (2) clinical information systems; (3) decision support; (4) delivery system design; (5) self-management support; and (6) community, which includes organizations and resources for patients (refer to Box 15.4 on page 280).[60-65] The individual components are not meant to be used in isolation, and experts recommended that practitioners employ at least two or more for the best care.[63] According to previous literature, the three components perceived as priorities in the primary health care setting are clinical information systems, decision support, and self-management support.[63] However, which CCM components are implemented and how they are implemented is unique to each health care facility, making it difficult to systematically determine their overall effectiveness.[58,64] It is unlikely that each component operates in isolation; rather, the components are likely synergistic. Therefore, testing the individual effects of CCM components is not recommended.[58,63] Research suggests that smaller primary care practices may be less likely to implement all components, as doing so is seen as financially challenging and labor-intensive for small clinics.[58] The CCM has been shown to improve health outcomes in people with chronic disease, with demonstrated improvements in hemoglobin A1c levels, blood pressure levels, BMI, low-density lipoprotein cholesterol levels, and treatment goals.[58,65] However, research on the model has been conducted primarily among people with type 2 diabetes and there is limited research on the effectiveness of the CCM for other chronic conditions, including obesity.[63,65]

The 2013 AHA/ACC/TOS guidelines propose a chronic disease management model for the treatment of overweight and obesity (refer to Figure 15.1 on page 281).[24] The model focuses on assessment by the primary care provider and possible interventions to be discussed with the client, embracing the CCM components of decision support, self-management support, and resources for patients.

In light of changes in health care practices in response to the COVID-19 pandemic, a team of researchers reviewed eHealth tools that are used to support the CCM and proposed a revised CCM, called the eHealth Enhanced Chronic Care Model (eCCM).[56] Their review also stressed the importance of a complete feedback loop when using eHealth-based interventions.[56,66] The five stages of the feedback loop include: (1) providing health status data to patients, (2) interpreting the health care data and information provided to patients, (3) addressing the unique needs of the patient, (4) ensuring the patient receives the information in a timely manner, and (5) ensuring there is consistent repetition of the health care information.[66]

Research Gaps for the Chronic Care Model

Despite the promising research on the eCCM, there is scant research on the management of chronic conditions through eHealth and telehealth.[57] A rapid

BOX 15.4

Components of the Chronic Care Model and Examples of Their Application for the Management of Obesity[60-65]

Chronic Care Model component	Description	Examples for obesity management
Health system or health organization[a]	Support from health care leaders, which stimulates organizational change	Changing policies to reduce the availability of ultraprocessed foods and hyperpalatable foods Expanding payment structures for obesity interventions and increasing access to weight management services
Clinical information systems	Implementation of clinical information systems for effective documentation and tracking of patients' health data	Using technology-based tools for remote monitoring of patients' diets, physical activity, and body measurements Expansion of electronic medical records to identify patients at risk, changes in BMI, and associated comorbidities that could be treated with interventions for obesity
Decision support[b]	Upskilling of health care professionals and patients so they are aware of the most current, evidence-based management of the chronic disease	Educating patients and health care professionals about metabolic adaptation and the importance of patient self-monitoring of diet, physical activity, body measurements, and appetite Utilizing interdisciplinary teams for multicomponent weight management services, recognizing the expertise of various disciplines
Delivery system design[c]	Design of the delivery systems used in health care facilities	Using technology-based tools for remote delivery of care, which may greatly enhance the feasibility and affordability of long-term support for weight loss maintenance
Self-management support[d]	Upskilling of patients so they have the confidence, knowledge, and skills to manage their own care	Embracing shared decision-making for client centered care Ensuring patients have the skills to use technology-based tools to support weight loss through self-monitoring of diet, physical activity, and body measurements, and providing real-time feedback of progress to the individual
Community, including organizations and resources for patients	Supporting patients' health through community-based resources and local health care policies	Ensuring a healthy physical environment, including the walkability, street connectivity, land-use mix, residential density, availability of public transportation, and availability of green space, among other factors Engaging in public policy initiatives for federal, state, and local policies that affect the obesogenic environment as well as food and health services for the underserved

[a] Refer to Chapter 19 for further details.
[b] Refer to Chapter 18 for further details.
[c] Refer to Chapter 17 for further details.
[d] Refer to Chapter 5 for further details.

FIGURE 15.1 Treatment algorithm: chronic disease management model for primary care of patients with overweight and obesity[24]

Evaluation

Treatment

Patient encounter → **Measure weight, height; calculate BMI** → BMI 25–29.9 (overwieght) or 30–34.9 (class 1 obesity) or 35–39.9 (class 2 obesity) or ≥40 (class 3 obesity)

Yes, BMI ≥25 → **Assess and treat risk factors for CVD- and obesity-related comorbidities** → **Assess weight and lifestyle histories** → Assess need to lose weight: BMI ≥30 or BMI 25–29.9 with risk factor(s)

No BMI 18.5–24.9 → **Advise to avoid weight gain; address and treat other risk factors**

No, insufficient risk ← from "Assess need to lose weight"

Yes → Assess readiness to make lifestyle changes to achieve weight loss

No, not yet ready → Advise to avoid weight gain box

Yes, ready → **Determine weight loss and health goals and intervention strategies** → **Comprehensive lifestyle intervention alone or with adjunctive therapies (BMI ≥30 or ≥27 with comorbidity)**

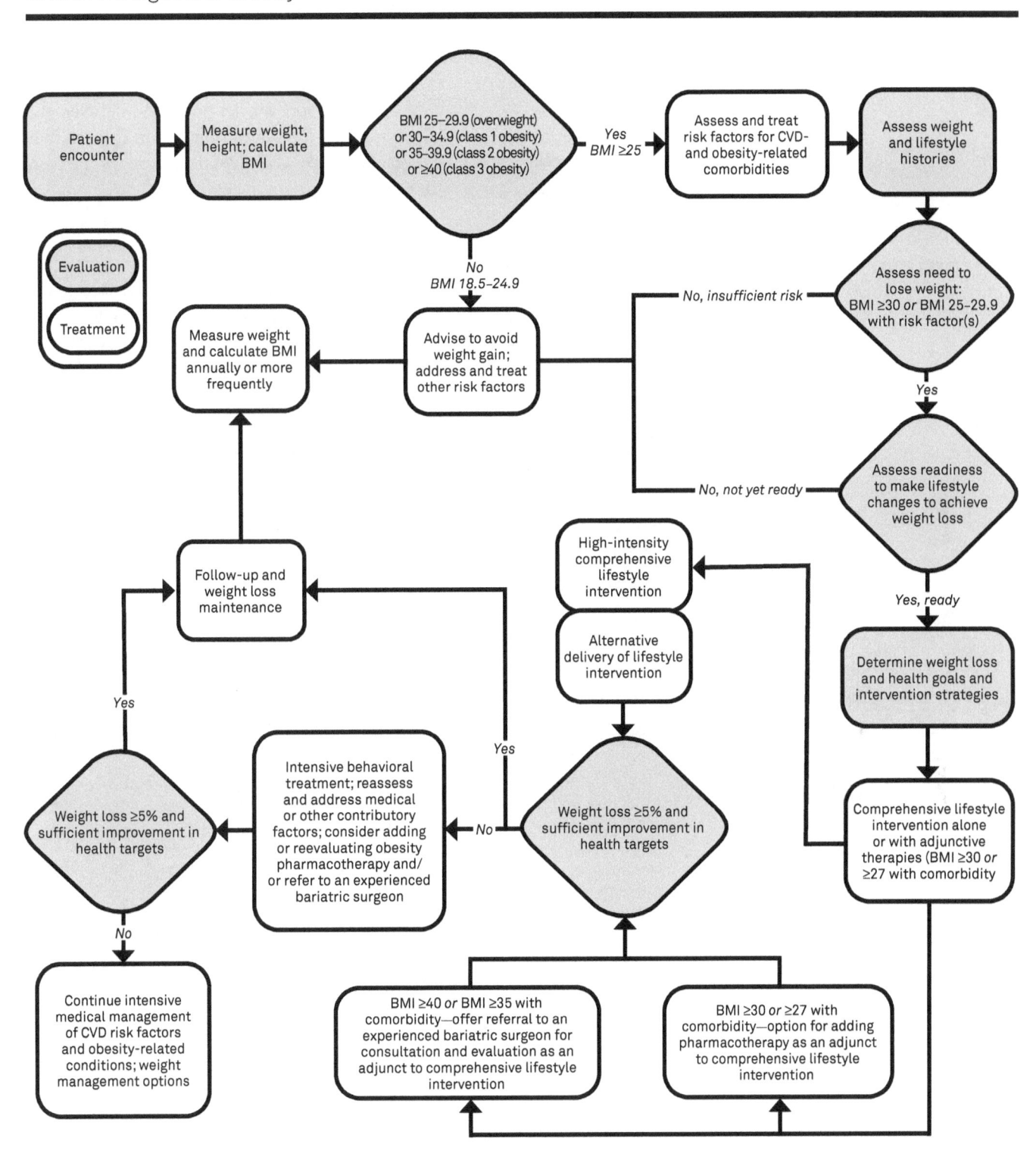

Measure weight and calculate BMI annually or more frequently ← Advise to avoid weight gain

Follow-up and weight loss maintenance ← High-intensity comprehensive lifestyle intervention / Alternative delivery of lifestyle intervention

Weight loss ≥5% and sufficient improvement in health targets
- Yes → Follow-up and weight loss maintenance
- No → **Intensive behavioral treatment; reassess and address medical or other contributory factors; consider adding or reevaluating obesity pharmacotherapy and/or refer to an experienced bariatric surgeon**

Weight loss ≥5% and sufficient improvement in health targets (left diamond)
- Yes → Follow-up
- No → **Continue intensive medical management of CVD risk factors and obesity-related conditions; weight management options**

BMI ≥40 or BMI ≥35 with comorbidity—offer referral to an experienced bariatric surgeon for consultation and evaluation as an adjunct to comprehensive lifestyle intervention

BMI ≥30 or ≥27 with comorbidity—option for adding pharmacotherapy as an adjunct to comprehensive lifestyle intervention

Abbreviation: CVD, cardiovascular disease.
Adapted with permission from Jensen MD, Ryan DH, Apovian CM, et al. 2013 AHA/ACC/TOS guideline for the management of overweight and obesity in adults: a report of the American College of Cardiology/American Heart Association Task Force on Practice Guidelines and The Obesity Society. *J Am Coll Cardiol.* 2014;63(25):2985-3023. doi:10.1016/j.jacc.2013.11.004.[24]

systematic review of the role of eHealth, telehealth, and telemedicine for patients with chronic disease during the COVID-19 pandemic found limited evidence for the effectiveness of these techniques for chronic disease management and concluded that further research is needed to provide clear frameworks for chronic disease management in primary care.[57]

Furthermore, future research on the CCM and eCCM is needed among smaller primary care clinics to assess how to best support smaller practices in implementing large organizational changes, particularly for chronic conditions that are difficult to treat, such as obesity. In addition, future studies on the efficacy of the CCM and eCCM among racial and ethnic minority groups are essential.[65]

Summary

Given the complexity of obesity, its management is multifactorial. This chapter addressed interventions for the lifelong management of obesity, including self-monitoring of lifestyle related behaviors, dietary recommendations, and physical activity recommendations. Despite the physiological and environmental barriers to weight loss maintenance, long-term weight loss is achievable but requires pervasive self-monitoring, self-belief, and support from families, health care professionals, and the community.

Use of the CCM has proven effective in improving the outcomes of other chronic diseases, such as type 2 diabetes. As obesity is a chronic disease that affects 42% of adults in the United States and is a risk factor for multiple other diseases, it follows that the CCM can assist with the delivery of best practices for lifelong management of obesity and, thus, should serve as a framework for lifelong management of overweight and obesity to reduce the health burden on society.

References

1. Wharton S, Lau DCW, Vallis M, et al. Obesity in adults: a clinical practice guideline. *CMAJ*. 2020;192(31):e875-e891. doi:10.1503/cmaj.191707
2. Sharma AM. M, M, M & M: a mnemonic for assessing obesity. *Obes Rev*. 2010;11(11):808-809. doi:10.1111/j.1467-789X.2010.00766.x
3. Kyle TK, Dhurandhar EJ, Allison DB. Regarding obesity as a disease: evolving policies and their implications. *Endocrinol Metab Clin North Am*. 2016;45(3):511-520. doi:10.1016/j.ecl.2016.04.004
4. Kirk SFL, Price SL, Penney TL, et al. Blame, shame, and lack of support: a multilevel study on obesity management. *Qual Health Res*. 2014;24(6):790-800. doi:10.1177/1049732314529667
5. Deparment of Veterans Affairs, Department of Defense. VA/DoD *Clinical Practice Guideline for the Management of Adult Overweight and Obesity*. Ver. 3.0. 2020. www.healthquality.va.gov/guidelines/CD/obesity/VADoDObesityCPGFinal5087242020.pdf
6. Puhl RM, Phelan SM, Nadglowski J, Kyle TK. Overcoming weight bias in the management of patients with diabetes and obesity. *Clin Diabetes*. 2016;34(1):44-50. doi:10.2337/diaclin.34.1.44
7. Egger G, Swinburn B. An "ecological" approach to the obesity pandemic. *BMJ*. 1997;315(7106):477-480.
8. Rosenbaum M, Hirsch J, Gallagher DA, Leibel RL. Long-term persistence of adaptive thermogenesis in subjects who have maintained a reduced body weight. *Am J Clin Nutr*. 2008;88(4):906-912. doi:10.1093/ajcn/88.4.906
9. Berthoud HR, Morrison C. The brain, appetite, and obesity. *Annu Rev Psychol*. 2008;59:55-92. doi:10.1146/annurev.psych.59.103006.093551
10. Rosenbaum M, Leibel RL. 20 years of leptin: role of leptin in energy homeostasis in humans. *J Endocrinol*. 2014;223(1):T83-96. doi:10.1530/JOE-14-0358

11. Speakman JR, Levitsky DA, Allison DB, et al. Set points, settling points and some alternative models: theoretical options to understand how genes and environments combine to regulate body adiposity. *Dis Model Mech*. 2011;4(6):733-745. doi:10.1242/dmm.008698
12. Speakman JR. Why lipostatic set point systems are unlikely to evolve. *Mol Metab*. 2018;7:147-154. doi:10.1016/j.molmet.2017.10.007
13. Wu T, Gao X, Chen M, van Dam RM. Long-term effectiveness of diet-plus-exercise interventions vs. diet-only interventions for weight loss: a meta-analysis. *Obes Rev*. 2009;10(3):313-323. doi:10.1111/j.1467-789X.2008.00547.x
14. Nunes CL, Jesus F, Francisco R, et al. Adaptive thermogenesis after moderate weight loss: magnitude and methodological issues. *Eur J Nutr*. 2022;61(3):1405-1416. doi:10.1007/s00394-021-02742-6
15. Piaggi P, Vinales KL, Basolo A, Santini F, Krakoff J. Energy expenditure in the etiology of human obesity: spendthrift and thrifty metabolic phenotypes and energy-sensing mechanisms. *J Endocrinol Invest*. 2018;41(1):83-89. doi:10.1007/s40618-017-0732-9
16. Müller MJ. About "spendthrift" and "thrifty" phenotypes: resistance and susceptibility to overeating revisited. *Am J Clin Nutr*. 2019;110(3):542-543. doi:10.1093/ajcn/nqz090
17. Aronne LJ, Hall KD, Jakicic JM, et al. Describing the weight-reduced state: physiology, behavior, and interventions. *Obesity (Silver Spring)*. 2021;29(suppl 1):S9-S24. doi:10.1002/oby.23086
18. Flanagan EW, Most J, Mey JT, Redman LM. Calorie restriction and aging in humans. *Annu Rev Nutr*. 2020;40:105-133. doi:10.1146/annurev-nutr-122319-034601
19. Sohal RS, Allen RG. Relationship between metabolic rate, free radicals, differentiation and aging: a unified theory. *Basic Life Sci*. 1985;35:75-104. doi:10.1007/978-1-4899-2218-2_4
20. Martins C, Roekenes J, Salamati S, Gower BA, Hunter GR. Metabolic adaptation is an illusion, only present when participants are in negative energy balance. *Am J Clin Nutr*. 2020;112(5):1212-1218. doi:10.1093/ajcn/nqaa220
21. Fothergill E, Guo J, Howard L, et al. Persistent metabolic adaptation 6 years after "The Biggest Loser" competition. *Obesity (Silver Spring)*. 2016;24(8):1612-1619. doi:10.1002/oby.21538
22. Rosenbaum M, Sy M, Pavlovich K, Leibel RL, Hirsch J. Leptin reverses weight loss-induced changes in regional neural activity responses to visual food stimuli. *J Clin Invest*. 2008;118(7):2583-2591. doi:10.1172/JCI35055
23. Gao Q, Horvath TL. Neurobiology of feeding and energy expenditure. *Annu Rev Neurosci*. 2007;30:367-398. doi:10.1146/annurev.neuro.30.051606.094324
24. Jensen MD, Ryan DH, Apovian CM, et al. 2013 AHA/ACC/TOS guideline for the management of overweight and obesity in adults: a report of the American College of Cardiology/American Heart Association Task Force on Practice Guidelines and The Obesity Society. *J Am Coll Cardiol*. 2014;63(25):2985-3023. doi:10.1016/j.jacc.2013.11.004
25. Wadden TA, Stunkard AJ, Day SC, Gould RA, Rubin CJ. Less food, less hunger: reports of appetite and symptoms in a controlled study of a protein-sparing modified fast. *Int J Obes*. 1987;11(3):239-249.
26. Martin CK, O'Neil PM, Pawlow L. Changes in food cravings during low-calorie and very-low-calorie diets. *Obesity (Silver Spring)*. 2006;14(1):115-121. doi:10.1038/oby.2006.14
27. Apolzan JW, Myers CA, Champagne CM, et al. Frequency of consuming foods predicts changes in cravings for those foods during weight loss: the POUNDS Lost study. *Obesity (Silver Spring)*. 2017;25(8):1343-1348. doi:10.1002/oby.21895
28. Swinburn B, Egger G, Raza F. Dissecting obesogenic environments: the development and application of a framework for identifying and prioritizing environmental interventions for obesity. *Prev Med*. 1999;29(6 Pt 1):563-570. doi:10.1006/pmed.1999.0585
29. Berthoud HR. Multiple neural systems controlling food intake and body weight. *Neurosci Biobehav Rev*. 2002;26(4):393-428. doi:10.1016/S0149-7634(02)00014-3
30. Berthoud HR, Münzberg H, Morrison CD. Blaming the brain for obesity: integration of hedonic and homeostatic mechanisms. *Gastroenterology*. 2017;152(7):1728-1738. doi:10.1053/j.gastro.2016.12.050
31. Hall KD, Ayuketah A, Brychta R, et al. Ultra-processed diets cause excess calorie intake and weight gain: an inpatient randomized controlled trial of ad libitum food intake. *Cell Metab*. 2019;30(1):67-77.e3. doi:10.1016/j.cmet.2019.05.008
32. Hall KD, Guo J, Courville AB, et al. Effect of a plant-based, low-fat diet versus an animal-based, ketogenic diet on ad libitum energy intake. *Nat Med*. 2021;27(2):344-353. doi:10.1038/s41591-020-01209-1
33. Lissner L, Levitsky DA, Strupp BJ, Kalkwarf HJ, Roe DA. Dietary fat and the regulation of energy intake in human subjects. *Am J Clin Nutr*. 1987;46(6):886-892. doi:10.1093/ajcn/46.6.886
34. Stubbs RJ, Harbron CG, Murgatroyd PR, Prentice AM. Covert manipulation of dietary fat and energy density: effect on substrate flux and food intake in men eating ad libitum. *Am J Clin Nutr*. 1995;62(2):316-329. doi:10.1093/ajcn/62.2.316
35. Monteiro CA, Cannon G, Moubarac JC, Levy RB, Louzada MLC, Jaime PC. The UN Decade of Nutrition, the NOVA food classification and the trouble with ultra-processing. *Public Health Nutr*. 2018;21(1):5-17. doi:10.1017/S1368980017000234

36. Enriori PJ, Evans AE, Sinnayah P, et al. Diet-induced obesity causes severe but reversible leptin resistance in arcuate melanocortin neurons. *Cell Metab.* 2007;5(3):181-194. doi:10.1016/j.cmet.2007.02.004

37. Fazzino TL, Rohde K, Sullivan DK. Hyper-palatable foods: development of a quantitative definition and application to the US food system database. *Obesity (Silver Spring).* 2019;27(11):1761-1768. doi:10.1002/oby.22639

38. Fazzino TL, Dorling JL, Apolzan JW, Martin CK. Meal composition during an ad libitum buffet meal and longitudinal predictions of weight and percent body fat change: the role of hyper-palatable, energy dense, and ultra-processed foods. *Appetite.* 2021;167:105592. doi:10.1016/j.appet.2021.105592

39. Anderson JW, Konz EC, Frederich RC, Wood CL. Long-term weight-loss maintenance: a meta-analysis of US studies. *Am J Clin Nutr.* 2001;74(5):579-584. doi:10.1093/ajcn/74.5.579

40. Wing RR, Phelan S. Long-term weight loss maintenance. *Am J Clin Nutr.* 2005;82(1):222 S-225 S. doi:10.1093/ajcn/82.1.222 S

41. Thomas JG, Bond DS, Phelan S, Hill JO, Wing RR. Weight-loss maintenance for 10 years in the National Weight Control Registry. *Am J Prev Med.* 2014;46(1):17-23. doi:10.1016/j.amepre.2013.08.019

42. Wyatt HR, Grunwald GK, Mosca CL, Klem ML, Wing RR, Hill JO. Long-term weight loss and breakfast in subjects in the National Weight Control Registry. *Obes Res.* 2002;10(2):78-82. doi:10.1038/oby.2002.13

43. Xie W, Lundberg DJ, Collins JM, et al. Association of weight loss between early adulthood and midlife with all-cause mortality risk in the US. *JAMA Netw Open.* 2020;3(8):e2013448. doi:10.1001/jamanetworkopen.2020.13448

44. Carlsson LMS, Sjöholm K, Jacobson P, et al. Life expectancy after bariatric surgery in the Swedish Obese Subjects Study. *N Engl J Med.* 2020;383(16):1535-1543. doi:10.1056/NEJMoa2002449

45. Varkevisser RDM, van Stralen MM, Kroeze W, Ket JCF, Steenhuis IHM. Determinants of weight loss maintenance: a systematic review. *Obes Rev.* 2019;20(2):171-211. doi:10.1111/obr.12772

46. Hall KD, Kahan S. Maintenance of lost weight and long-term management of obesity. *Med Clin North Am.* 2018;102(1):183-197. doi:10.1016/j.mcna.2017.08.012

47. Hall KD, Kahan S. Maintenance of lost weight and long-term management of obesity. *Med Clin North Am.* 2018;102(1):183-197. doi:10.1016/j.mcna.2017.08.012

48. Martin CK, Heilbronn LK, de Jonge L, et al. Effect of calorie restriction on resting metabolic rate and spontaneous physical activity. *Obesity.* 2007;15(12):2964-2973. doi:10.1038/oby.2007.354

49. Reyes NR, Oliver TL, Klotz AA, et al. Similarities and differences between weight loss maintainers and regainers: a qualitative analysis. *J Acad Nutr Diet.* 2012;112(4):499-505. doi:10.1016/j.jand.2011.11.014

50. Thomas JG, Bond DS, Phelan S, Hill JO, Wing RR. Weight-loss maintenance for 10 years in the National Weight Control Registry. *Am J Prev Med.* 2014;46(1):17-23. doi:10.1016/j.amepre.2013.08.019

51. Donnelly JE, Blair SN, Jakicic JM, et al. American College of Sports Medicine Position Stand: appropriate physical activity intervention strategies for weight loss and prevention of weight regain for adults. *Med Sci Sports Exerc.* 2009;41(2):459-471. doi:10.1249/MSS.0b013e3181949333

52. Hill JO, Peters JC, Wyatt HR. Using the energy gap to address obesity: a commentary. *J Am Diet Assoc.* 2009;109(11):1848-1853. doi:10.1016/j.jada.2009.08.007

53. Washburn RA, Szabo-Reed AN, Gorczyca AM, et al. A randomized trial evaluating exercise for the prevention of weight regain. *Obesity (Silver Spring).* 2021;29(1):62-70. doi:10.1002/oby.23022

54. Powell-Wiley TM, Baumer Y, Baah FO, et al. Social determinants of cardiovascular disease. *Circ Res.* 2022;130(5):782-799. doi:10.1161/CIRCRESAHA.121.319811

55. Dixon BN, Ugwoaba UA, Brockmann AN, Ross KM. Associations between the built environment and dietary intake, physical activity, and obesity: a scoping review of reviews. *Obes Rev.* 2021;22(4):e13171. doi:10.1111/obr.13171

56. Gee PM, Greenwood DA, Paterniti DA, Ward D, Miller LMS. The eHealth Enhanced Chronic Care Model: a theory derivation approach. *J Med Internet Res.* 2015;17(4):e86. doi:10.2196/jmir.4067

57. Bitar H, Alismail S. The role of eHealth, telehealth, and telemedicine for chronic disease patients during COVID-19 pandemic: a rapid systematic review. *Digit Health.* 2021;7:20552076211009396. doi:10.1177/20552076211009396

58. Dunn P, Conard S. Chronic Care Model in research and in practice. *Int J Cardiol.* 2018;258:295-296. doi:10.1016/j.ijcard.2018.01.078

59. LeBlanc ES, Patnode CD, Webber EM, Redmond N, Rushkin M, O'Connor EA. Behavioral and pharmacotherapy weight loss interventions to prevent obesity-related morbidity and mortality in adults: updated evidence report and systematic review for the US Preventive Services Task Force. *JAMA.* 2018;320(11):1172-1191. doi:10.1001/jama.2018.7777

60. Wagner EH. Academia, chronic care, and the future of primary care. *J Gen Intern Med.* 2010;25(S4):636-638. doi:10.1007/s11606-010-1442-6

61. Wagner EH. Chronic disease management: what will it take to improve care for chronic illness? *Eff Clin Pract.* 1998;1(1):2-4.

62. Wagner EH, Austin BT, Davis C, Hindmarsh M, Schaefer J, Bonomi A. Improving chronic illness care: translating evidence into action. *Health Affairs.* 2001;20(6):64-78. doi:10.1377/hlthaff.20.6.64

63. Yeoh EK, Wong MCS, Wong ELY, et al. Benefits and limitations of implementing Chronic Care Model (CCM) in primary care programs: a systematic review. *Int J Cardiol*. 2018;258:279-288. doi:10.1016/j.ijcard.2017.11.057
64. Davy C, Bleasel J, Liu H, Tchan M, Ponniah S, Brown A. Effectiveness of chronic care models: opportunities for improving healthcare practice and health outcomes: a systematic review. *BMC Health Serv Res*. 2015;15(1):194. doi:10.1186/s12913-015-0854-8
65. Stellefson M, Dipnarine K, Stopka C. The Chronic Care Model and diabetes management in us primary care settings: a systematic review. *Prev Chronic Dis*. 2013;10:120180. doi:10.5888/pcd10.120180
66. Jimison H, Gorman P, Woods S, et al. Barriers and drivers of health information technology use for the elderly, chronically ill, and underserved. *Evid Rep Technol Assess (Full Rep)*. 2008;(175):1-1422.

CHAPTER 16

Treatment of Obesity and Eating Disorders

Laura D'Adamo, MS
Molly Fennig, MA
Anne Claire Grammer, MA
Hiba Jebeile, APD, PhD
Ellen E. Fitzsimmons-Craft, PhD
Denise E. Wilfley, PhD

CHAPTER OBJECTIVES

- Discuss the evidence for the relationship between dieting and eating pathology.
- Describe the relationship between professionally delivered weight management programs and eating pathology.
- Identify treatment options for comorbid binge eating disorder and obesity.
- Provide recommendations for the assessment and monitoring of eating disorder risk in weight management programs.

Introduction

A substantial number of individuals with overweight or obesity also experience disordered eating.[1] The codevelopment of these conditions may result from shared etiological factors and relations between lifestyle behaviors, psychosocial processes, and weight regulation.[2-5] Despite evidence demonstrating that a sizable proportion of adults seeking weight management care have eating pathology, no guidance exists for health professionals regarding procedures for screening, intervention, and ongoing evaluation of eating pathology during weight management interventions.[6,7] This chapter attempts to aid health professionals in monitoring and addressing eating pathology in this population. Specifically, it aims to: (1) highlight the prevalence, shared etiological mechanisms, and presentations of comorbid overweight or obesity and eating disorders; (2) discuss the evidence regarding the risk for developing or exacerbating eating pathology during interventions for weight management; and (3) provide guidance for assessment, treatment, and continued monitoring of eating disorder risk during weight management interventions.

The Intersection of Overweight or Obesity and Eating Disorders

Patients with overweight or obesity who also have an eating disorder may face a greater health toll than that posed by either condition alone, warranting the need for early identification and treatment.[8] This section aims to aid health professionals in identifying and managing these comorbid concerns.

Overview of Eating Disorders and Disordered Eating

Defining Clinical Eating Disorders

Eating disorders are serious psychiatric disorders characterized by a substantial eating disturbance that impairs a person's physical health or psychosocial functioning.[9] The three main types of eating disorders are anorexia nervosa (AN), bulimia nervosa (BN), and binge eating disorder (BED). The key diagnostic criteria for these disorders, as outlined in the *Diagnostic and Statistical Manual of Mental Disorders*, Fifth Edition (*DSM-5*), are provided in Box 16.1.[9] A systematic review of 94 studies conducted between 2000 and 2018 found that the mean rates of lifetime eating disorder diagnosis were 8.4% for women and 2.2% for men[†], although the difference in proportions by gender is not as pronounced in BED.[10] Onset of AN and BN typically occurs during adolescence and young adulthood,[11] whereas BED has a broader age of onset, spanning from childhood to late adulthood.[12] The category of "other specified feeding or eating disorders" encompasses eating disorders that do not meet the full diagnostic criteria for any of the aforementioned diagnoses. Included in this category are atypical AN (AN with weight in the normal

† Study participants were described as men and women. Gender was not further specified.

BOX 16.1

Diagnostic Criteria for the Main Types of Eating Disorders[9]

Eating disorder	*Diagnostic and Statistical Manual of Mental Disorders*, Fifth Edition, diagnostic criteria
Anorexia nervosa	Restriction of food intake leading to lower-than-expected body weight
	Intense fear of weight gain or being fat
	Body-image disturbance, excessive influence of shape or weight on self-assessment, or not acknowledging the seriousness of low body weight
	Subtypes: restricting, binge/purge
Bulimia nervosa	Recurrent episodes of binge eating characterized by eating a very large amount of food within 2 hours and experiencing loss of control during the episode
	Recurrent compensatory behaviors (vomiting, laxative or diuretic use, excessive exercise, diet pills)
	Binge eating and compensatory behaviors occurring at least once per week for 3 months
	Self-evaluation unduly influenced by shape or weight
	Behaviors occurring distinctly apart from anorexia nervosa
Binge eating disorder	Recurrent episodes of binge eating characterized by eating a very large amount of food within 2 hours and experiencing loss of control during the episode
	Binge eating occurring at least once per week for 3 months
	Binge episodes that are associated with three of the following: eating more rapidly than normal; eating until overly full; eating large amounts of food when not hungry; eating alone because of embarrassment about quantity of food eaten; feeling emotionally bad after eating
	Distress about binge eating
	Binge eating that occurs in the absence of compensatory behaviors

range), BN of low frequency and/or limited duration, BED of low frequency and/or limited duration, purging disorder (purging behavior without binge eating), and night eating syndrome (recurrent episodes of night eating).

Well-established risk factors for AN include negative affect, low BMI, perfectionism, family weight and eating concerns, family history of AN, and impaired interpersonal functioning.[13,14] A leading risk-factor model of BN, BED, and purging disorder proposes that these three disorders have overlapping etiological and maintaining mechanisms that are somewhat distinct from those of AN. In this model, internalization of the "thin ideal" leads to body dissatisfaction. Body dissatisfaction predicts dieting behavior or negative affect (or both), which each predict the onset of an eating disorder.[15] Notably, negative affect and impaired interpersonal functioning are risk factors for all eating disorders.[14]

Defining Disordered Eating

Disordered eating refers to attitudes (eg, overvaluation of shape and weight) and behaviors (eg, binge eating, extreme weight-control behaviors) that characterize eating disorders but which do not occur at the frequency or duration required to meet *DSM-5* diagnostic criteria. One such form of disordered eating—binge eating—will be discussed at length in this chapter. Unlike overeating, binge eating refers to eating a very large amount of food *and* feeling a loss of control during eating episodes. Despite not qualifying for a diagnosis, disordered eating has detrimental effects and is important to detect and address. Importantly, it increases risk for the development of clinical eating disorders and weight gain.[5,16] Prospective research has shown that the risk factors predicting subthreshold eating disorders are generally the same risk factors that predict clinical eating disorders of the same type,[14] highlighting the need for early detection of risk factors for disordered eating and early intervention to prevent full-syndrome eating disorders.

Co-Occurrence of Overweight or Obesity and Eating Disorders

Prevalence of Co-Occurrence

Although a common perception is that eating disorders primarily affect individuals of lower body weight, the prevalence of eating disorders and disordered eating among adults with overweight or obesity is actually higher than it is among lower-weight adults.[1,17,18] In particular, overweight or obesity and binge-spectrum eating disorders (BN and BED) tend to co-occur. Data from the World Health Organization's World Mental Health Surveys show that 32.8% and 38.1% of respondents with lifetime BN and 12-month BN, respectively, and 36.2% and 41.7% with lifetime BED and 12-month BED, respectively, had obesity. Both sets of rates were markedly high compared to the percentage of individuals with no lifetime eating disorder who had obesity (15.8%).[19] The co-occurrence of BED and obesity is particularly well-documented. In a nationally representative sample of 36,306 adults in the United States, those with a lifetime or 12-month diagnosis of BED were more likely to have current class 1, 2, or 3 obesity than were individuals with no history of an eating disorder.[20] Individuals with BED are three to six times more likely to have obesity than those without an eating disorder.[19,21]

Distinguishing Features of Eating Disorders and Obesity

Although binge-spectrum eating disorders are highly associated with obesity, these disorders and obesity have distinguishing psychopathological features. Thus, not all individuals with obesity have BED or BN, and not all individuals with BED or BN have obesity, despite the substantial rate of co-occurrence. Box 16.2 presents the distinguishing characteristics associated with eating disorders and obesity.

BOX 16.2

Distinguishing Characteristics of Eating Disorders and Obesity

Eating disorders

Psychiatric disorders marked by persistent disturbance in eating behavior and associated distress that may impair physical functioning, psychosocial functioning, or both

Can occur in individuals of any weight; do not necessarily involve body weight being on the higher or lower end of the weight spectrum

Obesity

Multifactorial disease defined by elevated BMI

Does not necessarily involve pathological forms of eating (eg, binge eating)

Shared Risk and Maintenance Factors for Co-Occurrence

The common co-occurrence of overweight or obesity and binge-spectrum eating disorders may result from shared risk and maintenance factors for both conditions, which are summarized in Box 16.3. For example, both overweight or obesity and eating disorders are associated with body dissatisfaction, dieting, deficits in executive function, and general psychopathology.[2-4,17] Research has also supported a bidirectional relation between excess weight and eating pathology. For instance, binge eating and compensatory behaviors are risk factors for weight gain and may contribute to the development and maintenance of overweight and obesity.[5] In the other direction, high BMI has been shown to precede the development of eating disorder symptomology.[5,22,23] In a study of 9,713 young adults, higher weight was found to be the most consistent predictor of eating disorder symptoms; participants with excess weight showed greater eating disorder risk, binge eating, and compensatory behaviors than those with lower weights.[24] This correlation may be due to the psychosocial risk

---

BOX 16.3

Shared Risk Factors for Excess Weight and Binge-Spectrum Eating Disorders in Adults

Weight and shape concerns

Binge eating and compensatory behaviors (eg, excessive exercise)

Dieting

Depressive and anxiety symptoms

Weight stigma

Food-related impulsivity, negative affect, and deficits in interpersonal functioning

factors for eating disorders that individuals with higher body weight face, including body dissatisfaction and weight stigma.[25] These factors may lead individuals to diet or experience negative affects, which in turn may result in disordered eating. A large body of literature supports the notion that experiencing weight-based stigma and discrimination is associated with disordered eating, increased food intake, weight gain, and obesity.[26,27] This indicates that individuals with overweight or obesity may face heightened risk for disordered eating and further weight gain. The shared roles of negative affect, impaired interpersonal functioning, and food-related impulsivity in binge-spectrum eating disorders and obesity have also been demonstrated.[28-31] Shared maintenance factors of overweight or obesity and BED include sedentary behavior and preference for foods with a high energy content.[32,33] This is important for providers to recognize, as the similar lifestyle behaviors of individuals with each condition may make it difficult to detect BED. As discussed in the previous section, providers need to be able to distinguish between overeating and binge eating among patients seeking weight management interventions.

Presentations, Correlates, and Health Outcomes in Co-Occurrence

Patients with eating disorders and obesity differ in important ways from patients with eating disorders who do not have obesity; the distinct characteristics of those with co-occurrence are summarized in Box 16.4. For instance, individuals with BED and obesity tend to be older and have a longer duration of binge-eating problems compared to their lower-weight counterparts.[34] Similarly, individuals with eating disorders and obesity have a later age of onset for eating disorders, longer duration of eating disorders, greater eating pathology severity, and greater general psychopathology than do individuals without obesity.[35] Longer periods of eating disorder pathology may be a signal of delayed receipt of treatment for individuals with comorbid obesity, which is concerning given the detrimental physical and psychosocial correlates of these disorders. Delayed treatment may result from stereotypes about the types of individuals who have eating disorders. Furthermore, a study of university women with eating disorders found that participants with overweight or obesity had greater weight and shape concerns, perceived benefits of thinness, and general psychopathology than those without overweight or obesity, as well as higher rates of subclinical or clinical BED.[17]

BOX 16.4

Correlates and Features of Co-Occurrence of Overweight or Obesity and Eating Disorders

- Greater severity of eating pathology (eg, weight or shape concerns)
- Heightened general psychopathology (eg, depressive symptoms and anxiety)
- Later age of onset of eating disorder and longer duration of eating disorder
- Greater weight-related comorbidities (eg, type 2 diabetes and metabolic syndrome)
- Greater weight gain prior to the start of weight-management interventions

Individuals with eating disorders and excess weight also appear to be at greater risk for negative psychosocial and medical comorbidities than individuals with overweight or obesity but without eating disorders. For instance, women with BED and obesity report higher rates of depression, anxiety, and external and emotional eating than those with obesity but without BED.[8,36] BED is also associated with weight-related comorbidities, including metabolic syndrome and type 2 diabetes, and individuals with BED and obesity have an elevated risk of developing dyslipidemia and respiratory and gastrointestinal diseases.[37-39] Research has shown that compared to individuals with overweight or obesity but without BED, those in whom these conditions co-occur gain more weight in the year prior to weight management treatment.[40] In nonclinical samples, research has established that similar correlates of subclinical binge eating among individuals with overweight or obesity have emerged, including higher rates of impulsivity; inhibitory control deficits; depressive symptoms; greater weight, shape, and eating concerns; lower self-esteem; and lower satisfaction with one's appearance.[1,41,42]

On the whole, these data indicate that patients with comorbid overweight or obesity and eating disorders may have unique presentations and face greater risk for comorbidities than those with either condition alone. These patterns suggest an urgent need to detect and treat these comorbid concerns among individuals seeking interventions for weight management.

Stigma and Stereotypes as Barriers to Evidence-Based Care

To facilitate quality care for patients with excess weight and eating disorders, health professionals should be aware of the barriers to the recognition of these conditions and access to quality care, as well as clinical practices that may exacerbate them. As previously mentioned, weight stigma is a risk factor for disordered eating and excess weight, with effects that hold even when controlling for BMI.[26,43] At least 40% of adults in the United States report having experienced weight stigma.[44,45] Importantly, weight stigma is prevalent in health care settings.[46,47] A study published in 2021 found that, of individuals enrolled in weight management programs who reported a history of experiencing weight stigma, 67% reported experiencing weight stigma from physicians.[43] Participants who internalized stigmatizing messages about their weight reported greater avoidance of physician visits, greater perceived weight-based judgment from physicians, lower frequency of attending regular checkups, and lower quality of received health care.[43] This indicates that weight stigma may both preclude patients with comorbid excess weight and eating disorders from receiving quality care and exacerbate both conditions. Health professionals should use nonstigmatizing language when communicating about weight and eating disorders, acknowledge barriers to evidence-based care for obesity and eating disorders, respect the patient's right to decline discussing weight status or pursuing weight management, and enact health care training practices that do not promote stereotypes about obesity.[48]

Health professionals should also be aware of other common barriers that patients face when seeking and receiving treatment for eating disorders. First, eating disorders often go undetected in clinical settings, and very few individuals receive treatment for eating disorders.[49-52] Established barriers to receiving treatment include the social stigma surrounding eating disorders, which can cause patients to conceal their conditions; stereotypes about the types of patients who have eating disorders, which can cause physicians to fail to recognize such disorders; financial barriers; and proximity to treatment centers.[53] Stereotypes about people with eating disorders may even lead higher-weight patients to not recognize these conditions in themselves, which may interfere with seeking treatment. Evidence also suggests that patients who are ethnic minorities are less likely to be referred for treatment of eating disorders.[53] Moreover, individuals with excess weight and eating disorders more readily seek and receive treatment for overweight or obesity than for eating disorders.[54,55] Health professionals should be aware that patients may present with eating pathology that has persisted over time without treatment. They should aim to combat stigma and stereotypes surrounding eating disorders and complete routine screening to improve the rates of detection and treatment for eating disorders using evidence-based guidelines.

Relative Risk of Dietary Restriction

Self-Directed Dieting vs Professionally Delivered Weight Management Interventions

Dieting, the effort to restrict food intake to change one's weight or shape, is one of the most common strategies used by adults for weight management. Between 2010 and 2015, 40% of adults worldwide reported self-attempted weight loss in the preceding year.[56] Self-directed dieting is common across the life span, with women[†] and individuals with overweight or obesity showing the highest prevalence.[56-58] Prospective studies have established self-directed dieting as a risk factor for the development of eating disorders and disordered eating behavior.[5,59] This section discusses the psychological and behavioral processes involved in self-directed dietary restriction, the risk for eating disorders and weight gain implicated in common dieting practices, and recommendations for providing guidance to patients who aim to make dietary changes for weight management.

Of importance to health professionals is the distinction between dietary restriction prescribed in professionally delivered weight management interventions and self-directed dieting. Professionally delivered interventions typically promote dietary change, either with or without an energy prescription, for the reduction of excess adiposity. These prescriptions generally promote increased consumption of nutrient-dense foods (ie, foods high in vitamins, minerals, and fiber) and reduced consumption of energy-dense foods (ie, foods with a high energy content per volume or weight). In addition, dietary restriction in professionally delivered interventions is employed under supervision and is often coupled with either psychoeducation, comprehensive behavior-change techniques, or both. Features of specific forms of self-directed dieting and professionally delivered weight management treatment will be discussed.

Self-Directed Dieting for Weight Loss and the Risk for Eating Disorders

Self-directed dieting is well established as a risk factor for eating disorders and disordered eating. For instance, research has found that dieters are more likely to develop onset of binge eating than nondieters.[60-62] Binge eating can, in turn, contribute to weight gain, which may reinforce concerns about weight or shape

---

† Study participants were described as women. Gender was not further specified.

and perpetuate dieting. This idea is supported by longitudinal data that have consistently shown self-directed dieting behaviors to be associated with binge eating and weight gain.[63] However, research suggests that most individuals who diet will not develop symptoms of an eating disorder.[60] Some research suggests that the risk for developing a dieting-induced eating disorder may be greatest in the presence of other factors that increase vulnerability for the development of eating pathology. A study that monitored 1,272 young women[†] at high risk for developing an eating disorder for 3 years found dieting to be a predictor of BN and BED, alongside depression, internalization of the thin ideal, functional impairment, body dissatisfaction, and overeating.[14] Another study that monitored a sample of adolescents and young adults for 10 years found that depressive symptoms and self-esteem played a key role in the relationship between dieting and the onset of binge eating, in that they predicted binge-eating onset beyond the effects of dieting alone. However, these factors only predicted increased binge eating among dieters (compared to nondieters), suggesting that dieting alone remained a key risk factor.[60] On the whole, data suggest that self-directed dieting is a major mechanism for eating pathology, and risk may be greatest among dieters who have other psychopathology.

Disentangling the Dimensions of Dieting

Experts generally agree that dieting (ie, following a specific eating regimen for weight loss or maintenance), *dietary restraint* (the cognitive effort to limit energy intake), and *energy restriction* are related but distinct concepts.[64,65] However, the term *dieting* is often used to denote all processes and behaviors related to attempted energy restriction in response to a desire to lose weight or change body shape or dimensions, acknowledging the fact that restraint and restriction may both be involved in dieting. Dietary restraint, which a person can engage in even in the absence of true energy restriction, has received much attention for its link to eating disorder risk and weight management. Experts theorize that it promotes eating pathology by increasing feelings of self-deprivation and psychological pressure to eat restricted foods, thereby increasing the risk for binge eating and weight gain.[66] In weight management programs, however, engaging in dietary restraint is considered a primary goal of treatment, as attempting to limit food intake signifies adherence to a dietary regimen that requires self-regulatory effort.[67] A review of longitudinal studies of weight loss interventions found that increased restraint over time was associated with greater weight losses and weight loss maintenance outcomes.[68] To explain this discrepancy, experts have proposed that individuals can display either rigid or flexible characteristics of restraint, with flexible restraint allowing for healthy behavior and weight loss without inducing eating disorder risk.[69] For example, people with flexible restraint implement dietary rules in a way that allows them to enjoy food and participate in social aspects of eating (eg, eating a piece of cake at a birthday party). On the other hand, those who display rigid restraint adhere strictly to dietary rules and may feel guilty or employ compensatory behaviors to counteract breaking those rules.

A 2016 review[64] of the relationship between dietary restraint, weight trajectory, and the development of eating pathology explains that a number of self-regulatory efforts are needed to sustain healthy forms of dietary restraint: self-monitoring, self-evaluation of one's behavior relative to goals, and self-reinforcement of one's reactions to self-evaluation. Ineffective forms of self-regulation (eg, inaccurate self-monitoring, feelings of self-deprivation) interrupt this process and lead to dysregulated behaviors (eg, binge eating). For instance, a patient who completes irregular or inaccurate self-monitoring may set unrealistic weight loss goals and experience poor self-evaluation and self-reinforcement as a result, leading to disordered eating. The authors of the review also posit that the circumstances under which restraint is employed probably influence the likelihood of effective or ineffective self-regulation and, thus, the likelihood of success with weight management or disordered eating. For instance, they note that someone with obesity who is enrolled in a weight management program may be better equipped to display successful self-regulation (and thus healthy dietary restraint) than someone with lower weight who is pursuing self-directed weight loss.

A team of researchers has provided a classification paradigm for dieting phenomena, including behavioral and psychological indices and their presumed associations with eating pathology.[70] This paradigm, illustrated in Figure 16.1,[70] includes both behavioral dimensions (ranging from low to high, indicating the degree to which dieting behaviors are sufficient to produce change in body shape or weight) and psychological dimensions (ranging from negative to positive, indicating psychological approaches reflecting characteristics associated with either disordered eating and weight gain or flexibility and healthful dieting).

FIGURE 16.1 Psychobehavioral paradigm of dieting[70]

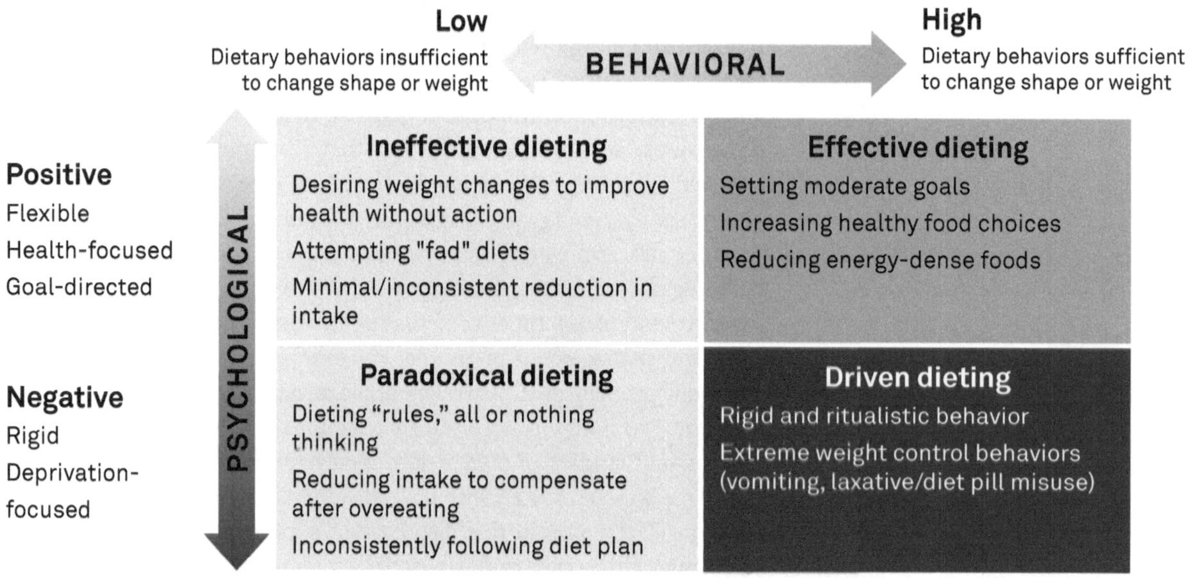

	Low — Dietary behaviors insufficient to change shape or weight	**High** — Dietary behaviors sufficient to change shape or weight
Positive — Flexible, Health-focused, Goal-directed	**Ineffective dieting** — Desiring weight changes to improve health without action; Attempting "fad" diets; Minimal/inconsistent reduction in intake	**Effective dieting** — Setting moderate goals; Increasing healthy food choices; Reducing energy-dense foods
Negative — Rigid, Deprivation-focused	**Paradoxical dieting** — Dieting "rules," all or nothing thinking; Reducing intake to compensate after overeating; Inconsistently following diet plan	**Driven dieting** — Rigid and ritualistic behavior; Extreme weight control behaviors (vomiting, laxative/diet pill misuse)

Driven dieting (behaviorally high, psychologically negative) refers to dietary restriction accompanied by negative psychological processes—for example, an "all or nothing" diet mentality—and is associated with risk for disordered eating.

Paradoxical dieting (behaviorally low, psychologically negative) encompasses processes captured by the construct of rigid dietary restraint, as seen in individuals who have intentions to diet that are not carried out, coupled with a rigid psychological focus on dieting.

Effective dieting (behaviorally high, psychologically positive), on the other hand, reflects characteristics of flexible dietary restraint, wherein individuals have intentions to diet and employ dieting behaviors that effectively reduce weight. Dieting behaviors are generally moderate and approached with psychological flexibility. As such, effective dieting is unlikely to lead to eating pathology.

Ineffective dieting (behaviorally low, psychologically positive) reflects characteristics of individuals with intentions to diet and a positive approach to dieting whose dieting behaviors are not sufficient to produce weight loss. Although weight is unlikely to change with this approach, ineffective dieters are likely to be protected from the risk of developing an eating disorder because the rigid psychological processes that promote eating pathology are absent.

Professionally Delivered Weight Management Programs and the Risk for Eating Disorders

Increasing recognition of the overlap between eating disorders and overweight or obesity, coupled with findings that support self-directed dieting as a risk factor for eating disorders, has led to concerns that professionally delivered interventions for weight management may promote risk for the development of eating disorders. Importantly, individuals who engage in binge eating are more likely to seek weight management treatment than individuals who do not binge eat.[6] Thus, it is essential for health professionals to know whether weight management interventions influence the risk for eating disorders. This section discusses eating disorder risk in professionally delivered interventions for weight management.

Lifestyle Interventions

Behavioral Weight Loss

Behavioral weight loss (BWL) interventions, which pair prescriptions to reduce energy intake and increase physical activity with behavior therapy, are recommended as the first line of intervention for adults with overweight or obesity.[71] In contrast with many forms of self-directed dieting, the structured form of BWL programs promotes gradual, sustainable changes to lifestyle behaviors to promote long-term maintenance of weight loss and health.[72,73] As such, BWL interventions may be considered a form of effective dieting within the aforementioned psychobehavioral paradigm (refer to Figure 16.1).[70] They effectively produce clinically significant weight losses, promote moderate behavioral changes (eg, gradual reduction in energy intake, moderate levels of physical activity), and promote a flexible psychological approach to weight loss behaviors.[48] Furthermore, as the previously discussed 2016 review article suggests, BWL therapy is employed under professional supervision and for individuals who may benefit from weight loss, making it more likely that a healthy approach to dieting is possible with a BWL intervention.[64]

Few studies have examined eating disorder outcomes following trials of BWL interventions in patients without BED. A 2017 systematic review found that two studies delivered in primary care, one evaluating a BWL program and one evaluating a motivational-interviewing intervention, reported reductions in binge eating following the interventions.[74] Another study of adults participating in a lifestyle intervention that included diet and exercise counseling found that individuals who successfully maintained a weight loss of at least 5% of their body weight showed reductions in uncontrolled eating and increased cognitive restraint.[75] A weight management intervention for individuals with class 3 obesity that included personalized combinations of lifestyle intervention, behavioral modification, dietary intervention, and pharmacotherapy found that the proportion of participants at high risk for an eating disorder decreased from 53% at baseline to 47% at 12 months; the intervention also produced improved global eating pathology, which was correlated with weight loss.[76] In addition, obesity prevention programs that promote lifestyle modification for adolescents and young adults with normal weight and overweight have been found to reduce symptoms of eating disorders.[77-79]

Low-Calorie Diet Prescriptions

Lifestyle interventions with restrictive dietary prescriptions, including the use of meal replacements, have been used to facilitate rapid weight loss. These programs differ from BWL programs, which promote moderate restriction and slower weight loss. The effects of clinically supervised interventions prescribing restrictive diets, including low-calorie diets (800–1,200 kcal/d) and very low-calorie diets (approximately 800 kcal/d), on disordered eating have been examined in a systematic review of 10 trials.[80] Findings from these trials were mixed. Participants with pretreatment BED generally reported a reduction in binge eating. One such study, which prescribed severe dietary restriction and then randomly assigned participants to either receive cognitive-behavioral therapy (CBT) for BED or receive no further treatment, found that reductions in binge eating did not differ between the CBT and control groups. For participants with subclinical symptoms of binge eating or no symptoms of binge eating, researchers report a reduction in symptoms, yet other studies reported no change or an increase; notably, two low-quality studies reported that 10% of participants developed BED.[80] Another study randomly assigned women[†] with obesity to one of three interventions: a 1,000-kcal/d diet with four servings per day of a liquid meal replacement (160 kcal per serving plus an evening meal), a 1,200 to 1,500-kcal/d balanced-deficit diet of typical foods, or a nondieting condition.[81] No significant differences in binge eating were observed over 20 weeks, and all three interventions produced reductions in hunger and disinhibition. However, by week 28, a significantly greater proportion of binge-eating cases were observed among individuals assigned to 1,000 kcal/d with meal replacement than among individuals in the other groups. More specifically, four participants reported one or two binge episodes by week 28, which remitted by week 40. One additional participant, who achieved a weight loss of 27% of initial body weight, reported four binge episodes by week 40 and then was lost to follow-up. At the 65-week follow-up mark, there were no differences in binge eating between the three groups, and at no time did any participant meet the diagnostic criteria for BED. Due to the small number of participants who experienced binge eating during the intervention period and one participant with persisting symptoms, the authors could not determine whether the binge eating occurred as a result of the restrictive diet, substantial weight loss, or other factors.

Recommendations: Lifestyle Interventions

Findings from these studies demonstrate that professionally delivered BWL interventions do not promote eating pathology and, in fact, have shown reductions in disordered-eating symptoms for most participants. However, most studies of obesity treatment have not included individuals with eating disorders. Several aspects of BWL therapy are congruent with gold-standard treatment for eating disorders, including the promotion of a structured, regular pattern of eating and meal planning.[48] In the cognitive-behavioral approach to treating eating disorders, regular eating is integral to reducing binge eating and is one of the first treatment components implemented. It has been found to mediate the effect of CBT on binge eating.[82] Eating regularly eliminates the chance of infrequent or delayed eating, two forms of dieting behavior known to trigger binge eating. As such, it theoretically prevents the psychological and physiological vulnerability

---

† Study participants were described as women. Gender was not further specified.

to binge eating caused by dietary restraint or restriction, thereby curbing patterns of binge eating. In turn, compensatory behaviors (eg, vomiting or misuse of laxatives or diuretics), which follow binge episodes, are likely to cease as well, making regular eating highly effective at disrupting binge-type eating disorders.[83] Given this, the prescription of regular eating in professionally delivered weight management programs may prevent patients with pretreatment binge eating from developing a full-syndrome binge-spectrum eating disorder.

In gold-standard obesity treatment, environmental changes and stimulus control are used to increase the accessibility of foods high in nutrients and low in energy and decrease the accessibility of foods with greater energy density and lower nutritional value.[72] This is a key component of treatment because excessive restriction of certain foods may make them more enticing, which could lead to binge eating or overeating when the foods become available. To prevent this and to promote a high-quality diet, evidence-based obesity treatments promote moderate restriction and do not prohibit specific foods.[48] This is also congruent with CBT for eating disorders, wherein patients who binge eat are instructed to use stimulus control strategies at the start of treatment to reduce accessibility of foods that trigger binge episodes.[83] Once regular eating is established, these foods can be systematically reintroduced into the patient's diet. Health professionals should encourage patients participating in weight management programs to adopt a varied diet, employ moderate energy restriction, and limit—rather than fully restrict—specific foods. According to the 2013 guidelines for managing overweight and obesity in adults issued by the American College of Cardiology/American Heart Association Task Force on Practice Guidelines and The Obesity Society, an energy deficit of 500 to 750 kcal/d is recommended to produce a weight loss of 1 to 1.5 lb (0.5–0.7 kg) per week.[84-86] Prescriptions typically recommend consumption of 1,200 to 1,500 kcal/d for females and 1,500 to 1,800 kcal/d for males. The 2013 guidelines recommend that patients participate in an intervention for at least 6 months to produce a clinically significant weight loss of at least 5% of initial body weight.[86]

Physical activity prescriptions are a key component of many professionally delivered weight management programs, as the literature has shown that physical activity is related to weight loss maintenance and health benefits.[87,88] Current guidelines for physical activity recommend engaging in 150 minutes of moderate-to-vigorous physical activity per week to improve health and 250 minutes per week for long-term maintenance of weight loss.[89,90] As such, recommendations for physical activity in BWL interventions range from 150 to 300 minutes per week.[6,89,91] These levels are generally considered healthy and do not represent excessive exercise. However, health professionals should be aware of ways that patients' physical activity patterns can indicate eating disorder risk, even when employed at recommended levels. For instance, the risk may be increased if patients use exercise to compensate for a binge-eating episode. Exercise may also become problematic if it is done excessively in terms of time or intensity, if patients feel compelled to exercise and feel guilty if they do not, or if a drive to exercise interferes with other areas of life. Physical activity levels should be self-monitored regularly and supervised by health professionals, particularly in patients at risk for an eating disorder. Health professionals should deter patients from using physical activity as a compensatory behavior and routinely assess patients' psychological attitudes toward exercise.

Interventions With Self-Monitoring Prescriptions

Self-monitoring, or regularly recording dietary intake, weight, and physical activity, is an integral component of behavioral treatments for weight loss.[92,93] For instance, in lifestyle-modification interventions, self-monitoring consistently predicts better weight loss outcomes.[94-96] However, experts have raised concerns that self-monitoring prescriptions in weight management interventions may promote eating disorder psychopathology (eg, preoccupation with weight changes). In one study, a cohort of 250 adults with overweight or obesity who were receiving dietary and exercise counseling were randomly assigned to self-weigh daily, log food intake in an app, or refrain from self-monitoring. No differences in eating pathology were observed between any groups at 12 months.[97] Another study evaluating a daily self-weighing intervention with diet and exercise components among individuals with overweight or obesity found that participants who self-weighed daily had *lower* body dissatisfaction and greater dietary restraint compared to participants in the control group.[98]

Recommendations for Self-Monitoring

These findings suggest that *supervised* self-monitoring does not promote, and may even reduce, risk for eating pathology in healthy individuals with overweight or obesity. Of note, some research has found associations between *self-directed* self-monitoring and increased eating disorder symptomatology among adolescents and young adults.[99-101] Lack of supervision during self-monitoring may allow for practices that are not recommended in evidence-based interventions (eg, obsessive self-weighing) and that may facilitate the development of risk factors for eating disorders, including overvaluation of shape and weight and extreme weight-control behaviors. As such, health professionals are encouraged to supervise self-monitoring, regularly review patients' self-monitoring records, and promote a flexible approach to monitoring. For example, self-monitoring may increase awareness of lapses in adherence to dietary rules. To prevent patients from feeling guilt in these instances, providers should explain that occasional dietary lapses do not substantially hinder weight loss progress and encourage patients to focus on overall trends in their behavior.

In line with evidence-based treatment approaches to obesity and eating disorders, experts recommend weekly weighing.[40] Although studies that support more frequent (eg, daily) self-weighing produces weight loss and does not increase risk for eating disorders among treatment-seeking adults with uncomplicated overweight or obesity (ie, free of comorbidities, including eating disorders),[102] research has not sufficiently examined its effects among treatment-seeking individuals with a history of eating pathology. Only one trial of a weight loss intervention with daily self-weighing recommendations included individuals with BED (20% of the sample at baseline); this trial showed greater weight losses, reduced disordered eating, and a reduction in odds of meeting BED criteria.[103] In addition, most research evaluating daily self-weighing has been conducted in the context of interventions that provide a detailed rationale for daily self-weighing to participants. For instance, in the aforementioned trial of a daily self-weighing intervention with diet and exercise components,[98] participants were informed that daily self-weighing serves as a measurement instrument that allows for awareness of how behaviors affect weight, which can improve self-regulation and inform decisions regarding behavior changes. Thus, research supports that providers may consider increasing self-weighing frequency for patients without increasing the risk for eating pathology, if the rationale for the utility of self-weighing is provided, along with psychoeducation.

For patients with low-level symptoms of an eating disorder who are embarking on treatment for weight management, weekly self-weighing is recommended. The cognitive-behavioral approach to treatment for eating disorders prescribes structured, weekly self-weighing because it prevents individuals from weighing too frequently or avoiding weighing, each of which can reinforce preoccupation with weight and shape.[83] Thus, weekly self-weighing may help with addressing low-level eating pathology during weight management interventions.

Regardless of the frequency of self-weighing prescribed, a patient-centered approach is advised; this includes monitoring patients for eating disorder risk and modifying the prescribed frequency of self-weighing if problematic attitudes or behaviors develop. If patients become discouraged by small weight gains, providers should offer psychoeducation about normal weight fluctuations and the many factors that influence the regulation of body weight. Patients should be encouraged to focus on long-term weight trends.

Addressing Binge Eating Disorder: Is Weight Management Appropriate?

BED and excess weight have a high degree of overlap, which can lead to detrimental health outcomes and weight-related comorbidities. BED is also associated with components of metabolic syndrome independent of weight, indicating an urgent need to address this disorder.[37,104] The leading treatments for BED are psychotherapies, including CBT and interpersonal psychotherapy (IPT).[105,106] These approaches target binge eating and associated eating disorders and general psychopathology; they are not intended to, and on average do not, produce weight loss.[7,107] However, because increased binge eating leads to weight gain, successfully eliminating binge eating can protect against future weight gain.[108,109] Treatment approaches for BED that aim to directly target excess weight include BWL therapy and bariatric surgery. Pharmacologic interventions for BED have also been studied. Box 16.5 on page 300 provides an overview of the efficacy of existing treatments for BED in adults, which will be discussed in this section.

Leading Psychotherapies for Binge Eating Disorder

Cognitive-Behavioral Therapy

The cognitive-behavioral theory of BED psychopathology proposes that the overvaluation of weight or shape drives individuals to engage in a cyclical pattern of extreme weight-control behaviors and binge eating. Experts posit that efforts at weight control mount psychological and physiological pressure to binge eat, which in turn reinforces the overvaluation of weight or shape and perpetuates the cycle of pathology. CBT aims to disrupt the disorder's maintaining mechanisms through cognitive and behavioral intervention strategies coupled with psychoeducation. After employing key behavioral changes to disrupt eating pathology (eg, regular eating vs cycles of binge eating and purging), patients achieve distance from their eating disorder, learn about the mechanisms that maintain it, and challenge the cognitions and beliefs that perpetuate their eating pathology.[110]

CBT for BED encompasses both therapist-led modalities and guided self-help modalities (in which patients access treatment materials on their own with the support of a therapist). Data support both modalities as efficacious therapies for BED that consistently produce clinically meaningful binge-eating abstinence and reduce the frequency of binge eating compared to placebo.[111,112] A 2017 systematic review failed to find consistent differences in efficacy between the modalities, whereas another suggested that guided self-help CBT may be most efficacious for

BOX 16.5

Efficacy of Existing Treatments for Binge Eating Disorder in Adults

Treatment	Efficacy for binge eating disorder (BED)	Efficacy for weight loss
Psychotherapies		
Cognitive-behavioral therapy (CBT)	Well-established treatment with high efficacy	Does not target weight loss
Interpersonal psychotherapy (IPT)	Well-established treatment with high efficacy Treatment outcomes comparable to CBT	Does not target weight loss
Third-wave therapies	Have been found to reduce binge eating and associated psychopathology but have not demonstrated superiority to first-line psychological treatments	Do not target weight loss
Weight-management treatments		
Behavioral weight loss therapy	Reduces binge eating with lower efficacy than CBT and IPT	Produces short-term weight loss
Bariatric surgery	May improve BED pathology immediately after surgery, but eating pathology may subsequently return and increase	Produces weight losses that are sustained over time Data on whether BED attenuates weight loss are inconsistent
Pharmacologic interventions		
Lisdexamfetamine	Produces improvements in binge eating	Not indicated for weight loss

patients without additional psychopathology (eg, negative affect).[112,113] Notably, the overvaluation of shape and weight, which is present in about 50% of BED cases and is associated with more severe disorder, may respond best to CBT, which targets overconcern for weight or shape.[107,114] A study published in 2020 proposed integrating enhanced CBT for BED and CBT for obesity as a way to dually target BED and excess weight with a cognitive-behavioral approach, but this approach has not yet been tested.[115] In sum, CBT is an efficacious intervention for patients with BED that should be recommended as a first-line treatment. Guided self-help CBT is currently recommended as the first-line treatment for BED and BN by the UK National Institute for Health and Care Excellence.[116]

Interpersonal Psychotherapy

The theoretical model of BED for IPT holds that problems with interpersonal relationships result in negative affect, which in turn leads to binge eating.[117] Indeed, research has shown that poor interpersonal functioning and negative affect are key risk factors for BED and BN.[14] IPT, therefore, seeks to improve the patient's interpersonal relationships to alleviate distress and BED psychopathology.[118] This is done by clarifying the interpersonal contexts from which the psychopathology's onset and maintenance arise and making changes to improve problem areas.[117,119]

From its development, IPT has been supported by research as an effective treatment for adults with BED.[117,120] When compared to CBT, IPT has consistently shown comparable reductions in binge eating and recovery rates that hold up over long periods of follow-up.[105,106,121] For example, two studies comparing group CBT and group IPT found that the interventions produced equivalent rates of abstinence from binge eating over 1-year and 5-year follow-up.[106,121] IPT also has the advantage of being more acceptable to patients than CBT, and it shows higher efficacy for patients with low self-esteem and more severe eating pathology.[122] Furthermore, it is a transdiagnostic treatment with efficacy at addressing depression, anxiety, and posttraumatic stress disorder and is highly acceptable to therapists, making it a "best buy" treatment.[51,123-126] On the whole, these data suggest that IPT should be recommended as a first-line intervention for BED alongside CBT.

Third-Wave Therapies

Third-wave therapies for BED include dialectical behavior therapy, acceptance and commitment therapy, compassionate mind training (compassion-focused therapy), mindfulness-based interventions, functional analytic therapy, metacognitive therapy, and schema therapy. A 2017 systematic review of the efficacy of CBT, schema therapy, acceptance and commitment therapy, mindfulness-based interventions, and compassion-focused therapy for the treatment of eating disorders found that each third-wave intervention produced symptom improvement relative to controls, but none was superior to other psychotherapies.[127] A more recent study comparing dialectical behavior therapy, which targets emotion regulation, to an intensive form of CBT for individuals with BED and obesity echoed these results, finding that dialectical behavior therapy was less effective than intensive CBT at reducing eating disorder psychopathology, frequency of objective binge-eating episodes, and low self-esteem.[128] However, outcomes between the two interventions were comparable at the end of treatment and at a 6-month follow-up.[128] Taken together, research suggests that third-wave therapies, particularly dialectical behavior therapy, may be efficacious, albeit they have not garnered enough research support to be recommended as first-line treatments.

Addressing Excess Weight in Binge Eating Disorder

Behavioral Weight Loss

As previously described, BWL therapy promotes comprehensive behavior-change techniques with strategies for moderately reducing energy intake and increasing energy expenditure. Rather than targeting binge eating directly, BWL therapy aims to improve diet and physical activity habits through gradual lifestyle changes, thereby reducing binge eating. Findings regarding the efficacy of BWL interventions are mixed, though a sizable body of literature indicates that they are not as effective at reducing binge eating as CBT or IPT.[113] A 2017 systematic review found that CBT was superior to BWL therapy at reducing binge eating, whereas BWL treatment was more efficacious at producing weight loss.[112] However, in another review, the advantageous effect of BWL therapy diminished at follow-up.[111] Several studies support that CBT improves the effects of BWL therapy, but CBT alone tends to be superior, highlighting its efficacy as a stand-alone treatment.[129,130] In a study comparing CBT vs BWL therapy vs CBT plus BWL therapy in a sequential approach, the greatest reductions in binge eating were seen with CBT, followed by CBT plus BWL, but the BWL intervention also saw reductions in binge eating that persisted through 12-month follow-up (51% for CBT, 36% for BWL, and 40% for CBT plus BWL).[130]

In a study comparing BWL treatments of varied doses (ie, number of sessions), all doses produced improved BED outcomes, but patient groups undergoing moderate doses (16 sessions) and high doses (24 sessions) of treatments reported significantly greater reductions in binge-eating severity than did those in the low-dose (eight sessions) or control groups, indicating that a moderate or high dose of treatment may be required for clinically significant BED outcomes.[131] Reductions in binge eating were also associated with treatment adherence and weight loss, and patients treated with BWL therapy who achieved clinically significant reductions in the severity of their binge eating also attained greater weight losses than those who did not. Overall, BWL interventions have not garnered enough consistent evidence to be recommended as first-line therapy for BED. However, they may produce beneficial outcomes for some patients, particularly those who respond rapidly to treatment.[132]

Bariatric Surgery

Bariatric surgery is an effective treatment for class 2 and class 3 obesity.[133,134] A large body of literature has demonstrated that candidates for bariatric surgery show higher rates of eating disorders compared to individuals seeking nonsurgical methods of weight management.[135] Thus, there is growing interest in how eating pathology influences weight loss outcomes and how bariatric surgery influences eating pathology. For instance, much research has investigated preoperative BED as a barrier to sustained weight loss following bariatric surgery. This work has led the International Federation for the Surgery of Obesity and Metabolic Disorders to develop guidelines calling for the assessment of key psychological factors when identifying bariatric surgery candidates.[136] However, existing data in this area are mixed. A 2021 systematic review of 19 studies found no differences in the percentage of total weight lost between patients with and without BED, and another systematic review reported inconsistent findings regarding the effects of preoperative binge eating on weight loss across 20 studies.[137,138] Mixed findings are likely a result of inconsistency in the use of eating pathology measures and the length of follow-up.[139] Also, most measures employed by researchers were not developed for use with patients seeking bariatric surgery.[140] Of note, the Eating Disorder Examination Questionnaire—Bariatric Surgery Version (EDE-Q-BSV) is recommended for screening with this population. Thus, health professionals should regularly assess eating disorder symptoms following surgery, especially in patients with preoperative eating pathology.[141] The use of psychological interventions (eg, CBT) shortly after bariatric surgery is garnering support to prevent the development of both disordered eating and weight regain.[142,143]

Although the presence of eating pathology *before* bariatric surgery does not reliably predict weight loss outcomes, the presence of eating pathology *after* surgery has been shown in numerous studies to more consistently hinder postsurgery weight loss.[140,144-148] However, data are limited on whether eating pathology decreases after bariatric surgery. A 2021 meta-analysis of seven studies indicated that the rate of postoperative eating disorders was 8%, with 4% of those being BED cases.[149] There is also evidence that disordered eating can return after surgery among patients who had preoperative eating disorders or disordered eating.[141,150] One study that monitored patients for 7 years after surgery found that the proportion of patients with BED initially declined following surgery but then gradually increased each year thereafter. However, at 7 years, the presence of BED remained lower than at baseline (12.7% vs 4%).[151] Another study echoed these findings, adding that substantial risk for eating pathology may arise between the first and third years following surgery.[152] A possible explanation is that patients transition to eating smaller amounts of food and eating more frequently due to the inability to eat large portions in the postoperative phase.[153] This explanation is supported by a study that found that patients with preoperative BED began reporting grazing and subjective binge eating in the postoperative period.[154] As patients who have undergone bariatric surgery may not report eating large amounts of food after surgery, most eating disorder measures may not accurately capture their symptoms in the postoperative phase.[152]

Pharmacologic Interventions

Pharmacologic interventions for BED may be considered when comorbid psychiatric conditions or obesity are present, psychotherapy is not available, or patients do not respond to psychotherapy.[155,156] Lisdexamfetamine dimesylate is currently the only drug approved by the US Food and Drug Administration for the treatment of BED.[157] Since its approval in 2015, lisdexamfetamine dimesylate has shown consistent efficacy in treating BED in short-term studies.[158] Experts find it produces lower risk of binge-eating relapse, fewer binge-eating days per week, and greater binge-eating cessation compared to placebo.[159-161] However, its long-term efficacy has not yet been documented. Lisdexamfetamine dimesylate is not intended for weight loss, and research has not yet established its safety for the treatment of obesity, though it has been shown to produce weight loss.[162,163]

Generally, combining pharmacologic and psychological interventions may have advantages, but research on this has produced mixed results. Adding medications to CBT or BWL therapy has shown better outcomes than treatment with medication alone in some studies, but such combinations are not superior to CBT or BWL therapy without medication.[164] On the other hand, a 2021 review of 12 randomized controlled trials found that only two trials (both of which tested antiseizure medications) reported reductions in binge eating and weight, calling into question the potential benefits of additive pharmacotherapy for BED.[165] For patients seeking assistance with weight management, topiramate and orlistat may slightly improve weight loss outcomes when paired with psychotherapy.[163]

Recommendations for the Assessment and Monitoring of Eating Disorder Risk in Weight Management Programs

Initial Risk Assessment for Eating Disorders

Health professionals providing weight management interventions may serve as initial detectors of patients' eating disturbances. Providers should be trained to recognize and monitor patients for symptoms of disordered eating behaviors or attitudes and intervene if they emerge. Thus, conducting an initial risk assessment for eating disorders in all patients before initiating interventions for weight management is advised.[54] Recommended procedures for the initial screening are described in Figure 16.2. These recommendations are indicated for weight management programs that prescribe moderate energy restriction (eg, BWL therapy). The Eating Disorder Examination Questionnaire with instructions (EDE-Q-I)—a version of the Eating Disorder Examination Questionnaire that includes descriptions of binge episodes to assist patients with responding—assesses the frequency of binge eating, extreme weight-control behaviors, and overevaluation of weight or shape.[166,167] The EDE-Q-I demonstrates high accuracy at assessing the frequency of binge eating and has excellent convergent validity with the gold-standard Eating Disorder Examination[133] clinical interview.[168,169] Providers are advised to use an abbreviated version of the EDE-Q-I (refer to Box 16.6 on page 306) for initial screening and ongoing monitoring of risk for eating disorders. The standard form of the EDE-Q-I assesses symptoms occurring within the previous 28 days. Because an accurate count of the number of binge-eating episodes during the previous 3 months is needed for diagnostic assessment of BED, the adapted version of the EDE-Q-I includes an assessment of binge eating for the preceding 3 months.

If no symptoms are present, or if a patient reports subclinical levels of binge eating (fewer than 12 episodes in the previous 3 months) or subclinical levels of overevaluation of weight or shape (a score of less than 4 on the "importance of shape/weight" item in the previous 28 days), providers should to begin a program of weight management and conduct ongoing monitoring of the patient's risk status, with monthly assessments and monitoring at each session. Patients who report *any* self-induced vomiting or misuse of laxatives or diuretics (ie, one or more times in the past 3 months) at the initial screening should be excluded from weight management interventions and be referred for further evaluation and specialized care. Providers should also refer the following patients who screen positive at a clinical level for an eating disorder for further evaluation and specialized care: patients who report moderate (four to seven binge episodes per week), severe (eight to 13 episodes per week), or extreme (14 or more episodes per week) levels of binge eating, as well as those who report mild levels of binge eating (one to three episodes per week) *and* overevaluation of weight or shape. When eating pathology warrants further evaluation, providers should supply the telephone number and website address for the National Eating Disorders Association helpline to assist patients in accessing treatment options. With patients who report mild binge eating in the absence of overevaluation of weight or shape, a patient-centered approach to determining a treatment course is appropriate. As discussed previously, BWL and specialized psychological treatments (ie, CBT and IPT) each have shown beneficial effects in the treatment of BED. The appropriate treatment approach may differ from patient to patient based on factors such as the individual's treatment goals, access to specialized care, and medical comorbidities. Providers should assess patients for potential risk factors as needed, including excessive weight gain the past year, depression, and anxiety, and should discuss these factors and treatment options with patients before jointly formulating a treatment plan.

FIGURE 16.2 Recommended procedures for screening and monitoring for eating disorder risk

```
                    ┌─────────────────────────────────────────────────┐
                    │ Screening and Monitoring Assessment for Eating  │
                    │                Disorder Risk                     │
                    └─────────────────────────────────────────────────┘
```

No symptoms	Subclinical symptoms	Extreme weight control behavior	Clinical eating disorder
Patient screens negative for eating disorders or elevated risk status	Patient reports subclinical binge eating, weight or shape concern, dietary restraint, or compensatory exercise	Patient reports *any* self-induced vomiting or laxative/diuretic misuse	Patient screens positive for a *DSM-5* eating disorder at a clinical level

Begin weight management, monitor risk, and target risk factors or symptoms during treatment

Monthly assessments and session monitoring
If symptoms present at intake: have symptoms improved?
If no symptoms present at intake: is patient still symptom free?

Symptom absence or improvement
Continue weight management and monitoring of sessions

Presence of extreme weight control behaviors, excessive weight loss, or clinical levels of binge eating; cease weight management

Mild binge eating, no weight or shape overevaluation

Moderate, severe, or extreme binge eating or mild binge eating and weight or shape overevaluation

Determine treatment course (specialized treatment or weight management) based on treatment goals, access to care, and medical comorbidities

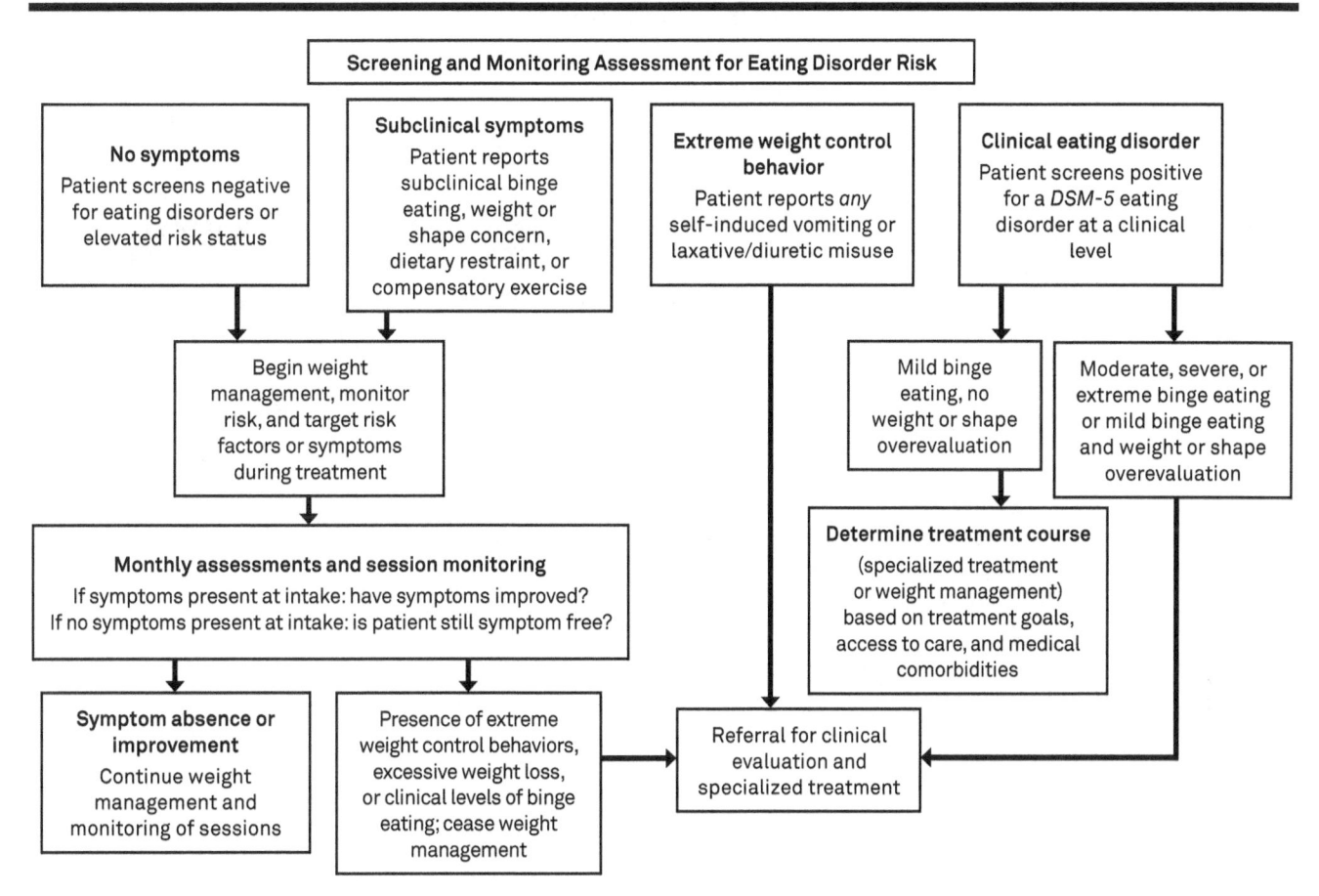

Referral for clinical evaluation and specialized treatment

Abbreviation: *DSM-5*, *Diagnostic and Statistical Manual of Mental Disorders*, Fifth Edition.

Monitoring Risk During Weight Management Interventions: Monthly Assessments and Session Monitoring

Ongoing monthly risk assessment for eating disorders, using a 1-month version of the adapted EDE-Q-I (refer to Box 16.6 on page 306), is recommended during weight management interventions. Ongoing assessments serve to ensure that eating pathology does not persist or worsen during treatment.[170] If extreme weight-control behaviors (ie, self-induced vomiting or misuse of laxatives or diuretics) emerge or if clinical levels of binge eating emerge or persist, providers should cease weight management interventions and refer patients for specialized eating disorder treatment. Excessive weight loss also warrants ceasing weight management interventions.

If patients report subclinical binge eating at their initial assessment, providers should target the binge eating as part of the treatment plan by identifying triggers for binge episodes, promoting regular eating and flexible dietary restraint, and adjusting behavioral goals as necessary. Reviewing food records and identifying areas for intervention are also recommended. Providers may also offer psychoeducation about the causes of binge eating according to the cognitive-behavioral approach, and patients may benefit from reading self-help material in this approach.[171] Providers should be asking to see if patients veer from dietary recommendations in favor of a more restrictive diet or engage in compensatory behaviors (eg, exercise)

BOX 16.6

Initial Screening, Monthly Assessment, and Session Monitoring for Eating Disorders

Initial screening questions

In the past 3 months, were there times when you ate a very large amount of food?

> If "Yes": In the past 3 months, were there times when you felt a loss of control over eating or that you just could not stop eating once you had started?
>
> If "Yes": Have you ever eaten a very large amount of food when you felt out of control while eating?
>
> If "Yes": How many times did you eat a very large amount of food AND felt out of control with your eating in the past month? In [month 2]? In [month 3]?

Over the past 28 days, has your weight or your shape made a difference in how you think about yourself as a person?

> (Scale of 0–6: 0 = not at all; 2 = a little bit; 4 = a lot; 6 = very, very much)

In the past 3 months, have you thrown up?

> If "Yes": Have you thrown up to control your weight or shape in the past 3 months? How many times?

In the past 3 months, have you taken laxatives or diuretics?

> If "Yes": Have you taken these medicines to control your weight or shape in the past 3 months? How many times?

Monthly assessment questions

In the past month, were there times when you ate a very large amount of food?

> If "Yes": In the past month, were there times when you felt a loss of control over eating or that you just could not stop eating once you had started?
>
> If "Yes": Have you eaten a very large amount of food when you felt out of control while eating in the past month?
>
> If "Yes": How many times did you eat a very large amount of food AND felt out of control with your eating in the past month?

Over the past 28 days, has your weight or your shape made a difference in how you think about yourself as a person?

> (Scale of 0–6: 0 = not at all; 2 = a little bit; 4 = a lot; 6 = very, very much)

In the past month, have you thrown up?

> If "Yes": Have you thrown up to control your weight or shape in the past month? How many times?

In the past month, have you taken laxatives or diuretics?

> If "Yes": Have you taken these medicines to control your weight or shape in the past month? How many times?

BOX 16.6 (CONTINUED)

Areas of risk to monitor at each session

Excessive energy restriction (below the healthy range of 1,200–1,500 kcal/d)

Excessive weight loss (substantially more than 0.5–0.7 kg, or 1.0–1.5 lb, per week)

Rigid dietary restraint (eg, fasting, elimination of food groups, skipping meals)

Excessive exercise (excessive duration or intensity as a way to influence shape or weight)

Eating behaviors (eg, chaotic patterns, binge eating)

Excessive self-weighing (more frequently than prescribed)

Exacerbation or onset of eating disorder symptoms (loss of control while eating, purging, concerns about weight or shape) or risk factors (depression, anxiety, weight-related stigma, elevated eating-disorder attitudes or behaviors)

Obsessive attitudes regarding any aspects of the treatment program

---

after eating. Provider intervention is called for if such behaviors emerge during weight management interventions. If patients develop weight or shape concerns, providers should emphasize the importance of health-related weight loss, ensuring not to promote idealization of a particular body type. In line with leading treatments for eating disorders, patients are to be encouraged to develop an acceptable weight range to target during treatment, rather than a particular weight.[83,172] If patients display a rigid focus on achieving a specific weight, psychoeducation and further evaluation of related psychopathology may be needed. Patients may also benefit from a discussion with their provider about the ways in which weight stigma enforces the idea that a BMI of less than 25 is ideal, which may not be the case for all patients.[48] In addition to monthly assessments, it is recommended that providers monitor self-reported behaviors that may signal potential eating-disorder attitudes and behaviors at each session. Areas to monitor are listed in Box 16.6. If a patient self-reports a concerning behavior at a given session, the provider may conduct a formal assessment with the adapted version of the EDE-Q-I to further evaluate risk.

Summary

This chapter aimed to provide guidance to health professionals for the detection and management of the risk for eating disorders in patients with overweight or obesity who are seeking professional help with weight management. Box 16.7 on page 308 summarizes the key practice tips for providers. Future needs in this area include the critical need for research to inform the development of formal guidelines for the assessment, treatment, and continued evaluation of eating disorder risk during weight management interventions. Specifically, more investigation into the utility of existing screening tools for eating disorders in this patient population is needed. In addition, the consistent use of measures for the assessment of eating pathology is needed in order to draw conclusions about the impacts of some weight management interventions on eating disorder risk. By following the recommendations in this chapter, health professionals will be equipped to provide early intervention to address comorbid eating pathology and excess weight in their patients.

BOX 16.7

Weight Management and Disordered Eating: Practice Tips for Providers[a]

Providers should consider early assessment for and ongoing monitoring of eating disorder risk in all patients seeking weight-management interventions for obesity.

Self-directed dieting and the risk for eating disorders

Self-directed dieting in individuals with obesity has been associated with disordered eating and is a risk factor for eating disorders. Dietary change and self-monitoring of diet, weight, and physical activity during weight-management interventions should be supervised and supported by health professionals.

Risk may be greatest for patients with other forms of psychopathology.

Health professionals should monitor and supervise all dietary changes and promote dietary practices that align with evidence-based obesity treatment.

Weight-management interventions and the risk for eating disorders

Professionally delivered, multicomponent, behavioral treatment of obesity has not been shown to increase the risk for developing eating disorders. However, most studies of obesity treatment have not included individuals with eating disorders.

Promoting regular eating during weight-management interventions is recommended and may be protective against eating disorders.

Interventions that include low-calorie diet prescriptions have mixed effects on eating pathology. Moderate energy restriction (energy deficit of 500–750 kcal/d) is recommended.

Current exercise guidelines (150–300 minutes of moderate-to-vigorous physical activity per week) indicate a healthy level of exercise. Exercise should be self-monitored and supervised.

Self-monitoring and the risk for eating disorders

Supervised self-monitoring of dietary intake, physical activity, and weight during weight-management interventions is key for successful outcomes and is not associated with increased risk for eating disorders.

Health professionals are encouraged to review patients' self-monitoring records and behaviors and assess for signs of risk (eg, rigid tracking).

Binge eating disorder and weight management

Specialized psychological treatments are the most effective treatment for binge eating disorder. Behavioral weight loss treatments produce reductions in binge eating to a lesser degree, as well as short-term weight losses. Bariatric surgery and pharmacologic interventions for weight management may improve binge eating in the short term, but long-term outcomes are unclear.

The presence of binge eating disorder may hinder successful weight management. In bariatric surgery candidates, binge eating should ideally be targeted before surgery. Postoperative binge eating is a consistent predictor of poor weight loss and should be targeted with psychotherapy early in the postoperative phase if not addressed before surgery.

[a] Supporting references can be found in the text.

References

1. Nightingale BA, Cassin SE. Disordered eating among individuals with excess weight: a review of recent research. *Curr Obes Rep*. 2019;8(2):112-127. doi:10.1007/s13679-019-00333-5
2. Aspen V, Weisman H, Vannucci A, et al. Psychiatric co-morbidity in women presenting across the continuum of disordered eating. *Eat Behav*. 2014;15(4):686-693. doi:10.1016/j.eatbeh.2014.08.023
3. Goldschmidt AB, Wall M, Choo TH, Becker C, Neumark-Sztainer D. Shared risk factors for mood-, eating-, and weight-related health outcomes. *Health Psychol*. 2016;35(3):245-252. doi:10.1037/hea0000283
4. Hayes JF, Eichen DM, Barch DM, Wilfley DE. Executive function in childhood obesity: promising intervention strategies to optimize treatment outcomes. *Appetite*. 2018;124:10-23. doi:10.1016/j.appet.2017.05.040
5. Neumark-Sztainer D, Wall M, Guo J, Story M, Haines J, Eisenberg M. Obesity, disordered eating, and eating disorders in a longitudinal study of adolescents: how do dieters fare 5 years later? *J Am Diet Assoc*. 2006;106(4):559-568. doi:10.1016/j.jada.2006.01.003
6. Look AHEAD Research Group; Wadden TA, West DS, et al. The Look AHEAD study: a description of the lifestyle intervention and the evidence supporting it. *Obesity (Silver Spring)*. 2006;14(5):737-752. doi:10.1038/oby.2006.84
7. Giel KE, Bulik CM, Fernandez-Aranda F, et al. Binge eating disorder. *Nat Rev Dis Primers*. 2022;8(1):16. doi:10.1038/s41572-022-00344-y
8. da Luz FQ, Hay P, Touyz S, Sainsbury A. Obesity with comorbid eating disorders: associated health risks and treatment approaches. *Nutrients*. 2018;10(7):829. doi:10.3390/nu10070829
9. American Psychiatric Association. *Diagnostic and Statistical Manual of Mental Disorders*. 5th ed. American Psychiatric Association; 2013.
10. Keski-Rahkonen A. Epidemiology of binge eating disorder: prevalence, course, comorbidity, and risk factors. *Curr Opin Psychiatry*. 2021;34(6):525-531. doi:10.1097/YCO.0000000000000750
11. Stice E, Marti CN, Rohde P. Prevalence, incidence, impairment, and course of the proposed DSM-5 eating disorder diagnoses in an 8-year prospective community study of young women. *J Abnorm Psychol*. 2013;122(2):445-457. doi:10.1037/a0030679
12. Favaro A, Busetto P, Collantoni E, Santonastaso P. The age of onset of eating disorders. In: de Girolamo G, McGorry P, Sartorius N, eds. *Age of Onset of Mental Disorders*. Springer; 2019:203-216.
13. Hilbert A, Pike KM, Goldschmidt AB, et al. Risk factors across the eating disorders. *Psychiatry Res*. 2014;220(1-2):500-506. doi:10.1016/j.psychres.2014.05.054
14. Stice E, Gau JM, Rohde P, Shaw H. Risk factors that predict future onset of each DSM-5 eating disorder: predictive specificity in high-risk adolescent females. *J Abnorm Psychol*. 2017;126(1):38-51. doi:10.1037/abn0000219
15. Stice E, Van Ryzin MJ. A prospective test of the temporal sequencing of risk factor emergence in the dual pathway model of eating disorders. *J Abnorm Psychol*. 2019;128(2):119-128. doi:10.1037/abn0000400
16. Striegel-Moore RH, Bulik CM. Risk factors for eating disorders. *Am Psychol*. 2007;62(3):181-198. doi:10.1037/0003-066X.62.3.181
17. Balantekin KN, Grammer AC, Fitzsimmons-Craft EE, et al. Overweight and obesity are associated with increased eating disorder correlates and general psychopathology in university women with eating disorders. *Eat Behav*. 2021;41:101482. doi:10.1016/j.eatbeh.2021.101482
18. Kass AE, Jones M, Kolko RP, et al. Universal prevention efforts should address eating disorder pathology across the weight spectrum: implications for screening and intervention on college campuses. *Eat Behav*. 2017;25:74-80. doi:10.1016/j.eatbeh.2016.03.019
19. Kessler RC, Berglund PA, Chiu WT, et al. The prevalence and correlates of binge eating disorder in the World Health Organization World Mental Health Surveys. *Biol Psychiatry*. 2013;73(9):904-914. doi:10.1016/j.biopsych.2012.11.020
20. Udo T, Grilo CM. Prevalence and correlates of DSM-5-defined eating disorders in a nationally representative sample of U.S. adults. *Biol Psychiatry*. 2018;84(5):345-354. doi:10.1016/j.biopsych.2018.03.014

21. Hudson JI, Hiripi E, Pope HG Jr, Kessler RC. The prevalence and correlates of eating disorders in the National Comorbidity Survey Replication. *Biol Psychiatry*. 2007;61(3):348-358. doi:10.1016/j.biopsych.2006.03.040
22. Burrows A, Cooper M. Possible risk factors in the development of eating disorders in overweight pre-adolescent girls. *Int J Obes Relat Metab Disord*. 2002;26(9):1268-1273. doi:10.1038/sj.ijo.0802033
23. Kessler RC, Shahly V, Hudson JI, et al. A comparative analysis of role attainment and impairment in binge-eating disorder and bulimia nervosa: results from the WHO World Mental Health Surveys. *Epidemiol Psychiatr Sci*. 2014;23(1):27-41. doi:10.1017/S2045796013000516
24. Lipson SK, Sonneville KR. Eating disorder symptoms among undergraduate and graduate students at 12 U.S. colleges and universities. *Eat Behav*. 2017;24:81-88. doi:10.1016/j.eatbeh.2016.12.003
25. Hay P, Mitchison D. Eating Disorders and obesity: the challenge for our times. *Nutrients*. 2019;11(5):1055. doi:10.3390/nu11051055
26. Hunger JM, Dodd DR, Smith AR. Weight discrimination, anticipated weight stigma, and disordered eating. *Eat Behav*. 2020;37:101383. doi:10.1016/j.eatbeh.2020.101383
27. Puhl R, Suh Y. Stigma and eating and weight disorders. *Curr Psychiatry Rep*. 2015;17(3):552. doi:10.1007/s11920-015-0552-6
28. Giel KE, Teufel M, Junne F, Zipfel S, Schag K. Food-related impulsivity in obesity and binge eating disorder—a systematic update of the evidence. *Nutrients*. 2017;9(11):1170. doi:10.3390/nu9111170
29. Lo Coco G, Sutton R, Tasca GA, Salerno L, Oieni V, Compare A. Does the interpersonal model generalize to obesity without binge eating? *Eur Eat Disord Rev*. 2016;24(5):391-398. doi:10.1002/erv.2459
30. Haedt-Matt AA, Keel PK. Revisiting the affect regulation model of binge eating: a meta-analysis of studies using ecological momentary assessment. *Psychol Bull*. 2011;137(4):660-681. doi:10.1037/a0023660
31. Masheb RM, Grilo CM. Emotional overeating and its associations with eating disorder psychopathology among overweight patients with binge eating disorder. *Int J Eat Disord*. 2006;39(2):141-146. doi:10.1002/eat.20221
32. Hrabosky JI, White MA, Masheb RM, Grilo CM. Physical activity and its correlates in treatment-seeking obese patients with binge eating disorder. *Int J Eat Disord*. 2007;40(1):72-76. doi:10.1002/eat.20323
33. Vancampfort D, Vanderlinden J, De Hert M, et al. A systematic review on physical therapy interventions for patients with binge eating disorder. *Disabil Rehabil*. 2013;35(26):2191-2196. doi:10.3109/09638288.2013.771707
34. Goldschmidt AB, Le Grange D, Powers P, et al. Eating disorder symptomatology in normal-weight vs. obese individuals with binge eating disorder. *Obesity (Silver Spring)*. 2011;19(7):1515-1518. doi:10.1038/oby.2011.24
35. Villarejo C, Fernandez-Aranda F, Jimenez-Murcia S, et al. Lifetime obesity in patients with eating disorders: increasing prevalence, clinical and personality correlates. *Eur Eat Disord Rev*. 2012;20(3):250-254. doi:10.1002/erv.2166
36. Schulz S, Laessle RG. Associations of negative affect and eating behaviour in obese women with and without binge eating disorder. *Eat Weight Disord*. 2010;15(4):e287-e293. doi:10.1007/BF03325311
37. Hudson JI, Lalonde JK, Coit CE, et al. Longitudinal study of the diagnosis of components of the metabolic syndrome in individuals with binge-eating disorder. *Am J Clin Nutr*. 2010;91(6):1568-1573. doi:10.3945/ajcn.2010.29203
38. Roehrig M, Masheb RM, White MA, Grilo CM. The metabolic syndrome and behavioral correlates in obese patients with binge eating disorder. *Obesity (Silver Spring)*. 2009;17(3):481-486. doi:10.1038/oby.2008.560
39. Thornton LM, Watson HJ, Jangmo A, et al. Binge-eating disorder in the Swedish national registers: somatic comorbidity. *Int J Eat Disord*. 2017;50(1):58-65. doi:10.1002/eat.22624
40. Ivezaj V, Kalebjian R, Grilo CM, Barnes RD. Comparing weight gain in the year prior to treatment for overweight and obese patients with and without binge eating disorder in primary care. *J Psychosom Res*. 2014;77(2):151-154. doi:10.1016/j.jpsychores.2014.05.006
41. de Zwaan M. Binge eating disorder and obesity. *Int J Obes Relat Metab Disord*. 2001;25 suppl 1:S51-S55. doi:10.1038/sj.ijo.0801699
42. Schag K, Schonleber J, Teufel M, Zipfel S, Giel KE. Food-related impulsivity in obesity and binge eating disorder—a systematic review. *Obes Rev*. 2013;14(6):477-495. doi:10.1111/obr.12017
43. Puhl RM, Lessard LM, Himmelstein MS, Foster GD. The roles of experienced and internalized weight stigma in healthcare experiences: perspectives of adults engaged in weight management across six countries. *PLoS One*. 2021;16(6):e0251566. doi:10.1371/journal.pone.0251566
44. Himmelstein MS, Puhl RM, Quinn DM. Intersectionality: an understudied framework for addressing weight stigma. *Am J Prev Med*. 2017;53(4):421-431. doi:10.1016/j.amepre.2017.04.003
45. Puhl RM, Latner JD, O'Brien K, Luedicke J, Danielsdottir S, Forhan M. A multinational examination of weight bias: predictors of anti-fat attitudes across four countries. *Int J Obes (Lond)*. 2015;39(7):1166-1173. doi:10.1038/ijo.2015.32
46. Phelan SM, Burgess DJ, Yeazel MW, Hellerstedt WL, Griffin JM, van Ryn M. Impact of weight bias and stigma on quality of care and outcomes for patients with obesity. *Obes Rev*. 2015;16(4):319-326. doi:10.1111/obr.12266
47. Tomiyama AJ, Carr D, Granberg EM, et al. How and why weight stigma drives the obesity "epidemic" and harms health. *BMC Med*. 2018;16(1):123. doi:10.1186/s12916-018-1116-5

48. Cardel MI, Newsome FA, Pearl RL, et al. Patient-centered care for obesity: how health care providers can treat obesity while actively addressing weight stigma and eating disorder risk. *J Acad Nutr Diet*. 2022;122(6):1089-1098. doi:10.1016/j.jand.2022.01.004
49. Becker AE, Thomas JJ, Franko DL, Herzog DB. Disclosure patterns of eating and weight concerns to clinicians, educational professionals, family, and peers. *Int J Eat Disord*. 2005;38(1):18-23. doi:10.1002/eat.20141
50. Fitzsimmons-Craft EE, Balantekin KN, Graham AK, et al. Results of disseminating an online screen for eating disorders across the U.S.: reach, respondent characteristics, and unmet treatment need. *Int J Eat Disord*. 2019;52(6):721-729. doi:10.1002/eat.23043
51. Kazdin AE, Fitzsimmons-Craft EE, Wilfley DE. Addressing critical gaps in the treatment of eating disorders. *Int J Eat Disord*. 2017;50(3):170-189. doi:10.1002/eat.22670
52. Mond JM, Hay PJ, Rodgers B, Owen C. Health service utilization for eating disorders: findings from a community-based study. *Int J Eat Disord*. 2007;40(5):399-408. doi:10.1002/eat.20382
53. Thompson C, Park S. Barriers to access and utilization of eating disorder treatment among women. *Arch Womens Ment Health*. 2016;19(5):753-760. doi:10.1007/s00737-016-0618-4
54. Hart LM, Granillo MT, Jorm AF, Paxton SJ. Unmet need for treatment in the eating disorders: a systematic review of eating disorder specific treatment seeking among community cases. *Clin Psychol Rev*. Jul 2011;31(5):727-735. doi:10.1016/j.cpr.2011.03.004
55. Palavras MA, Hay P, Filho CA, Claudino A. The efficacy of psychological therapies in reducing weight and binge eating in people with bulimia nervosa and binge eating disorder who are overweight or obese—a critical synthesis and meta-analyses. *Nutrients*. 2017;9(3):299. doi:10.3390/nu9030299
56. Santos I, Sniehotta FF, Marques MM, Carraca EV, Teixeira PJ. Prevalence of personal weight control attempts in adults: a systematic review and meta-analysis. *Obes Rev*. 2017;18(1):32-50. doi:10.1111/obr.12466
57. Neumark-Sztainer D, Wall M, Larson NI, Eisenberg ME, Loth K. Dieting and disordered eating behaviors from adolescence to young adulthood: findings from a 10-year longitudinal study. *J Am Diet Assoc*. 2011;111(7):1004-1011. doi:10.1016/j.jada.2011.04.012
58. Slof-Op 't Landt MCT, van Furth EF, van Beijsterveldt CEM, et al. Prevalence of dieting and fear of weight gain across ages: a community sample from adolescents to the elderly. *Int J Public Health*. 2017;62(8):911-919. doi:10.1007/s00038-017-0948-7
59. Stice E, Marti CN, Durant S. Risk factors for onset of eating disorders: evidence of multiple risk pathways from an 8-year prospective study. *Behav Res Ther*. 2011;49(10):622-627. doi:10.1016/j.brat.2011.06.009
60. Goldschmidt AB, Wall M, Loth KA, Le Grange D, Neumark-Sztainer D. Which dieters are at risk for the onset of binge eating? A prospective study of adolescents and young adults. *J Adolesc Health*. 2012;51(1):86-92. doi:10.1016/j.jadohealth.2011.11.001
61. Field AE, Austin SB, Taylor CB, et al. Relation between dieting and weight change among preadolescents and adolescents. *Pediatrics*. 2003;112(4):900-906. doi:10.1542/peds.112.4.900
62. Polivy J. Psychological consequences of food restriction. *J Am Diet Assoc*. 1996;96(6):589-592; quiz 593-594. doi:10.1016/S0002-8223(96)00161-7
63. Neumark-Sztainer DR, Wall MM, Haines JI, Story MT, Sherwood NE, van den Berg PA. Shared risk and protective factors for overweight and disordered eating in adolescents. *Am J Prev Med*. 2007;33(5):359-369. doi:10.1016/j.amepre.2007.07.031
64. Schaumberg K, Anderson DA, Anderson LM, Reilly EE, Gorrell S. Dietary restraint: what's the harm? A review of the relationship between dietary restraint, weight trajectory and the development of eating pathology. *Clin Obes*. 2016;6(2):89-100. doi:10.1111/cob.12134
65. Stewart TM, Martin CK, Williamson DA. The complicated relationship between dieting, dietary restraint, caloric restriction, and eating disorders: is a shift in public health messaging warranted? *Int J Environ Res Public Health*. 2022;19(1):491. doi:10.3390/ijerph19010491
66. Polivy J, Herman CP. Dieting and binging: a causal analysis. *Am Psychol*. 1985;40(2):193-201. doi:10.1037//0003-066x.40.2.193
67. Appelhans BM, French SA, Pagoto SL, Sherwood NE. Managing temptation in obesity treatment: a neurobehavioral model of intervention strategies. *Appetite*. 2016;96:268-279. doi:10.1016/j.appet.2015.09.035
68. Johnson F, Pratt M, Wardle J. Dietary restraint and self-regulation in eating behavior. *Int J Obes (Lond)*. 2012;36(5):665-674. doi:10.1038/ijo.2011.156
69. Westenhoefer J, Broeckmann P, Munch AK, Pudel V. Cognitive control of eating behaviour and the disinhibition effect. *Appetite*. 1994;23(1):27-41. doi:10.1006/appe.1994.1032
70. Haynos AF, Field AE, Wilfley DE, Tanofsky-Kraff M. A novel classification paradigm for understanding the positive and negative outcomes associated with dieting. *Int J Eat Disord*. 2015;48(4):362-366. doi:10.1002/eat.22355
71. Butryn ML, Webb V, Wadden TA. Behavioral treatment of obesity. *Psychiatr Clin North Am*. 2011;34(4):841-859. doi:10.1016/j.psc.2011.08.006
72. Bray GA, Fruhbeck G, Ryan DH, Wilding JP. Management of obesity. *Lancet*. 2016;387(10031):1947-1956. doi:10.1016/S0140-6736(16)00271-3
73. Looney SM, Raynor HA. Behavioral lifestyle intervention in the treatment of obesity. *Health Serv Insights*. 2013;6:15-31. doi:10.4137/HSI.S10474

74. Peckmezian T, Hay P. A systematic review and narrative synthesis of interventions for uncomplicated obesity: weight loss, well-being and impact on eating disorders. *J Eat Disord*. 2017;5:15. doi:10.1186/s40337-017-0143-5

75. Nurkkala M, Kaikkonen K, Vanhala ML, Karhunen L, Keranen AM, Korpelainen R. Lifestyle intervention has a beneficial effect on eating behavior and long-term weight loss in obese adults. *Eat Behav*. 2015;18:179-185. doi:10.1016/j.eatbeh.2015.05.009

76. Piya MK, Chimoriya R, Yu W, et al. Improvement in eating disorder risk and psychological health in people with class 3 obesity: effects of a multidisciplinary weight management program. *Nutrients*. 2021;13(5):1425. doi:10.3390/nu13051425

77. Austin SB, Field AE, Wiecha J, Peterson KE, Gortmaker SL. The impact of a school-based obesity prevention trial on disordered weight-control behaviors in early adolescent girls. *Arch Pediatr Adolesc Med*. 2005;159(3):225-230. doi:10.1001/archpedi.159.3.225

78. Stice E, Rohde P, Gau JM, et al. Enhancing efficacy of a dissonance-based obesity and eating disorder prevention program: experimental therapeutics. *J Consult Clin Psychol*. 2021;89(10):793-804. doi:10.1037/ccp0000682

79. Stice E, Rohde P, Shaw H, Gau JM. An experimental therapeutics test of whether adding dissonance-induction activities improves the effectiveness of a selective obesity and eating disorder prevention program. *Int J Obes (Lond)*. 2018;42(3):462-468. doi:10.1038/ijo.2017.251

80. da Luz FQ, Hay P, Gibson AA, et al. Does severe dietary energy restriction increase binge eating in overweight or obese individuals? A systematic review. *Obes Rev*. 2015;16(8):652-665. doi:10.1111/obr.12295

81. Wadden TA, Foster GD, Sarwer DB, et al. Dieting and the development of eating disorders in obese women: results of a randomized controlled trial. *Am J Clin Nutr*. 2004;80(3):560-568. doi:10.1093/ajcn/80.3.560

82. Sivyer K, Allen E, Cooper Z, et al. Mediators of change in cognitive behavior therapy and interpersonal psychotherapy for eating disorders: a secondary analysis of a transdiagnostic randomized controlled trial. *Int J Eat Disord*. 2020;53(12):1928-1940. doi:10.1002/eat.23390

83. Fairburn CG. *Cognitive Behavior Therapy and Eating Disorders*. Guilford Press; 2008.

84. US Preventive Services Task Force; Curry SJ, Krist AH, et al. Behavioral weight loss interventions to prevent obesity-related morbidity and mortality in adults: US Preventive Services Task Force recommendation statement. *JAMA*. 2018;320(11):1163-1171. doi:10.1001/jama.2018.13022

85. Wadden TA, Tronieri JS, Butryn ML. Lifestyle modification approaches for the treatment of obesity in adults. *Am Psychol*. 2020;75(2):235-251. doi:10.1037/amp0000517

86. Jensen M, Ryan, DH, Donato, KA, et al. Special issue: guidelines (2013) for managing overweight and obesity in adults. *Obesity (Silver Spring)*. 2014;22(S2):S1-S410.

87. Rhodes RE, Janssen I, Bredin SSD, Warburton DER, Bauman A. Physical activity: health impact, prevalence, correlates and interventions. *Psychol Health*. 2017;32(8):942-975. doi:10.1080/08870446.2017.1325486

88. Unick JL, Gaussoin SA, Hill JO, et al. Objectively assessed physical activity and weight loss maintenance among individuals enrolled in a lifestyle intervention. *Obesity (Silver Spring)*. 2017;25(11):1903-1909. doi:10.1002/oby.21971

89. Donnelly JE, Blair SN, Jakicic JM, et al. American College of Sports Medicine Position Stand. Appropriate physical activity intervention strategies for weight loss and prevention of weight regain for adults. *Med Sci Sports Exerc*. 2009;41(2):459-471. doi:10.1249/MSS.0b013e3181949333

90. US Department of Health and Human Services. *Physical Activity Guidelines for Americans*. 2nd ed. US Department of Health and Human Services; 2018. https://health.gov/paguidelines/second-edition/pdf/Physical_Activity_Guidelines_2nd_edition.pdf

91. Diabetes Prevention Program (DPP) Research Group. The Diabetes Prevention Program (DPP): description of lifestyle intervention. *Diabetes Care*. 2002;25(12):2165-2171. doi:10.2337/diacare.25.12.2165

92. Burke LE, Wang J, Sevick MA. Self-monitoring in weight loss: a systematic review of the literature. *J Am Diet Assoc*. 2011;111(1):92-102. doi:10.1016/j.jada.2010.10.008

93. Foster GD, Makris AP, Bailer BA. Behavioral treatment of obesity. *Am J Clin Nutr*. 2005;82(1 suppl):230S-235S. doi:10.1093/ajcn/82.1.230S

94. Butryn ML, Godfrey KM, Martinelli MK, Roberts SR, Forman EM, Zhang F. Digital self-monitoring: does adherence or association with outcomes differ by self-monitoring target? *Obes Sci Pract*. 2020;6(2):126-133. doi:10.1002/osp4.391

95. Carels RA, Selensky JC, Rossi J, Solar C, Hlavka R. A novel stepped-care approach to weight loss: the role of self-monitoring and health literacy in treatment outcomes. *Eat Behav*. 2017;26:76-82. doi:10.1016/j.eatbeh.2017.01.009

96. Harvey J, Krukowski R, Priest J, West D. Log often, lose more: electronic dietary self-monitoring for weight loss. *Obesity (Silver Spring)*. 2019;27(3):380-384. doi:10.1002/oby.22382

97. Jospe MR, Brown RC, Williams SM, Roy M, Meredith-Jones KA, Taylor RW. Self-monitoring has no adverse effect on disordered eating in adults seeking treatment for obesity. *Obes Sci Pract*. 2018;4(3):283-288. doi:10.1002/osp4.168

98. Steinberg DM, Tate DF, Bennett GG, Ennett S, Samuel-Hodge C, Ward DS. Daily self-weighing and adverse psychological outcomes: a randomized controlled trial. *Am J Prev Med*. 2014;46(1):24-29. doi:10.1016/j.amepre.2013.08.006

99. Hahn SL, Bauer KW, Kaciroti N, Eisenberg D, Lipson SK, Sonneville KR. Relationships between patterns of weight-related self-monitoring and eating disorder symptomology among undergraduate and graduate students. *Int J Eat Disord*. 2021;54(4):595-605. doi:10.1002/eat.23466
100. Neumark-Sztainer D, van den Berg P, Hannan PJ, Story M. Self-weighing in adolescents: helpful or harmful? Longitudinal associations with body weight changes and disordered eating. *J Adolesc Health*. 2006;39(6):811-818. doi:10.1016/j.jadohealth.2006.07.002
101. Simpson CC, Mazzeo SE. Calorie counting and fitness tracking technology: associations with eating disorder symptomatology. *Eat Behav*. 2017;26:89-92. doi:10.1016/j.eatbeh.2017.02.002
102. Steinberg DM, Tate DF, Bennett GG, Ennett S, Samuel-Hodge C, Ward DS. The efficacy of a daily self-weighing weight loss intervention using smart scales and e-mail. *Obesity (Silver Spring)*. 2013;21(9):1789-1797. doi:10.1002/oby.20396
103. LaRose JG, Fava JL, Steeves EA, Hecht J, Wing RR, Raynor HA. Daily self-weighing within a lifestyle intervention: impact on disordered eating symptoms. *Health Psychol*. 2014;33(3):297-300. doi:10.1037/a0034218
104. Mitchell JE. Medical comorbidity and medical complications associated with binge-eating disorder. *Int J Eat Disord*. 2016;49(3):319-323. doi:10.1002/eat.22452
105. Wilfley DE, Agras WS, Telch CF, et al. Group cognitive-behavioral therapy and group interpersonal psychotherapy for the nonpurging bulimic individual: a controlled comparison. *J Consult Clin Psychol*. 1993;61(2):296-305. doi:10.1037//0022-006x.61.2.296
106. Wilfley DE, Welch RR, Stein RI, et al. A randomized comparison of group cognitive-behavioral therapy and group interpersonal psychotherapy for the treatment of overweight individuals with binge-eating disorder. *Arch Gen Psychiatry*. 2002;59(8):713-721. doi:10.1001/archpsyc.59.8.713
107. Grilo CM. Psychological and behavioral treatments for binge-eating disorder. *J Clin Psychiatry*. 2017;78 suppl 1:20-24. doi:10.4088/JCP.sh16003su1c.04
108. Mourilhe C, Moraes CE, Veiga GD, et al. An evaluation of binge eating characteristics in individuals with eating disorders: a systematic review and meta-analysis. *Appetite*. 2021;162:105176. doi:10.1016/j.appet.2021.105176
109. Pacanowski CR, Mason TB, Crosby RD, et al. Weight change over the course of binge eating disorder treatment: relationship to binge episodes and psychological factors. *Obesity (Silver Spring)*. 2018;26(5):838-844. doi:10.1002/oby.22149
110. Fairburn CG, Cooper Z, Shafran R. Cognitive behaviour therapy for eating disorders: a "transdiagnostic" theory and treatment. *Behav Res Ther*. 2003;41(5):509-528. doi:10.1016/s0005-7967(02)00088-8
111. Berkman ND, Brownley KA, Peat CM, et al. *Management and Outcomes of Binge-Eating Disorder: Comparative Effectiveness Reviews No. 160*. Agency for Healthcare Research and Quality; 2015. AHRQ publication 15(16)-EHC030-EF.
112. Peat CM, Berkman ND, Lohr KN, et al. Comparative effectiveness of treatments for binge-eating disorder: systematic review and network meta-analysis. *Eur Eat Disord Rev*. 2017;25(5):317-328. doi:10.1002/erv.2517
113. Iacovino JM, Gredysa DM, Altman M, Wilfley DE. Psychological treatments for binge eating disorder. *Curr Psychiatry Rep*. 2012;14(4):432-446. doi:10.1007/s11920-012-0277-8
114. Grilo CM, Masheb RM, Crosby RD. Predictors and moderators of response to cognitive behavioral therapy and medication for the treatment of binge eating disorder. *J Consult Clin Psychol*. 2012;80(5):897-906. doi:10.1037/a0027001
115. Cooper Z, Calugi S, Dalle Grave R. Controlling binge eating and weight: a treatment for binge eating disorder worth researching? *Eat Weight Disord*. 2020;25(4):1105-1109. doi:10.1007/s40519-019-00734-4
116. National Institute for Health and Care Excellence. *Eating Disorders: Recognition and Treatment*. NICE guideline (NG69). National Institute for Health and Care Excellence; 2017.
117. Karam AM, Fitzsimmons-Craft EE, Tanofsky-Kraff M, Wilfley DE. Interpersonal psychotherapy and the treatment of eating disorders. *Psychiatr Clin North Am*. 2019;42(2):205-218. doi:10.1016/j.psc.2019.01.003
118. Wilfley DE, MacKenzie KR, Welch RR, Ayres VE, Weissman MM. *Interpersonal Psychotherapy for Group*. Basic Books; 2000.
119. Weissman MM, Markowitz, JC, Klerman G. *Comprehensive Guide to Interpersonal Psychotherapy*. Basic Books; 2008.
120. Wilfley D, Frank M, Welch R, Spurrell E, Rounsaville B. Adapting interpersonal psychotherapy to a group format (IPT-G) for binge eating disorder: toward a model for adapting empirically supported treatments. *Psychother Res*. 1998;8(4):379-391. doi:10.1080/10503309812331332477
121. Hilbert A, Bishop ME, Stein RI, et al. Long-term efficacy of psychological treatments for binge eating disorder. *Br J Psychiatry*. 2012;200(3):232-237. doi:10.1192/bjp.bp.110.089664
122. Wilson GT, Wilfley DE, Agras WS, Bryson SW. Psychological treatments of binge eating disorder. *Arch Gen Psychiatry*. 2010;67(1):94-101. doi:10.1001/archgenpsychiatry.2009.170
123. Cuijpers P, Donker T, Weissman MM, Ravitz P, Cristea IA. Interpersonal psychotherapy for mental health problems: a comprehensive meta-analysis. *Am J Psychiatry*. 2016;173(7):680-687. doi:10.1176/appi.ajp.2015.15091141
124. Markowitz JC, Petkova E, Neria Y, et al. Is exposure necessary? A randomized clinical trial of interpersonal psychotherapy for PTSD. *Am J Psychiatry*. 2015;172(5):430-440. doi:10.1176/appi.ajp.2014.14070908

125. Tanofsky-Kraff M, Wifley DE. Interpersonal psychotherapy for bulimia nervosa and binge-eating disorder. In: Grilo CM, Mitchell JE, eds. *The Treatment of Eating Disorders: A Clinical Handbook*. Guilford Press; 2010:271-293.
126. Weissman MM, Hankerson SH, Scorza P, et al. Interpersonal counseling (IPC) for depression in primary care. *Am J Psychother*. 2014;68(4):359-383. doi:10.1176/appi.psychotherapy.2014.68.4.359
127. Linardon J, Fairburn CG, Fitzsimmons-Craft EE, Wilfley DE, Brennan L. The empirical status of the third-wave behaviour therapies for the treatment of eating disorders: a systematic review. *Clin Psychol Rev*. 2017;58:125-140. doi:10.1016/j.cpr.2017.10.005
128. Lammers MW, Vroling MS, Crosby RD, van Strien T. Dialectical behavior therapy adapted for binge eating compared to cognitive behavior therapy in obese adults with binge eating disorder: a controlled study. *J Eat Disord*. 2020;8(1):27. doi:10.1186/s40337-020-00299-z
129. Devlin MJ, Goldfein JA, Petkova E, et al. Cognitive behavioral therapy and fluoxetine as adjuncts to group behavioral therapy for binge eating disorder. *Obes Res*. 2005;13(6):1077-1088. doi:10.1038/oby.2005.126
130. Grilo CM, Masheb RM, Wilson GT, Gueorguieva R, White MA. Cognitive-behavioral therapy, behavioral weight loss, and sequential treatment for obese patients with binge-eating disorder: a randomized controlled trial. *J Consult Clin Psychol*. 2011;79(5):675-685. doi:10.1037/a0025049
131. Ariel AH, Perri MG. Effect of dose of behavioral treatment for obesity on binge eating severity. *Eat Behav*. 2016;22:55-61. doi:10.1016/j.eatbeh.2016.03.032
132. Grilo CM, White MA, Wilson GT, Gueorguieva R, Masheb RM. Rapid response predicts 12-month post-treatment outcomes in binge-eating disorder: theoretical and clinical implications. *Psychol Med*. 2012;42(4):807-817. doi:10.1017/S0033291711001875
133. Carlsson LM, Peltonen M, Ahlin S, et al. Bariatric surgery and prevention of type 2 diabetes in Swedish obese subjects. *N Engl J Med*. 2012;367(8):695-704. doi:10.1056/NEJMoa1112082
134. Sjostrom L. Review of the key results from the Swedish Obese Subjects (SOS) trial—a prospective controlled intervention study of bariatric surgery. *J Intern Med*. 2013;273(3):219-234. doi:10.1111/joim.12012
135. Kalarchian MA, Marcus MD, Levine MD, et al. Psychiatric disorders among bariatric surgery candidates: relationship to obesity and functional health status. *Am J Psychiatry*. 2007;164(2):328-334; quiz 374. doi:10.1176/ajp.2007.164.2.328
136. De Luca M, Himpens J, Weiner R, Angrisani L. IFSO statement: credentials for bariatric surgeons 2015. *Obes Surg*. 2015;25(3):394-396. doi:10.1007/s11695-014-1553-y
137. Kops NL, Vivan MA, Fulber ER, Fleuri M, Fagundes J, Friedman R. Preoperative binge eating and weight loss after bariatric surgery: a systematic review and meta-analysis. *Obes Surg*. 2021;31(3):1239-1248. doi:10.1007/s11695-020-05124-9
138. Livhits M, Mercado C, Yermilov I, et al. Preoperative predictors of weight loss following bariatric surgery: systematic review. *Obes Surg*. 2012;22(1):70-89. doi:10.1007/s11695-011-0472-4
139. Parker K, Brennan L. Measurement of disordered eating in bariatric surgery candidates: a systematic review of the literature. *Obes Res Clin Pract*. 2015;9(1):12-25. doi:10.1016/j.orcp.2014.01.005
140. Williams-Kerver GA, Steffen KJ, Mitchell JE. Eating pathology after bariatric surgery: an updated review of the recent literature. *Curr Psychiatry Rep*. 2019;21(9):86. doi:10.1007/s11920-019-1071-7
141. de Zwaan M, Georgiadou E, Stroh CE, et al. Body image and quality of life in patients with and without body contouring surgery following bariatric surgery: a comparison of pre- and post-surgery groups. *Front Psychol*. 2014;5:1310. doi:10.3389/fpsyg.2014.01310
142. David LA, Sijercic I, Cassin SE. Preoperative and postoperative psychosocial interventions for bariatric surgery patients: a systematic review. *Obes Rev*. 2020;21(4):e12926. doi:10.1111/obr.12926
143. Galle F, Maida P, Cirella A, Giuliano E, Belfiore P, Liguori G. Does post-operative psychotherapy contribute to improved comorbidities in bariatric patients with borderline personality disorder traits and bulimia tendencies? A prospective study. *Obes Surg*. 2017;27(7):1872-1878. doi:10.1007/s11695-017-2581-1
144. Conceicao EM, Mitchell JE, Pinto-Bastos A, Arrojado F, Brandao I, Machado PPP. Stability of problematic eating behaviors and weight loss trajectories after bariatric surgery: a longitudinal observational study. *Surg Obes Relat Dis*. 2017;13(6):1063-1070. doi:10.1016/j.soard.2016.12.006
145. Fangueiro FS, Franca CN, Fernandez M, Ilias EJ, Colombo-Souza P. Binge eating after bariatric surgery in patients assisted by the reference service in a Brazilian hospital and the correlation with weight loss. *Obes Surg*. 2021;31(7):3144-3150. doi:10.1007/s11695-021-05372-3
146. Kalarchian MA, King WC, Devlin MJ, et al. Mental disorders and weight change in a prospective study of bariatric surgery patients: 7 years of follow-up. *Surg Obes Relat Dis*. 2019;15(5):739-748. doi:10.1016/j.soard.2019.01.008
147. Kalarchian MA, King WC, Devlin MJ, et al. Psychiatric disorders and weight change in a prospective study of bariatric surgery patients: a 3-year follow-up. *Psychosom Med*. 2016;78(3):373-381. doi:10.1097/PSY.0000000000000277
148. Meany G, Conceicao E, Mitchell JE. Binge eating, binge eating disorder and loss of control eating: effects on weight outcomes after bariatric surgery. *Eur Eat Disord Rev*. 2014;22(2):87-91. doi:10.1002/erv.2273
149. Taba JV, Suzuki MO, Nascimento FSD, et al. The development of feeding and eating disorders after bariatric surgery: a systematic review and meta-analysis. *Nutrients*. 2021;13(7):2396. doi:10.3390/nu13072396
150. Muller A, Mitchell JE, Sondag C, de Zwaan M. Psychiatric aspects of bariatric surgery. *Curr Psychiatry Rep*. 2013;15(10):397. doi:10.1007/s11920-013-0397-9

151. Smith KE, Orcutt M, Steffen KJ, et al. Loss of control eating and binge eating in the 7 years following bariatric surgery. *Obes Surg*. 2019;29(6):1773-1780. doi:10.1007/s11695-019-03791-x
152. Nasirzadeh Y, Kantarovich K, Wnuk S, et al. Binge eating, loss of control over eating, emotional eating, and night eating after bariatric surgery: results from the Toronto Bari-PSYCH cohort study. *Obes Surg*. 2018;28(7):2032-2039. doi:10.1007/s11695-018-3137-8
153. Conceicao EM, Utzinger LM, Pisetsky EM. Eating disorders and problematic eating behaviours before and after bariatric surgery: characterization, assessment and association with treatment outcomes. *Eur Eat Disord Rev*. 2015;23(6):417-425. doi:10.1002/erv.2397
154. Colles SL, Dixon JB, O'Brien PE. Grazing and loss of control related to eating: two high-risk factors following bariatric surgery. *Obesity (Silver Spring)*. 2008;16(3):615-622. doi:10.1038/oby.2007.101
155. Hay P, Chinn D, Forbes D, et al. Royal Australian and New Zealand College of Psychiatrists clinical practice guidelines for the treatment of eating disorders. *Aust N Z J Psychiatry*. 2014;48(11):977-1008. doi:10.1177/0004867414555814
156. McElroy SL, Guerdjikova AI, Mori N, O'Melia AM. Pharmacological management of binge eating disorder: current and emerging treatment options. *Ther Clin Risk Manag*. 2012;8:219-241. doi:10.2147/TCRM.S25574
157. FDA expands use of Vyvanse to treat binge-eating disorder. News release. US Food and Drug Administration. January 30, 2015. Accessed February 6, 2023. https://wayback.archive-it.org/7993/20170112222808/http://www.fda.gov/NewsEvents/Newsroom/PressAnnouncements/ucm432543.htm
158. Schneider E, Higgs S, Dourish CT. Lisdexamfetamine and binge-eating disorder: a systematic review and meta-analysis of the preclinical and clinical data with a focus on mechanism of drug action in treating the disorder. *Eur Neuropsychopharmacol*. 2021;53:49-78. doi:10.1016/j.euroneuro.2021.08.001
159. Fleck DE, Eliassen JC, Guerdjikova AI, et al. Effect of lisdexamfetamine on emotional network brain dysfunction in binge eating disorder. *Psychiatry Res Neuroimaging*. 2019;286:53-59. doi:10.1016/j.pscychresns.2019.03.003
160. Hudson JI, McElroy SL, Ferreira-Cornwell MC, Radewonuk J, Gasior M. Efficacy of lisdexamfetamine in adults with moderate to severe binge-eating disorder: a randomized clinical trial. *JAMA Psychiatry*. 2017;74(9):903-910. doi:10.1001/jamapsychiatry.2017.1889
161. McElroy SL, Hudson JI, Mitchell JE, et al. Efficacy and safety of lisdexamfetamine for treatment of adults with moderate to severe binge-eating disorder: a randomized clinical trial. *JAMA Psychiatry*. 2015;72(3):235-246. doi:10.1001/jamapsychiatry.2014.2162
162. Gasior M, Hudson J, Quintero J, Ferreira-Cornwell MC, Radewonuk J, McElroy SL. A phase 3, multicenter, open-label, 12-month extension safety and tolerability trial of lisdexamfetamine dimesylate in adults with binge eating disorder. *J Clin Psychopharmacol*. 2017;37(3):315-322. doi:10.1097/JCP.0000000000000702
163. Reas DL, Grilo CM. Pharmacological treatment of binge eating disorder: update review and synthesis. *Expert Opin Pharmacother*. 2015;16(10):1463-1478. doi:10.1517/14656566.2015.1053465
164. Grilo CM, Reas DL, Mitchell JE. Combining pharmacological and psychological treatments for binge eating disorder: current status, limitations, and future directions. *Curr Psychiatry Rep*. 2016;18(6):55. doi:10.1007/s11920-016-0696-z
165. Reas DL, Grilo CM. Psychotherapy and medications for eating disorders: better together? *Clin Ther*. 2021;43(1):17-39. doi:10.1016/j.clinthera.2020.10.006
166. Fairburn CG, Beglin SJ. Assessment of eating disorders: interview or self-report questionnaire? *Int J Eat Disord*. 1994;16(4):363-370.
167. Wilfley DE, Schwartz MB, Spurrell EB, Fairburn CG. Assessing the specific psychopathology of binge eating disorder patients: interview or self-report? *Behav Res Ther*. 1997;35(12):1151-1159.
168. Celio AA, Wilfley DE, Crow SJ, Mitchell J, Walsh BT. A comparison of the binge eating scale, questionnaire for eating and weight patterns-revised, and eating disorder examination questionnaire with instructions with the eating disorder examination in the assessment of binge eating disorder and its symptoms. *Int J Eat Disord*. 2004;36(4):434-444. doi:10.1002/eat.20057
169. Goldfein JA, Devlin MJ, Kamenetz C. Eating Disorder Examination-Questionnaire with and without instruction to assess binge eating in patients with binge eating disorder. *Int J Eat Disord*. 2005;37(2):107-111. doi:10.1002/eat.20075
170. Jebeile H, Gow ML, Baur LA, Garnett SP, Paxton SJ, Lister NB. Treatment of obesity, with a dietary component, and eating disorder risk in children and adolescents: a systematic review with meta-analysis. *Obes Rev*. 2019;20(9):1287-1298. doi:10.1111/obr.12866
171. Fairburn CG. *Overcoming Binge Eating: The Proven Program to Learn Why You Binge and How You Can Stop*. Guilford Press; 2013.
172. McIntosh VVW. Evidence-based treatments remain the best intervention for good long-term outcome of severe and enduring anorexia nervosa. *Int J Eat Disord*. 2020;53(8):1322-1323. doi:10.1002/eat.23325

CHAPTER 17

The Use of Technology in the Treatment of Obesity

Caitlin Martinez, MS, RD
Deborah F. Tate, PhD

CHAPTER OBJECTIVES

- Describe the categories of technology used in weight management assessments and interventions.
- Discuss the evidence base for the use of technology in weight management.
- List factors to consider when choosing a technology to use with a client.

Introduction

The COVID-19 pandemic has had a major effect on the use of technology for personal communication, work, and health care. The rapid increase in technology use and infrastructure growth has been called a digital surge or digitalization and has implications for the use of technology in practice settings in the postpandemic world.[1] The Pew Research Center reports that 90% of US adults considered technology important or essential during the COVID-19 outbreak, 40% used digital technologies in new ways compared to prepandemic uses, and more than 80% made video calls to family, coworkers, or providers.[2] Although debate continues over how this pandemic-induced digitalization will affect life in the future, some experts believe that new sensors and devices will allow for more and better remote monitoring of patient health and diagnostics, and that advances in therapeutics will promote unprecedented convenience and access. Others fear that economic inequalities may worsen and that misinformation will proliferate.[3] Nevertheless, it is clear that health care services—including those for weight management—will include digital components or be entirely remote for some patients moving forward due to limited access to services or patient preference.

Technology had been increasing in popularity with consumers and providers of weight management services even before the COVID-19 pandemic.[4] Many terms have been used to describe technology-based approaches, including *digital health*, *electronic health (eHealth)*, *connected health*, *internet health*, *web-based health*, and *mobile health (mHealth)*.[5] Several of these terms—such as digital health, connected health, and eHealth—describe large categories of interventions that use some form of technology. Others signal specific ways an intervention is delivered—for example, via websites or other internet sites meant to be accessed from a desktop computer or laptop, or via mobile-friendly apps or text messages meant to be accessed using a cell phone. As mobile internet access has increased, these distinctions have become less rigid; however, it is thought that cell phones offer more convenient access and may lend themselves to more frequent intervention touch points.[6]

For the purposes of changing behavior, it is important to distinguish the device or modality used *for* delivery from *what* is delivered via the device. For example, a mobile device, in itself, is not a behavior-change intervention; it is what the device is able to deliver that holds the power. Early work in internet interventions made clear that interventions delivered via the internet were not simply websites with patient information or handouts posted online. Rather, they contained key elements of evidence-based treatments, including structure, behavioral assessment or self-monitoring, feedback, and support or guidance for behavior change.[7]

A qualitative review of 21 efficacious technology-based weight loss interventions identified five key components considered to be crucial for weight loss: self-monitoring, counselor feedback and communication, social support, use of a structured program, and use of an individually tailored program.[8] In a follow-up review, 27 technology-based weight management interventions were screened for these five components; the researchers found that all interventions employing four or five of these components led to significant decreases in weight when compared to control interventions.[9] A separate metaregression looked at 122 (digital and nondigital) healthy-eating and physical-activity interventions and examined whether theoretically specified behavior-change techniques led to better outcomes. Intervention content was coded for inclusion of 26 different behavior-change techniques, including five techniques that CS Carver and MF Scheier's control theory suggests would lead to improved self-regulation and behavioral outcomes: prompt intention formation, prompt specific goal setting, provide feedback on performance, prompt self-monitoring behavior, and prompt review of behavioral goals.[10] The authors found that the specific technique of self-monitoring appeared most consistently related to positive outcomes, and interventions that combined self-monitoring with at least one other technique from control theory were significantly more effective.[11] In total, these reviews paint a consistent picture of the essential elements of digital health approaches.

Types of Technology Used for Weight Management

This section summarizes what is known about the different types of digital health interventions for weight management.

Interventions Delivered via the Internet

Since the first weight management studies were delivered via the internet in the early 2000s, internet use in the United States has increased from about 50% to 93% (based on data for 2000 and 2021).[12] Although internet use is nearly ubiquitous in some sociodemographic groups—such as young adults and high-income households—internet use does remain lower for older adults and individuals with lower incomes or educational achievement.[12]

Systematic reviews and meta-analyses of web-based weight management interventions suggest they are more effective than controls in producing short-term, modest weight loss. In these studies, control groups ranged from receiving no intervention to minimal intervention (predominantly in the form of written self-help materials or a single, face-to-face group session). Average weight losses were relatively small at approximately 3 kg (6.6 lb); however, outcomes varied across the literature, with some of the more intensive eHealth interventions achieving average weight losses of 5 kg to 8 kg (11 lb–17.6 lb) at the 6-month mark.[13-18]

Older studies suggest that technology-based treatments have been less effective in producing weight loss when compared with state-of-the-art behavioral treatments delivered in person. Estimates vary, but the average effect across studies of digital interventions appears to be about 2 kg (4.4 lb) less weight loss with digital vs in-person treatment.[15-17] However, few studies have allowed for head-to-head comparison; this is a notable limitation of the evidence, because differences in intervention design, dose, and modes of delivery can potentially confound findings. Yet, as digital treatments have improved and preferences for digital technologies have increased, it is possible that these differences may not hold today. For example, there is evidence that real-time video counseling can produce weight losses that are significantly greater than those produced with control interventions and at least as great as those produced with face-to-face counseling.[19-22] Although more evidence is needed in this area, it is clear that heterogeneity exists and these treatments work quite well for some and not so well for others, suggesting that a multitude of options may be needed to meet the diverse needs of patients.

Reviews suggest that weight losses via internet interventions can be enhanced with additional features, such as self-monitoring tools, feedback, reminders to engage with the program, email counseling, online group meetings or discussion groups, online lessons, text messages, and access to a smartphone app. Average weight losses in these "enhanced interventions" are about 1.5 kg (3.3 lb) more than those in standard eHealth groups.[18] Although some studies have tried to identify exactly which program components and features lead to this greater weight loss, more research is needed in this area. The strongest evidence for program components from systematic reviews and meta-analyses is for tailoring, though there is also evidence to support the beneficial effects of customized feedback, human feedback, health behavior theory, Short Message Service (SMS) reminders, goal setting, self-monitoring, and synchronous communication in eHealth interventions.[23-25]

Interventions Delivered via Cell Phones

In 2021, approximately 97% of Americans owned a cell phone and 85% owned a smartphone.[26] The proliferation of cell phones has presented new opportunities to reach individuals, especially now that people generally take their phones with them everywhere and can, therefore, access and participate in an intervention at any time. Research supports the acceptability of apps for health-seeking behavior in US adults. One study reported that 60% of adults found mHealth apps useful in achieving their health behavior goals, 35% found them helpful in making decisions about medical care, and 38% found them useful for asking their physicians new questions or seeking a second opinion.[27] It is possible that these numbers are higher in light of the COVID-19 pandemic.

The available evidence also supports the efficacy of mHealth interventions for weight management. Various systematic reviews and meta-analyses of randomized controlled trials suggest that interventions delivered by cell phones can produce a significant weight loss from a participant's baseline weight. Interventions delivered by cell phones have also been noted to produce significantly more weight loss than control interventions.[28-30] A 2017 review of 12 randomized controlled trials assessing weight loss interventions delivered by cell phone found that 10 of the 12 trials produced a significant change in body weight, and the average weight loss in these studies was 3.1 kg (6.8 lb).[28] Other meta-analyses of randomized controlled trials have suggested that, on average, participants randomly assigned to mHealth interventions may lose 1 to 2.5 kg (2.2 to 5.5 lb) more than control-group participants who receive no treatment or a treatment that does not involve a mobile electronic device.[29,30] In reviews that have attempted to assess the effect of individual treatment components, there is evidence to support the inclusion of the following: goal setting; self-monitoring; feedback on performance, including feedback that is personalized, actionable, and goal-oriented; and personal contact.[28,31-33] The evidence is inconsistent on whether adding other technologies to the interventions enhances their effectiveness.[28,32]

These mHealth interventions can be integrated with other technologies, specifically those that use text messages and connected devices as a part of the intervention.

Interventions Delivered via Text Messages

The use of text messages to deliver weight management interventions, either in full or in part, is of interest because most people with a cell phone are able to receive text messages. The other appeal of text messages is that they are pushed to the patient's cell phone and do not require the patient to log in or initiate the activity. Text messages are often used to send reminders, support, motivation, and feedback.

Text-messaging interventions for weight management have also been shown to produce better weight outcomes than control interventions. Across the six studies included in a 2015 systematic review and meta-analysis of interventions for weight management using text messaging, the weighted mean change in body weight in intervention participants was −2.56 kg (95% CI, −3.46 to −1.65 kg), compared to −0.37 kg (95% CI, −1.22 to 0.48 kg) in control-group participants (−5.64 lb [95% CI, −7.63 to −3.64 lb] vs −0.82 lb [95% CI, −2.69 to 1.06 lb]). However, the researchers were only able to combine the reported results over periods ranging from 8 to 12 weeks, highlighting the need for longer-term data on the efficacy of interventions delivered via text messages.[34]

Nutrition and weight loss interventions that employ text messages (SMS) are more efficacious when tailored to patients, with the most substantial effects perhaps occurring when messages are both tailored and targeted.[23,33] Text-message interventions that target weight loss have been tailored on measures such as stage of change, results of questionnaires that assessed food intake or psychosocial factors, and participant health goals; they have also been customized to meet participant preferences for day of the week, time of day, and preferred number of text messages.[33,35-37] Sufficient evidence is lacking to determine whether tailoring on one variable is more efficacious than tailoring on another. More research is needed to optimize tailoring and isolate its effect on outcomes in multicomponent interventions. Although some of the initial studies used static tailoring based on baseline measures, dynamic tailoring that assesses intervention variables prior to feedback holds some promise.[38]

Interventions Delivered via Interactive Voice Response

Some studies have incorporated interactive voice response (IVR) as an alternative or complementary strategy to text messages for weight management. Use of IVR is less common than use of text messages, and IVR has been employed more as an adjunct technology rather than as the primary intervention modality in weight management interventions.[39] In a 12-month randomized controlled trial of a digital health weight loss intervention delivered in a community health center system, IVR was used to support participant achievement of four tailored behavioral goals chosen for each participant.[40] Specifically, the IVR system's role was to support self-monitoring and feedback on behavior. The system called intervention participants weekly, prompted them to respond to questions (eg, "How many days did you drink sugary drinks last week?") via keypad, and then immediately provided automated, tailored feedback (eg, "You are doing better than last week. This week, try drinking flavored seltzer water instead of soda to save calories"). The IVR calls lasted 2 to 3 minutes, and messages were recordings made by professional actors rather than by a digitized voice. The participants who did not respond to IVR attempts were sent text messages to similarly support self-monitoring and feedback on behavior.

Emerging evidence suggests that such use of multiple modalities may support participant engagement over time. A study published in 2019 looked at the effects of introducing an additional reporting modality (email) to three existing modes (SMS, web, and mobile web) on self-reported weights of 312 participants, obtained through digital tools over 2 years. The data showed that adding a new modality increased weight reporting and that the use of several modes of reporting was associated with more weights being submitted (P <.01).[41]

Interventions Delivered via Connected Devices

Wearable Devices

Wearable devices, including fitness trackers such as pedometers, smartwatches, and armbands, offer objective tracking of physical movement and acceleration so that duration and intensity of different activities are recorded with minimal effort on the part of the wearer. However, weight loss interventions rarely rely on the use of a wearable device alone. Instead, data from wearables can be integrated with online programs and apps or reviewed by providers as part of behavioral counseling activities. In other words, they become part of a multicomponent intervention that involves a variety of behavior change-techniques, rather than just self-monitoring of physical activity alone.[42]

The evidence for wearables is less established than for other types of technology-based interventions. Evidence from systematic reviews of available studies is limited because reviews typically define *wearables* broadly (despite the variety of technologies included in this umbrella term) and there is great variation in the objectives, methods, and results of these studies. Although a 2020 systematic review of weight management interventions using wearable technology in adults with overweight or obesity for at least 12 months found that interventions delivered by wearable devices did not show a benefit over comparator interventions (though participants still lost weight over time), a second 2020 review that looked at Fitbit-based interventions with weight-related outcomes found a significant decrease in weight in intervention groups that used a Fitbit device, with a mean difference of −1.48 kg (−3.26 lb) in the Fitbit group, as compared to the group that did not use a Fitbit device.[43,44]

An important consideration is that wearables are most often one of many components in behavioral weight loss (BWL) studies, making it difficult to isolate the effect of the wearable so that its individual effect or additive effect on weight loss can be assessed. The extent to which wearables contribute to weight loss has yet to be determined. In one randomized controlled trial, 197 sedentary adults with overweight or obesity were randomly assigned to one of four treatment protocols during the 9-month study period: (1) a self-directed weight loss program via an evidence-based weight loss manual (standard care; control group), (2) a group-based BWL program, (3) a SenseWear Armband (a physical activity monitoring device worn on the upper arm) alone, or (4) the group-based BWL program plus the armband.[45] There was significant weight loss in all three intervention groups (group-based BWL program: 1.86 kg [4.10 lb], P=.05; armband alone: 3.55 kg [7.82 lb], P=.0002; group-based BWL program plus armband: 6.59 kg [14.52 lb],

$P<.0001$), but not in the standard-care group at 9 months. However, only the participants assigned to the group-based BWL program plus armband achieved significantly more weight loss at month 9 than the standard-care group, suggesting an additive benefit of an armband in group weight loss programs.

However, a second, larger (N=471) study from 2016 had different results.[46] The base intervention included a prescription to follow a low-calorie diet and increase physical activity, plus participate in group counseling sessions. At 6 months, participants were then randomly assigned to one of two self-monitoring conditions: (1) standard intervention, in which participants initiated self-monitoring of their diet and physical activity using a website; or (2) enhanced intervention, in which participants were provided with a wearable device and an accompanying website interface to monitor their diet and physical activity. Participants in both groups continued to attend group treatment sessions once a month during months 6 through 24 that were supplemented by brief (10-minute) individual telephone calls once a month and one to two text messages per week. In this study, the addition of a wearable technology device to a standard behavioral intervention resulted in less weight loss at 24 months.

This study took a step toward isolating the effect of a wearable device by looking at the additive benefit of the tracker after 6 months. Although the study did not find that the wearable device imparted any additional benefit compared to standard methods, the authors have posited that the hypothesized benefits of the wearable technology may not have been realized after 6 months because the behavioral counseling calls during the maintenance phase with the wearable technology may have been overly focused on wear time and adherence to the physical activity prescription, with less wholistic attention being paid to other problems, such as dietary adherence or lapses. This is likely an artifact of the manipulation being the addition of the armband (with the desire to test the effects of its usage) and might be less likely to occur outside of the research setting. Others have noted that an armband may be more intrusive than wrist-worn activity trackers. Additional research is needed to better understand the role of wearable activity monitors during active treatment, during maintenance, and in programs with less face-to-face and human telephone contact.

Smart Scales

Smart scales are internet-, Bluetooth-, or cellular-connected devices for measuring body weight and, in some instances, body fat. They are used primarily for assessment or self-monitoring of body weight. A benefit of smart scales is that they can be connected to a variety of health and weight management apps, or data can be shared with a provider if more frequent weight monitoring is desired without requiring the patient to enter data.[5] A 2013 study used daily self-monitoring of body weight via smart scales as the primary form of self-monitoring, without recommendations for formal monitoring of daily energy intake or physical activity tracking.[47] The intervention materials focused on teaching participants to use the daily fluctuations of their weight (up or down)—even by very small amounts—as indicators of whether their dietary intake and activity levels were promoting weight loss or not. If their efforts were resulting in weight loss, participants were advised to proceed with their current behaviors. If their efforts were resulting in weight gain, they were advised to eat a little less or exercise a little more the next day. Participants weighed themselves, on average, 6 days per week, and the weight losses were clinically significant (greater than 5%) on average after 6 months of following this approach. Some experts have suggested that this approach might be effective for patients who are unable or unwilling to use traditional diet-monitoring methods. A key component of this and other daily-weighing interventions has been to address the patient's view of weight measurements and the value placed on them so that the patient can begin to see weight measurements as being like other health indicators, such as blood glucose, blood pressure, or body temperature, as measurements that provide important information about how the body is functioning and not as indications of self-worth. For some patients, this approach may be difficult and unadvisable.

Commercial Mobile Apps for Weight Loss

Most studies that have explored the effects of eHealth and mHealth interventions on weight outcomes have employed interventions developed in research settings and which are not commercially available.

A few studies have attempted to assess the efficacy of commercially available apps. For example, one randomized controlled trial looked at the effectiveness of MyFitnessPal vs usual primary care in 212 adult primary care patients with overweight.[48] MyFitnessPal is one of the most popular apps for weight loss and has self-monitoring, goal-setting, and feedback features, among others. Researchers helped patients in the intervention group download the app, but these patients otherwise continued with usual primary care for 4 months. Research assistants told patients in the usual-care control group to "choose any activities you'd like to lose weight" and did not prescribe any specific weight-control approaches. After 6 months, weight change among participants was minimal, with no difference between the groups (mean between-group difference: 0.30 kg [0.66 lb]; 95% CI, 1.50–0.95 kg [3.30–2.09 lb]; $P=.63$). Compared with patients in the control group, those in the intervention group increased their use of a personal energy-intake goal, but other self-reported behaviors did not differ between groups. Although most users reported high satisfaction with MyFitnessPal, log-ins decreased sharply after the first month. By 3 to 6 months, median log-ins in the intervention group were zero.

A second study looked at factors related to sustained use of a free mobile app (The Eatery) that promoted healthy eating through photographic dietary self-monitoring and peer feedback.[49] The sample for this retrospective cohort study was 189,770 people who had downloaded the app and used it at least once between October 2011 and April 2012. The authors classified people who had taken more than one picture as users and people with one or no pictures as dropouts; they further classified users by the number of pictures they had taken as actives (at least 10 pictures taken plus at least 1 week of app use) and semiactives (two to nine pictures taken). They found that only 2.58% of app users were actives. Combined, these studies suggest that commercially available apps for weight loss alone may be insufficient for engagement in weight management programs.

One possible explanation for the limited effectiveness of commercially available apps and websites is that they may lack strategies that have been proven effective for weight loss in digital or in-person weight loss interventions. In one study, researchers coded 30 commercially available weight loss mobile apps (from the top 100 paid and free apps in the health and fitness category on Apple iTunes and Android Market, the primary sources of app downloads at the time) for whether they included any of 20 behavioral strategies from the Diabetes Prevention Program.[50] All apps included in the study were required to include dietary and weight self-monitoring features, given that self-monitoring is a key behavior change technique in evidence-based BWL programs and is the feature most common in apps. The apps reviewed contained a range of 5% to 65% of the strategies, and on average contained fewer than four of the strategies. Three strategies were included in most of the apps (weight loss goal [93.3%], dietary goal [90%], and discussion of energy balance [86.7%]), but all other strategies were found in 20% or fewer of the apps. In addition, seven strategies (including stress reduction, relapse prevention, management of negative thinking, social cues, development of a regular eating pattern, time management, and nutrition-label reading) were not found in any of the apps reviewed.

Another study looked at the overall quality of 23 popular weight management apps, rating them in four domains—engagement, functionality, aesthetics, and information quality—using the five-point Mobile App Rating Scale (MARS).[51] Overall, the apps were rated as being of average quality. Ratings were highest in the functionality domain, which largely focused on indicators of user experience (eg, app performance, ease of use, and navigation), suggesting that functionality may be a priority for users. The ratings were lowest for information quality, which encompassed factors such as how well the content was written, whether the app contained clearly defined behavior-change goals, and whether the app had been evaluated in randomized controlled trials (evidence base).

Evidence Base for the Use of Technology in Weight Management: Key Considerations

When looking at the evidence for digital obesity treatments, practitioners should keep in mind the following key considerations:

- **The evidence base largely focuses on weight loss interventions.** For example, in a 2015 review of 84 eHealth studies for the prevention and treatment of obesity, only 10 studies targeted weight loss maintenance, eight targeted weight-gain prevention, and five targeted weight loss and maintenance.[18] The limited evidence base—along with heterogeneity in the aims, samples, intervention designs, and study durations—make it difficult to pool findings and establish the efficacy of interventions for maintaining weight loss or preventing weight gain. More high-quality studies are needed in these areas.

- **It is difficult to disentangle the effects of individual technologies.** Most studies use technology as one component of multicomponent BWL interventions. The designs of these studies do not allow one to distinguish which components of the technology-based intervention were the most effective for promoting behavior change and weight loss. There is a need to discover the minimal intervention needed for change—that is, the lowest level of intervention intensity, expertise, and resources needed to achieve a clinically significant weight loss for a target population under a set of conditions.[52] This is important because additional technologies do not always lead to improved outcomes. For example, one study randomly assigned 301 participants to a basic condition (website plus email or SMS), an enhanced condition (website plus individualized feedback and email, SMS, or telephone reminders), or a wait-list control.[53] At 12 weeks, greater weight loss was seen in the two intervention groups than in the control group. However, there was no significant difference in mean weight loss between the basic condition vs the enhanced condition at 3 or 6 months.

- **Engagement with technologies is essential for behavior change.** Weight loss in digital health interventions is thought to stem from patient engagement with app components, which allows patients to receive behavior-change techniques that lead to changes in diet and physical activity behaviors and, subsequently, weight loss.[6] In many studies, participant engagement has been low, with many individuals dropping off in the first few weeks and few sustaining frequent regular engagement through 6 months—a time point traditionally associated with maximum weight loss in BWL interventions.[5,6] Some researchers have hypothesized that engagement naturally declines over time as patients learn new behaviors and have less need for the information, skills, or self-monitoring resources that the intervention provides. However, the use of key digital tools such as self-monitoring, goal setting, and social support has been consistently associated with better outcomes.

- **Experts do not yet know how sociodemographic factors may affect the types of interventions that patients need.** There is a growing interest in delivering the right intervention to the right person at the right time. However, the current evidence base does not allow for making these determinations. Studies attempting to identify baseline predictors of success in weight loss studies have not consistently found any sociodemographic factors (eg, age, socioeconomic status, self-identified race, or ethnicity) that predict success. The most consistent predictor of long-term success is early success, meaning weight lost in the first 3 to 6 weeks has been predictive of success at 12 to 18 months, even in digital programs.[54-57] Across studies of digital interventions, about 40% to 60% of participants achieve clinically meaningful weight losses, which means that 40% to 60% of participants do not.[54-56] Researchers hypothesize that greater individual tailoring of treatment approaches might improve these percentages. Experts and practitioners are also aware that more evidence is needed regarding the efficacy of digital health interventions among individuals who self-identify as members of racial or ethnic minority populations, as these populations have been underrepresented in early eHealth and mHealth interventions, yet they bear a disproportionate burden of the obesity epidemic.[58]

- **Experts and practitioners need evidence on readily available consumer apps.** As already noted, evidence for the effectiveness of commercial apps is needed for consumers and practitioners alike, as it is directly relevant to health care providers interested in recommending digital BWL interventions to patients. To date, most studies compare apps to no-treatment control groups or usual care; however, direct comparisons of apps are also needed, and transparency about for whom they are effective will be important.

Considerations for Using Technology With Patients

This section reviews key factors for practitioners to consider when deciding whether or not to use a specific digital support tool in practice and how to choose the right digital tools for their patients. Overall, the goal when using technology for weight management interventions is to find an evidence-based tool that is the right match for a patient's resources, comfort level with technology, health goals, and readiness to change.

Consideration 1: The Evidence Base

When trying to identify the appropriate weigh-management app for a patient, practitioners must consider the available evidence for the app or, in the absence of dedicated research on the specific app, for the strategies the app uses to elicit behavior change. If studies of the app are available, the practitioner should review each study publication, asking the following questions: Was the app used alone or in combination with other technologies or human support? For what length of time was it used? In what population? Was the app effective in producing weight loss? If studies on the specific app are not available, the next best thing is to determine what evidence-based behavior change techniques are included in the app. In a review of available data for 23 popular weight management apps, inclusion of a combination of effective behavior-change techniques (goal setting, feedback, self-monitoring) was the only app feature associated with higher scores for information quality, suggesting this as a possible strategy for identifying apps with higher-quality information.[51] It is also helpful to consider how the technology can complement current clinical expertise: Will the clinician refer patients to use specific apps or websites for behavior change? Or between sessions? Or alongside clinician guidance and feedback? Answering such questions can help clinicians identify key behavior change techniques to deliver and which strategies the technology can help deliver.

Consideration 2: Cost (Financial and Time)

Two separate reviews of commercially available apps found that app cost (free vs paid) made no difference to app quality (by MARS rating) or the number of evidence-based behavior-change strategies included in the app, though both reviews noted (as previously discussed) that the apps were lacking some behavior change features.[50,51] If considering a paid app, the practitioner should determine whether the cost would be directly incurred by the patient or whether the provider can pay a fee that would then allow patients to access the app for free. Such provider fees can be bundled into the overall cost for weight-management counseling services.

"Cost" often entails more than just financial cost. One can also think of cost in terms of time—that is, the amount of time the patient has to dedicate to using the app. Some apps contain technology-enhanced features that may reduce the amount of time the patient needs to invest in order to engage with an important behavior change strategy (eg, self-monitoring) or may prompt the patient to use the strategy. Examples of such features include barcode scanners, online social networks (for social support), reminders to eat a meal, tools for tracking negative thoughts or stress, calendars for scheduling exercises, or flags for lapses in dietary-goal adherence.[50] Because patients often need to engage with the technology to receive key behavior change strategies, finding a tool that is consistent with the money and time patients are able to commit to behavior change is important.

Consideration 3: Patient Access to and Interest in Technology

Sociodemographic considerations can affect the choice of weight management apps for a patient. Not all patients have the same level of comfort with or interest in engaging with technology, and the type of access a patient has to the internet or a smartphone may play a role in their desire or ability to engage. One consideration is a patient's mobile data plan. Most apps require data access, so having to turn off data access because of data limits or cost could affect the effectiveness of the technology.

Many apps have yet to be tested in diverse populations or at different literacy and health-literacy levels. Consequently, it is important for providers to try to make the best match between the usability and requirements of a specific app and a particular patient. Some patients might be comfortable using SMS or social media but may be less at ease with downloading and using apps. Furthermore, patients sometimes unintentionally turn off data permissions, disconnect from Bluetooth, or get signed out of an app and are unable to log in again. These are all real-world occurrences that can influence the effectiveness of an intervention delivered through a particular technology. Therefore, providers must consider how a patient might best be able to self-monitor, report information, and receive feedback and encouragement when deciding whether an app is the best option or if a simpler form of digital communication might be more appropriate.

Consideration 4: Existing Technologies vs Provider-Created Technologies

Whether providers opt to use existing technologies for weight management or create their own can depend on factors such as budget, level of technical knowledge and skills, the desire to control the content of the program recommendations, and the need to track patient utilization of the technology and progress. Customizing technologies can be a lot of work, can feel very costly, and, in some instances, can feel like reinventing the wheel. For example, commercial technologies for self-monitoring are readily available and are often free, so it might not make sense to create a new tool for self-monitoring. However, creating a simple web-based form for reporting progress and setting goals, videos or text-based lessons that provide weekly skills training and evidence-based information, or a closed online discussion board or social media group to provide patients with social support might be easy, cost-effective, and more specific to the goals of a weight management program than using existing resources. In many cases, customized technology also allows providers to better track patient use of the technology and patient data.

Summary

A digital tool is not, in and of itself, a behavior-change intervention. Rather, it is the behavior change intervention that the device is able to deliver that holds the power. Although new technologies offer many opportunities and advantages, they have their disadvantages too, and Box 17.1 summarizes the different types of technology discussed in this chapter and the pros and cons of each for weight management interventions. A comprehensive nutrition assessment remains paramount to determining whether a particular technology should be used in an intervention and, if so, what role the evidence-based tool should play, either independently of, or as an adjunct to, the clinician. Finding the right technology fit for a patient can help build clinician-patient rapport by extending the scope and effectiveness of the weight management intervention.

BOX 17.1

Summary of Technologies for Weight Management Interventions

Technology category	Key functions or components	Advantages	Disadvantages
Wearable devices	Self-monitoring	Lower patient burden Abundant data Objective data	Costly Large amounts of data for patient and provider to interpret
Self-monitoring apps	Self-monitoring	Well-established technology supported by extensive databases On-demand access via smartphone	Risk of inaccurately crowdsourced foods and portion sizes "Extra" information (ie, information that is not needed) Can be difficult for provider to access patient records
Short Message Service (SMS) messages (ie, text messages)	Content delivery Provider support Feedback Limited self-monitoring	Convenient Ability to push messages to the patient's phone without patient initiation or log-in Already used by most patients	Cumbersome and time-consuming if not automated
Social media sites	Social support Content delivery	Free, existing platforms that are already used by some patients daily to communicate with friends and family	Hesitancy among some patients to use Messages easily missed in a crowded feed Usually asynchronous Difficult to predict patient engagement May require regular monitoring
Videos	Content delivery Demonstration of behavior Encouragement and motivation	Easy to record Good for patients with lower literacy levels Preferred by some patients	Time-consuming and costly if higher production quality is desired Lack of appeal to patients who prefer written communication
Video chat services	Content delivery Provider support Feedback	Live, synchronous, human support	Provider time and resource input
Emails	Content delivery Provider support Feedback	Widely accessible Free	Less appealing to younger age groups May not be checked regularly by patients

References

1. De' R, Pandey N, Pal A. Impact of digital surge during Covid-19 pandemic: a viewpoint on research and practice. *Int J Inf Manage*. 2020;55:102171. doi:10.1016/j.ijinfomgt.2020.102171
2. McClain C, Vogels EA, Perrin A, Sechopoulos S, Rainie L. The internet and the pandemic. Pew Research Center. September 1, 2021. Accessed January 13, 2022. www.pewresearch.org/internet/2021/09/01/the-internet-and-the-pandemic
3. Anderson J, Rainie L, Vogels EA. Experts say the "new normal" in 2025 will be far more tech-driven, presenting more big challenges. Pew Research Center. February 18, 2021. www.pewresearch.org/internet/2021/02/18/experts-say-the-new-normal-in-2025-will-be-far-more-tech-driven-presenting-more-big-challenges
4. Nikolaou CK, Lean MEJ. Mobile applications for obesity and weight management: current market characteristics. *Int J Obes*. 2017;41(1):200-202. doi:10.1038/ijo.2016.186
5. Sim I. Mobile devices and health. *N Engl J Med*. 2019;381(10):956-968. doi:10.1056/NEJMra1806949
6. Pellegrini CA, Pfammatter AF, Conroy DE, Spring B. Smartphone applications to support weight loss: current perspectives. *Adv Health Care Technol*. 2015;1:13-22. doi:10.2147/AHCT.S57844
7. Ritterband LM, Gonder-Frederick LA, Cox DJ, Clifton AD, West RW, Borowitz SM. Internet interventions: in review, in use, and into the future. *Professional Psychology: Research and Practice*. 2003;34(5):527-534. doi:10.1037/0735-7028.34.5.527
8. Khaylis A, Yiaslas T, Bergstrom J, Gore-Felton C. A review of efficacious technology-based weight-loss interventions: five key components. *Telemed J E Health*. 2010;16(9):931-938. doi:10.1089/tmj.2010.0065
9. Raaijmakers LCH, Pouwels S, Berghuis KA, Nienhuijs SW. Technology-based interventions in the treatment of overweight and obesity: a systematic review. *Appetite*. 2015;95:138-151. doi:10.1016/j.appet.2015.07.008
10. Carver CS, Scheier MF. Control theory: a useful conceptual framework for personality-social, clinical, and health psychology. *Psychol Bull*. 1982;92(1):111-135. doi:10.1037//0033-2909.92.1.111
11. Michie S, Abraham C, Whittington C, McAteer J, Gupta S. Effective techniques in healthy eating and physical activity interventions: a meta-regression. *Health Psychol*. 2009;28(6):690-701. doi:10.1037/a0016136
12. Demographics of internet and home broadband usage in the United States. Pew Research Center. April 2021. Accessed January 12, 2022. www.pewresearch.org/internet/fact-sheet/internet-broadband
13. Hartmann-Boyce J, Jebb SA, Fletcher BR, Aveyard P. Self-help for weight loss in overweight and obese adults: systematic review and meta-analysis. *Am J Public Health*. 2015;105(3):e43-e57. doi:10.2105/AJPH.2014.302389
14. Sorgente A, Pietrabissa G, Manzoni GM, et al. Web-based interventions for weight loss or weight loss maintenance in overweight and obese people: a systematic review of systematic reviews. *J Med Internet Res*. 2017;19(6):e229. doi:10.2196/jmir.6972
15. Gilmartin J, Murphy M. The effects of contemporary behavioural weight loss maintenance interventions for long term weight loss: a systematic review. *J Res Nursing*. 2015;20(6):481-496. doi:10.1177/1744987115599671
16. Neve M, Morgan PJ, Jones PR, Collins CE. Effectiveness of web-based interventions in achieving weight loss and weight loss maintenance in overweight and obese adults: a systematic review with meta-analysis. *Obes Rev*. 2010;11(4):306-321. doi:10.1111/j.1467-789X.2009.00646.x
17. Webb TL, Joseph J, Yardley L, Michie S. Using the internet to promote health behavior change: a systematic review and meta-analysis of the impact of theoretical basis, use of behavior change techniques, and mode of delivery on efficacy. *J Med Internet Res*. 2010;12(1):e4. doi:10.2196/jmir.1376
18. Hutchesson MJ, Rollo ME, Krukowski R, et al. eHealth interventions for the prevention and treatment of overweight and obesity in adults: a systematic review with meta-analysis. *Obes Rev*. 2015;16(5):376-392. doi:10.1111/obr.12268

19. Byaruhanga J, Atorkey P, McLaughlin M, et al. Effectiveness of individual real-time video counseling on smoking, nutrition, alcohol, physical activity, and obesity health risks: systematic review. *J Med Internet Res*. 2020;22(9):e18621. doi:10.2196/18621
20. Ahrendt AD, Kattelmann KK, Rector TS, Maddox DA. The effectiveness of telemedicine for weight management in the MOVE! program. *J Rural Health*. 2014;30(1):113-119. doi:10.1111/jrh.12049
21. Taetzsch A, Gilhooly CH, Bukhari A, et al. Development of a videoconference-adapted version of the community diabetes prevention program, and comparison of weight loss with in-person program delivery. *Mil Med*. 2019;184(11-12):647-652. doi:10.1093/milmed/usz069
22. Johnson KE, Alencar MK, Coakley KE, et al. Telemedicine-based health coaching is effective for inducing weight loss and improving metabolic markers. *Telemed J E Health*. 2019;25(2):85-92. doi:10.1089/tmj.2018.0002
23. Lustria MLA, Noar SM, Cortese J, Van Stee SK, Glueckauf RL, Lee J. A meta-analysis of web-delivered tailored health behavior change interventions. *J Health Commun*. 2013;18(9):1039-1069. doi:10.1080/10810730.2013.768727
24. Lau Y, Chee DGH, Chow XP, Cheng LJ, Wong SN. Personalised eHealth interventions in adults with overweight and obesity: a systematic review and meta-analysis of randomised controlled trials. *Prev Med*. 2020;132:106001. doi:10.1016/j.ypmed.2020.106001
25. Ryan K, Dockray S, Linehan C. A systematic review of tailored eHealth interventions for weight loss. *Digit Health*. 2019;5:2055207619826685. doi:10.1177/2055207619826685
26. Demographics of mobile device ownership and adoption in the United States. Pew Research Center. June 2019. Accessed October 2, 2019. www.pewinternet.org/fact-sheet/mobile
27. Bhuyan SS, Lu N, Chandak A, et al. Use of mobile health applications for health-seeking behavior among US adults. *J Med Syst*. 2016;40(6):153. doi:10.1007/s10916-016-0492-7
28. Schippers M, Adam PCG, Smolenski DJ, Wong HTH, de Wit JBF. A meta-analysis of overall effects of weight loss interventions delivered via mobile phones and effect size differences according to delivery mode, personal contact, and intervention intensity and duration. *Obes Rev*. 2017;18(4):450-459. doi:10.1111/obr.12492
29. Park S-H, Hwang J, Choi Y-K. Effect of mobile health on obese adults: a systematic review and meta-analysis. *Healthc Inform Res*. 2019;25(1):12-26. doi:10.4258/hir.2019.25.1.12
30. Khokhar B, Jones J, Ronksley PE, Armstrong MJ, Caird J, Rabi D. Effectiveness of mobile electronic devices in weight loss among overweight and obese populations: a systematic review and meta-analysis. *BMC Obes*. 2014;1:22. doi:10.1186/s40608-014-0022-4
31. Schembre SM, Liao Y, Robertson MC, et al. Just-in-time feedback in diet and physical activity interventions: systematic review and practical design framework. *J Med Internet Res*. 2018;20(3):e106. doi:10.2196/jmir.8701
32. Schoeppe S, Alley S, Van Lippevelde W, et al. Efficacy of interventions that use apps to improve diet, physical activity and sedentary behaviour: a systematic review. *Int J Behav Nutr Phys Act*. 2016;13(1):127. doi:10.1186/s12966-016-0454-y
33. Head KJ, Noar SM, Iannarino NT, Grant Harrington N. Efficacy of text messaging-based interventions for health promotion: a meta-analysis. *Soc Sci Med*. 2013;97:41-48. doi:10.1016/j.socscimed.2013.08.003
34. Siopis G, Chey T, Allman-Farinelli M. A systematic review and meta-analysis of interventions for weight management using text messaging. *J Hum Nutr Diet*. 2015;28 suppl 2:1-15. doi:10.1111/jhn.12207
35. Allman-Farinelli M, Partridge SR, McGeechan K, et al. A mobile health lifestyle program for prevention of weight gain in young adults (TXT2BFiT): nine-month outcomes of a randomized controlled trial. *JMIR Mhealth Uhealth*. 2016;4(2):e78. doi:10.2196/mhealth.5768
36. Haapala I, Barengo NC, Biggs S, Surakka L, Manninen P. Weight loss by mobile phone: a 1-year effectiveness study. *Public Health Nutr*. 2009;12(12):2382-2391. doi:10.1017/S1368980009005230
37. Patrick K, Raab F, Adams MA, et al. A text message-based intervention for weight loss: randomized controlled trial. *J Med Internet Res*. 2009;11(1):e1. doi:10.2196/jmir.1100
38. Krebs P, Prochaska JO, Rossi JS. A meta-analysis of computer-tailored interventions for health behavior change. *Prev Med*. 2010;51(3-4):214-221. doi:10.1016/j.ypmed.2010.06.004
39. Burke LE, Ma J, Azar KMJ, et al. Current science on consumer use of mobile health for cardiovascular disease prevention: a scientific statement from the American Heart Association. *Circulation*. 2015;132(12):1157-1213. doi:10.1161/CIR.0000000000000232
40. Foley P, Steinberg D, Levine E, et al. Track: a randomized controlled trial of a digital health obesity treatment intervention for medically vulnerable primary care patients. *Contemp Clin Trials*. 2016;48:12-20. doi:10.1016/j.cct.2016.03.006
41. Tate DF, Crane MM, Espeland MA, Gorin AA, LaRose JG, Wing RR. Sustaining eHealth engagement in a multi-year weight gain prevention intervention. *Obes Sci Pract*. 2019;5(2):103-110. doi:10.1002/osp4.333
42. Lyons EJ, Lewis ZH, Mayrsohn BG, Rowland JL. Behavior change techniques implemented in electronic lifestyle activity monitors: a systematic content analysis. *J Med Internet Res*. 2014;16(8):e192. doi:10.2196/jmir.3469
43. Ringeval M, Wagner G, Denford J, Paré G, Kitsiou S. Fitbit-based interventions for healthy lifestyle outcomes: systematic review and meta-analysis. *J Med Internet Res*. 2020;22(10):e23954. doi:10.2196/23954

44. Fawcett E, Van Velthoven MH, Meinert E. Long-term weight management using wearable technology in overweight and obese adults: systematic review. *JMIR Mhealth Uhealth*. 2020;8(3):e13461. doi:10.2196/13461
45. Shuger SL, Barry VW, Sui X, et al. Electronic feedback in a diet- and physical activity-based lifestyle intervention for weight loss: a randomized controlled trial. *Int J Behav Nutr Phys Act*. 2011;8:41. doi:10.1186/1479-5868-8-41
46. Jakicic JM, Davis KK, Rogers RJ, et al. Effect of wearable technology combined with a lifestyle intervention on long-term weight loss: the IDEA randomized clinical trial. *JAMA*. 2016;316(11):1161-1171. doi:10.1001/jama.2016.12858
47. Steinberg DM, Tate DF, Bennett GG, Ennett S, Samuel-Hodge C, Ward DS. The efficacy of a daily self-weighing weight loss intervention using smart scales and e-mail. *Obesity (Silver Spring)*. 2013;21(9):1789-1797. doi:10.1002/oby.20396
48. Laing BY, Mangione CM, Tseng C-H, et al. Effectiveness of a smartphone application for weight loss compared with usual care in overweight primary care patients: a randomized, controlled trial. *Ann Intern Med*. 2014;161(10 suppl):S5-S12. doi:10.7326/M13-3005
49. Helander E, Kaipainen K, Korhonen I, Wansink B. Factors related to sustained use of a free mobile app for dietary self-monitoring with photography and peer feedback: retrospective cohort study. *J Med Internet Res*. 2014;16(4):e109. doi:10.2196/jmir.3084
50. Pagoto S, Schneider K, Jojic M, DeBiasse M, Mann D. Evidence-based strategies in weight-loss mobile apps. *Am J Prev Med*. 2013;45(5):576-582. doi:10.1016/j.amepre.2013.04.025
51. Bardus M, van Beurden SB, Smith JR, Abraham C. A review and content analysis of engagement, functionality, aesthetics, information quality, and change techniques in the most popular commercial apps for weight management. *Int J Behav Nutr Phys Act*. 2016;13:35. doi:10.1186/s12966-016-0359-9
52. Glasgow RE, Fisher L, Strycker LA, et al. Minimal intervention needed for change: definition, use, and value for improving health and health research. *Transl Behav Med*. 2014;4(1):26-33. doi:10.1007/s13142-013-0232-1
53. Collins CE, Morgan PJ, Hutchesson MJ, Callister R. Efficacy of standard versus enhanced features in a Web-based commercial weight-loss program for obese adults, part 2: randomized controlled trial. *J Med Internet Res*. 2013;15(7):e140. doi:10.2196/jmir.2626
54. Nackers LM, Ross KM, Perri MG. The association between rate of initial weight loss and long-term success in obesity treatment: does slow and steady win the race? *Int J Behav Med*. 2010;17(3):161-167. doi:10.1007/s12529-010-9092-y
55. Unick JL, Jakicic JM, Marcus BH. Contribution of behavior intervention components to 24-month weight loss. *Med Sci Sports Exerc*. 2010;42(4):745-753. doi:10.1249/MSS.0b013e3181bd1a57
56. Miller CK, Nagaraja HN, Weinhold KR. Early weight-loss success identifies nonresponders after a lifestyle intervention in a worksite diabetes prevention trial. *J Acad Nutr Diet*. 2015;115(9):1464-1471. doi:10.1016/j.jand.2015.04.022
57. Wadden TA, West DS, Neiberg RH, et al. One-year weight losses in the Look AHEAD study: factors associated with success. *Obesity (Silver Spring)*. 2009;17(4):713-722. doi:10.1038/oby.2008.637
58. Bennett GG, Steinberg DM, Stoute C, et al. Electronic health (eHealth) interventions for weight management among racial/ethnic minority adults: a systematic review. *Obes Rev*. 2014;15 suppl 4:146-158. doi:10.1111/obr.12218

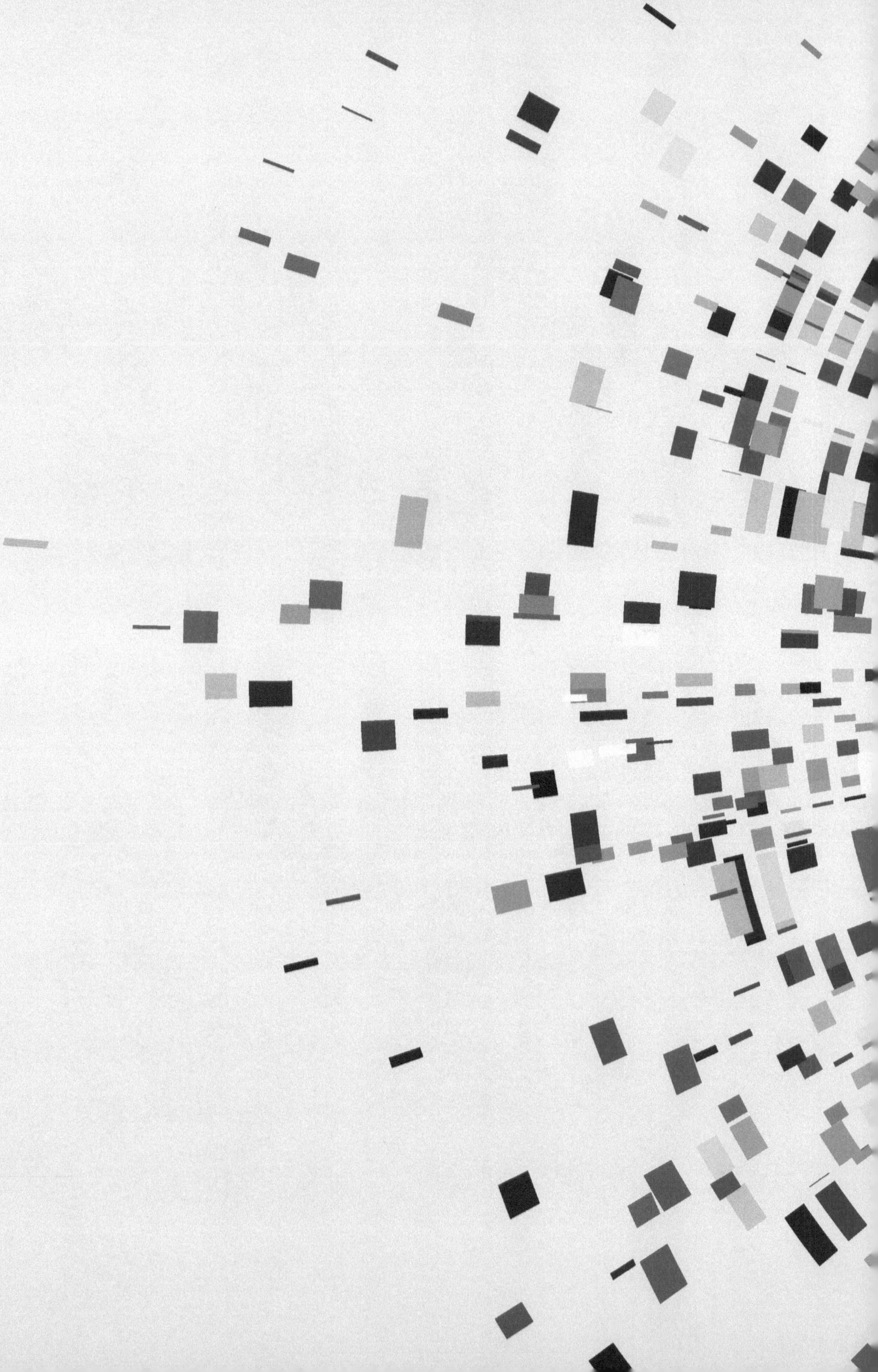

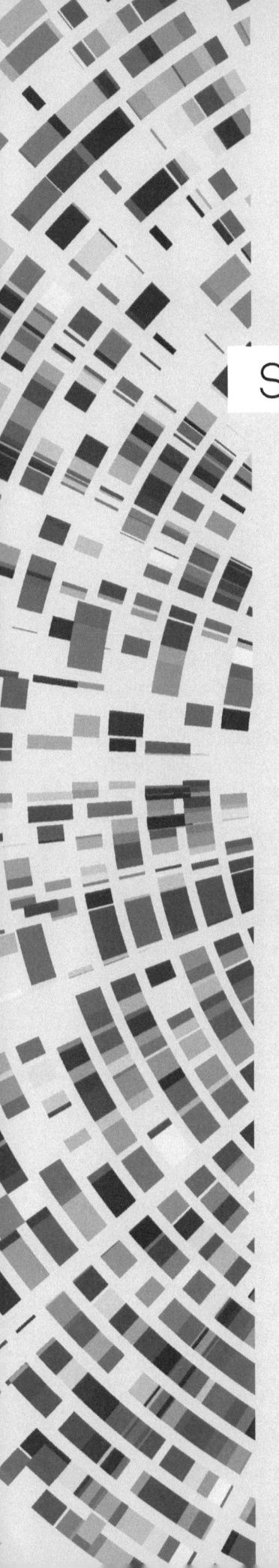

SECTION 4

Models and Insurance Coverage for the Treatment of Obesity

CHAPTER 18 Interprofessional Teams and Models of Practice | 334

CHAPTER 19 Health Care Systems, Policies, and the Coverage of Services | 346

CHAPTER 18

Interprofessional Teams and Models of Practice

Colleen Tewksbury, PhD, RD

CHAPTER OBJECTIVES

- Identify the roles of interdisciplinary team members in a multicomponent weight management team.
- Describe the scope of practice related to weight management for each health care discipline represented on the team.
- List credentials and certifications available to providers to establish expertise in treatment of overweight and obesity.
- Discuss care team models for the delivery of weight management services.

Introduction

Obesity is a complex disease requiring comprehensive treatment that incorporates multilevel, staged approaches beyond the first-line therapies of diet, exercise, and behavioral intervention.[1] As with other chronic diseases, comprehensive treatment for obesity encompasses the complete spectrum of available services and requires the involvement of multiple providers from different disciplines over an extended period of time.[2] No single clinician can treat obesity in one interaction; therefore, the primary goal of any interaction within obesity treatment is to keep the patient engaged in care. As negative or stigmatizing interactions can cause patients with excess weight or obesity to avoid care altogether, all members of the team must be acutely aware of implicit and explicit weight bias, as well as internalized bias (refer to Chapter 3). Furthermore, because individuals entering weight management programs tend to have higher weight loss goals than the treatment is expected to achieve,[3,4] it is essential that treatment facilitate continued participation and support from the entire care team. All team members must participate in expectation setting, utilizing appropriate behavioral techniques and combating weight bias in order to maximize the patient's use of services and ongoing care.

A health care team is defined as two or more people working interdependently toward a common health-related goal.[5] Interprofessional care teams have been a fixture of many areas of health care for decades (eg, oncology, transplantation, orthopedics). As the understanding of body weight and metabolism advances, so does the need to incorporate more team members for optimal patient-centered care. Specifically, clinicians on interprofessional teams tend to endorse the importance of improved care coordination, communication, and reinforced care, compared to those in independent practice.[6] Health care practitioners also have highlighted interprofessional care as a way to address inconsistencies in or disagreements with treatment plans and coordination, and health information systems have been developed to address this.[7,8] However, a frequently cited challenge to interprofessional teams is the lack of defined roles for team members[7]; therefore, greater clarity around team dynamics is essential for the practical analysis of team-based weight management care.

Members of the Interprofessional Team

Health care practitioners, researchers, and patients agree that weight management care should be multifaceted and that an interdisciplinary team, as illustrated by Figure 18.1, is required to deliver patient-centered care.[9]

Medical Providers

Physicians, advanced practice providers (eg, nurse practitioners, physician assistants), and nurses are an integral part of the health care team. Medical assessment and interventions for obesity are discussed in Chapters 6 and 14. Because of the higher-level scope granted to these positions by state licensing boards, physicians are often viewed as the leaders within weight management teams. However,

FIGURE 18.1 Types of interprofessional team members and specific examples[9]

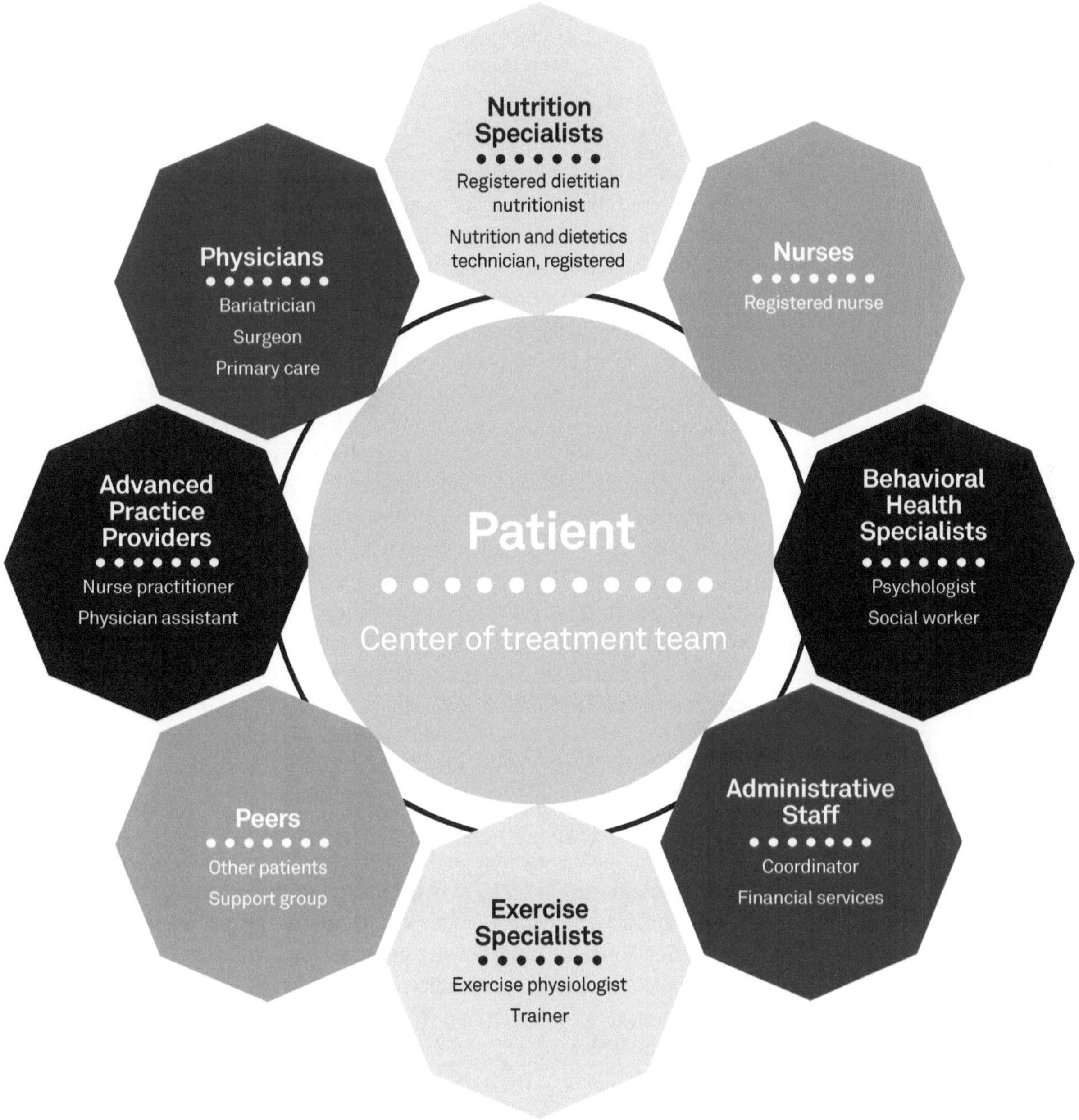

- **Nutrition Specialists**: Registered dietitian nutritionist; Nutrition and dietetics technician, registered
- **Physicians**: Bariatrician; Surgeon; Primary care
- **Nurses**: Registered nurse
- **Advanced Practice Providers**: Nurse practitioner; Physician assistant
- **Behavioral Health Specialists**: Psychologist; Social worker
- **Peers**: Other patients; Support group
- **Exercise Specialists**: Exercise physiologist; Trainer
- **Administrative Staff**: Coordinator; Financial services
- **Patient**: Center of treatment team

traditional medical school education continues to provide suboptimal training in obesity treatment. Notably, only 10% of medical schools report that their graduates are "very prepared" to manage patients with obesity.[10] In addition, one-third of medical schools report that they have no obesity education program in place and no plans to develop one. Specifically, primary care providers perceive their knowledge of nutrition and obesity treatment to be suboptimal, despite the fact that primary care is often the first line of treatment for weight management.[11] While the lack of expertise in obesity medicine presents itself as a gap in education and training, it also highlights the need for complementary specializing physicians with advanced training and expertise. Specialized training varies depending on the provider, as physicians specializing in pharmacotherapy or endoscopic treatments for obesity often have completed fellowships and hold board certifications in endocrinology, gastroenterology, or bariatric and minimally invasive surgery. Nursing care, as an extension of medical care, is also a critical component of obesity treatment. One study in an academic medical center found that more than half of physicians and nurses reported having inadequate training in obesity care.[12] Nurses report having limited basic training and express a strong desire for additional information on obesity to be included in standardized curricula.[13]

Nutrition Specialists

Diet modification is a component of all weight management interventions, making the registered dietitian nutritionist (RDN) an indispensable part of the weight management care team. RDNs receive extensive training in nutrition; at minimum, they must currently have a bachelor's degree (requirements will be updated in 2024 to a minimum of a master's degree), undergo supervised practice, and take an examination to qualify for registration.[14] Nutrition and dietetics technicians, registered (NDTRs) must have completed at least an associate degree with supervised practice and taken an examination to qualify for registration. Continuing professional education is required to maintain registration for each credential.

Nutrition assessment and intervention are described in Chapters 7 and 11. NDTR team members can provide screenings, conduct portions of the assessment, and provide nutrition education. Medical nutrition therapy (MNT), nutrition care for the purpose of disease management, is the primary intervention used by RDNs. In a comparison of different treatment options, when MNT provided by an RDN was included in the weight loss intervention, participants lost significantly more weight.[15] RDN involvement is key to optimizing any weight management program. Specific to bariatric surgery, postoperative nutrition counseling is associated with greater weight losses up to 2 years after surgery.[16-18]

The Academy of Nutrition and Dietetics standards of practice (SOP) and standards of professional performance (SOPP) in adult weight management explicitly outline the scope of an RDN in this field.[19] While state licensure and practice acts may have more specific requirements, individual scope of practice is determined by measured competency rooted in the Dreyfus model of skill acquisition (eg, competent, proficient, expert). The SOP in adult weight management describe four individual standards (nutrition assessment, diagnosis, intervention, and monitoring), and the SOPP include the following six domains of professionalism: quality in practice; competence and accountability; provision of services; application of research; communication and application of knowledge; and utilization and management of resources. The SOP and SOPP outline indicators for each standard along with indicators at varying levels of practice. Each indicator level is determined not by the task itself but by how the task is performed. The SOP and SOPP are updated every 7 years and are a means by which RDNs in adult weight management can assess their competency in a standardized manner and determine progressive steps for practice advancement.

Exercise Specialists

Exercise specialists represent a range of levels of physical activity expertise, from exercise physiologist or physical therapist to certified fitness trainer. The American College of Sports Medicine offers multiple certifications, including group exercise instructor (GEI), certified personal trainer (CPT), clinical exercise physiologist (CEP), and registered clinical exercise physiologist (RCEP).[20] The National Strength and Conditioning Association also offers certifications specific to different areas of physical activity.[21] Each certification has a specific definition and scope of practice appropriate for the level of prerequisites and care provided. Within the designated scope, exercise specialists assess a patient, develop activity programs to address the primary exercise diagnosis, and support and monitor the individual throughout the intervention. Although exercise specialists do not typically have the authority to diagnose diseases, a clinician such as an RCEP is able to conduct in-depth medical and physical assessments to determine an exercise-specific diagnosis and prescription. As described in Chapters 8 and 12, the level of assessment and treatment needs of the patient determine the type of exercise specialist that is most appropriate to include on the care team.

Behavioral Health Specialists

Behavioral health specialists include those with prescriptive authority (eg, psychiatrists or psychiatric nurse clinical specialists) and those who deliver counseling—namely, licensed clinical social workers (LCSW), psychologists, licensed mental health counselors (LMHC), licensed professional counselors (LPC), and licensed marriage and family therapists (LMFT). Like other health professionals, mental health professionals receive minimal training in weight management or weight sensitivity. However, they can employ general behavior change strategies and obtain advanced training in weight management or adjacent fields, such as health psychology. Specific behavioral assessment and intervention strategies are reviewed in Chapters 9 and 13.

Having an expert in counseling and behavior change on the care team is critical for effective treatment. Patients undergoing bariatric surgery who receive postoperative counseling experience greater weight losses up to 3 years after surgery.[22] In addition, many untreated or uncontrolled psychiatric diagnoses are contraindications to most weight management interventions.[1] Although the majority of patients seeking weight management services do not meet the criteria for a psychiatric diagnosis, a high prevalence of past mental health diagnoses along with previous trauma have been reported in patients with obesity.[23] As discussed in Chapter 9, although many of the behavioral health screenings can be conducted by other members of the interprofessional team, more complex assessment and diagnosis are often required because of this increased prevalence.[24]

Peers

Peer support is an often overlooked component of weight management. Social modeling is a core element of the social cognitive theory and the underpinning for many behavioral weight loss interventions.[25] Being able to observe one's peers and relate to others in a similar situation helps bolster self-efficacy and sustainable behavior change. Peers have been integrated into different models in various ways, including through training community leaders to deliver key behavioral interventions and group behavioral treatment. The most common way that peer support is incorporated into weight management interventions is through support groups, which provide a means for individuals undergoing similar treatment to share their experiences and provide each other with relatable support.[24] For instance, bariatric surgery patients who attend structured support groups often achieve more favorable weight loss outcomes in both the short and long term.[26] In addition, many peer support systems have expanded into online networks, leveraging an easily accessible communication platform to promote even greater interaction.[27] Patients with stronger support systems, whether in-person or virtual, often have higher rates of self-efficacy, experience better quality of life, and achieve more favorable weight loss outcomes.

Administrative Staff Members

Administrative staff are also often overlooked as core members of the care team, but they are essential in providing patients with accessible, quality care. This group includes individuals in nonclinical positions who, although they may not directly interact with patients, play a key role in facilitating care. Examples are front desk staff, quality managers, data managers, and operations leadership. Many weight management interventions require multiple office visits or extensive testing. Administrative support is necessary not only to coordinate the scheduling of these visits but also to assist in navigating the financial components of care. Third-party payer coverage of obesity treatments is variable, so having financial experts assist the clinical team and the patient with navigating coverage and payment options is critical. In addition, quality management teams in health care systems are essential for optimizing patient care, including in the area of weight management. For example, the American College of Surgeons' Metabolic and Bariatric Surgery Accreditation and Quality Improvement Program (MBSAQIP) acknowledges the importance of administrative support in providing quality care and requires bariatric surgery centers to have specific administrative positions (director, coordinator, clinical reviewer), structured quality improvement programs, and explicit documentation of institutional support in order to achieve and maintain their accreditation.[28] The people in these positions work with the clinical team and patients (directly or indirectly) in order to provide effective weight management treatment.

Establishing Weight Management Expertise and Credentialing

Because weight and BMI are key metrics for assessing health risk, the field of weight management intersects with most areas of health care. Therefore, even if health care practitioners do not explicitly work in a traditional weight management setting, they can establish extensive knowledge, experience, and expertise in the field. The most common mechanisms for doing so involve advanced credentialing or completing advanced training in weight management care. Box 18.1 details the various avenues for establishing weight management expertise.

BOX 18.1

Ways to Establish Weight Management Expertise Within the Interprofessional Team

Board Certified Specialist in Obesity and Weight Management (CSOWM)

Eligible team members	Advanced practice providers, exercise physiologists, psychologists, licensed clinical social workers, pharmacists, physical therapists, registered dietitian nutritionists
Issuing organization	Commission on Dietetic Registration
Website address	www.cdrnet.org/interdisciplinary

American Board of Obesity Medicine certification (ABOM)

Eligible team members	Physicians
Issuing organization	American Board of Obesity Medicine
Website address	www.abom.org

Fellow of the American Society for Metabolic and Bariatric Surgery (FASMBS)

Eligible team members	Surgeons
Issuing organization	American Society for Metabolic and Bariatric Surgery
Website address	https://asmbs.org/become-fellow-asmbs

Certified Bariatric Nurse (CBN)

Eligible team members	Licensed nurses
Issuing organization	American Society for Metabolic and Bariatric Surgery
Website address	https://asmbs.org/professional-education/cbn

Certificate of Training in Obesity for Pediatrics and Adults (noncredentialed)

Eligible team members	Registered dietitian nutritionists; nutrition and dietetics technicians, registered
Issuing organization	Commission on Dietetic Registration
Website address	www.cdrnet.org/obesity-pediatrics-adults

Box continues

BOX 18.1 (CONTINUED)

NP/PA Certificate of Advanced Education in Obesity Medicine (noncredentialed)

Eligible team members	Advanced practice providers
Issuing organization	Obesity Medicine Association
Website address	https://obesitymedicine.org/education/certificate-advanced-education

Abbreviation: NP/PA, nurse practitioner/physician assistant.

The Commission on Dietetic Registration (CDR) is the credentialing agency for the Academy of Nutrition and Dietetics; they offer a wide range of credentials. In the fall of 2016, CDR launched its first interdisciplinary weight management credential—Board Certified Specialist in Obesity and Weight Management (CSOWM).[29] Advanced practice providers, exercise physiologists, psychologists, licensed clinical social workers, pharmacists, physical therapists, and RDNs are eligible to take the exam after at least 2 years of maintaining their credential and 2,000 hours of practice in weight management. This credential is valid for 5 years, after which the candidate must provide documentation of continued hours and retake the exam to maintain their credential. The CSOWM credential is a recognition of documented experience and competence in weight management and is a mechanism for health care practitioners to differentiate their expertise on the team.

The American Board of Obesity Medicine (ABOM) offers a certification for physicians in the United States or Canada. Certification starts with a minimum of 60 continuing medical education credits over a 3-year period prior to completing an examination.[30] This credential designates a physician as having advanced knowledge and expertise in all areas of obesity treatment and weight management.

Physicians specializing in bariatric surgery can demonstrate their expertise in one of two ways. The American Society for Metabolic and Bariatric Surgery (ASMBS) offers a fellowship with corresponding credential (FASMBS).[31] Surgeons with this credential must be regular members of ASMBS, perform a minimum number of bariatric surgeries per year, and complete regular continuing medical education specific to metabolic and bariatric surgery. In addition, MBSAQIP, as a part of accreditation, offers bariatric surgeon verification with similar requirements, which all bariatric surgery center directors must maintain in order to retain their center's MBSAQIP accreditation.[28] As a part of this accreditation, bariatric surgery centers are also able to designate an obesity medicine director to oversee nonsurgical obesity medicine services provided to patients.

Nursing care for persons undergoing bariatric surgery has also been established as an area of expertise. ASMBS offers the Certified Bariatric Nurse (CBN) program to acknowledge the specific competence of bariatric nursing. Licensed nurses who have at least 2 years of experience in caring for patients who have undergone bariatric surgery and patients with severe obesity are eligible to take the exam.[32]

Although individual team members have the opportunity to establish their expertise through individual certifications, several weight management recognitions exist for entire teams or programs as well. Most notably, MBSAQIP offers levels of distinction (ie, designations) for centers that perform bariatric surgery, including designations for comprehensive surgical care, ambulatory care, adolescent surgical care, and obesity medicine.[28] MBSAQIP accreditation is given to specific entities that perform surgery, not to individuals or multisite programs. The base designation is MBSAQIP Comprehensive Center. Specialized designations include MBSAQIP Comprehensive Center with Obesity Medicine Qualifications, for centers offering pharmacotherapy interventions, and MBSAQIP Comprehensive Center with Adolescent Qualifications, for programs with a pediatric component. Ambulatory centers and low acuity centers can also apply for accreditation. Accreditations in bariatric surgery serve as independent verification of care provided and are associated with lower rates of postoperative mortality and complications.[33] Centers can also apply for participation in third-party payer distinctions. These designations are often used to identify preferred weight management and surgical programs based on quality outcomes and cost and are often required for coverage of services.

Aside from these certifications and credentials, many certificate-of-training programs are available for health care practitioners to advance their skills in weight management. CDR routinely offers such certificate programs, which range in format from short online training modules to more comprehensive trainings with live, facilitated components. The Academy of Nutrition and Dietetics Weight Management dietetic practice group hosts regular continuing education events and provides a vast array of training resources. The Obesity Medicine Association offers a certificate of training for advanced practice providers as well. Each of the weight management professional organizations, including The Obesity Society and ASMBS, hosts regular symposia and conferences. In addition, longstanding interdisciplinary trainings, such as the Blackburn Course in Obesity Medicine and the Bariatric Summit, offer consistent, high-quality training for clinicians looking to advance their knowledge and skills specific to medical or surgical treatment of obesity.[34,35]

Each of these credentials, certifications, and certificates of training serves multiple purposes for both clinicians and patients. For clinicians, an obesity and weight management care designation allows for clear delineation of expertise. Although this is often a component of professional development, as described for RDNs in the SOPP in adult weight management, it also clearly communicates the specialized nature of weight management care separate from general practice. This gives a level of assurance to referring practitioners and patients that the information and care being provided is of the highest quality.

Care Team Models

Various systems of providing team care are employed in weight management. The most common care team models are primary care, specialty services, and service line care. For day-to-day collaborative care, clinicians are employing systems such as interprofessional review and shared visits. These approaches have both benefits and challenges for the clinical team and the patient.

Primary Care

Primary care is the first line of treatment for weight management. Because of current limitations put forth by the Centers for Medicare and Medicaid Services (CMS), billing for intensive behavioral therapy for weight management must be done through a primary care group. These groups are often the only viable option for providing nonsurgical obesity interventions. Many primary care offices, therefore, have added allied health providers, such as RDNs, exercise specialists, and behavioral health providers to their clinical staff in order to adhere to current CMS reimbursement requirements. Although primary care faces many challenges in terms of staffing and providing adequate patient support, studies have shown that primary care offices can be ideal locations for weight management care.[36-38] Resources are available for primary care providers to better integrate weight management services into their practice and to develop forward-thinking models of weight management care.[39] Methods of integration include adding systems for screening and diagnosis, providing a built environment that is weight inclusive, and establishing training and policies for staff regarding obesity and weight bias.[40]

Service Line Models

A service line model is an approach to care in which the provision of health services is organized by the type of disease. In this model, all the clinicians who serve as a part of the patient care team are housed within the same administrative system or department according to the disease being treated. This type of care is most commonly seen in fields such as oncology, transplantation, or orthopedics. Service line approaches center the patient experience in one place, unlike traditional health care models that require patients to visit multiple providers in different locations (each with their own administrative support).[41] With the recognition of obesity as a complex metabolic disease, more health care systems are shifting to this model for obesity care, thus allowing all members of the care team to work and communicate in the same space and eliminating many of the administrative hurdles of siloed interprofessional care. In comprehensive, dedicated weight management centers, multiple services (nutrition, physical activity, behavioral health, surgery, pharmacotherapy) are offered to patients in one system or location. This model can be extended to create similar systems within private practice groups, by having complementary health care providers partner with each other within the practice. This can take the form of shared partnership or ownership of the practice, shared physical space, or even coordinated locations and referral systems.

Shared Medical Appointments

In a shared medical appointment, an individual patient sees more than one health care practitioner during a single encounter. This may include any mix of members of the health care team. Shared appointments are most commonly employed in the bariatric-surgery setting, where patients may often see an RDN, a behavioral health provider, and an exercise specialist all during their scheduled appointment with their surgeon or surgical advanced practice provider. This model promotes improved communication, greater patient satisfaction, and greater weight loss.[42] A study comparing 2-year weight loss outcomes of patients who attended individual obesity-treatment visits vs shared visits (involving multiple providers and group visits) at an academic medical center found that patients attending shared visits experienced 1.5% to 1.6% greater total weight loss compared to patients who saw care team members individually.[42] However, practitioners should be aware of the increased complexity of shared visits and be able to adjust their approach to align with care being provided simultaneously by other team members. In addition, clinicians should work with their administrative teams to optimize billing practices, as many payers do not reimburse for multiple visits in the same practice on the same day.

Interdisciplinary Review

Interdisciplinary review of care is an adjunctive model and can take many forms, including rounds, clinical huddles, and review boards. Rounds within weight management care are typically used to review the current treatment of patients for a specific period of time (eg, the current day or the past week). Clinical huddles are informal interactions for the purpose of coordinating care for a specific patient. Review boards are formal, interdisciplinary reviews of patients deemed to be at high risk with the goal of agreeing on a treatment plan and coordinating care. Within the field of bariatric surgery, interdisciplinary review of care has been established as vital for standardizing care and minimizing surgical complications.[43] In one study, health care practitioners identified clear communication, a focus on patients, and holistic care planning as the primary benefits of rounds.[6] In the same study, clinicians reported that the primary challenges to employing interdisciplinary review approaches were time, staffing, and interprofessional coordination issues. These benefits and challenges should be assessed and addressed when developing an interdisciplinary review program in order to balance competing priorities.

Future Models of Care for Weight Management

It is estimated that approximately four in five US adults will have overweight or obesity by 2030.[44] Because of the impending increase in the demand for care and the cross-cutting nature of weight management, health care practitioners must continue to work creatively toward offering weight management care in areas of need. Depending on the payment model, care can often be provided by bringing treatment directly to the target populations. In the face of the COVID-19 pandemic, many weight management and obesity treatment centers were able to continue care while keeping staff and patients safe by utilizing telehealth.[45]

In addition, certain populations who may be at higher risk for overweight and obesity and who are already engaged in specific health care systems for treatment of a condition (eg, cancer) can be targeted for weight management care through the systems in which they are already engaged. For example, cancer survivors with weight-related cancers often participate in survivorship groups, which are well-established networks for those in remission, and these can be ideal settings in which to offer weight management interventions and support.[46] Similarly, pregnancy and the postpartum period are important periods of weight gain and weight loss, respectively, and have been shown to be practical and effective times to introduce weight management interventions[47]; therefore, as is done in other disciplines, weight management professionals can be integrated into obstetrics care to improve access for this population.

Summary

Interprofessional care teams for weight management bring together different disciplines to provide the highest quality of care to patients. Each team member plays an integral role in care management. Clinicians have various mechanisms by which they can advance their training and skills in obesity and weight management care and also earn credentials to validate their level of expertise. Though there are currently several effective ways to structure the provision of weight management care, such as service line systems and shared medical visits, ample opportunity exists to develop more forward-facing models, reduce barriers to providing and accessing interdisciplinary care, and further establish weight management as a subspecialty.

References

1. Jensen MD, Ryan DH, Apovian CM, et al. 2013 AHA/ACC/TOS guideline for the management of overweight and obesity in adults: a report of the American College of Cardiology/American Heart Association Task Force on Practice Guidelines and The Obesity Society. *J Am Coll Cardiol.* 2014;63(25 pt B):2985-3023. doi:10.1016/j.jacc.2013.11.004
2. Foster D, Sanchez-Collins S, Cheskin LJ. Multidisciplinary team–based obesity treatment in patients with diabetes: current practices and the state of the science. *Diabetes Spectr.* 2017;30(4):244-249. doi:10.2337/ds17-0045
3. Lent MR, Vander Veur SS, Peters JC, et al. Initial weight loss goals: have they changed and do they matter? *Obes Sci Pract.* 2016;2(2):154-161. doi:10.1002/osp4.45
4. Phelan SM, Burgess DJ, Yeazel MW, Hellerstedt WL, Griffin JM, van Ryn M. Impact of weight bias and stigma on quality of care and outcomes for patients with obesity. *Obes Rev.* 2015;16(4):319-326. doi:10.1111/obr.12266
5. Babiker A, El Husseini M, Al Nemri A, et al. Health care professional development: working as a team to improve patient care. *Sudan J Paediatr.* 2014;14(2):9.
6. Walton V, Hogden A, Long JC, Johnson JK, Greenfield D. How do interprofessional healthcare teams perceive the benefits and challenges of interdisciplinary ward rounds. *J Multidiscip Healthc.* 2019;12:1023-1032. doi:10.2147/JMDH.S226330
7. Aboueid S, Pouliot C, Hermosura BJ, Bourgeault I, Giroux I. Dietitians' perspectives on the impact of multidisciplinary teams and electronic medical records on dietetic practice for weight management. *Can J Diet Pract Res.* 2019;81(1):2-7. doi:10.3148/cjdpr-2019-015
8. Kuziemsky CE, Borycki EM, Purkis ME, et al. An interdisciplinary team communication framework and its application to healthcare "e-teams" systems design. *BMC Medical Infom Decis Mak.* 2009;9(1):43. doi:10.1186/1472-6947-9-43
9. Cochrane AJ, Dick B, King NA, Hills AP, Kavanagh DJ. Developing dimensions for a multicomponent multidisciplinary approach to obesity management: a qualitative study. *BMC Public Health.* 2017;17(1):814. doi:10.1186/s12889-017-4834-2
10. Butsch WS, Kushner RF, Alford S, Smolarz BG. Low priority of obesity education leads to lack of medical students' preparedness to effectively treat patients with obesity: results from the US medical school obesity education curriculum benchmark study. *BMC Med Educ.* 2020;20(1):23. doi:10.1186/s12909-020-1925-z
11. Aboueid S, Bourgeault I, Giroux I. Nutrition and obesity care in multidisciplinary primary care settings in Ontario, Canada: short duration of visits and complex health problems perceived as barriers. *Prev Med Rep.* 2018;10:242-247. doi:10.1016/j.pmedr.2018.04.003
12. Bucher Della Torre S, Courvoisier DS, Saldarriaga A, Martin XE, Farpour-Lambert NJ. Knowledge, attitudes, representations and declared practices of nurses and physicians about obesity in a university hospital: training is essential. *Clin Obes.* 2018;8(2):122-130. doi:10.1111/cob.12238
13. Fruh SM, Golden A, Graves RJ, Hall HR, Minchew LA, Williams S. Advanced Practice Nursing student knowledge in obesity management: a mixed methods research study. *Nurse Educ Today.* 2019;77:59-64. doi:10.1016/j.nedt.2019.03.006
14. Academy of Nutrition and Dietetics. About RDNs and NDTRs. eatRIGHT website. Accessed April 2, 2023. www.eatright.org/about-rdns-and-ndtrs
15. Williams LT, Barnes K, Ball L, Ross LJ, Sladdin I, Mitchell LJ. How effective are dietitians in weight management? A systematic review and meta-analysis of randomized controlled trials. *Healthcare.* 2019; 7(1):20. doi:10.3390/healthcare7010020
16. Sarwer DB, Moore RH, Spitzer JC, Wadden TA, Raper SE, Williams NN. A pilot study investigating the efficacy of postoperative dietary counseling to improve outcomes after bariatric surgery. *Surg Obes Relat Dis.* 2012;8(5):561-568. doi:10.1016/j.soard.2012.02.010
17. Endevelt R, Ben-Assuli O, Klain E, Zelber-Sagi S. The role of dietician follow-up in the success of bariatric surgery. *Surg Obes Relat Dis.* 2013;9(6):963-968. doi:10.1016/j.soard.2013.01.006
18. Andromalos L, Crowley N, Brown J, et al. Nutrition care in bariatric surgery: an Academy Evidence Analysis Center systematic review. *J Acad Nutr Diet.* 2019;119(4):678-686. doi:10.1016/j.jand.2018.08.002

19. Tewksbury C, Nwankwo R, Peterson J. Academy of Nutrition and Dietetics: revised 2022 standards of practice and standards of professional performance for registered dietitian nutritionists (competent, proficient, and expert) in adult weight management. *J Acad Nutr Diet.* 2022;122(10):1940-1954. doi:10.1016/j.jand.2022.06.00
20. American College of Sports Medicine. *ACSM's Guidelines for Exercise Testing and Prescription.* 9th ed. Lippincott Williams and Wilkins; 2013.
21. National Strength and Conditioning Association certification. National Strength and Conditioning Association. Accessed December 10, 2021. www.nsca.com/certification-overview
22. Rudolph A, Hilbert A. Post-operative behavioural management in bariatric surgery: a systematic review and meta-analysis of randomized controlled trials. *Obes Rev.* 2013;14(4):292-302. doi:10.1111/obr.12013
23. Avila C, Holloway AC, Hahn MK, et al. An overview of links between obesity and mental health. *Curr Obes Rep.* 2015;4(3):303-310. doi:10.1007/s13679-015-0164-9
24. Mechanick JI, Apovian C, Brethauer S, et al. Clinical practice guidelines for the perioperative nutrition, metabolic, and nonsurgical support of patients undergoing bariatric procedures–2019 update: cosponsored by American Association of Clinical Endocrinologists/American College of Endocrinology, The Obesity Society, American Society for Metabolic and Bariatric Surgery, Obesity Medicine Association, and American Society of Anesthesiologists. *Endocrine Practice.* 2019;25:1-75. doi:10.4158/GL-2019-0406
25. Bandura A. Social cognitive theory: an agentic perspective. *Annu Rev Psychol.* 2001;52(1):1-26. doi:10.1146/annurev.psych.52.1.1
26. Andreu A, Jimenez A, Vidal J, et al. Bariatric support groups predicts long-term weight loss. *Obes Surg.* 2020;30(6):2118-2123. doi:10.1007/s11695-020-04434-2
27. Athanasiadis DI, Carr RA, Smith C, et al. Social support provided to bariatric surgery patients through a Facebook group may improve weight loss outcomes. *Surg Endosc.* 2022;36(10):7652-7655. doi:10.1007/s00464-022-09067-3
28. American College of Surgeons. *Optimal Resources for Metabolic and Bariatric Surgery: 2019 Standards.* American College of Surgeons; 2019. Accessed April 2, 2023. www.facs.org/quality-programs/accreditation-and-verification/metabolic-and-bariatric-surgery-accreditation-and-quality-improvement-program/standards
29. CDR's Interdisciplinary Obesity and Weight Management Certification. Commission on Dietetic Registration. Accessed April 2, 2023. www.cdrnet.org/interdisciplinary
30. American Board of Obesity Medicine certification. American Board of Obesity Medicine. Accessed December 10, 2021. www.abom.org/cme-certification-pathway-eligibility-and-requirements-2
31. Fellow of the American Society for Metabolic and Bariatric Surgery. American Society for Metabolic and Bariatric Surgery. Accessed December 10, 2021. https://asmbs.org/become-fellow-asmbs
32. Certified Bariatric Nurse Program. American Society for Metabolic and Bariatric Surgery. Accessed December 10, 2021. https://asmbs.org/professional-education/cbn
33. Gebhart A, Young M, Phelan M, Nguyen NT. Impact of accreditation in bariatric surgery. *Surg Obes Relat Dis.* 2014;10(5):767-773. doi:10.1016/j.soard.2014.03.009
34. The Blackburn Course in Obesity Medicine. Harvard Medical School. Accessed December 10, 2021. https://obesity.hmscme.com
35. Bariatric Summit. Accessed December 10, 2021. https://bariatricsummit.com
36. Wadden TA, Volger S, Sarwer DB, et al. A two-year randomized trial of obesity treatment in primary care practice. *NEJM.* 2011;365(21):1969-1979. doi:10.1056/NEJMoa1109220
37. Fitzpatrick SL, Wischenka D, Appelhans BM, et al. An evidence-based guide for obesity treatment in primary care. *Am J Med.* 2016;129(1):115.e1-7. doi:10.1016/j.amjmed.2015.07.015
38. Tsai AG, Remmert JE, Butryn ML, Wadden TA. Treatment of obesity in primary care. *Med Clin North Am.* 2018;102(1):35-47. doi:10.1016/j.mcna.2017.08.005
39. Kahan SI. Practical strategies for engaging individuals with obesity in primary care. *Mayo Clin Proc.* 2018;93(3): 351-359. doi:10.1016/j.mayocp.2018.01.006
40. Puhl RM, Phelan SM, Nadglowski J, Kyle TK. Overcoming weight bias in the management of patients with diabetes and obesity. *Clin Diabetes.* 2016;34(1):44-50. doi:10.2337/diaclin.34.1.44
41. Lee D. A model for designing healthcare service based on the patient experience. *Int J Healthc Manag.* 2019;12(3):180-188. doi.org/10.1080/20479700.2017.1359956
42. Shibuya K, Ji X, Pfoh ER, et al. Association between shared medical appointments and weight loss outcomes and anti-obesity medication use in patients with obesity. *Obes Sci Pract* 2020;6(3):247-254. doi:10.1002/osp4.406
43. Rebibo L, Maréchal V, De Lameth I, et al. Compliance with a multidisciplinary team meeting's decision prior to bariatric surgery protects against major postoperative complications. *Surg Obes Relat Dis.* 2017;13(9):1537-1543. doi:10.1016/j.soard.2017.05.026
44. Ward ZJ, Bleich SN, Cradock AL, et al. Projected US state-level prevalence of adult obesity and severe obesity. *NEJM.* 2019;381(25):2440-2450.
45. Tewksbury C, Deleener ME, Dumon KR, Williams NN. Practical considerations of developing and conducting a successful telehealth practice in response to COVID-19. *Nutr Clin Pract.* 2021;36(4):769-774. doi:10.1056/NEJMsa1909301
46. Demark-Wahnefried W, Schmitz KH, Alfano CM, et al. Weight management and physical activity throughout the cancer care continuum. *CA Cancer J Clin.* 2018;68(1):64-89. doi:10.3322/caac.21441
47. Lim S, Liang X, Hill B, Teede H, Moran LJ, O'Reilly S. A systematic review and meta-analysis of intervention characteristics in postpartum weight management using the TIDieR framework: a summary of evidence to inform implementation. *Obes Rev.* 2019;20(7):1045-1056. doi:10.1111/obr.12846

CHAPTER 19

Health Care Systems, Policies, and the Coverage of Services

Marsha Schofield, MS, RD, LD, FAND
Hannah E. Martin, MPH, RDN

CHAPTER OBJECTIVES

- Summarize the current health care systems and policies that determine the coverage of weight management services.
- Discuss the payment structures for weight management services and how to demonstrate, to payers and employers, the value of these services.
- Identify barriers to accessing weight management services.
- Propose solutions to improve access to weight management services.

Introduction

In the US health care system, access to weight management services depends as much on the specifics of health insurance plans as it does on the availability of high-quality providers. It is incumbent upon health care providers to understand the nuances of the health care systems and various policies that determine the coverage of weight management services to ensure they are helping their patients access care to the fullest extent possible.

This chapter discusses the overall health coverage landscape for weight management services—particularly, coverage of intensive behavioral therapy and medical nutrition therapy for obesity under Medicare, Medicaid, state employee health plans, and private-payer plans. In some cases, as with Medicare, coverage of services is fairly straightforward and providers can know with relative ease what services will and will not be covered, for which patients, for which diagnoses, by which provider types, and for how many hours or visits at what reimbursement rates along with any copayment or deductible requirements. In other cases, particularly with employer-provided or other types of private coverage, providers have to work harder to determine in advance what services each patient will have access to and the details of that coverage. This chapter also reviews the various federal and state policies that govern coverage decisions by each payer type, the policy levers that can be used to effect change and improve coverage for patients, and several suggested starting points for engaging in this type of advocacy.

This chapter also provides a practical summary of payment structures for weight management services and estimated revenues when providing care to patients with Medicare. Evidence is provided for demonstrating value to payers and providers in fee-for-service environments and value-based payment environments. Actionable tips for explaining the value proposition for weight management services to other medical providers, health systems, and payers are also discussed.

Although coverage is a key requirement for access, many other factors influence patients' ultimate degree of access to high-quality weight management services. Potential barriers to care are outlined at the provider, system, and patient levels, and solutions are offered to address these barriers, with a focus on actionable advice for providers.

Coverage of Weight Management Services

Medicare

Medicare is the federal health insurance program covering more than 60 million adults over the age of 65, as well as individuals with end-stage renal disease and certain individuals with disabilities.[1,2] Medicare consists of several parts: Medicare Part A covers hospital and other institutional expenses; Medicare Part B covers physician and other provider visits; Medicare Part D covers prescription drugs; and Medicare Part C is the Medicare Advantage program, through which individuals enroll in a private health plan that provides coverage that is equal to or better than original Medicare (Parts A and B) coverage.[2]

Medicare covers intensive behavioral therapy (IBT) for obesity under its Part B medical insurance program.[3] The benefit allows for up to 22 visits per year, distributed as follows:

- one visit every week for the first month
- one visit every other week for months 2 through 6
- one visit every month for months 7 through 12

Medicare also requires that patients achieve 3 kg (6.6 lb) of weight loss by month 6 in order to be eligible for coverage of the visits in months 7 through 12. In the absence of sufficient weight loss, providers must cease care and wait at least 6 months to reevaluate the patient's "readiness to change" and restart IBT at that time, if deemed appropriate. Billing for IBT for obesity through Medicare is limited to primary care providers: physicians, physician assistants, nurse practitioners, or clinical nurse specialists working in a primary care setting. The services, however, can be provided by others, including registered dietitian nutritionists (RDNs), and billed "incident to" the primary care provider, as long as the services are rendered in the primary care setting. A discussion of billing and payment for IBT for obesity can be found later in this chapter.

Medicare covers a variety of bariatric surgery procedures through Medicare Parts A and B.[4] This benefit came into effect in 2006 and currently covers five types of surgical procedures.[5] Patients are eligible for bariatric surgery if they have a BMI of 35 or higher, at least one comorbid condition related to obesity, and a history of not succeeding with medical treatment for obesity. This reimbursement is limited to aspects of care directly related to the surgical procedure, and Medicare does not cover any RDN visits for preoperative or postoperative care.

Because of legal restrictions, Medicare Part D does not cover antiobesity medications when they are used to treat obesity in the absence of other comorbid conditions for which they are approved. More will be said about these restrictions elsewhere in the chapter.

Medicaid

Medicaid is a joint state and federal program in which states administer their own Medicaid programs in accordance with certain federal requirements. The program provides coverage to more than 75 million low-income adults, children, and people with disabilities, and costs are shared between state and federal governments.[6]

The federal government does not require state Medicaid programs to cover obesity care services; thus, Medicaid coverage for counseling, medications, and surgery varies widely from state to state. The Strategies to Overcome and Prevent

(STOP) Obesity Alliance at George Washington University maintains the most comprehensive and up-to-date information on coverage of obesity care services among state Medicaid programs.[7] According to the alliance's most recent review (2016–2017), out of 50 states and the District of Columbia[7]:

- 41 cover at least one obesity screening and counseling visit;
- 20 cover at least one visit specifically for nutrition counseling;
- 49 cover at least one type of bariatric surgery procedure; and
- 16 cover US Food and Drug Adminstration (FDA)-approved antiobesity medications.

State Employee Health Plans

State employee health plans are also highly variable across states. The STOP Obesity Alliance tracks coverage provided by these plans and reports that, as of the 2020–2021 plan year, out of 50 states[8]:

- all cover at least one obesity screening and counseling visit;
- 42 cover at least one visit specifically for nutrition counseling;
- 42 cover at least one type of bariatric surgery procedure; and
- 16 cover FDA-approved antiobesity medications.

Private Payers

Data on coverage of weight management services by private payers (ie, commercial insurance companies) are much harder to ascertain due to the sheer volume of payers and plans available in the public market and the myriad plans offered by employers. Though the exact prevalence of coverage is not known, research conducted by the Academy of Nutrition and Dietetics in 2018 found that adult overweight or obesity was the second most common diagnosis for which RDNs received reimbursement from third-party payers (public or private payers), indicating at least modest coverage for weight management services.[9] Overall, private coverage is inconsistent across states and plans; providers need to assess coverage within each plan individually and should not assume that patients are aware of the coverage details of their policies, given how difficult it is for some patients to obtain this information.[10]

Federal and State Policies Governing Change

Medicare

Coverage for IBT for obesity under Medicare originated in 2011, pursuant to the Patient Protection and Affordable Care Act (the Affordable Care Act, for short).[11] That law requires that Medicare cover preventive services that have received a grade A or B from the US Preventive Services Task Force (USPSTF), and coverage must be without cost-sharing and not subject to patients' deductibles. Since 1996, the USPSTF has recommended obesity screening and counseling for patients with a BMI of 30 or higher; the latest iteration of the recommendation was published in 2018.[12] At the time that the original Medicare benefit for IBT for obesity was created, the prevailing USPSTF recommendation for obesity screening and counseling was from 2003. In that older recommendation, USPSTF recommended that clinicians *offer* counseling, language that has since been updated to "offer or refer" in subsequent versions. This detail is potentially important, as it was cited as a reason why the benefit can only be provided by, or "incident to," a primary care provider.[13] Unfortunately, there are no laws or policies in place that require Medicare to update its coverage determinations based on revised USPSTF recommendations, even when those updates include fundamental changes to the underlying recommendations that would reasonably be expected to affect coverage.

The focus on the IBT for obesity benefit rather than the medical nutrition therapy (MNT) benefit is because MNT is not covered by Medicare when the patient is referred for a diagnosis of obesity. The Medicare MNT benefit was created by Congress in 2000 and specified coverage for MNT to treat diabetes or renal disease.[14] The law did not give Medicare the authority to cover MNT for additional diseases or conditions, therefore the service cannot be covered for obesity without a change in legislation.

As previously noted, Medicare is also precluded by law from covering antiobesity medications in its Part D prescription drug program. This policy severely restricts patients' access to these medications, some of which are covered if the patient has diabetes but not if the patient has a diagnosis of obesity without co-occurring diabetes. Due to the greater flexibility afforded to the program, Medicare Advantage plans (ie, Medicare Part C) are allowed to cover antiobesity medications, and some plans have chosen to do so; therefore, knowing the details of a patient's insurance status—even when the patient is over 65 years of age—is important in determining a plan of care.

Medicaid

Although Medicaid programs were originally intended to be state run, more than two-thirds of Medicaid beneficiaries are now enrolled in "managed-care plans" run by private payers that contract with the state Medicaid agency to provide care to enrollees.[15] Rather than offering a single program, states may maintain a series of different Medicaid plans (or managed-care contracts) to accommodate the legal requirements and special health care needs of various beneficiary populations, such as pregnant women, children, individuals with disabilities, low-to-middle-income adults eligible through Medicaid expansion under the Affordable Care Act, and others.

As previously mentioned, coverage of weight management services under Medicaid varies considerably from state to state. Also highly variable are the policies and procedures that govern what each state covers. States typically have some form of shared decision-making arrangement between their legislative branch and their executive branch. This serves as a framework to determine what is covered by their plans or what minimum benefits must be covered under any managed-care contracts, with subsequent discretion given to the managed-care organization to determine the specifics of the benefit.

State Employee Health Plans

As with Medicaid, each state designs its own unique state employee health plan, with differing levels of authority given to the state legislature vs the administration and with differing administrative agencies having involvement. For example, a state legislature could pass a law requiring that certain benefits be included in the state employee health plan, but it is unlikely that this is the primary or preferred method for designing the state's benefit plans. Some states may also have separate plans for their teaching workforce vs other state employees because teachers' unions may independently negotiate salaries and benefits for educators or because of how a state's employee benefit system was originally created.

Private Payers

On paper, many private health insurance plans are legally required to cover behavioral interventions for obesity. Like the Medicare coverage requirement, this requirement stems from the Affordable Care Act, which stipulates that private plans must cover preventive services that have received a grade A or B from the USPSTF.[16] Other than a shrinking number of "grandfathered" plans that have not changed their coverage policies since 2010, any plan sold on a state or federal health insurance exchange and any employer-sponsored plan, including self-insured plans, must cover behavioral interventions for obesity.[17]

Unfortunately, the Affordable Care Act's preventive service requirement has translated poorly into coverage of behavioral interventions for obesity among commercial and employer-sponsored plans. One suspected barrier is that the USPSTF recommendation regarding obesity does not specify what counts as an *intensive*, *multicomponent*, or *behavioral intervention*. Instead, it is left up to the insurance companies to make such determinations, with enforcement authority resting with states' insurance regulators. The federal government could issue guidance for how to translate USPSTF recommendations into coverage and benefit design but has declined to do so.

Policy Levers for Improving Coverage

Medicare

At the federal level, the Treat and Reduce Obesity Act seeks to both improve the Medicare Part B benefit for IBT for obesity and instate coverage in Medicare Part D for antiobesity medications. Supported by a broad coalition of organizations, convened as the Obesity Care Advocacy Network, the act would[18,19]:

- allow RDNs, psychologists, and other qualified providers to independently provide and bill Medicare Part B for IBT for obesity;
- create Medicare Part B coverage for evidence-based, community-based weight management interventions; and
- provide Medicare Part D coverage for FDA-approved antiobesity medications.

The bill has consistently achieved broad, bipartisan cosponsorship in both the US House of Representatives and the US Senate over the last few congressional sessions. It has yet to receive a budgetary analysis score from the Congressional Budget Office or be the subject of a congressional hearing or markup. Providers who are interested in advocating for the passage of the Treat and Reduce Obesity Act should contact their respective professional associations to engage with ongoing advocacy efforts.

There are also regulatory avenues that the Centers for Medicare and Medicaid Services could pursue to improve benefits without passage of new legislation. Reconsideration—or updating—of the rules for determining coverage of IBT for obesity is fully within the purview of the agency. Since 2006, the rules for determination of coverage for bariatric surgery procedures have been reconsidered three times.[4] In contrast, the guidelines governing coverage determination for IBT for obesity have never been reconsidered, despite the USPSTF's having issued two updated recommendations in the decade since the Medicare benefit for IBT for obesity was first created.[3,12]

There is also legislation addressing the lack of coverage within Medicare for MNT when treating obesity. The Medical Nutrition Therapy Act would address this by expanding the existing Medicare MNT benefit to include obesity and a number of other diagnoses.[20,21]

Medicaid

Coverage determinations within state Medicaid plans are far from standardized across the United States. Some states have laws on the books that specifically add individual services for specific diseases. In other states, the executive branch of the government may have more authority in making these decisions. For example, a state legislature could pass a law instructing the state's Medicaid program to cover IBT for beneficiaries with obesity, and then the state Medicaid agency would determine the specific eligibility criteria, referral requirements, benefit design, billable providers, and so on. Or, a state could have less-specific laws already on the books that allow the state's Medicaid agency to use its discretion in determining which benefits are appropriate to cover within the program, in which case the state's benefit-design department would be the target of advocacy.

Understanding the nexus of power within a state's Medicaid program is the first step in devising an advocacy strategy for expanding coverage of weight management services. Advocates should be aware that a successful campaign to expand coverage may ultimately involve working with the legislature, state Medicaid agency, and relevant managed care organizations to ensure full coverage for the continuum of services being sought.

State Employee Health Plans

To address the coverage policies of a state employee health plan, the first step is to understand who the decision makers are. Similar to state Medicaid plans, there may be involvement from the legislature or an executive branch office. In some states, there may be union representation involved as well. The second step is to determine what processes are used to make annual changes to the state employees' health insurance benefit for obesity and how to influence those processes.

Private Payers

Private-payer health plans are regulated at the state level; therefore, advocating for changes in coverage and benefit design is a grassroots effort that may involve the state legislature, the executive branch, individual payers, and individual employers' human resources departments or benefits managers.

Although legislative action can be a slow and resource-intense process, the end result can be the creation of a legal requirement for minimum coverage. These laws, however, do not typically apply to employer-funded plans. In 2021, an estimated 64% of covered workers had an insurance plan that was wholly or partially funded by their employer, limiting the reach of legislation in improving private-payer coverage.[22]

Another avenue for advocating for better obesity-care coverage from a private payer is through employers. As individual health care consumers, health care practitioners can speak to their human resources departments or unions, if applicable, about including coverage for weight management services in their own organization's health plan. This strategy is likely to be most successful with employers that fund their own health plans, because they determine the benefit design and offerings. In the case of smaller employers, which are more likely to buy predesigned plans, the insurance companies they buy from may not have plans for sale that include coverage of weight management services, and a smaller organization may not have the bargaining power to request a modified plan or to persuade an insurance company to modify its standard options.

One can also approach a private payer directly as a health care provider to advocate for new or expanded coverage of weight management services. As noted in the discussion of state employee health plans, advocates need to identify the decision makers and the process used to make changes in benefits. Partnering with other providers in such efforts can be an effective strategy, as a request made by a group that includes multiple provider types often carries more weight with a payer. While this type of advocacy is neither easy nor straightforward, influencing policy at the private-payer level can have a trickle-down effect on all the plans that a payer sells in the individual market or to employers, including the baseline benefits they recommend for large, self-insured employers.

Finally, an often overlooked stakeholder is the benefits consultant. Benefits consultants advise business clients (ie, employers) on what health insurance and benefits packages will help them attract and retain employees. Convincing a benefits consultant of the value of offering a comprehensive weight management benefit can have an impact on numerous employers and individuals in a particular marketplace.

Payment Structures and Demonstrating Value

Many health care providers and stakeholders operate under the belief that using RDNs to provide weight management services is not financially viable. As a result, either services are not offered or money is left on the table that could otherwise contribute to an organization's bottom line. This belief is a misconception, however, as medical and nutrition practices have reported success in leveraging both fee-for-service and value-based payment structures to deliver medically necessary, patient-centered care to individuals with obesity or overweight.[23]

The following information describes opportunities for payment for weight management services and provides examples of business arrangements between medical providers and RDNs that can enhance access to team-based care for persons with obesity or overweight.

Fee-for-Service

For practices that have fee-for-service payment arrangements with payers, it is important to know how to leverage individual benefits and coverage in order to provide patients with care from an RDN and then get paid or reimbursed for that care. Depending on a payer's policies, benefit design, and coverage, RDNs may be able to bill public or private payers directly for individual or group weight management services or render and bill for services "incident to" a physician or other medical provider. Payment may be available for in-person and telehealth services. Under Medicare, when an RDN is integrated into a primary care practice, the practice may be able to capture the time the RDN spends providing MNT as part of monthly billing for care management services under the following Current Procedural Terminology (CPT) codes: for chronic care management, codes 99439 and 99490; for complex chronic care management, codes 99487 and 99489; and for principal care management, codes 99426 and 99427.

Box 19.1 illustrates projected revenues for a 6-month course of weight management services using 2023 national payment rates for MNT CPT codes in the nonfacility setting under the Medicare Physician Fee Schedule. Box 19.2 on page 354 illustrates projected revenues when utilizing RDNs to deliver the Medicare benefit for IBT for obesity in the primary care setting using 2023 national payment rates.[24] Note that other payers often structure their benefits in alignment with Medicare coverage.

Health care providers should ask private payers about payments for the group-MNT codes, telephonic and electronic assessment and follow-up by the RDN, and MNT via telehealth, as all these modalities can be used to improve patients' access to care and maximize efficiency. Practices may consider a hybrid model of in-person and virtual interventions to improve the frequency of intervention, maintain patient engagement, and better comply with clinical guidelines for efficacy of treatment.

BOX 19.1

Estimated Revenues for Registered Dietitian Nutritionist–Provided Medical Nutrition Therapy for Obesity or Overweight[24]

Nutrition intervention	Length of intervention	Current Procedural Terminology codes	Registered dietitian nutritionist billing revenue
Initial assessment	60 min	97802 × 4 units[a]	$125.60
Follow-up at 2, 4, 6, and 8 weeks	30 min	97803 × 2 units × 4	$218.89
Monthly follow-up (months 3–6)	30 min	97803 × 2 units × 4	$218.89
Telephonic follow-up	10 to 30 min	98966 through 98968	Inquire with private payers
Online digital assessment and management	5 to 21 min or more	98970 through 98972	Inquire with private payers
Group medical nutrition therapy (2–10 people)	30 to 60 min	97804 × 1 to 2 units	$14.40 to $28.80
Estimated payments for individual medical nutrition therapy			$563.38 per patient

[a] Medical nutrition therapy Current Procedural Terminology codes are defined as "each [X] minutes" of service and may be billed multiple times for the same service based on the face-to-face time spent with the patient. In contrast, for telephone and online services, different Current Procedural Terminology codes exist that are billed once per date of service based on the number of minutes spent with the patient.

> **BOX 19.2**
>
> **Estimated Revenues for Intensive Behavioral Therapy for Obesity Services for Medicare Beneficiaries**[24]
>
> **Individual sessions**
>
> *Current Procedural Terminology code G0447*
>
> $25.75 per unit (15 min) × 22 sessions
>
> $566.50 per patient per year
>
> Note: Medicare may pay up to 2 units per date of service.
>
> **Group sessions**
>
> *Current Procedural Terminology code G0473*
>
> $12.54 per unit (30 min) per patient × 22 sessions
>
> $275.88 per patient per year

Additional tips for practices with fee-for-service payment arrangements with payers include the following:

- If obesity or overweight is an excluded diagnosis under an individual plan or if coverage is limited, consider submitting a "medical necessity" request.[25]
- Do not let denied claims stop the pursuit of payment. Both providers and payers make mistakes submitting and processing claims. These mistakes are often easy to fix and can lead to payment success.
- Manage the practice's payer mix (the percentage of revenue coming from private insurance companies vs government insurance programs vs patients that pay out-of-pocket) to ensure a healthy bottom line. For example, you can do so by negotiating fees when possible with payers who pay less and targeting a higher number or percentage of patients for your practice from higher-paying payers.

Value-Based Payments

Health care payments are shifting from volume-based (ie, fee-for-service) to value-based payments, in which provider payments are tied to cost and quality targets. There are four main types of value-based payment models, all of which share the same four goals: better outcomes, lower costs, improved patient experiences, and better clinical experiences. This shift away from fee-for-service offers opportunities to structure new, financially viable models for MNT services for obesity and overweight. For example, "per member, per month" payments can be used to fund RDN positions on the weight management team.[26] Bundled payments, shared savings, and quality incentive programs offer other mechanisms for covering nutrition services, as MNT provided by RDNs has been shown to improve clinical outcomes (eg, weight, BMI, waist circumference, hemoglobin A1c, blood glucose, lipids) and lower costs of care.[27,28] Practices and institutions participating in alternative payment models, such as episode or bundled payments for orthopedic procedures,[29] can consider building the cost of presurgical and postsurgical weight loss interventions provided by the RDN into the total cost of care. Pilot programs conducted by the Centers for Medicare and Medicaid Services Innovation Center, such as the Comprehensive Primary Care Initiative Plus (CPC+)[30] and Primary

Care First,[31] represent other opportunities to leverage available payment streams to offset nonbillable provider time (eg, MNT) and support the integration of RDNs into the care team. Other opportunities to tap into innovative payment models are available on a state-by-state basis.[32] Many excellent references are available for readers looking to learn more about value-based payments.[33-38]

Business Arrangements

Medical providers and RDNs should consider several options for collaborative business arrangements to support the delivery of weight management services, as well as other services within the RDN scope of practice[39] that bring value to a practice. Beyond MNT, RDNs can provide the following services based on business needs and on the nutrition-related conditions of the patients served:

- care management for patients with multiple chronic conditions
- collection and reporting of quality-measures data
- management of patient registries
- quality-improvement initiatives
- group cooking classes
- Diabetes Prevention Program oversight and delivery
- annual wellness visits as stipulated and covered by Medicare
- shared medical appointments
- health and well-being coaching

The basic business models for RDNs working in a multidisciplinary medical practice include the following:

- traditional employee (part-time or full-time)
- independent paid contractor
- independent private contractor

Box 19.3 on page 356 describes these models in more detail.[40] The Academy of Nutrition and Dietetics offers several resources to support the integration of RDNs into medical practices and partnerships for the purpose of providing weight management services; these resources include a discussion of factors for RDNs to consider when entering contractual business relationships.[40-44]

The Value Proposition

Although there is strong evidence to support the cost-effectiveness of MNT provided by RDNs for weight management, access to such services will not improve without RDNs' "selling" the message to key stakeholders such as payers, medical providers, and health care administrators. These stakeholders want to know the *value proposition*. A value proposition articulates why a stakeholder should use a service (ie, what's in it for them) and should be formulated with the stakeholder's needs and perspective in mind. This section outlines some key talking points for RDNs to use as leverage in conversations with stakeholders about weight management services. Other talking points and "leave-behinds" for stakeholders are available through the Academy of Nutrition and Dietetics.[45] Data from the Evidence Analysis Library[46] along with data from the RDN's own practice, can be used to support these talking points.

BOX 19.3

Business Models for Registered Dietitian Nutritionists in Multidisciplinary Practices[40]

	Traditional employee	**Independent paid contractor (not private practice)**	**Independent private contractor**
Office space	In primary care physician's (PCP's) office complex	In PCP's office complex Rented at reasonable rate from PCP	Registered dietitian nutritionist (RDN) pays for own office space
Who bills	PCP's office	PCP's office	RDN bills for patients seen (or hires billing service)
Billing methods			
Intensive behavioral therapy (IBT)	"Incident to" PCP	"Incident to" PCP	Cannot provide IBT benefit in RDN office
Medical nutrition therapy (MNT) private payers	"Incident to" as authorized by each insurer: PCP's office needs to check with each private insurer to determine if "incident to" billing is allowed for RDN's services	"Incident to" as authorized by each insurer: PCP's office needs to check with each private insurer to determine if "incident to" billing is allowed for RDN's services	Provides MNT as authorized and contracted with private payers RDN uses own credentialing number and tax ID
MNT Medicare	Service billed under RDN's Medicare provider number. The RDN has reassigned their reimbursement back to their employer-physician (note: this situation is not considered "incident to" billing)	Service billed under RDN's Medicare provider number. The RDN has reassigned their reimbursement back to their employer-physician (note: this situation is not considered "incident to" billing)	Provides MNT for patients with diabetes or chronic kidney disease if RDN is Medicare provider RDN uses own national provider identifier
Compensation	Billing revenue goes to PCP's office RDN paid an hourly rate	Billing revenue goes to PCP's office RDN is paid a negotiated rate per patient seen	Billing and patient out-of-pocket revenue goes to RDN
Taxes	PCP withholds taxes from RDN's paycheck	No withholding from PCP office; RDN pays all taxes as self-employed	RDN pays all taxes as self-employed
Pros	Hours and salary are regular RDN potentially receives benefits (vacation, sick time) No office expense No need for business plan and marketing Do not have to bill	Flexible working schedule No need for business plan and marketing Higher rate of compensation Do not have to bill	Flexible schedule Highest revenue potential

BOX 19.3 (CONTINUED)

	Traditional employee	Independent paid contractor (not private practice)	Independent private contractor
Cons	Set schedule may be too restrictive for some RDNs	No benefits (vacation/sick time)	No benefits (vacation, sick time)
	Hourly rate lower than other models due to benefits and salary stability	Need to negotiate office space costs	Responsible for all business expenses (office space, billing, marketing)
		Reimbursement not as high as private practice	

Adapted with permission from Academy of Nutrition and Dietetics. *Intensive Behavioral Therapy for Obesity: Putting It Into Practice*. 2nd ed. Academy of Nutrition and Dietetics; 2017. Accessed December 15, 2021. www.eatrightstore.org/product-type/toolkits/intensive-behavioral-therapy-for-obesity-putting-it-into-practice[40]

Talking points for conversations with payers: RDNs should remind payers that the National Academy of Medicine (formerly the Institute of Medicine) describes RDNs as "the single, identifiable professional with the standardized education, clinical training, continuing education, and national credentialing requirements necessary to be directly reimbursed as a provider of nutrition therapy."[47] They should also inform payers that studies have shown that MNT provided by RDNs[48-50]:

- improves health outcomes,
- decreases the total cost of care,
- achieves increased satisfaction, and
- provides an increased focus on prevention.

Talking points for conversations with physicians and medical practices: RDNs should remind physicians and practices that RDNs are uniquely qualified to provide counseling for health behavior change and have extensive training in nutrition therapy. They should also inform these stakeholders that studies have shown that MNT provided by RDNs[48,49,51]:

- improves patient health outcomes;
- provides a positive return on investment;
- decreases medication use;
- increases patient satisfaction;
- allows physicians to spend more time focusing on medical care of their patients; and
- supports higher performance in value-based models of care (eg, through improved quality measures and reduced overall total cost of care).

Talking points for conversations with health care administrators: As with payers, RDNs should remind health care administrators that the National Academy of Medicine describes RDNs as "the single, identifiable professional with the standardized education, clinical training, continuing education, and national credentialing requirements necessary to be directly reimbursed as a provider of nutrition therapy."[47] They should also inform administrators that studies have shown that MNT provided by RDNs[48-50]:

- improves patient outcomes,
- decreases hospital admissions and total cost of care,
- improves patient metrics, and
- increases patient satisfaction.

Barriers to Accessing Weight Management Services

Despite the implementation of payment and coverage policies that are designed to provide access to weight management services, optimal access to and utilization of such services has yet to be achieved for many reasons. Although research into the underutilization of MNT services provided by RDNs for patients with obesity or overweight remains scant, research in other areas—namely, access to weight management services in general, access to weight management services specific to the Medicare benefit for IBT for obesity, anecdotal reports, low utilization of diabetes self-management training,[52-54] and low utilization of the Medicare Part B benefit for patients with chronic kidney disease[55,56]—has identified numerous barriers. These barriers can be characterized as either provider barriers, systems barriers, or patient barriers.

Provider Barriers

Both medical providers and RDNs often are unaware of existing coverage by third-party payers for weight management services.[9,55,57] Billing logistics may also create the perception that the services are not covered, especially when providers and billing staff do not know how to bill for MNT services.[9]

Medical providers often lack the skill set needed to support access to weight management services.[58] Many medical schools do not adequately train future physicians in obesity or nutrition issues.[59,60] Therefore, many medical providers are not comfortable discussing overweight or obesity with their patients[61] and are less likely to hold the conversations that must take place before a referral for services can be made. Obesity stigma and weight bias, as noted in Chapter 3, often lead to care discrimination or ineffective treatment.[62]

Insufficient cultural competence, communication barriers, and the inability to ensure shared decision-making have also been identified as provider barriers to the use of preventive services.[64] Even when medical providers recognize the need to make a referral, they may not know how to locate an RDN[64,65] or may need help in framing the message for an effective "handoff" of the patient. Providers' pessimistic views about the ability of patients to make lifestyle changes may also impede referrals for weight management services.[64] Finally, office locations (eg, accessible by public transportation, close to work or home, easy parking) and systems (eg, office hours, use of digital technologies) may not be convenient for the patient.[59]

Systems Barriers

The inconsistent landscape of coverage for MNT and nutrition counseling for weight management services creates several system-level barriers. First, both patients and providers may find it difficult to understand plan benefits and so may not seek out or refer for care.[52] Medical practices, especially those that are not part of a hospital system, often lack the administrative resources or capacity to verify health insurance benefits for each individual patient. Low reimbursement rates may cause providers to not offer weight management services because of concerns about financial viability.[9,55,65] Third-party payers may limit the site of service or what types of providers can bill for weight management services; for example, Medicare stipulates certain limitations in its benefit for IBT for obesity, and some state Medicaid programs only credential RDNs who are employed by hospital outpatient clinics.

Too few medical practices include RDNs on-site.[66,67] This requires patients to visit separate offices to access their nutrition care. For those practices with RDNs on-site, payer policies related to credentialing and billing may not support encounters with both a medical provider and an RDN on the same day; for example, if a payer does not credential RDNs, weight management services have to be billed "incident to" physician services, using evaluation or management CPT codes.

Patient Barriers

Patients themselves may create their own barriers to accessing weight management services. They may consider weight and weight loss a personal responsibility rather than a medical issue.[64] After a referral to an RDN is made, the patient must understand the value of the RDN's expertise and follow through with scheduling an initial visit if the scheduling is not done by the provider's office at the time of the referral. Patients may cancel or not show up for appointments if they operate under a mistaken belief that because they have not been successful in meeting their weight management goals, they should not meet with the RDN. Some patients may be embarrassed by what they perceive to be personal failure rather than recognize the need for additional support. In addition, health literacy and functional limitations may impede patients' utilization of weight management services.[52,68]

Solutions for Overcoming Barriers to Access

Many of these barriers are not insurmountable. Although achieving universal, robust access to MNT for overweight and obesity will require considerable action by policy makers, medical providers and RDNs can take action to increase patients' access to weight management services. Box 19.4 offers some solutions.[40,41,43,44,67,69-82]

BOX 19.4

Solutions for Overcoming Barriers to Accessing Weight Management Services[40,41,43,44,67,69-82]

Provider barriers	Solutions
Lack of knowledge of existing coverage by third-party payers	Medical providers and registered dietitian nutritionists (RDNs) should become familiar with existing coverage via the online resources from the Academy of Nutrition and Dietetics[69,70] and the Strategies to Overcome and Prevent (STOP) Obesity Alliance.[71]

Box continues

BOX 19.4 (CONTINUED)

System barriers	Solutions
Lack of knowledge of coding and billing procedures for weight management services	Medical providers and RDNs can access coding and billing resources from the Academy of Nutrition and Dietetics, including the following: • referrals to a Registered Dietitian Nutritionist Primary Care Referral Toolkit[44] • a guide for RDNs to credentialing and billing in the private payer market[72] • a list of the common ICD-10 CM codes related to nutrition services[73] • a list of the Current Procedural Terminology (CPT) codes frequently used by RDNs[72]
Inadequate provider self-efficacy or skill set	Providers should enhance patient-centered care and shared decision-making around the medical nutrition therapy (MNT) referral (refer to Chapter 5). Medical providers and RDNs can advocate within their professions for the following: • continuing education opportunities in obesity care • improvements in educational standards regarding obesity care
Lack of knowledge of how to find an RDN or make an effective referral	Medical providers can locate RDNs through the Find a Nutrition Expert tool from the Academy of Nutrition and Dietetics.[74] The tool includes listings for RDNs that offer services via telehealth. Other ways for providers to locate RDNs include the following: • checking the online provider directories of health insurance plans • contacting their state affiliate of the Academy of Nutrition and Dietetics • creating collaborative relationships with an RDN in their community[75] Providers can use the Academy of Nutrition and Dietetics toolkit for primary care providers on how to make referrals to RDNs.[44]
Unsuitable office design	Practices should consider taking the following measures to make their offices and services more accessible to patients with overweight or obesity: • Offer MNT via telehealth. Telenutrition services have been successfully utilized for weight management services.[76-78] • Purchase waiting room furniture and exam room tables that accommodate persons of larger body size. • Offer early morning, evening, and weekend office hours to meet the needs of working patients and families. • Offer weight management services via telehealth. • When identifying a new office location, consider accessibility by public transportation and availability of easy and free parking.
Inadequate resources for verifying patient benefits for weight management services	Measures that medical providers and RDNs can take to overcome or reduce this barrier include the following: • Advocate for additional resources based on potential return on investment (ie, potential ability to recoup money being "left on the table"). • Ask patients to verify their benefits. Tools are available to support patients in doing so.[72]

BOX 19.4 (CONTINUED)

System barriers	Solutions
Lack of (or uncertain) financial viability	Measures that medical providers and RDNs can take to overcome or reduce this barrier include the following: • Offer group MNT and intensive behavioral treatment (IBT) sessions or shared medical appointments, or both. Group services have been successfully employed in diabetes care.[79,80] • Find out if their state utilizes community health teams that incorporate RDNs, which can provide shared resources to practices that cannot afford to employ the full team of health care providers necessary to meet the needs of the populations served.[81,82] • Calculate potential revenues (see Payment Structures and Demonstrating Value section). • Leverage value-based payment models (see Payment Structures and Demonstrating Value section). • Advocate for federal legislation, such as the Medical Nutrition Therapy Act and the Treat and Reduce Obesity Act.
Lack of integration of RDNs into medical practices	Medical providers can co-locate an RDN within their medical practice.[67] The Academy of Nutrition and Dietetics offers resources to help implement this solution.[40,41,43]

Summary

Since the passage of the Affordable Care Act, the health care policy landscape at both the federal and state levels has broadened access to weight management services. However, more work needs to be done to achieve consistent, comprehensive coverage to address the obesity epidemic. In addition to advocacy efforts to improve coverage for evidence-based care for persons with obesity or overweight, providers can and should take actions to address other barriers to access within their control. Currently, providers and patients are not maximally utilizing existing coverage and benefits under fee-for-service or value-based payments systems. The value proposition for access to weight management services provided by RDNs is strong and should be leveraged to build a robust, cost-effective system of care.

References

1. Centers for Medicare and Medicaid Services. What's Medicare? Medicare.gov. Accessed December 22, 2021. www.medicare.gov/what-medicare-covers/your-medicare-coverage-choices/whats-medicare
2. An overview of Medicare. Kaiser Family Foundation. February 13, 2019. Accessed December 22, 2021. www.kff.org/medicare/issue-brief/an-overview-of-medicare
3. Intensive behavioral therapy for obesity. National Coverage Determinations (NCD) Manual, section 210.12. Centers for Medicare and Medicaid Services. Effective November 29, 2011. Accessed December 22, 2021. www.cms.gov/medicare-coverage-database/view/ncd.aspx?NCDId=353
4. Bariatric surgery for treatment of co-morbid conditions related to morbid obesity. National Coverage Determinations (NCD) Manual, section 100.1. Centers for Medicare and Medicaid Services. Effective September 24, 2013. Accessed December 22, 2021. www.cms.gov/medicare-coverage-database/view/ncd.aspx?NCDId=57

5. Bariatric surgery for the treatment of morbid obesity. National Coverage Analysis (NCA), CAG-00250R, decision memo. Centers for Medicare and Medicaid Services. February 21, 2006. Accessed December 22, 2021. www.cms.gov/medicare-coverage-database/view/ncacal-decision-memo.aspx?proposed=N&ncaid=160
6. Centers for Medicare and Medicaid Services. Medicaid. Medicaid.gov. Accessed November 23, 2021. www.medicaid.gov/medicaid/index.html
7. Coverage for obesity treatment services: state Medicaid programs, 2016-2017. Strategies to Overcome and Prevent (STOP) Obesity Alliance. Accessed December 22, 2021. https://stop.publichealth.gwu.edu/coverage/medicaid
8. Our updated review of state employee health plan obesity coverage. Strategies to Overcome and Prevent (STOP) Obesity Alliance. July 29, 2022. Accessed March 6, 2023. https://stop.publichealth.gwu.edu/LFD-jul22
9. Jortberg BT, Parrott JS, Schofield M, et. al. Trends in registered dietitian nutritionists' knowledge and patterns of coding, billing, and payment. *J Acad Nutr Diet*. 2020;120(1):134-145. doi:10.1016/j.jand.2019.05.008
10. Fast facts—obesity care coverage. Strategies to Overcome and Prevent (STOP) Obesity Alliance. Accessed December 22, 2021. https://stop.publichealth.gwu.edu/fast-facts/obesity-care-coverage
11. Removal of barriers to preventive services in Medicare. Patient Protection and Affordable Care Act, Pub L No. 111-148, §4104. March 23, 2010.
12. Weight loss to prevent obesity-related morbidity and mortality in adults: behavioral interventions. US Preventive Services Task Force. September 18, 2018. Accessed December 22, 2021. www.uspreventiveservicestaskforce.org/uspstf/recommendation/obesity-in-adults-interventions
13. Intensive behavioral therapy for obesity. National Coverage Analysis (NCA), CAG-00423 N, decision memo. Centers for Medicare and Medicaid Services. November 29, 2011. Accessed December 22, 2021. www.cms.gov/medicare-coverage-database/view/ncacal-decision-memo.aspx?proposed=N&NCAId=253
14. Coverage of medical nutrition therapy services for beneficiaries with diabetes or a renal disease. Consolidated Appropriations Act, 2001, Pub L No. 106-554, §105. December 21, 2000.
15. Medicaid Managed Care Market Tracker. Kaiser Family Foundation. Updated 2021. Accessed December 22, 2021. www.kff.org/data-collection/medicaid-managed-care-market-tracker
16. Coverage of preventive health services. Patient Protection and Affordable Care Act, Pub L No. 111-148, §2713. March 23, 2010.
17. Preventive services covered by private health plans under the Affordable Care Act. Kaiser Family Foundation. Oct. 26, 2022. Accessed March 28, 2023. www.kff.org/health-reform/fact-sheet/preventive-services-covered-by-private-health-plans
18. Treat and Reduce Obesity Act, HR 1577, 117th Cong (2021).
19. Treat and Reduce Obesity Act, S 596, 117th Cong (2021).
20. Medical Nutrition Therapy Act, HR 3108, 117th Cong (2021).
21. Medical Nutrition Therapy Act. S1536, 117th Cong (2021).
22. Kaiser Family Foundation. *Employer Health Benefits: 2021 Annual Survey*. Kaiser Family Foundation; 2021. https://files.kff.org/attachment/Report-Employer-Health-Benefits-2021-Annual-Survey.pdf
23. Amanatullah DF, Ohanisian L, Ivanov D, Schofield M, Beseler L. Pre-operative weight loss—plan for stepwise incorporation of registered dietitian nutritionists into an orthopaedic practice. *Int J Orth*. 2019;2(2):44-48.
24. Physician Fee Schedule Look-Up Tool. Centers for Medicare and Medicaid Services. Accessed March 18, 2022. www.cms.gov/Medicare/Medicare-Fee-for-Service-Payment/PFSlookup
25. Bujnowski M. How can providers get payment for medical nutrition therapy when the diagnosis is not explicitly covered? *J Acad Nutr Diet*. 2018;118(4):788. doi:10.1016/j.jand.2018.02.003
26. Wang QC, Chawla R, Colombo CM, Snyder RL, Nigam S. Patient-centered medical home impact on health plan members with diabetes. *J Public Health Manag Pract*. 2014;20(5):e12-20. doi:10.1097/PHH.0b013e3182a8eb3d
27. Jortberg BT, Fleming MO. Registered dietitian nutritionists bring value to emerging health care delivery models. *J Acad Nutr Diet*. 2014;114(12):2017-2022. doi:10.1016/j.jand.2014.08.025
28. Academy of Nutrition and Dietetics. MNT: cost effectiveness, cost-benefit, or economic savings of MNT (2009): What is the evidence to support the cost-effectiveness, cost benefit or economic savings of outpatient MNT services provided by an RDN? Evidence Analysis Library. Accessed December 22, 2021. www.andeal.org/topic.cfm?menu=4085&cat=4085
29. Bundled Payments for Care Improvement Advanced Model. Centers for Medicare and Medicaid Services. Accessed December 15, 2021. https://innovation.cms.gov/innovation-models/bpci-advanced
30. Comprehensive Primary Care Plus. Centers for Medicare and Medicaid Services. Accessed December 15, 2021. https://innovation.cms.gov/initiatives/comprehensive-primary-care-plus
31. Primary Care First Model Options. Centers for Medicare and Medicaid Services. Accessed December 15, 2021. https://innovation.cms.gov/innovation-models/primary-care-first-model-options
32. Where innovation is happening. Centers for Medicare and Medicaid. Accessed December 15, 2021. https://innovation.cms.gov/innovation-models/map
33. Academy of Nutrition and Dietetics. Different payment models. eatrightPro.org. Accessed March 29, 2023. www.eatrightpro.org/career/payment/how-rdns-are-paid-for-services/different-payment-models

34. Kaiser Family Foundation. Medicaid delivery system and payment reform: a guide to key terms and concepts. KFF.org. Accessed March 29, 2023. www.kff.org/medicaid/fact-sheet/medicaid-delivery-system-and-payment-reform-a-guide-to-key-terms-and-concepts
35. Rajkumar R, Conway PH, Tavenner M. CMS—engaging multiple payers in payment reform. *JAMA*. 2014;311(19):1967–1968. doi:10.1001/jama.2014.3703
36. Bethke M, Guest D, Lowry A, Bailey R, Fleisher D and Weger J. Value based health care models in shifting economy. Deloitte Consulting LLP. December 2020. Accessed March 29, 2023. www2.deloitte.com/us/en/pages/life-sciences-and-health-care/articles/value-based-care-payment-models.html
37. Plante J. What is value-based payment, and what does it mean for healthcare? christenseninstitute.org. Accessed March 29, 2023. www.christenseninstitute.org/blog/what-is-value-based-payment-and-what-does-it-mean-for-healthcare
38. APM Framework. Health Care Payment Learning & Action Network. hcp-lan.org. Accessed March 29 2023. https://hcp-lan.org/apm-framework
39. Academy Quality Management Committee. Academy of Nutrition and Dietetics: Revised 2017 Scope of Practice for the Registered Dietitian Nutritionist. *J Acad Nutr Diet*. 2018;118(1):141-165. doi:10.1016/j.jand.2017.10.002
40. Academy of Nutrition and Dietetics. *Intensive Behavioral Therapy for Obesity: Putting It into Practice*. 2nd ed. Academy of Nutrition and Dietetics; 2017. Accessed December 15, 2021. www.eatrightpro.org/career/payment/medical-nutrition-t/www.eatrightpro.org/-/media/files/eatrightpro/career/payment/ibt-for-obesity-putting-it-into-practice-rev-nov-201739.pdfherapy/additional-mnt-resources
41. Academy of Nutrition and Dietetics. RDNs in the new primary care: a toolkit for successful integration. eatrightPRO.website. 2016. Accessed March 6, 2023. www.eatrightpro.org/career/career-resources/rdns-in-the-new-primary-care-toolkit
42. Academy of Nutrition and Dietetics. Additional MNT resources. eatrightPRO website. Accessed April 3, 2023. www.eatrightpro.org/career/payment/medical-nutrition-therapy/additional-mnt-resources
43. Academy of Nutrition and Dietetics. Sample RDN/MD business agreement. eatrightSTORE website. 2019. Accessed December 15, 2021. www.eatrightstore.org/product-subject/mnt-references/sample-rdmd-business-agreement
44. Academy of Nutrition and Dietetics. Referrals to an RDN primary care referral toolkit. eatrightPRO website. 2020. Accessed April 3, 2023. www.eatrightpro.org/referrals-to-an-rdn-primary-care-provider-toolkit
45. Academy of Nutrition and Dietetics. Additional MNT resources: audience-specific marketing flyers. eatrightPRO website. Accessed December 15, 2021. www.eatrightpro.org/career/payment/medical-nutrition-therapy/additional-mnt-resources
46. Academy of Nutrition and Dietetics. Evidence Analysis Library. Medical nutrition therapy effectiveness (MNT) systematic review (2013-2015). Accessed April 3, 2023. www.andeal.org/topic.cfm?menu=5284&cat=3808
47. Institute of Medicine (US) Committee on Nutrition Services for Medicare Beneficiaries. *The Role of Nutrition in Maintaining Health in the Nation's Elderly: Evaluating Coverage of Nutrition Services for the Medicare Population*. National Academies Press; 2000.
48. Academy of Nutrition and Dietetics Evidence Analysis Library. Medical nutrition therapy (MNT) systematic review (2009). Evidence Analysis Library website. Accessed December 16, 2021. www.andeal.org/topic.cfm?menu=5284&cat=4171
49. Academy of Nutrition and Dietetics Evidence Analysis Library. MNT: weight management (2015). Evidence Analysis Library website. Accessed December 16, 2021. www.andeal.org/topic.cfm?menu=5284&cat=5230
50. van Baal PH, van den Berg M, Hoogenveen RT, Vijgen SM, Engelfriet PM. Cost-effectiveness of a low-calorie diet and orlistat for obese persons: modeling long-term health gains through prevention of obesity-related chronic diseases. *Value Health*. 2008;11(7):1033-1040. doi:10.1111/j.1524-4733.2008.00328.x
51. Wolf AM, Crowther JQ, Nadler JL, Bovbjerg VE. The return on investment of a lifestyle intervention: the ICAN Program. Accepted for presentation at the American Diabetes Association 69th Scientific Sessions (169-OR), June 7, 2009, New Orleans, LA.
52. Strawbridge LM, Lloyd JT, Meadow A, Riley GF, Howell BL. Use of Medicare's diabetes self-management training benefit. *Health Educ Behav*. 2015;42(4):530-538. doi:10.1177/1090198114566271
53. Powers MA, Bardsley J, Cypress M, et al. Diabetes Self-management Education and Support in Type 2 Diabetes: A Joint Position Statement of the American Diabetes Association, the American Association of Diabetes Educators, and the Academy of Nutrition and Dietetics. *Clin Diabetes*. 2016;34(2):70-80. doi:10.2337/diaclin.34.2.70
54. Vorderstrasse A, Shaw RJ, Blascovich J, Johnson CM. A theoretical framework for a virtual diabetes self-management community intervention. *West J Nurs Res*. 2014;36(9):1222-1237. doi:10.1177/0193945913518993
55. Jimenez EY, Kelley K, Schofield M, et al. Medical nutrition therapy access in CKD: a cross-sectional survey of patients and providers. *Kidney Med*. 2021;3(1):31-41. doi:10.1016/j.xkme.2020.09.005
56. Kramer H, Yakes Jimenez E, Brommage D, et al. Medical nutrition therapy for patients with non-dialysis-dependent chronic kidney disease: barriers and solutions. *J Acad Nutr Diet*. 2018;118(10):1958-1965. doi:10.1016/j.jand.2018.05.023
57. Mastrocola MR, Roque SS, Benning LV, Stanford FC. Obesity education in medical schools, residencies, and fellowships throughout the world: a systematic review. *Int J Obes (Lond)*. 2020;44(2):269-279. doi:10.1038/s41366-019-0453-6

58. Jacobs M, Harris J, Craven K, Sastre L. Sharing the "weight" of obesity management in primary care: integration of registered dietitian nutritionists to provide intensive behavioural therapy for obesity for Medicare patients. *Fam Pract.* 2021;38(1):18-24. doi:10.1093/fampra/cmaa006
59. Kris-Etherton PM, Akabas SR, Douglas P, et al. Nutrition competencies in health professionals' education and training: a new paradigm. *Adv Nutr.* 2015;6(1):83-87. doi:10.3945/an.114.006734
60. Butsch WS, Kushner RF, Alford S, Smolarz BG. Low priority of obesity education leads to lack of medical students' preparedness to effectively treat patients with obesity: results from the U.S. medical school obesity education curriculum benchmark study. *BMC Med Educ.* 2020;20(1):23. doi:10.1186/s12909-020-1925-z
61. National Academies of Sciences, Engineering, and Medicine; Health and Medicine Division; Food and Nutrition Board; Roundtable on Obesity Solutions. *The Challenge of Treating Obesity and Overweight: Proceedings of a Workshop.* National Academies Press; 2017. doi:10.17226/24855
62. Phelan S, Burgess D, Yeazel M, Hellerstedt W, Griffin J, van Ryn M. Impact of weight bias and stigma on quality of care and outcomes for patients with obesity. *Obes Rev.* 2015;16(4):319-326. doi:10.1111/obr.12266
63. Steeves JA, Liu B, Willis G, Lee R, Smith AW. Physicians' personal beliefs about weight-related care and their associations with care delivery: the U.S. National Survey of Energy Balance Related Care among Primary Care Physicians. *Obes Res Clin Pract.* 2015;9(3):243-255. doi:10.1016/j.orcp.2014.08.002
64. Kaplan LM, Golden A, Jinnett K, et al. Perceptions of barriers to effective obesity care: results from the national ACTION study. *Obesity.* 2018;26(1):61-69. doi:10.1002/oby.22054
65. Petrin C, Kahan S, Turner M, Gallagher C, Dietz WH. Current practices of obesity pharmacotherapy, bariatric surgery referral and coding for counselling by healthcare professionals. *Obes Sci Pract.* 2016;2(3):266-271. doi:10.1002/osp4.53
66. Sastre LR, Van Horn LT. Family medicine physicians report strong support, barriers and preferences for registered dietitian nutritionist care in the primary care setting. *Fam Pract.* 2021;38(1):25-31. doi:10.1093/fampra/cmaa099
67. Silberberg M, Carter-Edwards L, Mayhew M, et al. Integrating registered dietitian nutritionists into primary care practices to work with children with overweight. *Am J Lifestyle Med.* 2017;14(2):194-203. doi: 10.1177/1559827617726950
68. Green CA, Johnson KM, Yarborough BJ. Seeking, delaying, and avoiding routine health care services: patient perspectives. *Am J Health Promot.* 2014;28(5):286-293. doi:10.4278/ajhp.120702-QUAL-318
69. Academy of Nutrition and Dietetics. Medical nutrition therapy. eatrightPRO website. Accessed April 3, 2023. www.eatrightpro.org/career/payment/medical-nutrition-therapy
70. Academy of Nutrition and Dietetics. Private insurance. eatrightPRO website. Accessed April 3, 2023. www.eatrightpro.org/career/payment/private-insurance
71. Obesity treatment coverage. Strategies to Overcome and Prevent (STOP) Obesity Alliance. Accessed December 10, 2021. https://stop.publichealth.gwu.edu/coverage
72. Academy of Nutrition and Dietetics. RDNs complete guide to credentialing and billing. eatrightPRO website. 2021. Accessed April 3, 2023. www.eatrightpro.org/career/payment/coding-and-billing/rdns-complete-guide-credentialing-billing
73. Academy of Nutrition and Dietetics. ICD Codes. eatrightPRO website. 2021. Accessed April 3, 2023. www.eatrightpro.org/career/payment/coding-and-billing/icd-codes
74. Academy of Nutrition and Dietetics. Find a nutrition expert. eatRIGHT website. Accessed December 10, 2021. www.eatright.org/find-a-nutrition-expert
75. Liebhart J, Cook SR, Schofield M, Peterson LE, Radecki L. The Childhood Obesity Performance Improvement (COPI) Collaborative: a pilot to improve practice systems for children with overweight or obesity through enhanced care coordination, evidence-based practice, and use of the healthier generation benefit. *Pediatrics.* 2006;137(suppl 3). doi:10.1542/peds.137.Supplement_3.147A
76. Rollo ME, Hutchesson MJ, Burrows TL, et al. Video consultations and virtual nutrition care for weight management. *J Acad Nutr Diet.* 2015;115(8):1213-1225. doi:10.1016/j.jand.2015.03.016
77. Castelnuovo G, Manzoni GM, Cuzziol P, et al. TECNOB Study: Ad interim results of a randomized controlled trial of a multidisciplinary telecare intervention for obese patients with type-2 diabetes. *Clin Pract Epidemiol Ment Health.* 2011;7:44-50. Published 2011 Mar 4. doi:10.2174/1745017901107010044
78. Ahrendt AD, Kattelmann KK, Rector TS, Maddox DA. The effectiveness of telemedicine for weight management in the MOVE! Program. *J Rural Health.* 2014;30(1):113-119. doi:10.1111/jrh.12049
79. Hwee J, Cauch-Dudek K, Victor JC, et al. Diabetes education through group classes leads to better care and outcomes than individual counselling in adults: a population-based cohort study. *Can J Public Health.* 2014;105(3):e192-e197. doi:10.17269/cjph.105.4309
80. Lorig K, Ritter PL, Turner RM, et al. Benefits of diabetes self-management for health plan members: a 6-month translation study. *J Med Internet Res.* 2016;18(6):e164. doi:10.2196/jmir.5568
81. Bielaszka-DuVernay C. Vermont's blueprint for medical homes, community health teams, and better health at lower cost. *Health Aff (Millwood).* 2011;30(3):383-386. doi:10.1377/hlthaff.2011.0169
82. Dubard A. *Savings Impact of Community Care of North Carolina: A Review of the Evidence.* CCNC Data Brief no. 11. Community Care North Carolina; 2017.

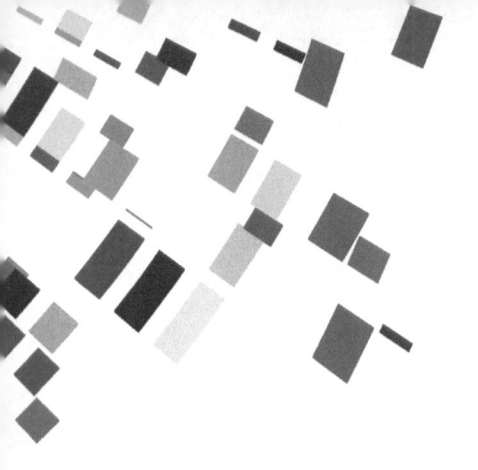

Continuing Professional Education

This edition of *Health Professional's Guide to Treatment of Overweight and Obesity* offers readers 11.75 hours of Continuing Professional Education (CPE) credit. Please check the expiration date at the link below. Readers may earn credit by completing the interactive online quiz at:

https://publications.webauthor.com/hpg_overweight_obesity

Index

Letters *b*, *f*, and *t* after page number indicate box, figure, and table, respectively.

A

abdominal examination, 89, 110*b*
abdominal fat, 82
    health problems associated with, 22, 82
    and lipid levels, 20, 202
    in menopause, 19
    in stress, 146
    waist circumference in, 86
ability, in change talk, 234, 234*b*
Academy of Nutrition and Dietetics
    on business models for RDNs, 357
    Care Manual of, 109
    Commission on Dietetic Registration as credentialing agency for, 32, 340
    continuing education programs of, 341
    on cultural foods, 109
    Evidence Analysis Library of, 63, 357
    on physical activity, 196*b*, 208, 210*b*, 212
    on private payer health plans, 348
    race and ethnicity of members, 32, 37
    on referrals to RDNs, 360*b*
    standards of, 336–337
acanthosis nigricans, 87, 87*f*, 110*b*
accelerometers in activity measurement, 123, 131
acceptance and commitment therapy, 225–231
    in binge eating disorder, 231, 301
    population considerations in, 230–231, 245
    treatment format and structure in, 229, 246
acceptance-based behavioral therapy, 226, 227–231
    integration with other approaches, 244–245
    practitioner skills and training on, 244
    treatment format and structure in, 229, 246
access to health care, barriers to. *See* barriers in access to health care
acne, in polycystic ovary syndrome, 87
ActiGraph device, 121*t*, 124
Action for Health in Diabetes Look AHEAD study, 166, 175–179, 222
active embodiment, 238, 240
Active Living Research, 130
Active People, Healthy Nation initiative, 210*b*
Activities Completed Over Time in 24 Hours, 119
activity space assessment, 128–132
activPAL wearable device, 121*t*, 124

addiction, food, 149, 154, 157*t*
additive model on physical activity and energy expenditure, 199–200, 201*f*
adherence with therapy, 190
    in bariatric surgery, 34, 265
    in cognitive-behavioral therapy, 224
    cultural factors affecting, 108
    in Diabetes Prevention Program, 170
    in drug therapy, 258
    food diaries increasing, 104
    in Look AHEAD, 176
    in physical activity strategies, 204
    in portion-controlled diets, 184
    racial and ethnic bias on, 34
    satisfaction with diet affecting, 110
    in shared decision-making, 70
    stress affecting, 224
    unrealistic expectations affecting, 100
    weight bias and stigma affecting, 50
adipose tissue. *See* fat, body
administrative staff in interprofessional team, 338
adolescence
    behavioral health assessment in, 159
    body mass index and obesity in, 18
    peer victimization in, 46
    prevalence of obesity in, 16, 18
    self-directed dieting and binge eating in, 293
    weight stigma and bias in, 46
adrenal insufficiency, 88
Adult Weight Management Evidence-Based Nutrition Practice, 63–64
advocacy, in Health at Every Size, 241, 243
aerobic exercise, 83
    and appetite, 198
    blood pressure reduction in, 202
    guidelines on, 196*b*, 197*b*, 204
    history-taking on, 83
    and lipid levels, 202
    minimum amount recommended, 206
    prescription of, 206, 207*b*
    and resistance training, 205, 207*b*
    in weight gain prevention, 204, 207*b*
    in weight loss, 205, 206, 207*b*
    in weight maintenance, 207*b*
affirmations, in motivational interviewing, 232, 233*b*
Affordable Care Act, 348, 349, 350, 361
Agency for Healthcare Research and Quality, 70
age-related changes. *See* life span changes
agouti-related peptide, 10, 11*f*

AHA/ACC/TOS guidelines. *See* American Heart Association/American College of Cardiology/The Obesity Society (AHA/ACC/TOS) guidelines
air-displacement plethysmography, 90
Alaska Native individuals
    antiobesity medications in, 31
    in Diabetes Prevention Program, 167
    as health care providers and researchers, 32
    prevalence of obesity in, 26
    racism experienced by, 28
    socioeconomic status and food insecurity of, 28–29
Albright hereditary osteodystrophy, 84
alcohol use
    assessment of, 106*b*
        history-taking in, 85
        questionnaires in, 152, 158*t*
    and bariatric surgery, 266, 266*b*
    motivational interviewing on, 231, 236
Alcohol Use Disorder Identification Test, 152, 158*t*
allergies to foods, 106*b*, 110
allostatic load in weight bias and stigma, 49
American Association of Clinical Endocrinologists, 264
American Board of Obesity Medicine
    certification from, 32, 37, 339*b*, 340
    evidence-based guidelines of, 37
    race and ethnicity of members, 32
American College of Cardiology guidelines. *See* American Heart Association/American College of Cardiology/The Obesity Society (AHA/ACC/TOS) guidelines
American College of Endocrinology, 264
American College of Sports Medicine, 118, 212
    certification of exercise specialists, 337
    on physical activity, 197*b*, 208, 210*b*
American College of Surgeons Metabolic and Bariatric Surgery Accreditation and Quality Improvement Program, 338, 340, 341
American Diabetes Association, 64*b*, 65
American Heart Association, on ultraprocessed foods, 108
American Heart Association/American College of Cardiology/The Obesity Society (AHA/ACC/TOS) guidelines, 64*b*
    on body mass index, 254
    on chronic disease management, 279, 281*f*
    on duration of interventions, 275
    on energy deficit for weight loss, 183, 297
    on high-protein diets, 185
    on lifestyle interventions, 166–167
    on low-carbohydrate diets, 185
    on low-fat diets, 184
    on Mediterranean-style diet, 186, 187
    on mode of care delivery, 278
    on physical activity, 196*b*
    on prevention of weight regain, 277
    on vegetarian-style diets, 186, 187
American Indians
    access to health care resources, 31
    antiobesity medications in, 31
    in culturally sensitive lifestyle interventions, 33
    health care provider bias on, 33
    as health care providers and researchers, 32
    prevalence of obesity in, 26
    racism experienced by, 28
    socioeconomic status and food insecurity of, 28–29

American Medical Association, on obesity as disease, 80, 253, 270
American Society for Metabolic and Bariatric Surgery (ASMBS), 92, 261
    Centers of Excellence designation from, 264
    continuing education programs of, 341
    fellowship and credential from, 339*b*, 340
American Society of Anesthesiologists, 264
amylin, 15*f*
anabolic pathway, 9–10, 10*f*, 11*f*
Analysis Grid for Environments Linked to Obesity, 135
anemia, 88
animal studies
    on menopause, 19
    on ultraprocessed foods, 273
    on weight regulation, 3–6, 4*f*–6*f*, 273
anorexia nervosa, 286
    age of onset, 287
    atypical, 287
    brain regions in, 12
    diagnostic criteria on, 287*b*
    questionnaires in assessment of, 149
    risk factors for, 288
anthropometric measurements, 85–86, 89
    in bariatric surgery, 92
    in transgender patients, 91*b*
antidepressant drugs, weight gain associated with, 84, 146, 212, 259*b*
antidiabetes medications, 258
    dual benefits of, 260
    weight gain associated with, 84, 212, 259, 259*b*
antiepileptic drugs, weight gain associated with, 259, 260*b*
antiobesity drugs. *See* drug therapy, in weight management
antipsychotic drugs, weight gain associated with, 84, 146, 212, 260*b*
antiretroviral drugs, 84, 87
anxiety
    assessment of, 145, 148, 150, 156*t*, 158*t*
    and binge eating, 83
    and binge eating disorder, 291
    interpersonal psychotherapy in, 301
    physical activity in, 203–204
    sleep affecting, 152
    in weight bias and stigma, 48
apnea in sleep, obstructive. *See* obstructive sleep apnea
Apnea Risk Evaluation System, 152, 159*t*
appetite, 9, 11–12
    drugs affecting, 257
    genetic influences on, 13
    physical activity affecting, 198–199
    questionnaires in assessment of, 149
    sleep affecting, 152
    ultraprocessed foods affecting, 108
    weight loss affecting, 14, 16, 272, 276
applied behavior analysis, 226
apps for cell phones, 318, 322–323, 324
    cost of, 325
    evidence on, 325
    patient access to and interest in, 325–326
Archimedes principle in hydrostatic weighing, 89
arcuate nucleus, 10, 11*f*
armband devices in physical activity monitoring, 320–321
arthritis, 20, 21*f*

activity limitations in, 209
bariatric surgery in, 91
physical examination in, 88
Asians
    body mass index in, 3t, 86
    in Diabetes Prevention Program, 167, 170, 171f
    disordered eating behaviors in, 35
    as health care providers and researchers, 32
ASMBS. *See* American Society for Metabolic and Bariatric Surgery
assessment
    behavioral health, 145–160. *See also* behavioral health assessment
    of diet, 98–112. *See also* diet, assessment of
    of eating disorder risk, 304–307
    history of patient in, 81–85. *See also* history of patient
    in holistic approach, 81, 98, 109–110, 152
        factors considered in, 111b–112b
    interprofessional team in, 81, 335
    medical, 80–92. *See also* medical issues, assessment of
    of physical activity, 116–139. *See also* physical activity, assessment of
    of social determinants of health, 34–35, 37, 84–85
    in transgender patients, 82, 90, 91b
atherosclerosis, 202
Atkins diet, 185
attuned eating, 239–240
audit-based tools in activity space assessment, 129, 130, 132
Automated Self-Administered 24-Hour Dietary Assessment Tool, 102b, 104
autonomy of patients, 35, 51, 231

B

Banting, William, 80
Bardet-Biedl syndrome, 84
bariatric surgery, 31, 260–267
    accreditation in, 338, 340, 341
    in binge eating disorder, 299, 300b, 302–303, 308b
    body mass index in, 90, 254, 254t, 260, 347
    Centers of Excellence in, 264
    contraindications to, 264
    counseling in, 336, 337
    health insurance coverage for, 347, 348, 350
    interprofessional team approach in, 264, 336, 337, 338
        expertise in, 340
        and interdisciplinary review, 343
    life expectancy in, 274–275
    peer support in, 338
    perioperative care in, 264–265
    and physical activity, 212, 267b
    postoperative care in, 212, 265, 337
        and adherence to therapy, 34, 265
        recommendations on, 266b
    preoperative assessment in, 264, 264b, 303
        dietary, 92, 110b, 264, 264b
        medical and physical, 90–92
        psychosocial, 92
    race and ethnicity in, 31–32
        and bias of health care providers, 34
        and research inequities, 32
    referrals for, 34, 260–261
    revision procedures in, 267
    shared medical appointments in, 342
    side effects of, 267
    types of procedures in, 31, 261, 262t–263t
    weight loss in, 262t–263t, 265
        average, 262t–263t, 266
        in binge eating disorder, 302, 303
        in interprofessional team approach, 336, 337, 338
        and nutrition counseling, 336
        and peer support, 338
        and physical activity, 212
        in shared medical appointments, 342
    weight regain in, 260, 266–267, 266b
barriers in access to health care, 346–347, 358–362
    insurance coverage in, 31, 346
    patient-related, 361
    provider-related, 358–359, 359b
    systemic, 30–34, 359–360, 360b–361b
    weight bias and stigma in, 33–34, 291–292, 359
Barriers to Being Active quiz, 135
basal metabolic rate, 7f, 7–8, 199
    and energy requirements, 98, 99
    in lean body mass, 8, 13, 98, 101, 102
    in weight loss, 13, 14, 98, 101
Beck Anxiety Inventory, 148, 156t
Beck Depression Inventory-II (BDI-II), 147, 148, 156t
behavioral change. *See* change
behavioral health assessment, 145–160
    anxiety in, 145, 148, 156t
    depression in, 145–146
    eating behaviors in, 145–146, 148–150, 155, 156t–157t
    food insecurity in, 155, 159, 159t
    health literacy in, 155, 158t
    interprofessional team specialists in, 337
    mood in, 145, 147–148, 156t
    motivation and readiness to change in, 153–154, 158t
    physical activity in, 153, 155
    psychological factors in, 146–151, 147b
    quality of life in, 151, 158t
    sleep in, 146, 152–153, 159t
    sociocultural factors in, 155, 159
    strategies in, 154–155, 159
    stress in, 146, 150, 158t
    substance use in, 152, 158t
    suicidality in, 156t
    trauma history in, 150, 158t
    weight history in, 148–150
    weight stigma in, 150–151, 158t
behavioral health specialists, 337
Behavioral Risk Factor Surveillance System, 16
behavioral therapy, 230
    acceptance-based, 226, 227–231, 244–245, 246
    cognitive-behavioral therapy. *See* cognitive-behavioral therapy
    intensive. *See* intensive behavioral therapy
behavioral weight loss interventions, 295–296, 304
    in binge eating disorder, 295, 299, 302, 304
        and drug therapy, 303
        efficacy of, 300b, 302
    technology use in, 320–321, 323

behavior analysis, applied, in acceptance and commitment therapy, 226
beige fat, 13
Bem, Daryl, 232
biases, 30
    on race and ethnicity, 33–34
    selective daily mobility bias, 131–132
    social desirability bias, 102b, 119, 120t, 130
    on weight, 33–34, 44–53. *See also* weight bias and stigma
The Biggest Loser (television show), 272
biliopancreatic diversion with duodenal switch, 261, 263t
binge eating, 243, 288, 296–297
    assessment of, 305
        questionnaires in, 149, 154, 156t, 157t, 304
        social history in, 85
        weight history in, 83, 148
    attuned eating in, 239
    behavioral weight loss therapy in, 295
    definition of, 288
    drug therapy in, 260
    in food insecurity, 155
    in internalization of weight stigma, 48
    intuitive eating in, 238
    low-calorie diet in, 296
    meditation in, 240
    mindful-eating in, 240
    in self-directed dieting, 292–293
    in sleep disturbances, 152
    unconditional permission to eat in, 240
    weight gain in, 289
binge eating disorder, 287–288, 299–303
    acceptance and commitment therapy in, 231, 301
    age of onset, 287
    bariatric surgery in, 299, 300b, 302–303, 308b
    behavioral weight loss therapy in, 295, 299, 302, 304
        and drug therapy, 303
        efficacy of, 300b
    cognitive-behavioral therapy in, 296, 299–301, 302, 303
        efficacy of, 299, 300b, 301
    co-occurrence with overweight or obesity, 288, 289, 290
    diagnostic criteria on, 149, 287b
    drug therapy in, 299, 300b, 303
    interpersonal psychotherapy in, 299, 300b, 301, 302, 304
    low-calorie diet in, 296
    mindful eating in, 237
    psychosocial and medical comorbidities in, 291
    questionnaires in assessment of, 149, 154, 304
    risk factors for, 288, 290, 293
    self-monitoring in, 298
    in trauma history, 150
    weight management in, 300b, 302–303, 308b
Binge Eating Scale, 149, 157t
bioimpedance methods in fat measurement, 90
Biological, Environmental, Social/Psychological, and Timing model, 154
biomarkers in diet assessment, 103b, 104–105
Blackburn Course in Obesity Medicine, 341
Blacks
    in acceptance-based behavioral therapy, 230, 245
    antiobesity medications in, 31
    bariatric surgery in, 31, 32, 34
    body mass index in, 5f
    in cognitive-behavioral therapy, 245
    in culturally sensitive interventions, 33, 245
    in Diabetes Prevention Program, 167, 170, 171f
    disordered eating behaviors in, 35
    food insecurity of, 28–29
    health care provider bias on, 33, 34
    as health care providers and researchers, 32
    in Look AHEAD, 179
    prevalence of obesity in, 16, 17f, 26, 31, 245
        built environment as factor in, 30
        and socioeconomic status, 28–29, 30
    racism experienced by, 28
    systemic barriers affecting, 31–32, 33
blame, in weight bias and stigma, 44, 49
blood pressure, 86–87, 254–255
    in Chronic Care Model, 279
    in Health at Every Size, 242
    in hypertension. *See* hypertension
    in Look AHEAD, 176, 177, 178t, 179
    in metabolic syndrome, 89, 112b
    physical activity reducing, 200–202
BMI. *See* body mass index
body composition profile, 89–90, 200
body dissatisfaction, 27, 48
    cognitive restructuring in, 224
    eating disorders in, 288, 289, 290, 293, 298
    in internalization of thin ideal, 288
    promotion of positive body esteem in, 241
    sociocultural factors affecting, 27
body mass, lean. *See* lean body mass
body mass index (BMI)
    in acceptance-based behavioral therapy, 230
    in bariatric surgery, 90, 254, 254t, 260, 347
    in childhood, 18
    in Chronic Care Model, 279
    in cognitive-behavioral therapy, 225
    in definition of obesity, 2–3, 3t, 18, 80
    in Diabetes Prevention Program, 167
    in eating disorders, 307
    in emerging adulthood, 18
    in emotional eating, 146
    and ethnicity, 3, 3f, 5f
    genetic influences on, 13
    and health insurance coverage, 45, 51, 347, 348
    ideal range in, 20, 265, 307
    in intensive behavioral interventions, 166
    in Look AHEAD, 175
    and medical complications, 3t, 20, 86, 254
        mortality risk in, 20, 21f, 85, 86f
        type 2 diabetes in, 20, 22f, 167
    in physical examination, 85–86, 112b
    in selection of treatment options, 253–254, 254t
    sleep affecting, 146
    trajectory of. *See* weight history
    in transgender patients, 91b
body weight. *See* weight
Body Weight Planner, 100–102, 101f, 182, 183b
bone density measurement, 89, 110b
brain
    in appetite regulation, 9, 272

in energy balance, 9
    in response to food-related stimuli, 12, 146
        in mindful eating, 237
        weight loss affecting, 14–16, 272
    in set point theory on body fat, 271
breast cancer, 21f, 22
buffers in geographic information system-based assessment, 131
built environment
    food access and availability in, 27, 30, 35, 107–108
    physical activity in, 29, 30, 35, 128–132, 134–135
        walkability affecting, 30, 129, 130, 277, 278
    as social determinant of health, 27, 30, 34–35
bulimia nervosa, 287
    age of onset, 287
    co-occurrence with overweight or obesity, 288, 289
    diagnostic criteria on, 149, 287b
    questionnaires in assessment of, 149
    risk factors for, 288, 293, 301
bullying behaviors, weight-based, 46, 47
    cyberbullying in, 45
    laws and policies on, 45
    mental health outcomes in, 48
bupropion
    and naltrexone, 31, 256t, 257
    off-label use of, 261b

C

calorimetry, indirect, 99, 118–119, 121t, 127f
    in planning dietary interventions, 100
    wearable devices used with, 124
cancer
    as complication of obesity, 20, 21f, 22, 81, 82, 91
    Diabetes Prevention Program Outcomes Study on, 172–173
    history-taking on, 111b
    physical activity affecting risk for, 200, 203
    screening for, 50, 92, 264b
    shared decision-making in, 70
    and social determinants of health, 27
    survivor groups in, 343
carbohydrates
    in hyperpalatable foods, 273, 274b
    in ketogenic diets, 185
    in low-carbohydrate diets, 185
cardiometabolic benefits of physical activity, 200–203
cardiorespiratory fitness, 203, 209
cardiovascular disorders, 20–22
    Diabetes Prevention Program Outcomes Study on, 172–173
    electrocardiography in, 89
    family history of, 84, 111b
    lipid levels in, 20, 86, 202
    in Look AHEAD, 177, 177f
    physical activity affecting risk for, 200, 202
    weight loss affecting risk for, 274
CART (cocaine and amphetamine-related transcript), 10, 11f
Carver, C. S., 317
case managers in Diabetes Prevention Program, 169
catabolic pathway, 10, 10f, 11f
cell phones/smartphones, 316, 318–319
    apps for, 318, 322–323, 324, 325–326
    in counseling interventions, 246, 247
    in diet assessment, 104
    in internet interventions, 318
    in mobile health interventions, 318–319, 322
    patient access to and interest in, 325–326
    in physical activity assessment, 125
    in text-messaging interventions, 319
Centers for Disease Control and Prevention, 210b, 212
    Barriers to Being Active quiz, 135
    on body weight categories, 85
    National Diabetes Prevention Program, 173
    on weight-for-age of children, 18
Centers for Medicare and Medicaid Services, 264
    Innovation Center programs, 354
    on intensive behavioral therapy, 350
    on obesity as disease, 80
    on primary care, 341, 342
Centers of Excellence in bariatric surgery, 264
central adiposity. *See* abdominal fat
certificate-of-training programs, 341
certification and credentials. *See* credentials and certification
Certified Bariatric Nurse, 339b, 340
Certified Specialist in Obesity and Weight Management, 339b, 340
change
    commitment to, 234–235
    counseling approaches for, 220–250
    and motivational interviewing, 69, 153–154, 231–236, 244
    readiness for, 153–154, 158t, 235, 347
    resistance to, 235
    stages of, 153, 154, 232
    in technology-based interventions, 323–324, 325
    transtheoretical model of, 153, 232
change talk
    in motivational interviewing, 154, 231, 232, 234, 235, 234b
    in patient-centered approach, 75
childhood
    body mass index in, 18
    environmental risk factors for obesity in, 85
    genetic factors in, 83–84
    prevalence of obesity in, 16, 18, 80
    trauma history in, 150, 158t
    weight stigma and bias in, 46, 47, 50
Childhood Trauma Questionnaire, 150, 158t
cholelithiasis, 89
cholesterol levels. *See* lipid and lipoprotein levels
Chronic Care Model, 279–282
chronic disease
    as consequence of obesity, 99, 110
        and weight stigma, 47f, 49
    obesity as, 270–282
        American Medical Association on, 80, 253, 270
        body weight regulation in, 2, 3–16, 270–271
        Chronic Care Model in, 279–282
        dietary guidelines in, 186
        implications of, 13–14
        lifestyle interventions in, 13–14, 166
        long-term management in, 274–282
        medical and surgical interventions in, 253, 258
        pathophysiology in, 270–274
        physical activity in, 203, 204

training of health care providers on, 37
physical activity benefits in, 203, 204
circadian timing of physical activity, 117b, 138
classical conditioning, 221, 226
class 1 obesity
   in binge eating disorder, 288
   body mass index in, 2, 3t, 85
   gestational weight gain in, 18
   history of patient in, 82
class 2 obesity
   bariatric surgery in, 302
   in binge eating disorder, 288, 302
   body mass index in, 2, 3t, 85
   gestational weight gain in, 18
   history of patient in, 82
class 3 obesity
   bariatric surgery in, 90-92, 212, 302
   behavioral weight loss therapy in, 295
   in binge eating disorder, 288, 302
   body mass index in, 2, 3t, 85
   cognitive-behavioral therapy in, 225
   gestational weight gain in, 18
   multidisciplinary interventions in, 180
   physical activity in, 212
   prevalence of, 16, 17f
   resting energy expenditure in, 99
clinical huddles in interdisciplinary review, 343
clinical information systems, 279, 280b
clustering-focused analysis of physical activity, 137
cocaine and amphetamine-related transcript (CART), 10, 11f
cognitive-behavioral therapy, 31, 65, 220-225
   acceptance-based behavioral therapy compared to, 230
   cognitive restructuring in, 223
   in eating disorders, 296, 297, 299-301, 302, 303.305
   empirical support of, 224-225
   goal setting in, 222
   integration with other approaches, 244
   population considerations in, 225, 245
   practitioner skills and training on, 244
   problem-solving in, 222
   relapse prevention in, 223
   self-monitoring in, 221-222, 225
   social support in, 223
   stimulus control in, 222-223, 228, 229, 232, 297
   theoretical framework in, 221
   treatment format and structure in, 224, 246
   weight maintenance in, 16, 225
cognitive defusion in acceptance-based behavioral therapy, 228, 229, 244
cognitive dissonance, 231-232, 244
cognitive restructuring, 223, 244
Columbia Suicide Severity Rating Scale, 148, 156t
Commission on Dietetic Registration, 32, 339b, 340, 341
commitment to change, 235
communication in patient-provider relationship, 67-76
   as barrier to service, 359
   in group setting, 72-73
   in motivational interviewing, 69, 72, 153-154, 231-236
   nonverbal language in, 72, 75
   on patient goals, 35, 68, 154
   in shared decision making, 69-72

community
   in Chronic Care Model, 279, 280b
   in participatory research, 33
compassion-focused therapy in binge eating disorder, 301
compensatory behaviors after eating, 289, 289b, 293, 297
   assessment of, 148, 149, 304, 305
      questionnaires in, 156t, 157t
   in binge eating, 297
   in bulimia nervosa, 287b
   physical activity as, 149, 287b, 289b, 297, 305
compliance with therapy. See adherence with therapy
conditioning
   classical, 221, 226
   operant, 221, 226
confidence and importance ruler, 75, 234
connected health, 316
constrained model on energy expenditure, 199-200, 201f
consumer-grade wearable devices in activity measurement, 121t, 122, 124, 125, 127f
Consumer Technology Association, 128
contextualism, functional, in acceptance and commitment therapy, 226
control
   in acceptance-based behavioral therapy, 229
   and loss-of-control eating. See loss-of-control eating
   stimulus control
      in acceptance-based behavioral therapy, 244
      in cognitive-behavioral therapy, 222-223, 228, 229, 232, 297
cooking skills, as factor in dietary assessment, 106b, 110
coping behaviors, 48, 49, 52
coronary artery disease, 20, 21f, 84
correlates and determinants of physical activity, 133, 134, 136
corticosteroid therapy, weight gain in, 84, 260b
cortisol in stress response, 28, 49
cost considerations
   in body composition assessment, 90
   in Diabetes Prevention Program, 172, 173
   in energy expenditure measurement, 118, 119
   in evidence-based guidelines, 62, 63
   in food choices, 29, 105, 110
   in intensive lifestyle interventions, 179
   in nutrition assessment, 102b, 104
   in patient-centered care, 68, 76
   in physical activity assessment, 122, 127, 128, 138, 139
      comparison of methods in, 120t-121t, 127t
   in physical activity engagement, 135, 136, 155
   in technology-based interventions, 325
counseling, 220-250
   acceptance and commitment-based approaches in, 225-231
   in bariatric surgery, 336, 337
   cognitive-behavioral, 220-225
   future directions in, 246-247
   health insurance coverage for, 347, 348
   in life stages, 245, 247
   in long-term weight maintenance, 276
   motivational interviewing in, 69, 72, 231-236
   nondiet approaches in, 237-243
   and physical activity monitoring, 320, 321
   population characteristics in, 245-246
   real-time video technology in, 318
   selection and integration of approaches in, 243-245

INDEX   371

treatment format and structure in, 246
coverage of services. *See* health insurance coverage
COVID-19 pandemic, 37, 278, 279, 282
    technology use in, 278, 279, 282, 316, 318, 343
cravings, 149, 157*t*, 272
credentials and certification, 338-341
    of exercise specialists, 337
    organizations providing, 32, 37, 337, 338, 339*b*-340*b*, 340-341
    of registered dietitian nutritionists, 336, 357, 358
criterion measures of energy expenditure, 118-119, 121*t*, 124, 127*f*, 128
Crossing the Quality Chasm (Institute of Medicine), 68
cultural and social influences. *See* sociocultural factors
Current Procedural Terminology codes, 352-353, 353*b*, 354*b*, 359*b*, 360
Cushing syndrome, 84, 87, 87*f*

D

DARN strategy, 234, 234*b*
decision-making
    autonomy of patients in, 35, 51, 231
    in Chronic Care Model, 279, 280*b*
    on dietary interventions, 183, 190
    environment affecting, 30
    in evidence-based practice, 59, 63-64, 69
    goals and motivation of patients in, 35, 69-70
    informed, 35-36, 63, 68, 69-70
    mindful, 228
    in patient-centered care, 67-76
    on physical activity assessment, 125, 126*f*, 127, 127*f*
    shared, 63, 69-72, 73*b*-74*b*, 76
        lack of, as barrier to care, 359, 360*b*
defended weight, 6, 14
definition of obesity, 2-3
    body mass index in, 2-3, 3*t*, 18, 80
degenerative joint disease, 20, 22
depression
    acceptance-based behavioral therapy in, 230
    assessment of, 145-146, 147-148, 154
        questionnaires in, 147, 148, 150, 156*t*, 158*t*
    and binge eating, 83
    and binge eating disorder, 291
    drug therapy in, 146, 258, 259*b*
    eating behaviors in, 83, 145-146, 148, 293
    interpersonal psychotherapy in, 301
    and obesity, 20, 145-146, 147
    physical activity in, 203-204
    in racism, 27
    sleep affecting, 152
    suicidality in, 148
    in weight bias and stigma, 48
Depression, Anxiety, and Stress Scale, 150, 158*t*
desire, in change talk, 234, 234*b*
Determinants of Physical Activity Questionnaire, 135
device-based measures of activity. *See* wearable devices in activity measurement
diabetes mellitus
    drug therapy in, 258, 349
        weight gain associated with, 84, 259, 259*b*
    family history of, 84, 111*b*
    gestational, 82
    laboratory tests in, 89
    medical nutrition therapy in, 349
    type 2. *See* type 2 diabetes mellitus
Diabetes Prevention Program, 166, 167-174
    cognitive-behavioral therapy in, 222
    evidence-based lifestyle interventions in, 222
    maintenance phase in, 170
    mobile apps using strategies from, 322
    National, 174
    Outcomes Study in, 172-174
    publications on, 172
Diagnostic and Statistical Manual of Mental Disorders, 149, 157*t*
    on eating disorders, 287, 287*b*, 288
dialectical behavior therapy in binge eating disorder, 301
diaries
    on diet, 102*b*, 104, 105
    on physical activity, 119, 120*t*
diet, 9-13, 182-190
    in acceptance and commitment therapy, 226, 228, 229-230
    animal studies of, 3, 4, 4*f*, 6
    and appetite. *See* appetite
    assessment of, 98-112
        energy requirements in, 98-102
        food access and food security in, 105-108
        history-taking in, 82-83, 102-105, 106*b*
        laboratory tests in, 88
        nutritional knowledge as factor in, 106*b*, 110
        nutrition specialists in, 336
        physical examination in, 88, 98, 109-110, 110*b*-112*b*
        preoperative, in bariatric surgery, 92, 110*b*, 264, 264*b*
        screening tools in, 103*b*, 105
        self-reports in, 9, 102*b*-103*b*, 102-105
        sociocultural factors in, 105, 106*b*, 108-109, 155
        summary of additional elements in, 105, 106*b*-107*b*
        in transgender patients, 91*b*
        types of foods in, 83, 106*b*, 108
    in bariatric surgery
        postoperative, 264-267, 266*b*
        preoperative assessment of, 92, 110*b*, 264, 265*b*
    in behavioral weight loss therapy, 295, 302
    in cognitive-behavioral therapy, 220-225
    in Diabetes Prevention Program, 168*b*, 169-170, 172
    in eating disorders, 292, 294-299
        self-directed dieting in, 292-293
        self-monitoring of, 298
    and energy balance, 100-102, 182-190
    energy density of foods in. *See* energy density of foods
    energy intake in. *See* energy intake
    evidence-based guidelines on. *See* evidence-based guidelines, on diet
    in Finnish Diabetes Prevention Study, 174
    in Health at Every Size, 238
    hyperpalatable foods in, 272-274, 274*b*, 277
    hypothalamic regulation of, 9-10, 10*f*
    in intermittent-fasting, 187-188
    in intuitive eating, 237-238
    ketogenic, 185
    in long-term weight management, 275-277
    in Look AHEAD, 175, 176, 178, 179

low-calorie, 64, 184, 296, 321
low-carbohydrate, 185
low-fat, 184–185
meal replacement products in. *See* meal replacement products
Mediterranean-style, 186, 187
in motivational interviewing, 236
in multicomponent interventions, 65, 166–180, 183, 187
   with physical activity, 205, 208
portion control in, 184
protein in. *See* protein, dietary
restraint in, 293–295
self-monitoring of. *See* self-monitoring
in technology-based interventions, 319–320
thermic effect of foods in, 7, 7f, 8, 15f, 98, 199
ultraprocessed foods in, 108, 272–274, 277
vegetarian and vegan, 106b, 110, 110b, 186, 187
very low-calorie, 184, 185, 272, 296
and weight regain, 6, 276
Dietary Approaches to Stop Hypertension (DASH), 186–187
Dietary Guidelines for Americans (2020–2025), 184, 186
Dietary Reference Intake, 91b, 99
diethylpropion, 255t, 261b
dieting
definition of, 292
driven, 294, 294f
effective, 294, 295, 294f
ineffective, 294f, 295
paradoxical, 294, 294f
rejecting culture of, 240–241
self-directed, 64, 292–293
   popular diets and weight loss products in, 188–189, 189b, 190b
   and risk for eating disorders, 292–293, 308b
dietitian nutritionists, registered. *See* registered dietitian nutritionists
Digital Clinical Measures Playbook, 127–128
digital health, 316. *See also* technology use
discrimination
racial and ethnic, 28, 29, 34, 35
weight-related, 44, 150–151
   advocacy in, 241
   as barrier to care, 359
   in health insurance coverage, 45, 51
   in interpersonal weight stigma, 46
   legal issues in, 45
   mental health in, 48, 203
   risk for disordered eating in, 290
   as social determinant of health, 47
   stress in, 48, 49, 151
disordered eating
assessment of, 148–150, 156t–157t, 304
binge eating in. *See* binge eating
co-occurrence with overweight or obesity, 288
definition of, 288
low-calorie diet in, 296
night eating in, 83, 148
nondiet approaches to, 243
patient goals and motivation in, 35
risk factors for, 288, 289–290
   in self-directed dieting, 292–293, 294
in sleep disturbances, 152

in social media content, 45
in weight bias and stigma, 45, 48, 290, 291
diuretic use, as compensatory behavior, 297
assessment of, 149, 304, 305
in bulimia nervosa, 287b
domestic domain of physical activity, 120t–121t, 128, 129b
dopamine, 12
doubly labeled water technique, 98–99, 118, 119, 128
compared to other activity measurement methods, 121t, 127f
and constrained model of energy expenditure, 200
Dreyfus model of skill acquisition, 336
driven dieting, 294, 294f
drug therapy
bariatric surgery affecting, 265
in binge eating disorder, 299, 300b, 303
in diabetes, 84, 258, 259, 259b, 349
health insurance coverage for, 258, 347, 348, 349, 350
weight gain associated with, 84, 146, 212, 246, 259, 265
   examples of drugs in, 259b–260b
   and weight-neutral alternatives, 259b–260b
in weight management, 255–260, 267
   adherence with, 258
   amount of weight loss in, 255t–257t, 258
   approved medications in, 31, 37, 255, 255t–257t, 258, 303
   in binge eating disorder, 299
   body mass index in, 254, 254t
   electrocardiography prior to, 89
   history-taking on, 107b
   initiation of, 258
   off-label uses of, 260, 261b
   and physical activity, 209, 212
   race and ethnicity in, 31–32
   research inequities on, 32
   selection of medications in, 258–259
   side effects of, 255t–257t, 258, 267
dual-energy x-ray absorptiometry scan, 89–90
duodenal switch procedures, 31, 261, 263t
dyslipidemia, 202, 203
in binge eating disorder, 291
as complication of obesity, 21f, 84, 86, 260, 267
diet recommendations in, 110
laboratory tests in, 88
low-density lipoprotein levels in, 202
waist circumference measurement in, 86

E

eating behaviors
in acceptance and commitment therapy, 226–227, 228, 230
in anxiety, 148
attuned, 239–240
in behavioral health assessment, 145–146, 148–150, 155, 156t–157t
cognitive-behavioral approaches to, 220–225
compensatory. *See* compensatory behaviors after eating
in depression, 83, 145–146, 148, 293
in dietary assessment, 83, 106b
in dietary restraint, 293–294
disordered. *See* disordered eating

INDEX **373**

food insecurity affecting, 155
intermittent fasting in, 187–188
intuitive, 237–238, 238b, 239f, 239–243
in long-term weight maintenance, 276–277, 277b
loss-of-control in. *See* loss-of-control eating
mindful. *See* mindful eating
in night eating. *See* night eating
nondiet approaches to, 237–243
questionnaires in assessment of, 148–150, 156t–157t
on food frequency, 103b, 104–105
sleep affecting, 146, 152
snacking in, 83, 146, 149
sociocultural factors affecting, 155
in stress, 146, 240
unconditional permission in, 240
Eating Disorder Examination
interview version, 149, 157t, 304
questionnaire version, 149, 157t
in bariatric surgery, 303
with instructions, 304, 305
eating disorders, 286–308. *See also specific disorders.*
acceptance and commitment therapy in, 231, 301
age of onset, 287, 290, 290b
anorexia nervosa, 286, 287b
bariatric surgery in, 92, 299, 300b, 302–303
barriers to care in, 291–292
behavioral weight loss therapy in, 295–296, 299, 302
assessment in, 304
and drug therapy, 303
efficacy of, 300b, 302
binge eating disorder, 287, 287b, 299–303
brain areas in, 12
bulimia nervosa, 287, 287b
characteristics of, compared to obesity, 289, 289b
cognitive-behavioral therapy in, 296, 297, 299–301, 302, 303, 305
co-occurrence with overweight or obesity, 288–291
diagnostic criteria on, 287, 287b, 288
in internalization of weight bias and stigma, 48, 291
lifestyle interventions in, 295–297
nondiet approaches to, 243
practice tips for providers on, 307, 308b
professionally delivered interventions in, 292, 294–299
psychotherapy in, 299–301
risk factors for, 288, 289b, 289–290
assessment of, 304–307
in self-directed dieting, 292–293, 308b
screening for, 304, 305f
in monthly assessments, 306b–307b
preoperative, in bariatric surgery, 92, 303
self-monitoring in, 298–299, 308b
stereotypes on, 290
Eating Inventory, 148–149, 157t
ecological model in physical activity assessment, 132–133, 133f, 136, 139
ecological momentary assessment, 104, 122, 131
education of health care providers
of behavioral health specialists, 337
on cognitive-behavioral therapy, 244
of exercise specialists, 337
expertise and credentialing in, 338–341

on nutrition and obesity, 336, 358–359
in primary care, 336
of registered dietitian nutritionist, 336, 357, 358
on weight bias and stigma, 36, 37, 50, 51
education of patients
decision aids in, 70, 73b
on diabetes in Look AHEAD, 175, 178
in evidence-based practice, 63–64
in Health at Every Size, 238
and health literacy, 155, 158t
for informed decision-making, 35–36, 68, 69
online materials in, 36
in patient-centered care, 68, 69, 70, 73b
on popular diets and weight loss diets, 188–190, 189b
racial and ethnic discrimination affecting, 29
readability of materials in, 35–36
on realistic treatment outcomes, 35
weight bias and stigma affecting, 47
effective dieting, 294, 295f
eHealth. *See* electronic health
eHealth Enhanced Chronic Care Model, 279, 282
electrocardiography, 89
electronic health (eHealth), 246, 278, 282, 316
in Chronic Care Model, 279
commercial apps in, 322–323
motivational interviewing in, 235
sociodemographic factors in, 324
synchronous communication in, 318
weight loss in, 317, 323
electronic health records, 279, 280b
email, in technology-based interventions, 318, 320, 323, 327b
embodiment, active, 238, 240
emerging adulthood, prevalence of obesity in, 18
empathy in motivational interviewing, 69, 72, 73b, 74b, 231
employment
physical activity in, 120t–121t, 128, 129b, 134
and type 2 diabetes risk, 203
racial and ethnic discrimination in, 29
sleep disruptions related to, 85
in social history, 85, 111b
weight-based discrimination in, 46, 47
wellness and health programs in, 134
Endocrine Society, 266
endometrial cancer, 21f, 22
endoscopic therapy, 254t
energy balance, 2, 3
and appetite, 11
deficit in, 182–184
in dietary interventions, 100–102, 182–190
energy expenditure in. *See* energy expenditure
energy intake in. *See* energy intake
energy storage in, 182
hypothalamus in regulation of, 9–10, 10f, 11f
physical activity affecting, 198–200, 213
positive, 182
and weight gain, 2, 7, 14, 182
energy density of foods, 30, 107, 155, 292
in cognitive-behavioral therapy, 222, 223
in diet history, 83
in eating disorders, 297
in low-energy-density diet, 187

and physical activity, 199
    ultraprocessed, 108, 273
energy expenditure, 3, 7–9
    assessment of, 116–128
        criterion measures in, 118–119, 121*t*, 124, 128
        decision matrix on, 125, 126*f*
        device-based measures in, 119, 121*t*, 122–125, 128
        in Diabetes Prevention Program, 169
        doubly labeled water technique in, 98–99, 118, 119, 121*t*, 200
        exercise history in, 83
        indirect calorimetry in, 99, 118–119, 121*t*
        in nutrition assessment, 98–102
        questionnaires in, 119, 120*t*
        report-based measures in, 99, 119–122
        selection of method for, 125–128
        validity and reliability of methods in, 128
    basal metabolic rate in, 7*f*, 7–8, 14, 98, 99
    components of, 7, 7*f*
    definition of, 116
    and energy storage, 182
    hypothalamus in regulation of, 9–10, 10*f*, 11*f*
    and life span changes, 3, 19
    in Look AHEAD, 178
    metabolic equivalents in, 116–117, 136
    in physical activity, 3, 7, 8–9, 98, 198, 199–200, 213
        additive model on, 199–200, 201*f*
        assessment of, 116–128
        constrained model on, 199–200, 201*f*
        and efficiency, 8, 14
        estimation of, 99, 100*b*
        in Look AHEAD, 178
        performance model on, 199–200, 201*f*
        weight affecting, 9, 13, 14, 101
        in weight gain prevention, 204–205
        for weight loss, 100–102
    resting. *See* resting energy expenditure
    and resting metabolic rate, 116, 117
    self-monitoring of, 276
    and thermic effect of food, 7, 7*f*, 8, 98, 199
    total. *See* total energy expenditure
    in weight loss, 8, 13, 14, 15*f*, 100–102, 182
        in adaptive response, 14, 271–272, 275–276
        research trials on, 136–139
    in weight maintenance, 100–102, 277–278
energy intake, 3, 9–13
    animal studies of, 3–4, 4*f*, 6
    and appetite, 11–12, 198–199
    assessment of
        calculators in, 100–102, 182, 183*b*
        history-taking in, 82–83
        preoperative, in bariatric surgery, 92
        qualitative, 35
        self-reports in, 9, 102*b*–103*b*, 102–105
        in transgender patients, 91*b*
    in bariatric surgery, 92, 184
    in behavioral weight loss therapy, 295, 302, 304
    in cognitive-behavioral therapy, 222
    in DASH diet, 187
    in Diabetes Prevention Program, 168*b*, 169–170, 172
    in emotional eating, 146
    and energy density of foods. *See* energy density of foods
    and energy storage, 182
    evidence-based guidelines on, 63–64, 183, 184
    in Finnish Diabetes Prevention Study, 174
    in food insecurity, 29
    in intermittent fasting, 187–188
    internalization of weight stigma affecting, 48
    in ketogenic diets, 185
    in Look AHEAD, 176
    in low-calorie diets, 184, 296
    in low-carbohydrate diets, 185
    in low-fat diets, 184–185
    in Mediterranean-style diets, 186
    and physical activity, 198–199, 208
    in portion-controlled diets, 184
    regulation of, 9–13
    restriction of, 182–190
        in animal studies, 4, 4*f*, 6
        basal metabolic rate in, 102
        in behavioral weight loss therapy, 304
        compared to dietary restraint, 293
        in eating disorders, 296, 297
        in low-calorie diets, 184, 296
        metabolic adaptation in, 271
        physical activity in, 208
        prescription of, 183, 297
        in very low-calorie diets, 184, 296
    self-monitoring of, 169–170, 276
    sleep affecting, 85
    and thermic effect of food, 7, 7*f*, 8, 98
    from ultraprocessed foods, 108, 273, 274*b*
    in vegetarian diets, 186
    in very low-calorie diets, 184, 296
    and weight loss, 100–102, 182–190, 272
        calculators for planning on, 100–102, 182, 183*b*
        in metabolic adaptation, 275–276
    in Western diet, 81
energy requirements, 98–102
energy storage, 182
environmental factors, 81*f*, 85
    built environment in. *See* built environment
    in diet, 105, 107–108, 190. *See also* food environment
    and efficacy of treatment interventions, 32
    in motivational interviewing, 236
    obesogenic. *See* obesogenic environment
    in physical activity, 134–135, 277–278
        in activity spaces, 128–132
        assessment of, 35, 128–132, 134–135
        in domains of activity, 120*t*–121*t*, 128, 129*b*
        ecological model in assessment of, 132–133, 133*f*, 136
        and socioeconomic status, 29, 30
        walkability in, 30, 129, 130, 277, 278
    sensitivity to, 32–33
    as social determinant of health, 27, 30, 34–35, 85
Epworth Sleepiness Scale, 87, 152–153, 159*t*
estradiol, 19
ethical issues in activity space assessment, 131
ethnicity
    in acceptance-based behavioral therapy, 230
    in behavioral health assessment, 155
    and body mass index, 3, 3*t*, 5*f*, 86

INDEX **375**

in Chronic Care Model, research needed on, 282
in Diabetes Prevention Program, 167, 170, 171f
and food choices, 155
of health care providers and researchers, 32
and health inequities, 26–37
    actionable strategies in, 34–37
    in biases of health care providers, 33–34
    social determinants of, 27–30
    in systemic barriers, 30–34
    in treatment access and outcomes, 31–32
    in treatment research, 32–33
in nutrition-focused physical examination, 111b
and prevalence of obesity, 16, 17f, 26
    built environment as factor in, 30
    in childhood, 18
    socioeconomic status as factor in, 29
and referrals for eating disorders, 292
and sociocultural factors affecting diet, 108–109, 155
and technology-based interventions, 324
and waist circumference, 3t

European Association for the Study of Obesity, 197b, 204
evidence-based guidelines, 37, 59–65
    access to treatment based on, 31, 36, 37, 45
    on counseling, 220, 222
    decisions on treatment based on, 63–64, 69, 70
    development of, 59–63
    on diet, 63–64
        and energy deficit for weight loss, 183, 184
        graded recommendations in, 183, 184, 185, 186
        high protein, 185
        lack of, in popular diets and weight loss products, 188–189
        low carbohydrate, 185
        low fat, 184
        Mediterranean-style, 186, 187
        vegetarian-style, 186, 187
    on eating disorders, 291–292, 297
    graded recommendations in, 60b, 61, 62–63
        on diets, 183, 184, 185, 186
    history of, 59–61
    implementation of, 63–64
    organizations issuing, 64b, 65
    in patient-centered care, 67, 69, 70
    patient goals in, 35, 64
    on physical activity, 195, 196b–197b
    on technology use, 278, 317, 323–324, 325
    updates of, 61b, 65
exercise, 198. *See also* physical activity
experiential exercise activities in acceptance-based behavioral therapy, 229
explicit bias, 33, 34, 36, 37
    weight-related, 49, 50

F

facultative thermic effect of food, 7f, 8
family history, 84, 111b, 149
fast-food restaurants, 27, 30
fasting, intermittent, 187–188
fat, body

abdominal. *See* abdominal fat
and blood pressure, 202
in body composition profile, 89–90, 200
and body mass index, 2, 86
in definition of obesity, 80
and energy balance, 9, 10f, 11
excess, health consequences of, 20, 22, 82
gender differences in, 80, 82, 90
leptin in, 9, 12b, 270–271
and lipid levels, 20, 202
and lipostatic theory, 9
measurement methods, 89–90, 321
in menopause, 19
physical activity affecting, 83, 200, 202
in sarcopenia, 19, 82
stress affecting, 146
thermogenic (beige), 13
in transgender patients, 90, 91b
and waist circumference, 86
fat, dietary
    in Diabetes Prevention Program, 168b, 169–170, 172
    in Dietary Approaches to Stop Hypertension, 186, 187
    in Finnish Diabetes Prevention Study, 174, 175f
    in hyperpalatable foods, 274b
    in ketogenic diets, 185
    and lipid levels, 202
    in Look AHEAD, 176
    in low-fat diets, 184–185
    in Mediterranean diet, 186
fatty liver disease, 20, 21f, 22, 88, 91
fee-for-service arrangements, 352–354, 353b, 354b
Festinger, Leon, 231
fiber, dietary, 83, 174, 175f
Finnish Diabetes Prevention Study, 174, 175f
Fitabase, 125
Fitbit device, 320
flexibility
    in dietary restraint, 293
    psychological, in acceptance and commitment therapy, 225, 227
follicle-stimulating hormone, 19
food access and availability
    in eating disorders, 297
    energy-dense foods in, 30, 107, 108, 155, 199
    in food deserts, 27, 30, 107
    socioeconomic status affecting, 155
    supermarket access affecting, 30, 35, 107
    ultraprocessed foods in, 108, 272–274
food addiction, 149, 154, 157t
food allergies and intolerances, 106b, 110
Food and Drug Administration approved antiobesity medications, 31, 37, 255, 258
    in binge eating disorder, 303
    list of, 255t–257t
Food and Nutrient Database, 104, 273
food apartheid, 27, 30
food choices and preferences, 64, 110
    assessment of, 83, 106b
    in cognitive-behavioral therapy, 223
    in emotional eating, 146
    in food cravings, 149

in intuitive eating, 237–238
in mindful eating, 243
operant conditioning of, 221
physical activity affecting, 199
sociocultural influences on, 105, 106b, 107, 108–109, 111, 155
ultraprocessed foods in, 108, 272–274
unconditional permission to eat, 240
Food Craving Inventory, 149, 157t
food cravings, 149, 157t, 272
food deserts, 27, 30, 107
food diaries, 102b, 104, 105
food environment, 105, 107–108
    in acceptance-based behavioral therapy, 229, 230
    assessment of, 107–108
    energy-dense foods in, 30, 107, 108, 199
    as factor in dietary interventions, 190
    fast-food restaurants in, 27, 30
    in motivational interviewing, 236
    obesogenic, 230, 272–274
    supermarket access in, 30, 35, 107
    ultraprocessed foods in, 108, 272–274, 277
food frequency questionnaires, 103b, 104–105
food labels, 106b, 155, 225, 323
food photographs in dietary assessment, 103b, 104
food processing
    classification on extent of, 108, 273, 273b
    of ultraprocessed foods, 108, 272–274, 277
food security issues, 28–30, 34
    in behavioral health assessment, 155, 159, 159t
    definition of, 105
    economic factors in, 29, 29b, 85
    in nutrition assessment, 98, 105, 107, 107b, 108, 111b
14 Weeks to a Healthier You, 211b
Framingham Heart Study, 8, 12, 82
FTO gene, 13
functional contextualism in acceptance and commitment therapy, 226

G

Galen (Greek physician), 80
gastrectomy, sleeve, 31, 261, 261f, 262t
gastric banding, adjustable, 261, 262t
gastric emptying rate, 89, 199
gender
    and body fat percentage, 80, 82, 90
    in eating disorder diagnosis, 287
    and medical complications of obesity, 21f, 22f
    and peer victimization, 46
    and prevalence of obesity, 16, 17f, 29
    of research participants, 245
    and trajectory of body mass index, 5f
    and transgender patients, 82, 90, 91b
    and waist circumference, 86
    and weight-based bias and stigma, 46
Generalized Anxiety Disorder-7 (GAD-7), 148, 154, 156t
genetic factors, 2, 13
    in medical history, 83–84
    in thrifty phenotype, 8
    twin studies of, 13

in weight gain, 2, 4, 6, 13
genome-wide association studies, 13
geographic information systems in activity assessment, 129–132
    ethical concerns in, 131
    and modifiable areal unit problem, 131
    and uncertain geographic context problem, 131
Geriatric Depression Scale–Short Form, 147, 156t
geriatric population. *See* older adults
German National Cohort study, 122
gestational diabetes, 82
gestational weight gain, 18–19
ghrelin, in appetite and hunger, 11, 14, 15f
    food insecurity affecting, 29
    physical activity affecting, 199
    stomach as source of, 12b
Global Physical Activity Questionnaire, 119, 120t
global positioning system technology in activity assessment, 129–130, 132
glucagon-like peptide 1
    physical activity affecting, 199
    receptor agonists in drug therapy, 89, 256t, 257t
    in satiety, 11, 12b
glucose levels
    in drug therapy, 255, 258
    in Health at Every Size, 242
    in Look AHEAD, 177
    in metabolic syndrome, 88, 112b
    monitoring of, 255
    motivational interviewing improving, 236
glucose tolerance, impaired, 89, 174, 175f
glycemic index and load of diet, 64
glycogen, 11
goals
    in acceptance and commitment therapy, 226, 227, 228, 229
    on amount of weight loss, 35, 334
        in acceptance-based behavioral therapy, 229
        in bariatric surgery, 265
        in cognitive-behavioral therapy, 222, 224
        in Diabetes Prevention Program, 167, 168b, 168–169, 172
        in lifestyle interventions, 13
        in Look AHEAD, 175, 176
        in nondieting interventions, 52–53
        and physical activity recommendations, 208, 222
    assessment of, 107b, 154
    and clinician support of patients, 35, 154
    in cognitive-behavioral therapy, 222, 223, 224
    in Diabetes Prevention Program, 167, 168b, 168–169, 172
    on diet, 176
        in cognitive-behavioral therapy, 222
        in Diabetes Prevention Program, 168b, 169
        energy intake in, 100–101, 168b, 169, 172, 176, 183, 185
        food choices in, 64
        in Look AHEAD, 176
    in Finnish Diabetes Prevention Study, 174
    in lifestyle interventions, 13
    in Look AHEAD, 175, 176, 179
    in patient-centered care, 35, 53, 69–70, 71b, 75
    on physical activity, 136, 206
        amount of activity time in, 206, 209
        in cognitive-behavioral therapy, 222
        in Diabetes Prevention Program, 168b, 169, 172

energy expenditure in, 100–101
in Look AHEAD, 175, 176
in pregnancy, 19
and readiness for change, 107b, 154
realistic expectations in, 35, 275
shared decision-making on, 69, 70
in weight-inclusive or weight-neutral approaches, 53
grazing, 83, 149, 303
grip strength, 110b
group setting
acceptance-based behavioral therapy in, 229, 246
cognitive-behavioral therapy in, 224
Health at Every Size in, 241, 242
nondiet interventions in, 241, 242
patient-centered care in, 72–73
social support in, 241, 338
technology use in, 246
growth hormone deficiency, 84
guided self-help cognitive-behavioral therapy, in binge eating disorder, 299, 301
gynecologic abnormalities, 20, 21f

H

Harris-Benedict equations, 99
Hawaiian Natives, 32
head and face examination, 87, 110b
moon face appearance in, 87, 87f
health
inequities in, 26–37
and actionable strategies for achieving equity, 34–37
assessment of, 34–35, 37
in health education materials, 35–36
social determinants of, 27–30, 34–35
in systemic barriers, 30–34
in weight bias and stigma, 37
medical issues affecting. *See* medical issues
obesity affecting, 19–23, 84, 86
bariatric surgery in, 90–92
mortality risk in, 20, 21f
physical activity affecting, 200–204
social determinants of, 27–30, 34–35. *See also* social determinants of health
weight as indicator of, 238, 240–241
weight loss affecting, 167, 172, 253, 267, 274, 275
Health at Every Size, 53, 237, 238–243
compared to other approaches, 239f, 242
empirical support of, 242–243
population considerations in, 243, 245
tools and strategies in, 239–241
treatment format and structure in, 242
health behaviors, 151–154
built environment affecting, 30. *See also* built environment
counseling for change in, 220–250
determinants of, 27–30, 135
internalization of weight bias and stigma affecting, 48, 151
motivation and readiness to change in, 153–154, 158t
physical activity in, 135, 153
questionnaires in assessment of, 151–154, 158t–159t
racial and ethnic biases on, 33, 34

sleep in, 152–153, 159t
sociocultural factors affecting, 108–109, 135
substance use in, 152, 158t
in weight-inclusive or weight-neutral interventions, 53
health care
avoidance of, in weight bias and stigma, 37, 46, 50, 53, 151, 291, 334
barriers in access to. *See* barriers in access to health care
in Chronic Care Model, 279, 280b
insurance coverage for, 346–362
modes of care delivery in, 278
payment structures for services in, 352–358
primary care in. *See* primary care
service line models in, 342
shared medical appointments in, 342, 361b
technology use in. *See* technology use
weight bias and stigma in, 291–292
as barrier in access to services, 359
and health care avoidance, 37, 46, 50, 53, 151, 291, 334
patient experiences with, 50, 291
prevention and reduction of, 36, 37, 51–53, 291
health care facilities
design for overweight or obese patients, 50, 51, 360b
reading materials in, 35–36, 50
health care providers
actionable strategies for achieving equity in care, 34–36
education and training of. *See* education of health care providers
in interprofessional teams, 334–343
in patient-centered care, 67–76
and patient relationship. *See* patient–provider relationship
payment structures for services, 352–358
physical activity resources for, 208, 210b–211b, 212–213
practice tips on disordered eating, 307, 308b
in professionally delivered interventions, 292, 294–299
race and ethnicity of, 32, 36
racial and ethnic bias of, 33–34
readability of patient education materials from, 35–36
shared medical appointments with, 342, 361b
weight bias of, 49–51, 151, 291
as barrier in access to services, 359
intersection with racial/ethnic bias, 33–34
patient experiences in, 50, 291
prevention and reduction of, 36, 37, 51–53, 52b, 291
Health Eating Index, 104
health insurance coverage, 346–362
for bariatric surgery, 347, 348, 350
as barrier to health care access, 31, 359–360
body mass index criteria in, 45, 51, 347, 348
CPT codes in, 352–353, 353b, 359b, 360
for drug therapy, 258, 347, 348, 350
in Medicaid. *See* Medicaid
medical necessity requests in, 354
in Medicare. *See* Medicare
payment structures in, 352–358
policy levers for improvements in, 350–352
for primary care, 341, 342
in Medicare, 347, 348, 352, 353
in private payer plans, 346, 348, 350, 351–352
role of benefits consultants in, 352
in state employee health plans. *See* state employee health plans

health literacy, 326
    assessment of, 155, 158*t*
    in cognitive-behavioral therapy, 225
    as patient barrier to care, 361
heart rate monitors, 121*t*, 123–124, 127*f*, 128
height, and body mass index, 2, 85
Helicobacter pylori test, 92, 264*b*
hemoglobin HbA1c levels
    in Chronic Care Model, 279
    and duration of obesity, 82
    in Look AHEAD, 176, 178*t*
    in screening for diabetes, 89
high-density lipoprotein levels, 20, 202
    laboratory assessment of, 89, 112*b*
    in Look AHEAD, 177, 178*t*
    in metabolic syndrome, 89, 112*b*
high-intensity interval training, 198, 207*b*
    guidelines on, 197*b*, 204
    insulin sensitivity in, 202
    in weight loss, 205, 207*b*
high-protein diets, 185
hirsutism in polycystic ovary syndrome, 87
Hispanics
    body mass index in, 5*f*
    in culturally sensitive interventions, 33, 245
    in Diabetes Prevention Program, 167, 170, 171*f*
    health care provider bias on, 33
    as health care providers and researchers, 32
    in Look AHEAD, 179
    prevalence of obesity in, 16, 17*f*, 26
        built environment as factor in, 30
        in children, 18
        and food insecurity, 28–29
        socioeconomic status as factor in, 28–29, 30
    racism experienced by, 28
    social determinants affecting health of, 28–29, 30
    systemic barriers affecting, 31, 33
historical aspects
    of evidence-based guidelines, 59–61
    of obesity, 80
    of weight loss diets, 80
history of patient, 81–85
    duration of obesity in, 82
    eating behaviors in, 82–83, 148–150
        in transgender patients, 91*b*
    exercise in, 83
    family history in, 84, 111*b*, 149
    medical and surgical, 83–84
    social history in, 84–85
    weight history in, 148–150, 274
holistic approach
    assessment in, 81, 98, 109–110, 152
        factors considered in, 111*b*–112*b*
    to food security issues, 105
    interdisciplinary review in, 343
homeorhesis, 4
homeostasis, 270–271
    compared to homeorhesis, 4
    hypothalamus in, 9, 11, 270
hormones. *See also specific hormones*.
    in appetite and hunger, 11, 12*b*

physical activity affecting, 199
    weight loss affecting, 14, 15*f*, 272
medical history of alterations in, 84
in menopause, 19
in pregnancy, 82
in stress response, 28, 49, 146
in transgender patient therapy, 90, 91*b*
Human Activity Behavior Identification Tool and Data Unification System, 131
hunger, 8
    in food insecurity, 28
    hormones affecting, 11, 12*b*, 14
        in physical activity, 199
        in weight loss, 14, 15*f*, 272
    and intuitive eating, 237, 238, 239
    and mindful eating, 237, 240
    in older adults, 19
    sleep affecting, 85
hydrogen isotope, in doubly labeled water technique, 98–99, 118
hydrostatic weighing, 89, 90
hyperpalatable foods, 272–274, 274*b*, 277
hypertension
    bariatric surgery in, 91, 260, 266
    as complication of obesity, 19, 20–22, 84, 200
    diet in, 186–187
    family history of, 84, 111*b*
    measurement of blood pressure in, 86–87
    medical history of, 84, 111*b*
    physical activity affecting risk for, 200–202
    in racism experience, 28
hypothalamus
    in appetite and hunger, 11
    in body weight regulation, 9–10, 10*f*, 11*f*, 272
        anabolic pathway in, 9–10, 10*f*, 11*f*
        catabolic pathway in, 10, 10*f*, 11*f*
    in homeostasis, 9, 11, 270
hypothyroidism, 84, 87

I

ideal body weight, 27
    body mass index in, 20, 265, 307
    gender differences in, and peer victimization, 46
    and internalization of thin ideal, 288, 293
    patient expectations on, 275
    promoted in clinical reading materials, 50
    sociocultural influences on perception of, 27, 35, 51, 53, 109
Impact of Weight on Quality of Life-Lite, 151, 158*t*
implementation science, 33
implicit bias, 33, 34, 36, 37
    weight-related, 49–50
impulsivity, brain regions in, 12
Indigenous Americans, in Diabetes Prevention Program, 167, 170, 171*f*
indirect calorimetry, 99, 118–119, 121*t*, 127*f*
    in planning dietary interventions, 100
    wearable devices used with, 124
ineffective dieting, 294*f*, 295
Institute of Medicine
    on evidence-based guidelines, 59, 60*b*–61*b*, 61

on patient-centered care, 68
insulin, 10, 11, 11f, 14
    resistance to, 20, 22, 202
        acanthosis nigricans in, 87
        cancer risk in, 22
        in medical history, 84
        physical activity affecting, 202–203
        in pregnancy, 82
        and type 2 diabetes, 202–203
    as therapy, weight gain associated with, 212, 259b
insurance coverage. *See* health insurance coverage
insurance hypothesis on food insecurity and obesity, 29
intensive behavioral therapy, 346
    in bariatric surgery, 267
    barriers in access to, 31, 361b
    in binge eating disorder, 301
    body mass index in, 166, 253–254, 254t
    in business models, 356b
    in cognitive-behavioral therapy, 224
    in Diabetes Prevention Program, 166, 167–174
    energy deficit diet in, 183
    in Look AHEAD, 166, 175–179
    in Medicaid, 351
    in Medicare, 347, 348–349, 350, 353, 354b, 358, 359
    in motivational interviewing, 236
    in primary care, 341
    in private payer insurance, 350
    referrals for dietary counseling in, 105
    US Preventive Services Task Force on, 166, 253–254
interactive voice response, 319–320
intermittent-fasting, 187–188
internalization of weight stigma, 46, 48, 203–204, 334
    assessment of, 150–151, 158t
    eating disorders in, 48, 291
    health behaviors in, 48, 151
    mental health in, 46, 48, 52, 53
    nondiet interventions in, 243
    physical health in, 49
    prevention and reduction of, 51–53
International Federation for the Surgery of Obesity and Metabolic Disorders, 302
International Physical Activity Questionnaire, 119, 120t
internet use, 316, 317–318
    COVID-19 pandemic affecting, 278
    patient access to and interest in, 325–326
    reliability of health information in, 36
interpersonal psychotherapy in binge eating disorder, 299, 300b, 301, 302, 304
interprofessional teams, 334–343
    administrative staff in, 338
    in bariatric surgery, 264, 336, 337, 338
        expertise in, 340
        interdisciplinary review in, 343
    behavioral health specialists in, 337
    business arrangements in, 355, 356b–357b, 357
    care models, 341–343
    exercise specialists in, 337
    expertise and credentialing in, 337, 338–341
    interdisciplinary review in, 343
    in medical and physical assessment, 81, 335
    medical providers in, 335–336
    nutrition specialists in, 336–337
    in primary care setting, 342
    registered dietitian nutritionists in, 336–337, 352–362
    roles in, 334
    in service line models, 342
    shared medical appointments with, 342
interviews
    history-taking in, 81–85
    motivational, 153–154, 231–236. *See also* motivational interviewing
intuitive eating, 237–238, 239–243
    compared to other approaches, 239f, 242
    empirical support of, 242–243
    integration with other approaches, 244–245
    population considerations in, 243
    principles of, 238b
    tools and strategies in, 239–241
    treatment format and structure in, 242
isotemporal substitution in physical activity assessment, 137
isotopes in doubly labeled water technique, 98–99, 118

J

just-in-time interventions, 247

K

ketogenic diets, 185
kidney disorders, 88, 349

L

laboratory tests, 88–89, 112b
    in bariatric surgery, 82, 264–265, 264b
    resting energy expenditure measurement in, 98–99
    in transgender patients, 91b
laparoscopic adjustable gastric banding, 262t
lapse in behavior, 223, 278, 298
lateral hypothalamic area, 10, 11f
laxative use, as compensatory behavior, 297
    assessment of, 149, 304, 305
    in bulimia nervosa, 287b
lean body mass, 8, 21f
    basal metabolic rate in, 8, 13, 98, 101, 102
    energy expenditure in, 8, 13, 271
    in menopause, 19
    in older adults, 19
    and thrifty phenotype, 8
legal issues
    in health insurance, 348, 349, 350, 361
    in weight discrimination, 45
leisure time, physical activity in, 120t–121t, 128, 129b, 134
    and type 2 diabetes risk, 203
leptin, 9, 10, 11f, 12b, 270–271
    in adipose tissue, 9, 12b, 270–271
    mutations affecting, 13, 83, 258
    as satiety hormone, 14

in weight loss, 14, 272
leptin receptor, 13, 257t, 258
LGBTQAI+ communities
    Health at Every Size approach in, 243, 245
    transgender patients in, 82, 90, 91b
life span changes
    basal metabolic rate in, 8
    in childhood, 18. *See also* childhood
    counseling in, 245, 247
    in emerging adulthood, 18
    energy expenditure in, 3, 8
    in menopause, 19
    obesity prevalence in, 17f
    in older adults, 19–20, 82. *See also* older adults
    in pregnancy, 18–19, 82
    weight and body mass index in, 3, 4–6, 18–20
        history-taking on, 82–83, 148
    in young adults, 245
lifestyle coaches
    in Diabetes Prevention Program, 168, 168b, 170, 174
    in Look AHEAD, 176
lifestyle interventions, 31, 166–180, 183
    assessment of barriers in, 35
    in behavioral weight loss therapy, 295–296, 302
    in cognitive-behavioral therapy, 220, 222
    culturally-sensitive, 33
    in Diabetes Prevention Program, 166, 167–174, 222
    diet in, 166–180, 183
    in eating disorders, 295–297
    in Finnish Diabetes Prevention Study, 174
    health inequities in, 31–32, 33
    in Look AHEAD, 166, 175–179, 222
    patient goals in, 13
    physical activity in, 195
    self-monitoring in, 276
lipid and lipoprotein levels, 20
    in binge eating disorder, 291
    in cardiovascular disorders, 20, 86, 202
    in Chronic Care Model, 279
    in complications of obesity, 21f, 84, 86, 260, 267
    and diet recommendations, 110
    in Health at Every Size, 242
    high-density lipoprotein in. *See* high-density lipoprotein levels
    and insulin resistance, 20
    laboratory tests of, 88–89, 112b
    in Look AHEAD, 176, 177, 178t, 179
    low-density lipoprotein in. *See* low-density lipoprotein levels
    in metabolic syndrome, 88, 89, 112b
    in older age, 19
    physical activity affecting, 202, 203
    triglycerides in, 89, 112b, 178t, 202
    and waist circumference values, 86
    weight loss affecting, 202, 267
lipodystrophy, 87
lipoprotein levels. *See* lipid and lipoprotein levels
lipostatic theory, 9
lipotoxicity, 20
liraglutide therapy, 31, 209, 256t
lisdexamfetamine, 260, 261b, 300b, 303

listening
    in motivational interviewing, 69, 72, 154, 231
        in DARN strategy, 234
        in OARS strategy, 232–233
    in patient-centered care, 69, 72
literacy
    health-related, 326
        assessment of, 155, 158t
        in cognitive-behavioral therapy, 225
        as patient barrier to care, 361
        and reading nutrition labels, 106b, 155, 225, 323
        and reading patient education materials, 36
        and selection of diet assessment method, 102b, 105
        and technology use, 326, 327b
literature search, in development of evidence-based guidelines, 59, 61–62, 63
liver disorders
    fatty liver disease, 20, 21f, 22, 88, 91
    laboratory tests in, 88, 89
    steatosis, 89
long-term management of obesity, 274–282
    mode of care delivery in, 278
    physical activity in, 277–278
    in relapse, 278
Look AHEAD, 166, 175–179, 222
loss-of-control eating, 149, 154, 288
    assessment of, 156t, 306b, 307b
    in binge eating disorder, 287b
    in bulimia nervosa, 287b
low-calorie diets, 64, 184, 296, 321
low-carbohydrate diets, 185
low-density lipoprotein levels, 20
    in Chronic Care Model, 279
    laboratory assessment of, 112b
    in Look AHEAD, 176, 177
    in metabolic syndrome, 112b
    physical activity affecting, 202
low-fat diets, 184–185

M

magnetic resonance imaging, fat measurement in, 90
managed care plans in Medicaid, 349
marijuana, 85
meal replacement products
    in eating disorders, 296
    in Look AHEAD, 175, 176
    in portion-controlled diets, 184
    in very low-calorie diets, 184
media
    social media, 45, 327b
    weight stigma and bias in, 45, 50
Medicaid, 346, 347–348, 349
    managed-care plans in, 349
    policy levers for improvements in, 351
    state differences in, 347–348, 349, 351
medical appointments, shared, 342, 361b
medical issues, 19–23, 253–267
    assessment of, 80–92
        in bariatric surgery, preoperative, 90–92

history-taking in, 81–85, 111b
laboratory tests in, 88–89
physical examination in, 85–88
role of medical providers in, 335
in transgender patients, 90, 91b
bariatric surgery in, 90–92, 260–267. See also bariatric surgery
body mass index in, 86, 253–254
diabetes risk in, 167
drug therapy in. See drug therapy
monitoring for, 254–255
mortality risk in, 20, 21f. See also mortality risk
and paradox in protective effect of obesity, 23
physical activity in
benefits of, 200–204
limitations of, 209
safety of, 118, 209
selection of treatment plan in, 253–254
waist circumference in, 86
weight loss benefits in, 253
medical nutrition therapy, 336, 346, 352–362
barriers in access to, 358–362
in business models, 356b
cost-effectiveness of, 357
Current Procedural Terminology codes on, 352–353, 353b, 354b
in Medicare, 349, 351, 352–353, 353b, 354b, 356b
value-based payments in, 354–355
value proposition on, 357–358
Medical Nutrition Therapy Act, 351, 361b
Medicare, 346, 347, 348–349
Current Procedural Terminology codes in, 352–353, 353b, 354b
drug therapy in, 347, 350
intensive behavioral therapy in, 347, 348–349, 350, 353, 354b, 358, 359
medical nutrition therapy in, 349, 351, 352–353, 353b, 354b, 356b
policy levers for improvements in, 350–351
primary care in, 347, 348, 352, 353
Medicare Advantage, 349
Medicare Physician Fee Schedule, 353
medications. See drug therapy
meditation in mindful eating, 237, 239–240
Mediterranean-type diet, 186, 187
meglitinides, 212
melanocortin receptors, 13, 83, 257
α melanocyte-stimulating hormone, 10, 11f
menopause, 19
mental health
in bariatric surgery, preoperative evaluation of, 92
depression affecting. See depression
internalization of weight stigma affecting, 46, 48, 52, 53, 203–204
in nondiet approaches, 243
racism affecting, 27
in weight-inclusive or weight-neutral interventions, 53
Metabolic and Bariatric Surgery Accreditation and Quality Improvement Program, 338, 340, 341
metabolic disorders, 9, 13, 19, 49
metabolic equivalents, 116–117
corrected, 117
in sedentary behavior, 198
in weight loss trials, 136
metabolic rate
basal. See basal metabolic rate
and life span, 271
resting, 15f, 116, 117
metabolic syndrome, 84, 88–89, 112b
in binge eating disorder, 291, 299
metformin
in Diabetes Prevention Program, 168b
in Outcomes Study, 172, 173, 173t
results of, 170, 171f, 172
dual benefits of, 260
off-label use of, 261b
mHealth. See mobile health
microaggressions, weight-related, 45–46, 48
micronutrient deficiencies, assessment of, 88, 92, 110b
Mifflin-St. Jeor equations, 7, 99, 100
mindful eating, 228, 237, 239–243
in acceptance-based behavioral therapy, 228
in binge eating disorder, 301
compared to other approaches, 239f, 242
integration with other approaches, 244–245
meditation in, 237, 239–240
mineral supplementation in bariatric surgery, 265, 266b
Mobile App Rating Scale, 323, 325
mobile health (mHealth), 278, 316, 318–319
commercial apps in, 322–323
sociodemographic factors in, 324
weight loss in, 318
modifiable areal unit problem in activity assessment, 131
mood, assessment of, 145, 147–148, 156t
moon face appearance, 87, 87f
mortality risk
and body mass index, 20, 21f, 85, 86f
and cardiorespiratory fitness, 203
and duration of obesity, 82
and weight discrimination, 49
weight loss affecting, 274–275
motivational interviewing, 153–154, 231–236
behavioral weight loss therapy compared to, 295
change talk in, 154, 231, 232, 234, 235, 234b
empirical support of, 235–236
in Look AHEAD, 179
in patient-centered care, 69, 72, 76, 231, 235
case study on, 73b–74b
population considerations in, 236
practitioner skills and training on, 244
resistant behaviors in, 235
strategies in, 232–235
theoretical framework in, 231–232
treatment format and structure in, 235
motivation of patients
assessment of, 153–154, 158t
in evidence-based practice, 63
interview process on, 69, 153–154. See also motivational interviewing
and physical activity recommendations, 208
and realistic goals, 35
in social cognitive theory, 221
weight bias and stigma affecting, 48

motor abnormalities, physical examination in, 88
MOVE! program, 179-180
multicomponent interventions, 166-180, 183, 254. *See also* treatment interventions
    cognitive-behavioral therapy in, 224
    counseling in, 65, 220
    in Diabetes Prevention Program, 166, 167-174
    diet in, 65, 166-180, 183, 187, 254
        and physical activity, 205, 208
    drug therapy in, 65, 166, 167
        and physical activity, 209, 212
    evidence-based guidelines on, 65, 166-167, 183, 220
    in Finnish Diabetes Prevention Study, 174
    interprofessional team in, 334-343
    in Look AHEAD, 166, 175-179
    physical activity in, 65, 195, 254
        and diet, 205, 208
        and drug therapy, 209, 212
    in primary care, 342
    in private payer health insurance, 350
    service line models in, 342
    surgery in, 65, 167
    US Preventive Services Task Force on, 166, 167, 350
muscles
    lipid accumulation in, 20
    in sarcopenia, 19, 82, 203
    strength and resistance training for. *See* strength and resistance training
MyFitnessPal app, 322

N

naltrexone and bupropion, 31, 256*t*, 257
National Academies of Sciences, 99
National Academy of Medicine, 18, 59, 68, 358
National Association to Advance Fat Acceptance, 238
National Cancer Institute, 173
National Center on Health, Physical Activity, and Disability, 210*b*, 211*b*, 212
National Diabetes Prevention Program, 174
National Eating Disorders Association, 304
National Health and Nutrition Examination Survey, 16, 18, 104, 122
National Heart, Lung, and Blood Institute, 173
National Institute for Health and Care Excellence, 301
National Institute of Diabetes and Digestive and Kidney Diseases
    Body Weight Planner, 100-102, 101*f*, 182, 183*b*
    Diabetes Prevention Program funded by, 167, 174
    Look AHEAD study funded by, 175
National Quality Forum, 69
National Strength and Conditioning Association, 337
National Weight Control Registry, 16, 104, 274, 276, 277
neck circumference measurement in obstructive sleep apnea, 87
need, in change talk, 234-35, 234*b*
neighborhood
    built environment of, 30
    food access and availability in, 27, 30, 35, 107-108
    physical activity options in, 29, 30, 35
        assessment of, 128-132, 134-135
        socioeconomic status affecting, 29, 30
    walkability affecting, 30, 129, 130, 277, 278
    in weight maintenance, 277-278
Neighborhood Environment Walkability Scale, 130
neuropathy, physical examination in, 88
neuropeptide Y, 10, 11*f*
neurotransmitters in hunger, 12, 12*b*
Newest Vital Sign, 155, 158*t*
night eating, 83, 148, 288
    acceptance-based behavioral therapy in, 231
    drug therapy in, 260
    questionnaire in assessment of, 149, 154, 157*t*
Night Eating Questionnaire, 149, 154, 157*t*
nondieting interventions, 237-243
    active embodiment in, 240
    attuned eating in, 239-240
    empirical support of, 242-243
    Health at Every Size in, 238-239
    intuitive eating in, 237-238
    meditation in, 240
    mindful eating in, 237
    population considerations in, 243
    rejecting diet culture in, 240-241
    respect and positivity in, 241
    social support in, 241
    treatment format and structure in, 242
    unconditional permission to eat in, 240
    as weight-neutral or weight-inclusive, 52-53
nonexercise activity thermogenesis, 8
NOVA food classification system, 108, 273, 273*b*
nutrition, 98-112, 182-190. *See also* diet
nutrition and dietetics technicians, registered, 336
Nutrition Environment Measures Survey, 108

O

OARS strategy, 232-233, 233*b*
obesity
    bias and stigma in, 44-53. *See also* weight bias and stigma
    characteristics of, compared to eating disorders, 289, 289*b*
    as chronic disease, 270-282. *See also* chronic disease, obesity as
    co-occurrence with eating disorders, 288-291
    definition of, 2-3, 20
        body mass index in, 2-3, 3*t*, 18, 80
    and depression, 20, 145-146, 147
    evidence-based treatment guidelines in, 59-65
    family history of, 84
    and health inequities, 26-37
    medical issues in, 19-23. *See also* medical issues
    origin of term, 80
    paradox in protective effect of, 23
    prevalence of. *See* prevalence of obesity
    risk factors for, 81*f*
    severe. *See* class 3 obesity
    in transgender patients, 90, 91*b*
    treatment interventions in. *See* treatment interventions
    waist circumference in, 2, 3*t*, 80
Obesity Action Coalition, 51
Obesity Medicine Association, 340*b*, 341
obesity paradox, 23

INDEX **383**

obesogenic environment, 20, 32, 272–274
    acceptance-based behavioral therapy in, 230
    definition of, 272
    ultraprocessed and hyperpalatable foods in, 108, 272–274, 277
obligatory thermic effect of food, 7f, 8
obstructive sleep apnea, 20, 21f, 22
    bariatric surgery in, 91, 260
        postoperative outcomes in, 266
        preoperative evaluation in, 264, 264b
    medical assessment of, 84
    neck circumference measurement in, 87
    polysomnography in, 89
    questionnaire in assessment of, 152, 159t
    screening for, 87
occupation. *See* employment
off-label uses of weight management drugs, 260, 261b
olanzapine, weight gain associated with, 84, 260b
older adults, 19–20, 82
    behavioral health assessment in, 147, 156t, 159
    counseling of, 245
    depression in, 147, 156t
    physical activity recommendations for, 209
    sarcopenia in, 19, 82, 203
    strength and resistance training in, 203, 209
open-ended questions in motivational interviewing, 232, 233b
operant conditioning, 221, 226
orlistat, 31, 256t, 303
osteoarthritis, 88, 91, 209
overfeeding
    animal studies of, 3, 4f
    brain response in, 14, 16
    nonexercise activity thermogenesis in, 8
overweight
    bias and stigma in, 44–53. *See also* weight bias and stigma
    body mass index in, 2, 3t, 21f, 85
    co-occurrence with eating disorders, 288–291
    diabetes risk in, 167
    evidence-based treatment guidelines in, 59–65
    mortality risk in, 21f, 274
    prevalence of, 343
    in transgender patients, 90, 91b
    treatment interventions in. *See* treatment interventions
oxygen isotope in doubly labeled water technique, 98–99, 118

P

Pacific Islanders
    antiobesity medications in, 31
    in culturally sensitive lifestyle interventions, 33
    in Diabetes Prevention Program, 167
    as health care providers and researchers, 32
    prevalence of obesity in, 26
    racism experienced by, 28
paleo diet, 106b, 110
pancreatic beta cells, lipid accumulation in, 20
pancreatic polypeptide, physical activity affecting, 199
paradoxical dieting, 294, 294f
paradoxical effect of obesity, 23
paraventricular nucleus, 10, 11f

patient burden
    in behavioral health assessment, 145, 155
    in nutrition assessment, 102b, 103b, 104, 105
        and energy expenditure measurement, 98, 99
    in physical activity assessment, 122, 127, 128, 137
        comparison of methods, 120t–121t, 127f
        and energy expenditure measurement, 118, 119
        with wearable devices, 121t, 124
    in technology-based interventions, 325
patient-centered care, 67–76
    alignment of preferences and treatment in, 69–70, 73b–74b
    case study on, 73b–74b
    challenges in, 75, 76
    in Chronic Care Model, 279
    components of, 67
    in counseling, 244
    in eating disorders, 304
    empathy in, 69, 72, 73b, 74b
    goals in, 35, 53, 69–70, 71b, 75
    in group setting, 72–73
    for individual patients, 72, 73b–74b
    in long-term weight maintenance, 276
    motivational interviewing in, 69, 72, 73b–74b, 76, 231, 235
    origin of term, 67
    rapport and trust in, 68b, 68–69
    reflective listening in, 69, 72
    shared decision making in, 69–72, 73b–74b, 76
    weight sensitivity in, 51
Patient Health Questionnaire-2 (PHQ-2), 147
Patient Health Questionnaire-9 (PHQ-9), 147, 148, 154, 156t
Patient Protection and Affordable Care Act, 348, 349, 350, 361
patient–provider relationship, 208
    biases affecting, 33–34, 36, 37, 50, 359
        in eating disorders, 291–292
    in Chronic Care Model, 279
    communication in. *See* communication in patient–provider relationship
    concordance in race and ethnicity affecting, 32, 36
    in counseling, 244
    in motivational interviewing, 69, 72, 153–154, 231–236
    in patient-centered care, 67–76
    and physical activity recommendations, 208
payment structures, 352–358
    business arrangements, 355, 356b–357b, 357
    fee-for-service arrangements, 352–354, 353b, 354b
    value-based, 354–355
    value proposition on, 357–358
pedometers, 121t, 123, 127f, 320
peer support
    in cognitive-behavioral therapy, 223
    in Health at Every Size, 241, 242
    in interprofessional team approach, 338
peer victimization in weight stigma, 46
Pennington Biomedical Research Center Weight Loss Predictor Calculator, 182, 183b
peptide YY, 11, 12b, 14, 15f, 199
Perceived Stress Scale, 150, 158t
performance model on physical activity and energy expenditure, 199–200, 201f
periodic fasting, 186–187
Pew Research Center, 316
pharmacotherapy. *See* drug therapy

phentermine, 31, 89, 255t, 261b
    mechanism of action, 255t, 257
    with topiramate, 31, 256t
photoplethysmography, 123
physical activity, 195–213
    in acceptance and commitment therapy, 228, 230
    in active embodiment, 240
    aerobic. *See* aerobic exercise
    and appetite, 198–199
    assessment of, 116–139
        activity spaces in, 128–132
        in behavioral health assessment, 153, 155
        correlates in, 133, 134, 136
        criterion measures in, 118–119, 121t, 124, 127f, 128
        decision matrix on, 125, 126f, 127
        determinants in, 133, 134, 135
        device-based measures in, 119, 121t, 122–125, 127f, 128, 137, 320–321
        in dietary assessment, 107b
        ecological model in, 132–133, 133f, 136, 139
        energy expenditure in, 116–128
        environmental factors in, 35, 128–132, 134–135
        exercise history in, 83
        individual-level factors in, 134
        sedentary behavior in, 136–139
        selection of method in, 125–128
        self-reports in. *See* self-reports, on physical activity
        sociocultural factors in, 132–136, 139
        validity and reliability in, 128
        variables in, 116, 117b
        in weight loss trials, 136–139
    and bariatric surgery, 212, 266b
    barriers to, 35, 135–136
    in behavioral weight loss therapy, 295, 297, 302
    benefits of, 23, 198–204
    and blood pressure, 200–202
    and body fat, 83, 200, 202
    cardiorespiratory fitness in, 203, 209
    in cognitive-behavioral therapy, 222, 225
    as compensatory behavior, 149, 287b, 289b, 297, 305
    continuous, 117b, 138
        compared to short bouts, 206, 207b
    definition of, 116, 198
    determinants of, 133, 134, 135, 136
    in Diabetes Prevention Program, 168b, 169–170, 172
    dimensions of, 120t–121t, 127
    domains of, 120t–121t, 127, 128, 129b
    duration of, 117b, 120t–121t, 138
        in Diabetes Prevention Program, 169, 172
        in exercise history, 83
        guidelines on, 196b, 197b, 204, 277, 297
        and insulin sensitivity, 202
        in Look AHEAD, 176
        in weight loss, 198, 205, 206, 207b, 213
        in weight maintenance, 277, 297
    in eating disorders, 295, 297, 298
    energy expenditure in. *See* energy expenditure, in physical activity
    environmental factors affecting. *See* environmental factors, in physical activity
    and exercise specialists in interprofessional team, 337
    in Finnish Diabetes Prevention Study, 174, 175f
    guidelines on, 122, 195, 196b–197b, 204, 206, 208
        in bariatric surgery, 212
        on duration, 196b, 197b, 204, 277, 297
        for weight maintenance, 277
    in Health at Every Size, 238
    history-taking on, 83
    and insulin resistance, 202–203
    and lipid levels, 202
    in Look AHEAD, 176, 178, 179
        fitness outcome in, 177, 178t
        goal for, 175, 176
    and low-calorie diet, 321
    in menopause, 19
    metabolic equivalents in, 116–117
    in motivational interviewing, 236
    in multicomponent interventions, 65, 195, 254
        in Diabetes Prevention Program, 168b, 169
        with diet, 205, 208
        with drug therapy, 209, 212
        in Finnish Diabetes Prevention Study, 174
        in Look AHEAD, 175
    in older adults, 19
    in orthopedic limitations, 209
    overestimation of, 99
    personalized recommendations on, 208–212, 213
    prescription of, 195, 206–213, 295, 297
    regulation of, 8–9
    resources on, 208, 210b–211b, 212–213
    safety considerations in, 118, 209
    self-monitoring of, 206, 308b, 321
    sociocultural factors affecting, 12, 116, 132–136, 139, 155
    socioeconomic status affecting, 29, 30
    strength and resistance training in. *See* strength and resistance training
    temporal patterns in, 138, 198, 208
        circadian, 117b, 138
        guidelines on, 204
        for weekend warriors, 137
    and type 2 diabetes, 202–203
    volume and frequency of, 117b, 120t
    weight bias and stigma affecting, 48
    in weight gain prevention. *See* weight gain, physical activity in prevention of
    and weight loss. *See* weight loss, and physical activity
    in weight maintenance. *See* weight maintenance, physical activity in
Physical Activity Guidelines for Americans, 122, 195, 196b, 204, 208, 210b
Physical Activity Readiness Questionnaire for Everyone, 118
Physical Activity Toolkit for RDNs, 208, 210b
physical examination, 85–90
    anthropometrics in, 85–86, 89
        in transgender patients, 91b
    blood pressure in, 86–97
    body composition profile in, 89–90
    in nutrition assessment, 88, 98, 109–110, 110b–112b
Picker/Commonwealth Program for Patient-Centered Care, 67
PICO format, 61
Pittsburgh Sleep Quality Index, 152, 154, 159t
placebo group in Diabetes Prevention Program, 168b, 170
    in Outcomes Study, 172, 173, 173t
    results in, 171f

plant-based diets, 106b, 110, 110b, 186, 187
Playbook by the Digital Medicine Society, 127–128
plethysmography
    air-displacement, 90
    photoplethysmography, 123
polycystic ovary syndrome, 21f, 22, 84, 87, 111b
polysomnography in sleep apnea, 89
popular diets and weight loss products, 188–190, 189b
portion-controlled diets, 184
postpartum weight gain, 19
posttraumatic stress disorder, 301
posture in physical activity assessment, 116, 124, 136
poverty, 29, 30
Power of Food Scale, 149, 154, 157t
practice standards, 336–337
Prader-Willi syndrome, 13
prediabetes, 110, 170, 258
preference misdiagnosis, 70
prefrontal cortex, 12
pregnancy, 18–19, 82, 343
prescription
    of diet and energy intake, 167, 183, 184
        in behavioral weight loss, 295
        in eating disorders, 295, 297
        in weight maintenance, 276
    of drug therapy, 31, 37. *See also* drug therapy
    of exercise and physical activity, 195, 206–213, 295, 297
    of self-monitoring, 298–299
prevalence of obesity, 16, 17f, 80–81, 343
    in childhood, 16, 18, 80
    in emerging adulthood, 18
    and medical complications, 20
    racial and ethnic differences in, 16, 17f, 26
    socioeconomic status as risk factor in, 29, 80–81
primary care, 341–342
    business models in, 356b
    health insurance coverage for, 341, 342
        in Medicare, 347, 348, 352, 353
    interprofessional teams in, 342
    training of providers on nutrition and obesity, 336
private-payer health insurance, 346, 348, 350
    fee-for-service, 352
    policy levers for improvements in, 351–352
problem-solving skills
    in cognitive-behavioral therapy, 222
    in Look AHEAD, 179
processed foods, 108, 272–274
    classification of, 108, 273, 273b
    energy density of, 30, 107, 108, 273
    hyperpalatable, 272–274, 274b
    minimally processed, 108, 273b
    ultraprocessed, 108, 272–274, 277
professional performance standards, 336–337
pro-opiomelanocortin, 10, 11f, 13, 257
    deficiency of, 257t, 258
prostate cancer, 21f, 22
protein, dietary, 83, 184
    and appetite, 272
    in bariatric surgery, 34, 212, 266b, 267
    in high-protein diets, 184, 185
    in ketogenic diets, 185
    sociocultural influences on, 155
    supplementation of, 107b, 184
    for transgender patients, 91b
    in very low-calorie diets, 184, 272
psychological factors
    in acceptance and commitment therapy, 225, 227
    in behavioral health assessment, 146–151, 147b
psychosocial factors
    in bariatric surgery, preoperative assessment of, 92
    in determinants of health, 27, 28
psychotropic drugs, weight gain associated with, 84, 146, 212, 260
purging behavior and disorder, 287b, 288, 299

Q

qualitative assessment of health inequities, 35
quality of life
    assessment of, 151, 158t
    and mental health, 48, 203–204
    patient goals on, 35
    and physical activity, 203–204
    and physical health, 49, 203
quantitative assessment on social determinants of health, 34
Questionnaire on Eating and Weight Patterns-5 (QEWP-5), 149, 154, 156t
questionnaires
    in behavioral health assessment, 146–160
        list of, 155t–159t
    on eating disorders, 149, 157t, 303, 304, 305
    on food frequency, 103b, 104
    on physical activity, 119, 120t, 127f, 135
    on physical activity readiness, 118

R

race
    in acceptance-based behavioral therapy, 230
    in behavioral health assessment, 155
    and body mass index, 5f
    in Chronic Care Model, research needed on, 282
    of health care providers and researchers, 32
    and health inequities, 26–37
        actionable strategies in, 34–37
        in biases of health care providers, 33–34
        social determinants of, 27–30
        in systemic barriers, 30–34
        in treatment access and outcomes, 31–32
        in treatment research, 32–33
    in nutrition-focused physical examination, 111b
    and prevalence of obesity, 16, 17f, 26, 29, 30
    of research participants, 33, 245
    and sociocultural factors affecting diet, 155
    and technology-based interventions, 324
    and treatment outcomes, 245
racism, 27–28, 37
    and obesogenic environment, 30, 32
    and socioeconomic status, 29, 30
    stress in, 28, 35

radical behaviorism, 226
rapport and trust
    in counseling strategies, 244
    in patient-centered care, 68b, 68–69, 72
RDNs. *See* registered dietitian nutritionists
Reach Ahead for Lifestyle and Health-Diabetes (REAL-Diabetes), 179
readiness to change, 153–154, 158t, 234–235, 347
reading materials
    nutrition labels as, 106b, 155, 225, 323
    provided for patient education, 35–36
    weight stigma and bias in, 50
reason, in change talk, 234, 234b
referrals
    for bariatric surgery, 34, 260–261
    for eating disorders, 292
    to registered dietitian nutritionists, 105, 361
        barriers affecting, 359, 359b, 360b
reflective listening in motivational interviewing, 69, 72, 232–233, 233b
registered clinical exercise physiologist, 337
registered dietitian nutritionists (RDNs), 167, 352–362
    barriers in access to services of, 358–362
    in Diabetes Prevention Program, 168, 168b, 174
    in evaluation for bariatric surgery, 92
    in evidence-based approaches, 63–64
    health insurance coverage for services, 359–360
        Current Procedural Terminology codes in, 352–353, 353b, 354b, 359b, 360
        in Medicaid, 359
        in Medicare, 347, 350, 352–353, 353b, 354b
        in private payer plans, 348
    in interprofessional team, 336–337, 352–362
    medical nutrition therapy provided by, 336, 352–362
    in nutrition assessment, 105, 108–109
    payment structures for services, 352–358
        business arrangements, 355, 356b–357b, 357
        fee-for-service, 352–354, 353b, 354b
        value-based, 354–355, 361b
        value proposition on, 357–358
    physical activity resources for, 210b
    in primary care practice, 352
    race and ethnicity of, 32, 37
    referrals to, 105, 359, 359b, 360b, 361
    skills and training of, 244, 357, 358
    standards on, 336–337
regulation of body weight, 3–16
Regulation of Cues program, 154
relapse, 153, 223, 278
relational frame theory, 226–227
reliability of physical activity assessment methods, 128
religion, as factor in eating behaviors, 155
reproductive disorders as complication of obesity, 20, 21f, 22
research
    animal studies in. *See* animal studies
    on Chronic Care Model, 279, 282
    community-based participatory, 33
    diversity of participants in, 32–33, 245
    diversity of researchers in, 32
    evidence-based guidelines developed from, 59–65
    inequities in, 32–33
    on lifestyle interventions, 166
        in Diabetes Prevention Program, 166, 167–174
        in Finnish Diabetes Prevention Study, 174
        in Look AHEAD, 166, 175–179
    literature search on, 59, 61–62
    physical activity assessment methods in, 120t–121t, 128–132
        audit-based tools in, 130
        indirect calorimetry in, 118–119
        wearable devices in, 121t, 122, 124, 125, 127f
        in weight loss trials, 136–139
    on physical activity interventions, 195
    on popular diets and weight loss products, 188–190, 189b
resistance training. *See* strength and resistance training
resistant behaviors, motivational interviewing in, 234–235
resource scarcity hypothesis on food insecurity, 29
respect
    in patient-centered care, 67, 72, 76
    and positivity in nondiet approaches, 241
resting energy expenditure, 199
    estimation of, 99
    measurement of, 98–99, 119
    physical activity affecting, 199, 200
    and total energy expenditure, 99, 199
    weight loss affecting, 101
resting metabolic rate, 15f, 116, 117
restraint, dietary, 293–294
review boards, 343
reward system, food-related, 12, 240
    brain areas in, 12, 14–16, 146, 237, 272
    in mindful eating, 237
    and obesogenic environment, 272
    in operant conditioning, 221
    physical activity affecting, 199
    sleep affecting, 85
    stress affecting, 146
    weight loss affecting, 14–16, 272
righting reflex, 235
risperidone, weight gain associated with, 84, 260b
Rogers, Carl, 231
rounds in interdisciplinary review, 343
Roux-en-Y gastric bypass, 31, 261, 262f

S

safety issues in physical activity, 118, 209
sarcopenia, 19, 82, 203
satiety, 8, 11, 237
    in attuned eating, 239
    in bariatric surgery, 262t–263t
    drugs affecting, 146, 255, 257, 258
    in Health at Every Size, 238, 240, 242
    in high-protein diets, 185
    hormones in, 11, 14, 15f
        sleep affecting, 152
        weight loss affecting, 14, 15f, 276, 277
    in intuitive eating, 237, 238, 244
    and loss-of-control eating, 154
    in mindful eating, 237, 244
    ultraprocessed foods affecting, 108
Scheier, M. F., 317
schema therapy in binge eating disorder, 301

screening
    dietary, 103b, 105
    for eating disorders, 304, 305f
        in monthly assessments, 306b–307b
        preoperative, in bariatric surgery, 92, 303
    for obesity, 85, 166, 253
        health insurance coverage for, 348
    for obstructive sleep apnea, 87
    for safety in physical activity, 118
sedentary behavior
    assessment of, 116–139
        activity factor in, 99
        in behavioral health assessment, 153
        on circadian timing, 138
        on duration, 138
        metabolic equivalents in, 116, 117, 124, 136
        sociocultural factors in, 132–136
        variables in, 116, 117b
        in weight loss trials, 136–139
    definition of, 198
    guidelines on, 195, 196b, 197b, 204
    health consequences of, 200, 202, 203
    reducing time of, 206, 206b, 209
selective daily mobility bias, 131–132
self-directed dieting, 64, 292–293
    popular diets and weight loss products in, 188–190, 189b
    and risk for eating disorders, 292–293, 308b
self-esteem, internalization of weight stigma affecting, 46, 48
self-management in Chronic Care Model, 279, 280b
self-monitoring, 276
    in cognitive-behavioral therapy, 221–222, 225
    in Diabetes Prevention Program, 169–170
    in dietary restraint, 293–294
    and eating disorders, 298–299, 308b
    of physical activity, 206, 308b, 321
    technology in, 317, 319, 321, 326
        with apps, 322, 325
        with smart scales, 321–322
self-perception theory in motivational interviewing, 232
self-regulation
    in dietary restraint, 293–294
    in technology use, 317
self-reports
    in behavioral health assessment, 146–160
    on diet, 102b–103b, 102–105
        accuracy of, 9, 104
        social desirability bias in, 102b
    on physical activity, 99, 119–122, 127f
        accuracy of, 99, 119, 128, 130
        and activity spaces, 129, 130, 132
        questionnaires in, 119, 120t, 127f, 135
        and sedentary behavior, 137
        social desirability bias in, 119, 120t, 130
    prevalence of obesity in, 16
semaglutide, 31, 256t, 260
sensory abnormalities, physical examination in, 88
service line models, 342
set point in body weight, 4, 271
severe obesity. See class 3 obesity
shared decision-making, 63, 67–76
    alignment of preferences and treatment in, 69–70
    case study on, 73b–74b
    components of, 69
    decision aids in, 70, 73b
    lack of, as barrier to care, 359, 360b
    steps in, 70–71, 71b
shared medical appointments, 342, 361b
Short Form Health Survey, 151, 158t
Short Message Service (SMS), 318, 319, 320, 323, 326, 327b
SilverSneakers program, 211b
single anastomosis duodeno-ileal switch, 261, 263t
skin examination, 88
skinfold thickness, 89
sleep
    apnea in, obstructive. See obstructive sleep apnea
    assessment of, 106b, 146
        polysomnography in, 89
        questionnaires in, 152–153, 154, 159t
    and eating behaviors, 146, 152
    and obesity risk, 85
sleeve gastrectomy, 31, 261, 261f, 262t
smartphones. See cell phones/smartphones
smart scales, 321–322
smoking and tobacco use
    assessment of, 92, 106b, 152, 158t
    in bariatric surgery, 92, 264b, 266, 266b
snacks between meals, 83, 146, 149
SNAP-Ed physical activity programs, 211b
social and cultural factors. See sociocultural factors
social cognitive theory, 221, 223
social desirability bias, 102b, 119, 120t, 130
social determinants of health, 27–30
    assessment of, 34–35, 37, 84–85
    built environment in, 27, 30, 34–35
    racism in, 27–28
    socioeconomic status in, 27, 28–29, 47
    weight bias and stigma in, 47
social history, 84–85, 111b
social justice, in Health at Every Size approach, 238
social media, 45, 327b
social support
    in cognitive-behavioral therapy, 223
    in Health at Every Size, 241, 242
    in interprofessional team approach, 338
sociocultural factors, 12–13, 27–30, 190
    in behavioral health assessment, 155, 159
    in body ideals, 27, 35, 51, 53, 109
    in food choices, 105, 106b, 107, 108–109, 111, 155, 190
    in food security, 29–30, 98, 105, 107
    in physical activity, 12, 116, 132–136, 139, 155
    in prevalence of obesity, 16
    and rejection of diet culture, 240–241
    sensitivity to, in treatment interventions, 32–33, 245
socioeconomic status, 27, 28–30
    and food choices, 155
    in nutrition-focused physical examination, 111b
    and prevalence of obesity, 29, 80–81
    social history on, 85
    weight bias and stigma affecting, 47
sodium in hyperpalatable foods, 273, 274b
standards of practice and professional performance, 336–337
state employee health plans, 346, 348

policy levers for improvements in, 351
state differences in, 348, 349–350, 351
for teaching workforce, 349–350
statistical issues in physical activity assessment, 137
steatosis, hepatic, 89
step counting in activity assessment, 123, 125, 128, 222
stereotypes
in eating disorders, 290, 291–292
in weight bias and stigma, 44, 45, 46, 150
internalized, 48, 150–151
stigma and bias, weight-related. *See* weight bias and stigma
stimulus control
in acceptance-based behavioral therapy, 244
in cognitive-behavioral therapy, 222–223, 228, 229, 232, 297
STOP-BANG questionnaire, 87
Strategies to Overcome and Prevent (STOP) Obesity Alliance, 347–348
strength and resistance training, 83, 195
with aerobic exercise, 205, 207*b*
in bariatric surgery, 212
guidelines on, 196*b*, 197*b*, 204
health benefits of, 203
history-taking on, 83
for older adults, 203, 209
in weight loss, 206, 207*b*
stress, 28, 28*b*
assessment of, 35, 146, 150
questionnaires in, 150, 158*t*
social history in, 85
cognitive-behavioral therapy in, 224
meditation and mindful eating in, 240
in racism and discrimination, 28, 35
in weight bias and stigma, 48, 49
weight gain in, 146
structural racism, 27
substance use, assessment of, 85, 92, 152, 158*t*
suicidality
assessment of, 92, 148, 154, 156*t*
in weight bias and stigma, 48
sulfonylureas, weight gain associated with, 212, 259*b*
summary statements in motivational interviewing, 232, 233, 233*b*
supermarket access, 30, 35, 107
supplements, dietary, 107*b*
in bariatric surgery, 34, 265
evaluation of information on, 188–189
in very low-calorie diets, 184
surgery
bariatric. *See* bariatric surgery
cranial, medical history of, 84
sympathetic nervous system, 14, 22
systemic barriers to health care, 30–34, 359–360, 360*b*–361*b*

T

team approach, interprofessional, 334–343
technology use, 316–327
behavior change in, 323–324, 325
cell phones in. *See* cell phones/smartphones
commercial apps in, 322–323, 324, 327*b*
cost issues in, 325
in COVID-19 pandemic, 278, 279, 282, 316, 318, 343
in eHealth. *See* electronic health
email in, 318, 320, 323, 327*b*
engagement in, 323–324
evidence-based guidelines on, 278, 317, 323–324, 325
interactive voice response in, 319–320
internet in. *See* internet use
in long-term care delivery, 278
patient factors affecting, 324, 325–326
Short Message Service (SMS) in, 318, 319, 320, 323, 326, 327*b*
smart scales in, 321–322
sociodemographic factors in, 324, 325–326
wearable devices in. *See* wearable devices in activity measurement
telehealth, 278, 282, 343
in fee-for-service arrangements, 352, 353
motivational interviewing in, 234–235
text messaging, 319, 327*b*
The Eatery mobile app, 322
The Obesity Society, 264, 341
guidelines of. *See* American Heart Association/American College of Cardiology/The Obesity Society (AHA/ACC/TOS) guidelines
theoretical domains framework, 135
thermic effect of food, 7, 7*f*, 8, 15*f*, 98, 199
thermogenesis
nonexercise activity, 8
total daily activity, 15*f*
thermogenic fat, 13
thiazolidinediones, weight gain associated with, 84, 259*b*
Three-Factor Eating Questionnaire, 148
thrifty phenotype, 8
thyroid disorders, 84, 88, 111*b*
thyroid hormones, 14, 84, 88
time-restricted eating, 186, 187
Tobacco, Alcohol, Prescription medication, and other Substance use (TAPS) Tool, 152, 158*t*
tobacco use
assessment of, 106*b*, 152, 158*t*
in bariatric surgery, 92, 264*b*, 266, 266*b*
topiramate, 260, 261*b*
in binge eating disorder, 303
mechanism of action, 256*t*, 257
and phentermine, 31, 256*t*
total daily activity thermogenesis in weight loss, 15*f*
total energy expenditure, 7–9, 199
basal metabolic rate in, 7*f*, 7–8, 199
estimation of, 99, 100, 100*b*
in physical activity, 7, 7*f*, 8–9, 199–200
equations on, 99, 100*b*
resting energy expenditure in, 199
thermic effect of food in, 7, 7*f*, 8, 15*f*, 199
in weight loss, 8, 13–14, 15*f*, 100
trajectory of body mass index, 3, 4–6. *See also* weight history
transfer of stimulus functions in relational frame theory, 227
transgender patients, 82, 90, 91*b*
transportation domain in physical activity assessment, 120*t*–121*t*, 128, 129*b*
transtheoretical model of change, 153, 232
trauma history, 150, 158*t*
Treat and Reduce Obesity Act, 350, 361*b*
treatment interventions. *See also specific interventions*.

INDEX **389**

actionable strategies for equity in, 34–37
bariatric surgery in, 31, 90–92, 260–267
barriers in access to, 30–34, 358–362
biases of health care providers affecting, 33–34, 36, 37
body mass index as factor in, 45, 51, 253–254, 254t, 347, 348
counseling in, 220–250
culturally-sensitive, 32–33, 245
diet in, 182–190
drug therapy in, 31, 255–260, 267
in eating disorders, 286–308
evidence-based guidelines in, 59–65
health insurance coverage for, 31, 45, 346–362
history-taking on prior experiences, 82–83
implementation science in, 33
in lifelong management, 270–282
lifestyle in, 31, 166–180
long-term, 274–282
nondieting, 237–243
patient-centered care in, 67–76
patient goals in, 35, 52–53, 64, 68
physical activity in, 195–213
research inequities in, 32–33
and risk for eating disorders, 308b
selection of, 253–254
shared decision-making in, 68, 69–72
technology in, 316–327
weight-inclusive (weight-neutral), 53, 237, 241
triglyceride levels, 89, 112b, 178t, 202
trust and rapport
    in counseling strategies, 244
    in patient-centered care, 68b, 68–69, 72
24-hour recall in dietary assessment, 102b, 104
twin studies, body mass index in, 13
type 2 diabetes mellitus, 19, 20, 22, 82
    bariatric surgery in, 91, 260, 264b, 266
    in binge eating disorder, 291
    body mass index in, 20, 22f, 167
    Chronic Care Model in, 279
    cognitive-behavioral therapy in, 220
    drug therapy in, 258, 349
        weight gain associated with, 84, 259, 259b
    family history of, 84
    laboratory tests in, 89
    lifestyle interventions in, 166–180
        in Diabetes Prevention Program, 166, 167–174
        in Finnish Diabetes Prevention Study, 174
        in Look AHEAD, 166, 175–179
    medical assessment in, 84
    medical supervision in, 255
    physical activity affecting risk for, 202–203
    physical examination in, 110
    waist circumference measurement in, 86
    weight loss affecting risk for, 274

U

UK Biobank Study, 122
ultraprocessed foods, 108, 272–274, 277
    classification of, 108, 273, 273b
    definition of, 108, 273
    hyperpalatable, 272–274, 274b
uncertain geographic context problem in activity assessment, 131
underweight, 3t, 20, 85
United Nations Committee on World Food Security, 105
University of Rhode Island Change Assessment Scale, 153, 158t
urge surfing, 228, 229, 244
US Department of Agriculture, 104, 211b, 273
US Department of Health and Human Services, 195, 210b, 212
US Department of Veterans Affairs MOVE! program, 179–180
US Food and Drug Administration approved antiobesity medications, 31, 37, 255, 258
    in binge eating disorder, 303
    list of, 255t–257t
US Household Food Security Survey Module, 155, 159, 159t
US Preventive Services Task Force recommendations
    insurance coverage based on, 348–349, 350
    on multicomponent interventions, 166, 167, 350
    on obesity screening and counseling, 85, 253–254, 348–349

V

V 3 principle (verification, analytical validation, clinical validation), 128
validity of physical activity assessment methods, 127f, 128, 137, 138, 139
value-based payments, 354–355, 361b
value proposition on RDN services, 357–358
values
    definition of, 227
    and goals compared, 227
    in patient-centered approach, 75
    and value-congruent action in acceptance-based behavioral therapy, 227–228, 244
vegan diet, 106b, 110, 110b, 186
vegetarian diet, 186, 187
Venner, Thomas, 80
ventral stratum, 12
vertical sleeve gastrectomy, 261, 262t
very low-calorie diets, 184, 272, 296
    ketogenic, 185
video chat services, 327b
videos, in weight management interventions, 327b
vitamin deficiencies
    in bariatric surgery, 92, 265, 266b
    laboratory tests in, 88
    physical examination in, 88, 110b
vomiting, self-induced, as compensatory behavior, 297
    assessment of, 149, 304, 305
    in bulimia nervosa, 287b

W

WAGR syndrome, 83–84
waist circumference measurement, 2, 3t, 80, 86, 110b
    in transgender patients, 91b
walkability of built environment, 30, 129, 130, 277, 278
wearable devices in activity measurement, 119, 122–125, 247, 320–321
    accuracy of, 128

    in behavioral weight loss therapy, 320–321
    comparison of, 121t, 127f
    consumer-grade, 121t, 122, 124, 127f
    research-grade, 121t, 122, 124, 125, 127f
    and sedentary behavior, 137
    and sleep estimation, 152
    and weight loss, 320–321
weathering hypothesis, 28
web-based interventions, 316, 317–318, 326
weight
    and basal metabolic rate, 8, 13, 14, 98, 101
    categories of, 2, 3t
    defended, 6, 14
    and energy expenditure, 7–9, 13–14
        resting, 99
        total, 100b
    genetic factors in, 2, 4, 6, 13
    and height in body mass index, 2
    history of changes in. *See* weight history
    ideal. *See* ideal body weight
    as indicator of health, 238, 240–241
    and life span changes, 3, 4–6, 18–20
    lifestyle factors affecting, 2, 4, 5f, 13–14
    monitoring of
        in acceptance-based behavioral therapy, 229
        in cognitive-behavioral therapy, 221–222, 224, 299
        in eating disorders, 298–299, 308b
        frequency of, 299
        in long-term management, 276
        with smart scales, 321–322
    personal responsibility view of, 44, 45
    in physical examination, 85–86, 112b
    regulation of, 2, 3–16, 270–271
        in adaptive response to weight loss, 14–16, 271–272
        animal studies on, 3–6, 4f–6f, 273
        energy expenditure in, 3, 7–9
        energy intake in, 3, 9–13
        homeorhesis in, 4
        homeostasis in, 9, 11, 270–271
        hypothalamus in, 9–10, 10f, 11f, 272
        lipostatic theory of, 9
        obesity as disease of, 2, 13–14
    set point in, 4, 271
    social influences on, 12–13
Weight and Lifestyle Inventory, 154, 156t
weight bias and stigma, 44–53, 270
    assessment of, 150–151, 158t
    as barrier to care, 33–34, 291–292, 359
    bullying in, 45, 46
    definition and examples of, 44–46
    disordered eating in, 45, 48, 290, 291
    in eating disorders, 291–292, 307
    and Health at Every Size approach, 238, 241
    health care avoidance in, 37, 46, 50, 53, 151, 291, 334
    of health care providers, 49–51, 53, 291
        as barrier to care, 359
        prevention and reduction of, 36, 37, 51–53, 52b, 151
        race and ethnicity as compounding factors in, 33–34, 37
    health consequences of, 47f, 47–49, 270
    internalization of. *See* internalization of weight stigma
    interpersonal sources of, 45–46
    intrapersonal, 46
    in media, 45, 50
    personal responsibility view in, 44, 45
    questionnaires in assessment of, 151, 158t
    stereotypes in, 44, 45, 46, 150
        internalized, 48, 150–151
    structural, 45
Weight Bias Internalization Scale, 151, 158t
weight gain
    after weight loss. *See* weight regain
    animal studies of, 3, 4, 4f, 5f, 6
    compensatory behaviors for avoiding. *See* compensatory behaviors after eating
    and defended weight, 6, 14
    in depression, 146
    diabetes risk in, 167
    drugs associated with, 84, 212, 246, 259, 259b–260b, 265
        in depression, 146, 259b
    in emotional eating, 146
    energy balance in, 2, 7, 14, 182
    and energy expenditure, 8, 9, 200
    genetic factors in, 2, 4, 6, 13
    history-taking on, 82–83, 148–150
    hypertension in, 200, 202
    and life span changes, 3, 4, 5f, 18–19
    in menopause, 19
    physical activity in prevention of, 195, 198, 204–205, 213
        appetite and energy intake in, 199
        energy expenditure in, 200
        guidelines on, 196b–197b, 204
        in long-term management, 277–278
        minimum amount in, 206
        prescription of, 206, 207b
    postpartum, 19
    in pregnancy, 18–19, 343
    self-directed dieting as risk for, 292–293
    social influences on, 12
    in stress, 146
    and thermic effect of food, 8
    in thrifty phenotype, 8
    in young adults, 245
weight history, 3–6, 8, 274
    in animal studies, 3–6
    in behavioral health assessment, 148–150
    in family, 149
    in medical and physical assessment, 82–83
    race and ethnicity in, 5f
weight-inclusive approach, 53, 237, 241
weight loss, 4, 13–16, 253
    in acceptance-based behavioral therapy, 229–230
    adaptive response to, 14–16, 271–272, 275–276
    appetite changes in, 14, 16, 272, 276
    in bariatric surgery. *See* bariatric surgery, weight loss in
    basal metabolic rate in, 13, 14, 98, 101
    in behavioral weight loss therapy, 295, 302, 320–321
    brain response to food-related stimuli after, 14–16, 272
    in cognitive-behavioral therapy, 220, 222, 230
    and defended weight, 6, 14
    in Diabetes Prevention Program, 167, 168b, 168–169, 172
    in drug therapy, 255t–257t, 258
    energy expenditure in, 8, 13, 14, 15f, 100–102, 182

INDEX **391**

in adaptive response, 14, 271–272, 275–276
   in research trials, 136–139
energy intake in, 100–102, 182–190, 272
   in metabolic adaptation, 275–276
in evidence-based guidelines, 63–64
in Finnish Diabetes Prevention Study, 174, 175*f*
goals on. *See* goals, on amount of weight loss
health benefits of, 167, 172, 253, 267, 274, 275
historical approach to, 80
history-taking on, 82–83, 274
insulin action in, 20
leptin levels in, 14, 272
lipid levels in, 202, 267
in Look AHEAD, 175, 176
   results in, 176, 177, 177*f*, 178, 178*t*, 179
medical supervision of, 254–255
Medicare requirements on, 347
in motivational interviewing, 234–235, 236
motivation in, 13–14, 52–53
in MOVE! program, 179–180
in nondiet approaches, 52–53, 237–243
in older adults, 4, 5*f*, 19
in patient-centered care, 67–76
patient expectations on, 35, 100, 208, 275, 334
and physical activity, 136–139, 195, 198, 205, 213
   in aerobic exercise, 205, 206, 207*b*
   in bariatric surgery, 212
   Body Weight Planner on, 100–102, 101*f*
   in cognitive-behavioral therapy, 222
   in Diabetes Prevention Program, 172
   duration of activity in, 198
   energy intake in, 199
   guidelines on, 196*b*–197*b*, 204
   in Look AHEAD, 176, 178
   minimum amount in, 206
   patient expectations in, 208
   prescription of, 206, 207*b*
   in wearable device use, 320–321
plateaus in, 13–14, 267, 275
popular diets and products for, 188–190, 189*b*
self-directed dieting for, 188–189, 292–293
in technology-based interventions, 246, 317–325
weight regain after. *See* weight regain
Weight Loss Predictor Calculator, 182, 183*b*
weight maintenance, 16
   cognitive-behavioral therapy in, 16, 225
   energy expenditure adjustments in, 100–102
   history-taking on, 274
   in motivational interviewing, 236
   physical activity in, 100–102, 195, 205
      and bariatric surgery, 212
      and energy intake, 199
      guidelines on, 196*b*–197*b*, 204
      in long-term management, 277–278
      minimum amount in, 206
      prescription of, 206, 207*b*
   in pregnancy, 19
   self-monitoring in, 276
   social influences on, 12–13
weight-neutral approaches, 53, 240, 242
weight regain, 4, 6, 6*f*, 13

   in acceptance-based behavioral therapy, 230
   as adaptive response, 2, 14–16, 271–272, 275–276
   in animals and humans compared, 4, 5*f*
   in bariatric surgery, 260, 266–267, 266*b*
   in cognitive-behavioral therapy, 224–225
   in energy-restricted diet, 6
   history-taking on, 274
   in Look AHEAD, 179
   prevention of, 16, 277
Weight Self-Stigma Questionnaire, 151, 158*t*
whole-room indirect calorimetry, 118–119
willingness strategies in acceptance-based behavioral therapy, 228, 229
workplace. *See* employment
World Health Organization
   Mental Health Surveys, 288
   physical activity guidelines, 122, 195, 197*b*, 204, 208
   on weight categories, 85

Y

Yale Food Addiction Scale, 149, 154, 157*t*
YMCA, physical activity resources from, 211*b*
yoga, 205, 207*b*, 241

Z

zonisamide, 260, 261*b*